DIMENSIONS III
A Changing Concept of Health

DIMENSIONS III
A Changing Concept of Health

Third Edition

Kenneth L. Jones

Louis W. Shainberg

Curtis O. Byer

Canfield Press
San Francisco

A Department of Harper & Row, Publishers, Inc.
New York   Hagerstown   London

Interior and cover design: Christy Butterfield
Interior art: Donald Dean
Chapter opening art: Martha Weston
Layout and page make-up: Paul Quinn

DIMENSIONS III, A Changing Concept of Health
© 1972, 1974, 1976 by Kenneth L. Jones, Louis W. Shainberg and Curtis O. Byer

Library of Congress Cataloging in Publication Data

Jones, Kenneth Lamar, 1931-
    Dimensions III.

    First-2d ed. published under title: Dimensions.
    1. Hygiene. I. Shainberg, Louis W., joint
author. II. Byer, Curtis O., joint author.
III. Title. [DNLM: 1. Health. 2. Medicine—
Popular works. WB120 J77d]
QP36.J79 1974b   613   75-35782
ISBN 0-06-384372-2

76 77 78 10 9 8 7 6 5 4 3 2 1

To **Malvina Wasserman** who made it all happen

A Note from the Authors

The college health course has assumed a new vitality in recent years. This course must now come to terms with some of the most important aspects of humanity and the quality of life. Many of the major challenges facing the world today find their roots in the physical, emotional, and social health of people. This is a very unstable era in which all phases of life are changing at a rapid pace. Emotional health, interpersonal relationships, sexual behavior, health services, and the quality of our environment are now subject to pressures which can only be considered revolutionary. The most pressing problem has become survival—not just of the human species but of the individual human spirit as well.

At the focal point of this phenomenon is a changing definition of health. No longer is health defined as merely the absence of physical disease. Health is now regarded as a state of physical, emotional, and social well-being. The interdependence of a wide variety of factors in the determination of a healthful way of life is now generally acknowledged. As the concept of health has become more complex, it has perhaps become more difficult for each person to be well-informed, and to make personally valid decisions. Appropriate action on any matter must be based on accurate information.

We are constantly subjected to information about health from governmental commissions, private hospital groups, our casual and close friends, our families, and television and radio advertisements. It is essential to our development as human beings and to our relationships with others that we find a way of sorting out all of this information and advice. Today's health courses are designed to help accomplish just that, and we hope that this book will continue to make an important contribution to their success.

Dimensions is intended as a basic text for college health courses, to provide a broad background and, we hope, a stimulus for enlightened classroom discussion. We do not expect every reader to agree with everything here, since some of the material is, by its very nature, controversial. There are a few areas where not even all three of us agree, though our mutual respect remains intact.

In order to emphasize our view of health science today as a multidimensional subject, we have made some major departures from the traditional approaches. For example, there is a decided shift away from the anatomical and physiological, toward the behavioral and sociological aspects of health. Of course, biological material is introduced in some areas to provide a basis for understanding contemporary health issues, many of which have a biological foundation.

About this New Edition

This revision of *Dimensions* reflects our concept of health as a dynamic, rapidly changing field, reflecting not only advances in knowledge, but changes in the political and cultural environment as well.

In this edition, we have tried a new organization of the topics, based on the suggestions of users of the book. We have started with emotional health, since sound individual emotional health relates directly to physical health and the health of our society. The study of emotional health leads directly into an exploration of the use and abuse of substances—alcohol, tobacco, and other drugs— since substance abuse often relates to problems in emotional health. Continuing with substances, we discuss food and nutrition. Our discussion of calorie balance leads into a chapter on total fitness. Consumer health information follows, with an emphasis on selecting top quality health services. Sections then follow on human sexuality and reproduction, communicable and noncommunicable diseases, and the book concludes with a section on population and environmental quality.

We have added three new chapters: Emotional Health; Total Fitness; and Sexually Transmitted Diseases. In addition, there are extensive new sections on communication and intimacy, on new approaches to treating emotional problems, and on drug abuse. Throughout the book the reader will find evidence of the many factors which contributed to the up-dating of the book: extensive feedback from instructors and students over the past few years, helpful responses to a survey of users of the book, government publications, the popular media, and of course the exciting work being done in numerous areas of medical science.

We Would Like to Thank. . .

Throughout the history of this book, several people have contributed their time and ideas, providing thorough and constructive readings of the manuscript. For their contributions to previous editions, we would like to thank: Jack Brennecke, Mount San Antonio College; Barbara Combs, City College of San Francisco;

Janet Faurot, Long Beach City College; Kenneth Hurst, Merritt College; Allure Jefcoat, Diablo Valley College; Alfred Mathews, California State College at Hayward; James Pryde, American River College.

We also want to thank several people who helped in the preparation of the manuscript and production of this edition. We are particularly grateful to Abby Stitt of Bronx Community College, New York, for her in-depth review of both the second edition of *Dimensions* and the manuscript for this edition. We would particularly like to note her suggestion for the integration of Erikson's and Maslow's ideas into the new Chapter 2. For their critical assistance and commentary, we would also like to acknowledge the work of Michael Perrine of Portland Community College, and Victor Petreshene and James Webster, both of the College of Marin.

We especially thank Mary Fairfax for her contribution to the development of Section I, and her assistance throughout the preparation of the manuscript.

We also appreciate the efficiency and cooperation of the outstanding staff of Canfield Press, especially John Miller, editor; Mal Wasserman, developmental editor; and Tom Dorsaneo, production editor.

                                                              K.L.J.
                                                              L.W.S.
January, 1976   C.O.B.

CONTENTS

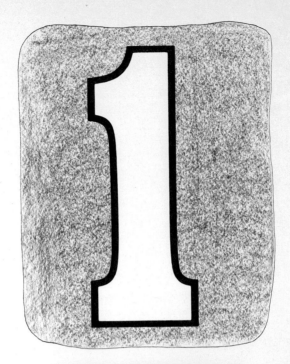

EMOTIONAL HEALTH

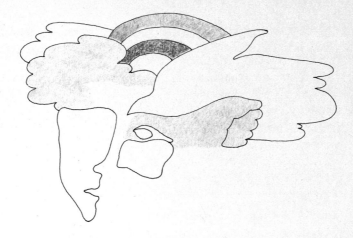

THE STRUCTURE OF PERSONALITY

We have chosen emotional health as the topic of the first section in this book because of our conviction that emotional health is basic to all health. Such problems as alcoholism and other substance dependencies can be thought of as reflections of the quality of our emotional health. Heart disease is often the direct result of emotional stresses. Problems in sexual response are almost always related to the emotions. Even resistance to infectious diseases may be reduced by emotional stress. It is safe to say that today, in terms of human welfare, the impact of emotional problems far exceeds that of all other health problems.

These three brief chapters are not intended to replace a good basic course in psychology. They may, however, provide a general overview of the subject with particular emphasis on the complex interaction between mind and body and the mutual dependency of physical and mental health.

Personality

A basic characteristic of all living things is their attempt to adjust to their environment. In human beings this adjustment is much more complicated than in the simpler animals, because we are capable of reasoning. We try to establish and maintain an equilibrium. Since the environment is constantly changing, our attempts at equilibrium demand constant attention.

The demands of our environment are further complicated by our inner needs, so that our life becomes a matter of constantly adapting to changes in the environment, while we still try to satisfy the basic inner needs. Very often we find that environmental situations make the satisfaction of inner needs difficult or even impossible. All of us are frustrated to some extent in our attempts to satisfy our needs. The ways in which we react to this frustration are indications of our emotional health, and vary with each personality.

Personality is made up of a number of behavior patterns, traits, attitudes, and all the other interactions we have with our environment. Everything that has ever happened to us has left some mark on our personality. As infants, we are born with a certain genetic makeup, and the personality we eventually develop depends both on our original genetic endowment and how the environment acts on that endowment. Our personality also includes the ways in which we interpret our environment and how we learn to deal with the conflicts between our basic inner needs and the obstacles to their fulfillment that are constantly presented by the outer world.

Thus, we find four forces that influence the personality: genetic makeup, environment, interpretation of the environment, and the learned ways of coping (the coping behavior). The first two forces are largely beyond our power of control. We have no control over those things we inherit, like basic intellectual capacity, body build, skin color, and so forth. We have limited ability to influence our environment. It is in the third and fourth categories—our interpretation of the environment and our methods of coping—that we can contribute to the healthy development of our personality.

Many attempts have been made to describe the makeup of personality. For example, pioneer psychoanalyst Sigmund Freud conceived of personality as being divided into three "processes": the *id*, which is unconscious; the *ego*, which is mostly conscious; and the *superego*, which has both conscious and unconscious elements. According to this scheme, the mind is like an iceberg, with the conscious mind visible and the great bulk of the unconscious mind below the surface.

Although psychoanalysis no longer enjoys the level of professional popularity it once held, the psychoanalytic concepts of id, ego, and superego may still serve to describe the structures of personality.

The Id The id, which is unconscious, is the most primitive of the three portions of the personality. It contains all the basic instinctive drives. These instincts, which are present at birth, represent the unconscious urges to survive and enjoy life. Throughout life, the id remains as the storage place for the primitive instincts.

Since the id works for the individual's biological survival, it is aggressive and selfish, and operates purely for pleasure and gratification. The id makes no distinction between good and evil, or between what is realistic and possible and what is not. Thus, aggression is seen by many authorities as a fundamental, inherent human characteristic, capable of being expressed in both harmful and beneficial ways. Competition, in business, politics, and sports, for example, is seen as an acceptable expression of basic human aggression. Harmful outlets of aggression include physical violence directed toward other persons or even self-directed, like suicide. It should be stressed that not all psychologists accept these concepts, especially the relationship of aggression to violence and suicide.

The Ego The ego represents the conscious mind, and acts as a moderator between the id and the outer world. It is in contact with the environment (reality) and with the id and the superego (judgments of goodness and worthiness). The ego must integrate all factors and determine appropriate behavior for the situation. The ego must decide which urges can be allowed satisfaction and which urges must be suppressed.

The ego is not present at birth; it develops gradually in response to experience and the pressures of society. The most important ego development occurs during the first years of life, but in the emotionally healthy person the ego continues to grow throughout life. New experiences constantly modify, strengthen, and enlarge the ego. The older person, with a more highly developed ego, is usually able to control and postpone instinct gratification. The infant, on the other hand, has only a weakly developed ego and is largely driven by id forces. Maturity can thus be measured by the degree to which the ego is able to control the id.

Even in the healthy, mature individual, the ego has a difficult task. But in the emotionally disturbed person, the ego is limited in strength and has increased difficulty in controlling the id and the superego.

The Superego The superego represents the judgment mechanisms regarding right and wrong, good and evil. It advises and threatens the ego. As very young children, we have little concept of what is right and wrong, but as codes and values of society are impressed upon us, we gradually develop our superegos. The main basis of the superegos of children is their concept of their parents. Children use their parents as a guide for their own behavior. Of course, their superego is based on their own *impression* of their parents, rather than on reality.

The attitudes that we as children perceived in our parents, and our interpretation of what we perceived, became our basis for judging the morality of situations. Since social values do change, these attitudes may be a source of trouble years after we have become adults. We may still be carrying childhood values that may have become outdated. Or we may have acquired overly strict or very lax ideals from our parents.

The word "conscience" is sometimes used to describe the superego, but actually the conscience is only part of the superego. It is this portion of the well-developed superego that makes cheating or stealing difficult or impossible for many persons, because they feel that these actions are wrong and know that they would feel guilty if they did them.

Another important element of the superego is the *ego-ideal*, which is a model of acceptability and worthiness, also gained from parents. It is important to realize that any violation of the judgment of the superego produces guilt, and that guilt is an extremely uncomfortable feeling. As a result, we will go to great lengths, both consciously and unconsciously, to avoid behavior that would produce guilt.

Or we may use certain ego-defense mechanisms to escape guilt, such as blaming our behavior on someone else or denying behavior that does not seem consistent with our ego-ideal.

Punishment is a way of dealing with guilt, so a person who feels guilt may unconsciously seek punishment in various disguised ways. Criminals sometimes deliberately leave clues so that they may be caught and punished. Accident-prone individuals may suffer from unconscious guilt, so they unconsciously allow "accidents" to happen to them to serve as punishment and release them from their guilt.

It is possible for a person with a weakly developed superego to live according to the principle of personal pleasure alone, without regard for the rights and privileges of others, yet suffer little or no guilt. On the other hand, it is possible for the superego to be so rigid and severe that it prevents almost all pleasure, regardless of the situation. The most healthy superego is one that fits within the demands of society and yet allows adequate individual pleasure.

The Self and Identity

The *self* is our individual awareness or perception of our own personality. It is a composite based on our own feelings about ourselves and on how we imagine other people to feel about us. Much of what we "know" about ourselves is based on our experiences with other people. Our chief sources of information about ourselves are the reactions of others to us. Of course, we evaluate these reactions subjectively. It is possible for us to see ourselves somewhat differently from the way others see us.

Many factors contribute to our self-image. The kinds of experiences that we have are very important in determining what our self-perception will be. We find that our appearance and personality elicit responses of acceptance or rejection, kindness or hostility, attention or indifference. We hear (or overhear) ourselves described by other people in terms of various personality traits. When these traits are consistently applied to us, we usually adopt them as descriptions of ourselves. Praise and attention help us to form a picture of ourselves as desirable persons. Rejection, indifference, criticism, or hostility can lead to a poor self-image, with resulting inferiority feelings.

The treatment that we receive from others may or may not reflect accurately our own traits and abilities. For example, we tend to react most positively to those whose traits are most like our own. Thus, people may meet with indifference or rejection merely on the basis of their racial, religious, or cultural background. As a result, many effective and pleasant people may come to perceive of themselves as inadequate, inferior, or undesirable in reflection of the prejudices or misconceptions of others. Conversely, children of overly admiring and doting parents who excessively praise even poor performance may grow up with a somewhat inflated self-image.

Knowing how people see themselves helps us to understand their behavior, especially when they see themselves much differently from the way others see them. Behavior is largely determined by how people perceive a situation with reference to themselves.

People whose self-images are too different from their true or objective personality may experience serious adjustment problems. They must constantly either explain or ignore circumstances that are inconsistent with their view of themselves. They rely on the ego-defense mechanisms, discussed later in this chapter. Consider, for example, a capable student whose self-esteem is so low that

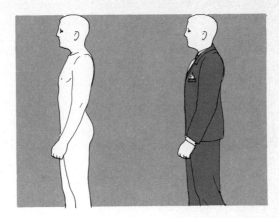

Often the apparel proclaims and explains the person. Little can be said of a person unadorned, other than that he or she has a unique face and body. Fully clothed, the person and personality often become clear. His or her bearing and expression take on a particular significance.

academic success would actually create anxiety by conflicting with his or her self-image. Such a student may purposefully, though unconsciously, create barriers to success.

A problem shared by the great majority of us is that we tend to underestimate our capabilities. We fall into the trap of feeling that our lives are completely structured for us by circumstances beyond our control and that we are impotent to make any significant change in their course. In reality, each one of us has an amazing ability to accomplish things, if we just accept and believe in this ability. This is the concept of *self-determination.*

Self-determination depends on two basic beliefs. First is a belief that human beings in general are self-determining and have considerable control over the courses of their lives. Second is a belief or confidence in your own personal ability to accomplish what you want. This belief in self is based on faith and experience. When people learn that they are successful in most of the things they attempt, they develop faith in themselves. Even their fail-

ures do not bother them excessively, because they have confidence in their ability to recover from failure. Through their experiences in living, they have learned what they can and cannot do and they have a basis for self-determination.

When people do not believe in themselves, they act in ways that are limiting or even self-destructive. When people "know" they are going to fail, their failure is assured. This concept is valid in every realm of life. It is true for the student in courses; for the athlete in competition; for anyone in his or her relations with people, especially in sexual relationships; and for the patient balanced between life and death with a critical illness.

An integral part of our concept of self is our sense of *identity.* This is our appraisal of who we are, what we mean to ourselves and others, and where we fit into the general scheme of things, especially in our relations with other people. This process of establishing identity is a source of much internal conflict for many people. By the time we reach our high school years we are deeply involved in the task of separating our identity from that of our parents and finding our own place in the world. But changes in identity (and identity crises resulting from conflicts in identity) can occur at any age throughout life. Since the development of personality continues from birth to death, it follows naturally that one's identity must also change. In the past, most people made only minor changes in their identity once they "found" their identity as adults. But the rate of change in all aspects of life has accelerated tremendously (and continues to accelerate) so that an identity that is satisfactory for a young adult today is very unlikely to remain satisfactory for a whole lifetime. In fact, even ten years from now, it would probably seem woefully inappropriate to his or her life situation at that

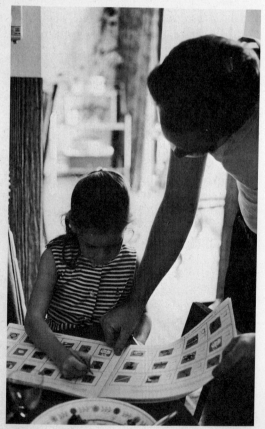

Photo © Alex Webb/Magnum

time. People who go through life with one career field and one spouse will probably be the exception, where once they were the majority.

Many people never do really discover their own identity. They may go through life hiding in a career, a marriage, organizations, or a succession of "causes." Or they identify themselves in terms of what they have, rather than what they are. Either of these approaches is just a way of dodging the difficult task of defining one's identity. But for a truly fulfilling life, each of us must find our own identity, as an individual. The rewards are well worth the cost.

Basic Human Needs

One of the first requirements for good emotional health is to know ourselves. Why do we feel the way we do? Why do we do the things we do? The answers to these questions will come largely from our understanding of our basic needs, the extent to which these needs are fulfilled in us, and how we react to the frustration of these needs.

We might expect all authorities on the subject to be in complete agreement on something as basic as the needs of people. But they are not in agreement. Perhaps the needs of all of us are not exactly the same, and each authority interprets and generalizes his or her own needs as being true for everyone.

Abraham H. Maslow, in his classic book *Motivation and Personality* (Harper & Row, 1970), made an interesting presentation of his interpretation of human needs. He arranged these needs in sequence from the most basic needs to the higher needs. Maslow believed that the higher needs develop only when the basic needs are fulfilled. For example, since food is a very basic need, people who are starving may have little interest in fulfilling higher needs such as pursuing knowledge or reaching their full artistic potential.

In the following discussion we shall examine some of the basic human needs presented by Maslow.

The Physiological Needs The most basic of human needs are the physical drives. Among them are hunger, thirst, sleep, sexuality, and many others. When someone's physiological needs are unsatisfied, he or she pushes all other needs into the background. Not only is immediate interest in the higher needs lost, but also the whole plan for the future is modified. For example, extremely hungry people may think of paradise merely as a place where there is plenty of food. They think that if only they were guaranteed enough to eat for the rest of their lives, they would never want anything more.

Victor Frankel's observations of behavior in a concentration camp suggest that among the physiological needs, those immediately related to survival dominate. (*Man's Search for Meaning*, 1963). Acts related to survival so dominated the individuals' thoughts and actions that no overt sexual activity was evident, and even dreams were reported to be free of sexual content typical of a more normal environment.

But what happens when the physiological needs are satisfied? Immediately, other and higher needs emerge and begin to dominate the person. As long as a need is satisfied, it has little effect on behavior. Behavior is governed much more by unsatisfied needs.

The Safety (Security) Needs Maslow rates the safety needs as second only to the physiological needs. After the physiological needs are fairly well satisfied, the safety needs emerge, and they make everything else appear less important. The safety needs are most easily seen in the fright reactions of infants and children, because adults in our society have been taught to hide or inhibit these reactions. Thus, even when some adults feel their security threatened, they are not likely to react in a visible manner, but rather with masked anxiety and such physical changes as increased heartbeat.

Actually, knowledge and experience in the adult should eliminate many of the fright reactions shown by the child. One of the most important functions of education is to neutralize apparent dangers through knowledge. Much unnecessary fear results from ignorance. For example, a sonic boom may be quite upsetting to someone who does not understand it. But one who understands sonic booms, while still not enjoying them, is not panic-stricken.

Parents must provide children with a feeling of security in the home. The relationship between parents is especially important to children. Quarreling, physical abuse, separation, or divorce may be particularly frightening to them. When the parents' anger is directed toward children, as in speaking harshly to them, handling them roughly, or administering physical punishment, children often react with such total terror that it is clear that their distress involves more than just the physical pain of the punishment. They fear that their parents' love will be taken from them.

Another indication of children's need for security is their preference for a certain amount of routine and ritual in the daily schedule of the family. They like a more predictable, orderly world. Young children seem to thrive under a system that has some structure and presents a framework of certain ground rules of conduct. They prefer and need freedom *within limits*, rather than total permissiveness. Consistency is more important, however, than the degree of rigidity or permissiveness. Children raised under a consistent system are happier and develop better emotionally than those who are not because they feel more secure. They know what their parents expect of them and how their parents will react to their behavior.

Adults in our society usually feel fairly secure as long as they believe their physical and emotional health are good and their source of income is reasonably stable. Many adults express their safety needs in such ways as looking for a job offering more security, saving money for emergencies, and maintaining various kinds of insurance.

Another result of the adult's need for security is the commonly seen preference for familiar rather than unfamiliar things—for the known rather than the unknown. This preference often increases with age, and it is one of the sources of the differences between generations, sometimes called the "generation gap." The older generation has often been dismayed by the new and unfamiliar actions, attitudes, clothing, and so forth, of the younger generation. A person who makes a conscious effort to overcome a rigid preference for familiar things should be able to face new ideas and challenges without fear.

The Needs for Love and Belonging

Maslow placed the needs for love and belonging (companionship) right after the physiological and safety needs. People whose physiological and safety needs are fulfilled rather consistently feel motivated to satisfy their needs for love and belonging. They feel a strong need for friends or a mate. They have a need for companionship with people in general, for a feeling of belonging and group acceptance, and a need to love and be loved.

A feeling of group belonging and acceptance has particular value to a person because social life generally centers around group activity. One of the greatest causes of unhappiness is the lack of this feeling of group acceptance. Along with the immediate social satisfaction derived from group belonging are other possible benefits to the individual, such as giving us the security needed to become more independent of our families, exposing us to values different from those of our parents, and providing us with experience in reacting as an equal with our peers. School, church, play, and work provide many opportunities for group involvement.

Our society has a rather inhibited and cautious attitude toward love and affection, and especially their possible expression in sexuality. This attitude has made it difficult for many people to establish close interpersonal relationships, including those in which sex would play no role. Love and sex are not synonymous. There may be strong love relationships in which sex is not involved, just as there may be sexual relationships in which love is not a factor. The most characteristic feature of love is a genuine concern for the welfare of the loved one.

It is of the utmost importance that parents be responsive to a child's love needs. Children who feel unloved and rejected by their parents may have a poor self-image; may endure and be the source of much trouble at home and at school; and may suffer emotional problems as adolescents and adults. Parental rejection can leave lifelong emotional scars in children. However, parents are not the only source of love and affection. Children often receive enough of these from others involved in their lives, such as relatives, neighbors, teachers, and leaders of community organizations. There are many opportunities for the growing child to learn that life is essentially what one makes of it and to go on to discover the richness of self-determination. The child, however, who has been totally rejected may later be reluctant to establish close personal relationships for fear of further rejection, and may never be able to give and receive love, thus going through life as a "loner." The person who has "loved and lost" may also withdraw because of fear of further rejection. But to a reasonably secure person, the fulfilling of love needs is worth the risk involved.

The Esteem Needs Every normal person has a need for self-esteem, which means a feeling of personal value or worth, of success, achievement, self-respect, and confidence in the face of the world. In order to attain this feeling, most people need respect or esteem from other people, as seen in their striving for status, dominance, attention, and appreciation.

We shall first consider the need for *self-esteem*. Satisfaction of this need leads to feelings of self-confidence, value, strength, adequacy, and usefulness. Inability to satisfy the self-esteem need produces feelings of dependence, inferiority, weakness, helplessness, and despair.

The most obvious way to build self-respect is to do something of value well—to excel. The specific area in which to excel should be determined by one's interests and ability. Anyone who makes the effort can find some constructive activity in which to excel. It is especially fortunate when people receive a feeling of satisfaction from their work, since they must devote a great amount of time to it. But a sport or hobby can be equally rewarding in building self-respect, as can social and love experiences. Thus, the feelings gained through satisfaction of the need for self-esteem are likely to give rise to accomplishments that further build self-respect. A person who suffers from a lack of self-respect and who feels helpless finds it difficult to accomplish anything that

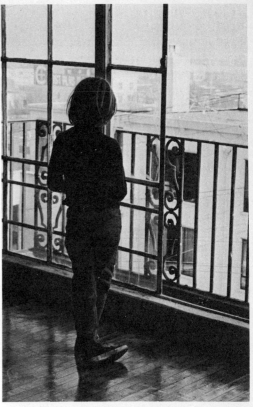

Alone.
Photo by David Bellak

will help build self-respect. Something must be done to break the cycle of insignificance and begin the building of self-esteem.

The second of the esteem needs concerns the desire for respect from *other* people, in the form of reputation or prestige. It seems that as a person's self-respect is strengthened, the need for the esteem of others diminishes. People who feel confident of their own worth are less dependent on the praise of others. It is certainly better to base self-respect on actual achievement rather than on the opinions of others, which often are either higher or lower than reality warrants.

The constant seeking of praise may suggest insecurity on the part of the seeker, but it is important in dealing with people to recognize that everyone has a need for some recognition from others. Sincere praise is one of the foundations of good interpersonal relationships. It is important to give praise when praise is due. Too often we tell people when we are annoyed with them, but forget to tell them when we are pleased.

The Need for Self-Actualization

The need for self-actualization is merely the need to do what one is capable of doing to achieve self-fulfillment. To be at peace with themselves, artists must paint, poets must write, and musicians must make music. Maslow said, "What a person can be, they must be." This statement means that in order to feel fulfilled, people must not only do the kind of thing they are able to do, but they must also do it as well as they are capable of doing. Most of us (Maslow said 99 percent) are not operating at this level. We are stuck at a lower level of need-satisfaction, sometimes through our own fault and sometimes through circumstances outside our control. According to Maslow we can best increase our level of self-actualization by discovering what we are really like inside.

The Need to Know and Understand

Among the higher needs of people are their impulses to satisfy curiosity, to know, to explain, and to understand. Curiosity is a natural rather than a learned characteristic. Children are naturally curious. They may lose this curiosity, however, through overly strict discipline or lack of encouragement at home or too much regimentation at school. The home and school must be careful not to destroy this valuable characteristic. When curiosity has already been suppressed, every effort should be made to restore it, for curiosity leads to creativity and invention.

Although many people can live fairly satisfying lives without much intellectual stimulation, these would not be highly fulfilling lives. People whose thoughts are confined to the mundane may become bored, feel constantly tired, and have little zest for life. In contrast, the satisfaction of the need to know and understand often gives people a bright, happy feeling of fulfillment in their emotional lives.

The Aesthetic Needs

Beauty is a subjective quality that defies any scientific measurement. But it is a basic need for many adults and probably for all normal children. Like curiosity, an appreciation of beauty may or may not be retained into adulthood.

Although beauty is often perceived through the senses (visual, auditory, tactile, and so on), this is not necessarily always the case. Beauty can also be a purely internal experience, such as feeling the beauty of ideas or philosophical concepts that are meaningful to us.

Most women and girls in our culture very readily show their appreciation of beauty. But many men and boys are embarrassed by their love of beauty, because they are afraid it may be an effeminate trait or be seen as such by their friends. Therefore, they may actually hide or suppress their enjoyment of beauty. But the male should realize that his love of beauty is perfectly natural and that he can enjoy beauty without risking his masculinity. He should be able to feel and express enjoyment of the beauty of a flower, a tree, a skillfully designed building, a well-designed car, or a beautiful landscape.

Sound Emotional Health

It would be very difficult to set up an exact standard by which an individual's level of emotional health could be judged. There certainly is no line that neatly divides the emotionally healthy from the emotionally ill. There are many different degrees of emotional health. The following characteristics are all signs of sound emotional health. But the lack of one or more of them in a person does not indicate emotional illness. Actually, no one has all the traits of emotional health at all times. At the very least, emotionally healthy, fully functioning, or self-actualizing people "feel good" and enjoy themselves and their personal existence.

Ability to Deal Constructively with Reality Healthy people accept reality, whether it is pleasant or not. They do not generally attempt to escape from reality through fantasies or by excessive use of alcohol or other drugs. Nor do they take the opposite path, becoming preoccupied with their own problems, and spending much time worrying or brooding.

Dealing constructively with reality means that people must learn to acknowledge and accept their own capabilities and limitations. Then, when a problem arises, they can do something about it (if the solution is within their ability) or else realistically accept the problem as beyond their ability to solve. In situations in which someone else has a greater ability to solve the problem, mature people do not hesitate to ask for help. When it is apparent that they are dealing with a problem that is impossible to solve even with help, they then adjust to the situation.

Healthy people set realistic goals for themselves. They try to make the fullest use of their natural abilities, but they also realize their natural limitations and do not frustrate themselves trying to do something that is obviously beyond their present ability. People usually are happiest when they are working at or near their full ability. They usually are not very happy when they are working far below their ability or when they are trying to work far above it.

It is unfortunate that many people in our society are unhappy, and therefore, not really healthy either. This is not always because they are unable to adjust to society's definitions and norms, but precisely because they are forced to do so. In adapting to the reality of the majority, a substantial part of individual reality may be surrendered.

For instance, in our society, reality is often defined in terms of material things. To achieve success as our society defines it, the individual often must limit his or her efforts towards those functions that are rewarded by our highly specialized, industrialized, and rationalized society. This choice may bring little personal satisfaction, but may be the only course that leads to acceptance and approval from others. From childhood, we are rewarded for developing those skills that are most likely to result in material gain. Education goes from the more generalized to the more specific. We learn more and more about less and less. Once a path has been chosen, it is often difficult to rechannel energies toward goals that might actually lead to a more satisfying life. Society too frequently rewards people for applying a limited range of skills, thus denying to many people the opportunity to develop their abilities to their fullest extent.

Another indication of emotional health is the acceptance of responsibility relative to ourselves as well as others. It should be recognized that responsibility to oneself is of primary importance. Unless one's own needs are met, very little can be accomplished for other people. It is important to remember that, except for the very young, the very old, or the severely handicapped, each person is individually responsible for his or her own actions and life.

Less healthy people may actually work harder at evasion of responsibility than they would if they accepted their responsibilities and did whatever was necessary to fulfill them. The more healthy person not only accepts responsibility, but also enjoys and needs a certain amount of it.

Ability to Adapt to Change   There is a natural tendency to resist change and even to fear the future. This results from the basic need for safety and security, as discussed previously. But healthy people are more confident of their ability to adapt to change. They realize that the world constantly changes, and they expect to change with it. They plan ahead and do not live in fear of the future.

Many aspects of maturity improve with increasing age, but one characteristic that is often gained at a young age and then lessened is the ability to adapt readily to change. Most young people welcome new experiences and new ideas. They should try to keep this open-minded approach to life as time passes. In past generations this adaptive ability was less important than it is now, because then conditions changed much more slowly than they do today.

Reasonable Degree of Autonomy

People in sound emotional health can function autonomously, think for themselves, and make the most of their own decisions. They can plan their lives and follow through with their plans. The inability to make decisions is very common in immature, insecure people. They may spend much time in confusion, not knowing what to do. They are afraid to face the consequences of whatever decisions they make, so they make as few as possible. Growth involves mistakes as well as successes.

Yet a certain amount of dependence is also desirable. People should not try to divorce themselves completely from the society in which they live and of which they are a part. For example, it is normal to enjoy being loved by another person (a form of dependence on that person). In our complex society we are dependent on other people in many ways. Healthy people enjoy this interdependency.

Ability to Cope with Stresses   All of us are subject to many stresses and tensions of both the everyday variety and the occasional crisis type. It is also perfectly

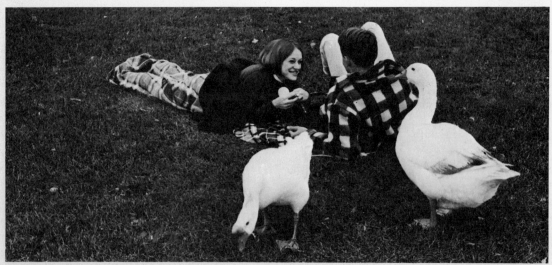

Photo © Roger Malloch/Magnum

normal to experience emotional reactions to these stresses and tensions. It is the type and degree of emotional response that indicates the state of our emotional health.

Emotionally healthy people are better able to control their emotions. They are not overpowered by fears, anger, hatred, jealousy, guilt, or worries. They can take life's disappointments in their stride, minimizing the unpleasant aspects. They have a more tolerant attitude toward themselves as well as toward others. They are inclined to look at the brighter side of life, rather than to concentrate on their troubles. They can laugh at themselves. This attitude tends to minimize problems and may make them more effectively solvable.

Good emotional control has two requirements: proper degree and desirable methods of control. These requirements are discussed later in this chapter.

Concern for Other People

The healthy personality combines self-respect with a concern for the rights and happiness of other people. Healthy people truly find as much satisfaction in giving as in receiving. They respect the differences they find among other people, accepting them as they are. They do not bully or use people unreasonably in achieving their own goals. They are careful in their words and actions to avoid offending others. They avoid saying things to build their own egos at the expense of others.

Satisfactory Relationships with Other People

People who enjoy better emotional health are able to relate to other people in a more consistent manner with mutual satisfaction and happiness. They like and trust most people and expect that people will like and trust them. Their relationships with others are satisfying and lasting. They have enough self-confidence to be able to feel a part of a group. They feel accepted and, conversely, make others feel accepted.

People who seem to have trouble dealing with others should examine their own attitudes and actions. They may mistakenly think that they are always right and that everyone else is wrong, or that they are being rejected by others when they have actually been hostile or inconsiderate themselves.

The Ability to Love

Mature people are able to express affection for other people. Even a rather immature person can receive love, but it takes a mature person to give love unselfishly. Although we refer to this type of love as "unselfish," it is actually very emotionally rewarding. It is one of the most fulfilling actions of humanity.

It must be stressed that the love to which we are referring is not just sexual love, but includes a love for children (not just our own, but all children) and for all people, regardless of their racial, religious, or cultural backgrounds. It is a love for humanity. Only the person with a well-developed sense of inner security can freely express such acceptance of others. Before people can love others, they must learn to accept and really love and respect themselves.

The Ability to Work Productively

It is widely agreed among authorities today that one of the prime indicators of good emotional health is the ability to work effectively and productively. The inability to be productive may be considered a symptom of emotional illness inasmuch as inner conflict requires a great amount of energy that would otherwise be available to an individual.

There are many examples. In school, it is often the students who have trouble completing their work who suffer from emotional conflicts. Chronically unemployed adults sometimes suffer from emotional problems that inhibit them from actively looking for a job, that work against them during job interviews, or that lower their productivity to the point where they repeatedly lose jobs. Of course, there are many cases where unemployment is the result of other factors such as economic conditions, lack of marketable skills, ethnic or sexual discrimination. But in an emotionally healthy individual, there is normally enough energy available to adapt to the situation, whatever it may be, so that productivity is not reduced.

At home, people may similarly reflect their emotional problems in their inability to keep up with housework or in the fact that routine household chores consume so much energy that they are able to do little else.

Emotional Maturity

We have now seen some of the characteristics of the emotionally mature person. But how does a person who lacks these characteristics develop them? For most of us, the passage of time and the gaining of various experiences bring on a degree of maturity. For example, we expect different levels of maturity in 3-, 10-, 16-, and 30-year-old people. But for various reasons, some people do not act at the level of maturity we expect of them, and there are times when everyone seems less mature than is desirable.

There are two basic forms of immaturity. One is called *fixation*, in which a person remains emotionally at an earlier level of development. A fixated person is one who has never grown up in certain attitudes, ideas or behaviors. The other type is called *regression*, a return to an earlier level of maturity. Many people show signs of regression temporarily while they are under stress. Some examples of their behavior during difficult periods might include pouting or throwing temper tantrums. During regression people display behavior patterns that are more characteristic of children than of adults. If a person's behavior seems to fit the description of either fixation or regression, we may wonder why and what can be done about it.

First, let us consider why people might be immature. It may be that they have never developed the traits of responsibility, courage, or the ability to view problems objectively. Sometimes people behave as though they want someone to protect them. They may be children of parents who have encouraged them to remain childlike by rewarding their immature behavior in devious ways. Such parents themselves fear and dislike adult life and may be trying to protect their children from it by keeping them immature.

Maturity is an ongoing process, rather than a condition finally reached. This process involves your relationship with others and with yourself as well. Maturity involves both actions and attitudes. The following suggestions may be of value in developing maturity:

1. Draw others out in conversation. In doing this, you are exposed to many new ideas and attitudes.

2. Accept the differences in others. Really accept these differences, do not just tolerate them, which is patronizing. Learn to appreciate and enjoy them!

3. Learn not to feel that you must establish a rightness or wrongness about everything. Most things (including beliefs and attitudes) are simply different, not necessarily better or worse than others. This does not mean that you should have no standards of your own. It is very important that you do have a set of values, but you should not believe that all values other than your own are wrong.

4. You can probably really learn about yourself only through exposure to

others. It is not enough to merely expose your intellectual ideas—you must expose your feelings as well. Such exposure of true feelings encourages others to reveal their feelings. People can hope to understand each other only when their true feelings are revealed. Emotions are normal and human.

Values Values are those things—acts, ideas, beliefs, traits—to which we attach worth. A value system is how we organize our values in such a way that they influence how we live our lives—it is actually a philosophy of life.

Most individuals hold many similar values. However, the order of importance placed on each varies considerably and ultimately affects the entire system. For example, honesty is a common value but some people give it higher priority than others do. Individuals who put honesty above other values are more likely to tell the truth regardless of personal consequences, while other people would not take the risk. Regardless of whether or not you have ever given the matter any conscious thought, you have some basic values that govern your life. These values are expressed in the way you spend your time and money and in all of your other actions.

Your philosophy of life is often more truthfully expressed by what you do than by what you say. We often meet people who express very lofty ideals, but whose actions reveal their true values.

Value systems range from the purely selfish to the overly idealistic. The person whose value system lies at either one of these extremes is likely to be unhappy and frustrated much of the time. The most emotionally rewarding philosophy lies somewhere between these extremes.

Your value system is influenced by many factors, some of which are beyond your own control. Each of the following factors have a degree of influence on your values:

1. Places you have lived.
   a. Nations.
   b. Regions.
   c. City, suburban, or rural areas.
2. Era in which you were born.
3. Values of your parents, as influenced by their
   a. Ethnic group.
   b. Religion.
   c. Economic level.
   d. Age.
   e. Occupation.
   f. Education.
4. Values of your age group and friends.
5. School experiences.
6. Religious training.
7. *Everything* that has happened to you in your entire life.

If you have never done so, it might be helpful for you to spend some time in an honest appraisal of your current value system. Does it seem adequate for the future you have planned for yourself—such as marriage, a career, and the raising of children? Is it even adequate for your current situation?

One characteristic of a truly successful value system is that it is never rigid. It is constantly being modified and changed as a person undergoes new experiences and gains in maturity, and as the world we live in continues to change. Change and flexibility are values too!

There is no cut-and-dried approach to developing a satisfying value system. Much depends on personal factors such as the philosophy of life that you accept and the many experiences that are exclusively your own. But a few general suggestions may be helpful.

1. *Draw on the experiences of others.*
   Spend some time reading the works of the great philosophers of the past as well as those of the present. Talk to more experienced people whose lives

you admire and study their value systems and how they express their values in their daily actions.

2. *Accept only that which is meaningful.* Evaluate what you read in respect to your own experiences. From all the conflicting ideas presented, you should accept only the ideas that seem personally meaningful and significant to you. It is not that some value systems are basically right and others wrong, but that ideas often conflict because a philosophy or value system is highly personal and individual. What is right for one person may be very wrong for another. You should not automatically accept the philosophy of another, regardless of how famous he or she may be. If your philosophy is not really your own, it is inadequate.

3. *Respect the rights of others.* A value system can work successfully only if it takes into consideration the reality that the freedom of the individual is limited by the rights and freedoms of others. A value system is unrealistic and will be unsuccessful as a guide through life if it demands rights and freedoms for one individual, while denying these same rights to others. For example, people who demand the right to freely express their own ideas must extend this same right to all others. This concept would seem to eliminate violence as a part of one's philosophy. Anyone who is willing to inflict violence upon another person should be equally willing to receive violence, and this seems rather unlikely.

Some value systems are totally self-centered. The pleasure and comfort of the individual is the only consideration. But such philosophies are self-defeating. It has been shown repeatedly that most people are happiest and their emotional health is best when their concern extends beyond their own material comfort to include the welfare of humanity in general. This type of value system indirectly leads to the greatest individual happiness, so it actually accomplishes that which the more selfish philosophies fail to produce. People who are totally occupied with the satisfaction of their own desires are destined for much frustration, because they must share this planet with billions of other people having similar desires and competing for the same goals. People who are satisfied with their fair share and who can feel satisfaction in the happiness of others will receive the greatest pleasure from life.

4. *Reevaluate your values periodically.* From time to time your philosophy should be reevaluated in the light of the kind of life it is producing for you. Are you truly satisfied with the way things are going? Perhaps your values are inadequate or could be on a higher plane. As you gain in wisdom and experience, it is normal to alter your value system accordingly. Values that are perfectly normal and acceptable for a 15-year-old could well seem immature and inappropriate for a 30-year-old person.

Emotional Stress The word *stress* appears in almost every discussion of emotional health, yet the word is used in many different ways. To avoid any misunderstanding, we will use the word in the following ways in this book:

1. *Stress*, in its most general sense, and as defined by the noted Canadian physiologist Hans Selye, is a group of nonspecific body responses induced by any harmful external force.

2. A *stressor* is any force that produces stress. It may be emotional conflict,

fear, fatigue, physical injury, disease, poison, radiation, or any other harmful force. In the urban environment, noise is one of the most prominent and harmful stressors.

3. *Emotional stress* is a condition involving tension, frustration, or conflict. Anxiety may or may not be present.

The General Adaptation Syndrome

Prolonged stress can have severe damaging effects on both the physical and emotional health of a person. A part of the nervous system reacts to emotional stress by preparing the body for emergency action. Among the many effects are increased speed and strength of heartbeat; diversion of the blood supply away from the digestive organs and to the body muscles; dilation of the pupil of the eye; changes in hormone levels; increase in blood sugar level; and inhibition of the digestive glands. Such effects, although useful while actually responding to emergencies, become harmful when continued over long periods of time.

Many aspects of contemporary life produce these severe kinds of emotional stress. Typical of these stress-producing factors are personal and domestic tensions, indecision over career goals, grades, the deteriorating urban environment with its housing and transportation problems, noise, threat of crime, and in general the effect of *novelty, diversity,* and *acceleration* on all aspects of our environment. Alvin Toffler, in his book *Future Shock* (Random House, 1970), describes these three forces as the significant factors that test the adaptational capacity of every member of a technological society.

If a person suffers from prolonged emotional stress, such as chronic conflict, anxiety, frustration, or hostility that smolders on month after month, then the resulting nervous stimulation can also continue without letup. A multitude of physical problems can result from such prolonged stress, including high blood pressure, asthma, peptic ulcers, skin disorders, impotence, and menstrual irregularities. Such disorders are termed *psychosomatic* (*psyche* meaning mind and *soma* meaning body), because they may be caused by psychological stresses. Of course, any of these disorders may also have purely physical causes, or be the result of a combination of both physical and psychological factors. Emotional stress, however, is the precipitating cause of many cases of these disorders.

Selye applied the term *general adaptation syndrome* (GAS) to the physical evidence of stress. (A syndrome is a group of symptoms.) Selye emphasized that the same reaction is elicited by any type of stressor to which we are subjected, be it emotional stress, physical injury, infection with disease organisms, fatigue, or exposure to extremes of heat or cold. The essence of stress is intense strain-producing anxiety. Anxiety is characterized by a variety of physiological and psychological responses that are no doubt familiar to all of us. They include rapid pulse, color changes like flushing or turning pale, changes in blood pressure, butterflies in the stomach, nausea and other gastrointestinal symptoms, fatigue, insomnia, and overall, generalized sensations of impending threat or danger.

The general adaptation syndrome includes three successive stages. The first is the *alarm reaction*, consisting of the immediate mobilization of the body's defense mechanisms just mentioned in the preceding paragraph. For example, an individual's alarm reaction could be triggered by the anticipation of taking an exam.

If the stress continues for some time, however, the person enters the second stage, called *resistance to stress*. This is the stage of maximum ability to withstand the stressor. It may continue for days, weeks, or even months, depending on the vitality of the person and the amount of rest the individual is able to obtain during this period of maximum effort. Sustained endurance, however, puts a considerable strain on the body's resources and often results in psychosomatic disorders. One of the causes of depression is related to stress in that emotional and physical stressors alike initially induce a state of psychological and somatic excitement that is followed by a secondary phase of depression. If the stress continues long enough, the third stage, *exhaustion*, may be reached, in which the person becomes progressively devitalized and the ability to resist stress diminishes. The internal resources for dealing with the continued assault have been exhausted. Every function of the body is weakened. Continued long enough, this stage inevitably results in death.

In returning to our example of the individual taking an exam, let us suppose that the person has taken on a very heavy course load. In addition to academic stresses he or she has also set high standards of achievement. In order to reduce the anxiety of possible failure to meet the self-imposed demands, a great amount of time and energy must be devoted to study. For a certain period of time the person is able to adapt and therefore realize the goal of good grades because of diligent study habits—the resistance to stress phase. However, now let us assume this person has, in addition to academic endeavors, other responsibilities such as a job and a family to support. The amount of time associated with meeting these demands is likely to reduce the time available for study, and grades begin to drop. Thus the person is no longer able to meet expectations of success. In order to compensate for lower exam scores, he or she tries to allow more time for study by sleeping less, and also by eliminating previous recreational diversions. It is only a matter of time until the person reaches the third stage—exhaustion. At this point certain symptoms are likely to appear: depression, guilt because of failure to live up to one's standards, and an array of physical disorders like ulcers, susceptibility to infectious organisms, high blood pressure, backaches, headaches, and so on. If the stresses are not alleviated, both body and mind will break down.

A key concept in the general adaptation syndrome is that, since all types of stressors produce the same reaction, exposure to any one type of stressor reduces our ability to defend ourselves against all other types of stressors. For example, prolonged emotional stress interferes with our ability to fight off infectious diseases. Thus we may become physically ill more readily while under a state of emotional stress. Or, conversely, physical illness lowers our ability to resist emotional stresses. Thus, the health of the body and of the mind are inseparably interrelated and interdependent. Because of this interdependence the full range of practices identified for the maintenance of "good health" serve as preventatives against physical and emotional stress. Conversely, their repeated neglect increases the potential for physical and emotional stress and illness.

Defense Mechanisms Stress situations are a part of every life and everyone develops methods for coping with them. The purpose of these coping methods is to avoid a conscious feeling of stress. These stress-preventing devices have been called "ego-defense mechanisms" or just "defense mechanisms."

There is no disagreement that defense mechanisms do exist. But there has been disagreement on how many of these defenses there are and to which defense mechanism a particular behavior pattern should be attributed. The problem has come about through efforts to neatly classify every type of behavior as the result of a particular mechanism. Actually, no such concrete classification is possible, since the same behavior can often result from any of several causes. Defense mechanisms are thought to be called into play whenever a situation or impulse or feeling comes up that is in conflict with the person's self-concept.

These defense mechanisms should not be thought of as abnormal. Everyone makes use of them. They are recognized by most authorities today as necessary and valuable in dealing with the stress situations that we all face throughout life. It is doubtful that anyone could successfully go through life without making use of them. However, excessive reliance upon them, or inability to acknowledge or accept them, can be a sign of low ego strength. This becomes difficult when we realize that most defense mechanisms are unconsciously motivated—that is, we don't know why we do them.

In examining a few of the more widely accepted defense mechanisms, we will make no attempt to classify these mechanisms as good or bad. In most cases, the value of a particular mechanism depends on the extent to which it is used. Used in moderation and in the proper situation, a mechanism might be of great value. Yet the same mechanism, used in excess or in inappropriate situations, might be definitely harmful.

Avoidance One of the simplest and most common methods of defense against anxiety is to avoid situations that produce it. We all use this defense to some extent. People who fear airplanes travel by car or train. People who are bothered by speaking in front of groups try to avoid situations in which they would be obliged to do

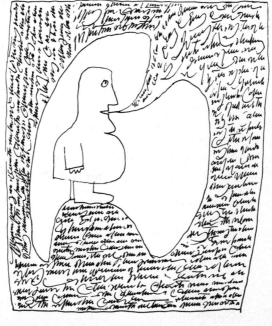

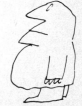

so. People who feel threatened by an intimate, caring relationship with another person often avoid this anxiety by keeping other people at emotional "arm's length."

Certainly, none of these examples of avoidance could be considered extreme or even unusual. But avoidance can become so intense that it does indicate a serious emotional conflict. Such would be the case if someone became so fearful that they refused to leave their house for any reason, or if they lacked the self-confidence to perform any kind of job at all. Thus it can be seen that the same defense mechanism can be normal and harmless or seriously disabling, depending on its degree of use.

Denial of Reality In using this mechanism, people protect their ego from a stressful situation by refusing to perceive it. Denial of reality is usually an unconscious process, or at least partly so. Individuals using this mechanism usually are not consciously aware that they are denying anything.

Denial appears in several forms. One is merely refusing to see or hear certain things that might lead to stress reactions, such as children "tuning out" their mother's calling them home. Another form is to deny the existence of a reality. Many people deny the risk of pregnancy, for example, and fail to take adequate precautions. Others deny the danger inherent in the street use of hard drugs or insist that only other, "stupid" people are victims of drug abuse.

Still another variation is the denial of inward feelings. We often deny our feelings of sexual desire for a person if we know we have no chance of winning them. We may even find something about them to criticize or ridicule. We also tend to react in the same way to material things that we believe are entirely out of our reach. We usually avoid anxiety by restricting our serious desire to that which is attainable, or nearly so.

Like avoidance, denial can be either a helpful or harmful defense, depending on the situation in which it is used and the extent to which it is used. For example, we must admit that the world is, to some extent, a dangerous place. Every day, each one of us faces the possibility of being cut down by fatal disease, war, murder, automobile accident, fire, flood, tornado, lightning, or building collapse, to name but a few of life's hazards. But the probability of anything happening to a given person on a given day is extremely remote. If we continually considered all the dangers we face, we would be in a constant state of anxiety. Through denial, we can ignore the remote dangers and live a normal life.

But denial can be harmful if it results in failure to take precautions against more immediate dangers. For example, some people fail to get immunizations or physical examinations because they deny the possibility of illness. Others fail to use automobile seat belts because they deny the possibility of an accident. When any clear and present danger is denied, that is obviously a misuse of the mechanism of denial.

Repression Repression is the process of forgetting (or more accurately, restricting to the unconscious mind) an event, feeling, or memory that would produce anxiety. The repressed material, though blocked from entering the conscious mind, continues to have an influence. It constantly seeks expression in some indirect way. It may cause tension in certain situations, or it may influence preferences, decisions, attitudes, or beliefs. It may require the use of other defense mechanisms in order to keep the material repressed and to prevent anxiety from rising to the conscious mind.

Material that is repressed is pushed back

into the unconscious mind much more rapidly than material that is ordinarily forgotten. It may happen almost immediately in response to the urgent need to defend the ego against the awareness of anxiety. This occurrence is especially true of frightening experiences in childhood, such as a bad fall or an attack by an animal. Adults similarly tend to repress such occurrences as accidents, attacks, socially unacceptable feelings or actions, and other frightening events. Interestingly, repression underlies most of the other defense mechanisms.

Psychologists use the term *cognitive dissonance* to describe the situation that exists when our knowledge, ideas, feelings, attitudes, and behavior are inconsistent or in conflict with each other. This creates a mental conflict that must be dealt with in some way. We either choose one of the alternatives that face us or we try to avoid or ignore the conflict. If we have two ideas that are dissonant (mutually inconsistent) we will attempt to take steps to reduce the inconsistency. For example, if an attitude pattern—such as prejudice against members of a specific ethnic group—is disrupted when we meet and befriend a member of that group, we have three choices. We can decide that we were wrong in our earlier prejudice. We can reassert the prejudice, and end the friendship. Or we can just try to ignore the differences between our prejudice and our personal experience with this good friend. Thus, the first two choices involve changing the attitude to match our desired behavior or changing our behavior to match our attitude.

The third choice (trying to ignore the dissonance) requires using repression as a defense mechanism against the anxiety that results when our behavior is in conflict with our attitudes. How we deal with our cognitive dissonances is really the foundation of many serious health problems. Too often, we change our attitude to fit our behavior, choosing to ignore established cause-and-effect health relationships. Or we take the third choice (which is really no choice at all) and continue with behavior that conflicts with what we know. This too often leads to both physical problems resulting from the behavior and emotional problems resulting from the continued conflict (dissonance) between what we know and what we do.

In the school of psychology called psychoanalysis, repressed conflicts are seen as the cause of much vague anxiety. Psychoanalysts make elaborate efforts to bring these conflicts from the unconscious mind into the conscious mind so that they can be rationally discussed and the anxiety of the patient relieved. This approach has been used much less frequently in recent years, although it still has followers and is of value in certain situations.

Projection Projection is the way in which people bolster their own self-image by unconsciously attributing their own feelings or characteristics to other people. This is generally done with some characteristic that we unconsciously consider to be undesirable. For example, people who lie, cheat, or steal usually believe that everyone lies, cheats, or steals. Thus, they can feel that their own behavior is really not too bad because "everybody does it." Very often the things that people accuse others of doing are exactly the things that they themselves are doing or would like to be doing.

Rationalization In rationalization, which is closely related to projection, people explain their behavior in such a way as to assign a socially acceptable motive to it and disguise the unacceptable motive their behavior actually expresses.

Rationalization is among the most commonly used of the defense mechanisms and we probably all use it to some extent. Students who fail exams or courses often blame the instructor, the curriculum—in fact, anything but their own lack of effort or ability. People who get fired from their job or get a traffic ticket similarly find someone or something else to blame. People using rationalization really believe what they are saying or thinking. They use this mechanism to protect their own opinion of themselves, not just the opinion that others have of them.

Regression   Regression occurs when, in times of acute stress, people unconsciously try to return to an earlier stage of life in order to escape their current anxiety. As we gain in age and maturity, we find that our responsibilities are equally increased. We become more responsible for the consequences of our own behavior and therefore must maintain a greater degree of control over our emotions and impulses. This naturally tends to produce some stress.

Most people can look back at the earlier stages of their lives as being less stressful than their current stage of development. This situation may be actually true, or it may be that the less pleasant aspects of the earlier ages have been forgotten or repressed. But when stress occurs, a person may behave in ways that were characteristic of the earlier period, often involving less responsibility and greater dependency.

Many examples of regression can be cited. The wife or husband who deserts a marriage and "goes home to mama" is demonstrating regression. The satisfaction received from sucking on a cigarette has been attributed to regression. A most extreme example of regression is the emotionally ill person who curls up, mute and withdrawn, into the fetal position (knees tucked under the chin).

Fixation   Fixation is closely related to regression. In fixation, however, people do not regress from an advanced point of development; they simply never reach it. They remain emotionally immature, either in all phases of personality or only in certain phases of it. Such people may never gain emotional maturity, or may gain it at a later than average age.

Sublimation   The word *sublimation* was used originally to indicate the process of satisfying frustrated sexual desires in nonsexual substitute activities. The term is now used more loosely by many authorities to include any substitution of higher need satisfaction for the satisfaction of a lower need.

Through sublimation, thoughts and actions that we consider to be undesirable can be repressed by developing forms of behavior that are more socially acceptable. Instead of expressing aggressive impulses toward others in the form of destructive acts or behavior that is not socially acceptable, we can express these impulses with socially acceptable forms of competition, as in sports, politics, and business.

Sublimation thus means converting basic emotional drives, sexual and otherwise, into acceptable and useful activities. Sublimation is considered by many authorities to be among the most constructive of the defense mechanisms. Though difficult to achieve, it can be both personally and socially beneficial, and can bring a social approval that strengthens the ego by satisfying one of the higher needs.

Sublimation can operate both unconsciously and as the result of conscious thought and effort. Unconsciously, it often keeps us from even being aware of undesirable motives. Most people would be very surprised to learn of the hostile and lustful impulses that they have been able to repress through the mechanism of sublimation. Through conscious effort, a person can sublimate conscious undesirable impulses and work toward more desirable personal and social goals.

Everyday Coping Devices The defense mechanisms as well as many similar mechanisms are necessary for the avoidance of anxiety. Yet, at the same time, the use of these mechanisms often creates a stress in itself.

The ability to tolerate this tension varies considerably among different individuals. Some can stand much more tension than others, but each has a limit. When the tension reaches this limit, it must be relieved in some personally satisfying way or the defense mechanisms will fail. Such a failure is commonly but incorrectly called a "nervous breakdown."

In order to obtain relief from tension, people use many types of behavior called "everyday coping devices" (Menninger, 1963). The purpose of these devices is to drain off the tension that may result from the use of the ego-defense mechanisms. According to Menninger, an important distinction between the defense mechanisms and the coping devices is that the defense mechanisms function on an unconscious level, while the coping devices are often consciously and purposely used to relieve tension. Some of these coping devices are as follows:

1. *Touch, rhythm, and sound.* These stimuli give pleasant sensations that relieve tensions. For example, playing, singing or listening to music is often useful in reducing tension. Dancing to rhythmic music is especially good.
2. *Eating, smoking, and chewing gum.* There are several theories on how these oral activities work to reduce tension. Obesity is often the result of tension.
3. *Alcohol and other drugs.* These work by dulling or altering one's perception and are among the least desirable coping devices.
4. *Laughing, crying, and swearing.* Such open expressions of tension may be very useful in relieving that tension.
5. *Sleeping.* This may be another device for escaping reality or boredom.
6. *Talking out a problem.* Discussing one's problems with a trusted person

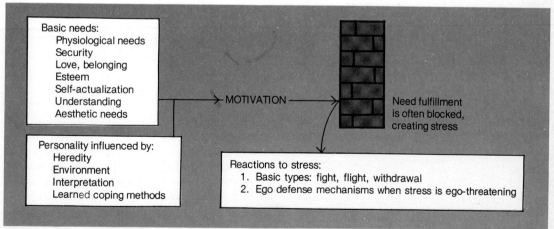

The personality adjustment process. Basic needs and personality create motivation, but the fulfillment of needs and motivations is often blocked, creating stress. Reaction to stress may then influence personality, possibly altering motivations.

can greatly relieve tension, even if the person does no more than listen. It reduces the sense of loneliness, even if the listener is a perfect stranger, as is often the case.

7. *Thinking through a situation.* Just a few minutes of clear, unemotional thinking can often place a problem in its proper perspective.

8. *Physical exercise.* It is now widely agreed that physical exercise is valuable in working off tension.

9. *Pointless activity.* This includes some of the less desirable tension-reducing devices, such as pacing the floor, hand wringing, nail biting, finger tapping, and scratching.

10. *Daydreaming.* Daydreaming is a retreat into fantasy, usually into a fantasy in which one's problems do not exist or have been solved. Occasional brief periods of daydreaming may be helpful in reducing tension, but it is easy to spend too much time in the retreat from reality.

11. *Familiar activities.* Doing something familiar so that it involves no threat or, perhaps, which is associated with comfort and satisfaction in the past (for example, working at a hobby, washing the car, working overtime).

Communication and Intimacy

Basic to many of our problems in human relations and personal emotional health is our frequent failure to communicate our thoughts, needs, and feelings openly and honestly. Lack of communication ranks high among the causes of sexual problems, family conflicts, and emotional problems of all kinds. Noncommunication and the resulting social isolation are implicated in many suicides and other emotional breakdowns.

Closely related to communication failure is the inability to establish or maintain intimate relationships. In essence, we all share the desire to develop various intimate associations through which we can satisfy our needs to belong, to give affection, to receive affection, and to maintain self-esteem.

To many people, the word *intimacy* is misunderstood as being synonymous with sexual intercourse. While sexual intimacy may imply a physical closeness, emotional intimacy is an important part of every close relationship in which one person feels free to communicate innermost feelings to another person and vice versa. It is quite possible to have emotional intimacy without sexual implications or to have sexual intercourse in the absence of true emotional intimacy.

Friendship, for example, provides more profound psychological uses than mere companionship or shared interests. Intimate friends help us deal with anxiety by lending us their support. They also enable us to keep our problems in perspective through sharing their troubles with us. And sometimes, just by listening to us in a nonjudgmental manner, friends assist in reducing emotional stress by verbalizing internal conflicts or sorting out possible solutions.

Relationships combining sexual as well as emotional intimacy, such as between married or otherwise committed persons, require the stimulation of effective, sensitive communication. Without it, these relationships eventually disintegrate by failing to fulfill the needs of the individuals.

Now let us look at some major factors in the communication process, and how we can relate to others more effectively. We will also discuss some of the common causes of communication failure.

Communication is not limited to spoken language. Our nonverbal behavior, commonly called *body language*, conveys much of our message, particularly its emotional content. Our true feelings are often more accurately perceived by others through facial expressions, posture, body gestures, clothing, and general appearance. In other words, feelings that we may not desire to or are unable to express verbally, can be otherwise communicated. The perception of our verbal messages is further influenced by the tone we use, volume, and inflection of words or sentences. Let us take for example the phrase "I love you too." Generally, we would say this sounds like a positive expression of caring for someone. However, try saying it in a sarcastic tone, squinting the eyes, pursing the lips, and clenching your fists—obviously the entire meaning is changed. Most of our nonverbal communication is not that dramatic. Rather, we reveal our emotions in numerous more subtle ways. For those who are interested in understanding body language, there are many excellent books available on the subject, including *How to Read A Person Like A Book* by Gerard Nierenberg and Henry Calero, and *Inside Intuition* by Flora Davis.

Successful communication requires at least two participants: one who honestly expresses a feeling and one who truly wants and tries to understand that feeling as well as hear the words. Many of us tend to view the speaker as taking an active role while the listener is passive. The listener is also an active participant of whom much is required for communication to be successful. Many people fail as listeners because they are so wrapped up in their own problems that they are unable to direct their attention and concern to the needs of others. The sounds may enter their ears and be transmitted as nerve impulses to their brain, but they do not hear the message. For example, a person may really be very unhappy and lonely but may attempt to cover up these feelings by talking excessively about trivia, by having many companions, or having too many social commitments. Unless listeners are being sincerely attentive, more than likely they will not receive the true meaning.

Sometimes people do hear, but fail to understand—or worse, misunderstand—what is being said to them. Often people take messages as being critical when in fact they were not intended as such. Little misunderstandings have a way of growing into big hostilities simply because we fail to ask for clarification of some ill-taken or vague statement. How often do people take remarks to be personal criticism when in fact they were merely a case of misplaced frustration? When someone makes a statement causing you to feel defensive or angry, these feelings should not be concealed in hopes they will disappear. Anger does not go away easily and most likely it will be expressed at another time—probably not an appropriate time.

In some instances, unsuccessful communication results from lack of adequate vocabulary, or the inability to express oneself in a particular area. In our society, sexual matters are frequently subject to flawed communication or even noncommunication because of the above inadequacies. Many people have difficulty finding the right words to explain their sexual feelings and desires. Sexual intercourse can easily become an unexciting, ritual chore simply because neither partner communicates what they would like to do. Fantasies should be shared; often it turns out both individuals were thinking similar things. When people are raised in homes where sex is an embarrassing topic, it is not always easy to overcome this feeling. However, it is not impossible to establish communication even if both partners are shy. The subject could be introduced in an academic way, or perhaps a book such as *The Joy of Sex*, by Alex Comfort, could be casually placed where the other person would see it. This is a form of communication.

Probably the greatest barrier to successful communication and the development of intimacy lies in the reluctance of so many people to make known their true feelings. There are many reasons why this is so. Men, for instance, have generally been raised to hide their emotions. Many have been taught to equate masculinity with strength and stonelike character. It is seen as unmasculine to reveal sadness in tears, to reveal fear by refusal to compete or strive, or to reveal love through tender words or gentle caresses. Whatever emotions we cannot let escape naturally will nevertheless surface, although they may be cleverly disguised or distorted. Frequently, men substitute material conveniences for verbal communication of affection. Expressions of love can also be displaced to objects such as cars or motorcycles or to sports because these are acceptable as love outlets for the masculine image.

Women also hide their feelings. This is particularly true when it comes to feelings of hurt and rejection. Rather than saying "I feel you are rejecting me" and asking "What do you think makes me feel this way?" resentment builds up and communication becomes hostile.

These are just a few examples of how ineffective communication becomes established. One insensitive response is likely to be met with another, and the consequences are a tangled mess of negative emotions: hurt, frustration, rejection, anger, resentment, hostility, and so forth. In time, communication is viewed as a waste of effort and finally there may be no real communication whatsoever. Many people withdraw ever deeper into themselves, silently directing hate at others or even toward themselves.

There is, however, no reason why communication cannot be successful. Initially, we must know as much as possible about our own true feelings; then it is necessary to risk exposing such emotions to another person. Without this risktaking, it is impossible to communicate honestly. Intimacy or closeness can only develop in such an atmosphere. When defenses are lowered, we are vulnerable and it is easy for someone, as part of their own ego-defense, to aim a hurt directly at one of our vulnerable areas.

Communication is further enhanced by the ability of both persons to remain as nonjudgmental as possible. Such an attitude allows for continued honesty and provides assurance that their vulnerability will not be taken advantage of. People can thus feel free to present themselves as they truly are, not as they would like to be or would like others to see them as being.

Intimacy requires a mutual concern for the welfare and happiness of each individual that can only develop and be maintained so long as communication remains open and honest. It also requires the mutual acceptance of each person for what they are so that each can lower any barrier-producing ego-defense mechanisms that may be in the way. Many of the problems we will be considering in the following pages could be avoided if such barriers to open communication could be lowered.

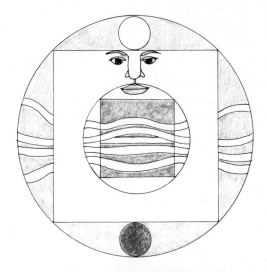

2

EMOTIONAL HEALTH

Each of us is conceived with a certain genetic potential for our physical and mental development. The extent to which this potential is realized is heavily dependent on environmental, psychological, and sociological factors. Few people are lucky enough to come even close to achieving their full potential.

Environmental factors begin their influence even before conception. Exposure of the ovaries or testes to radiation or to certain chemicals, for example, may result in genetic damage that severely limits the potential of offspring. During pregnancy diet, drugs, diseases, and hormonal factors exert lifelong influences on development. The experiences of early childhood are extremely important in our development—many basic lifetime personality characteristics are formed before the age of four years. Important influences continue throughout the school years and, in fact, until death. As young adults, we are faced with choices (and sometimes lack of choices) concerning life-styles, careers, and our emerging adult identities.

Continued emotional health requires an ongoing process of adjustment to our ever-changing life situation. Not only does the world around us change constantly, frequently presenting new barriers to the fulfillment of our basic needs, but also our own physical and mental selves are in a state of perpetual transition. Hopefully, we continue to gain in insight and understanding throughout life, though some of our new insights may in themselves threaten our sense of emotional security. Finally, every one of us faces the unavoidable reality of the physical aging process and the ultimate challenge of death itself. Unfortunately, we live in a society that has been largely unsuccessful in dealing with the psychological aspects of aging and

death, even though the number of elderly people has greatly increased and will continue to do so.

In this chapter, we will examine the stages of human personality development as presented by Erik Erikson in his classic *Childhood and Society* (1950 and 1963), relating Erikson's concepts to Maslow's thoughts on human needs and to our own discussion of intimacy and need fulfillment. We will then explore in somewhat greater depth some emotional factors that affect college students and ways of dealing with these factors. The chapter will conclude with an exploration of an area of rapidly growing interest—the psychological factors in aging and death.

In Erikson's concept of development, each phase of the human life cycle is characterized by a specific developmental task that must be resolved in some way before the individual proceeds to the next level. The success with which each task is resolved may have lasting effects on the

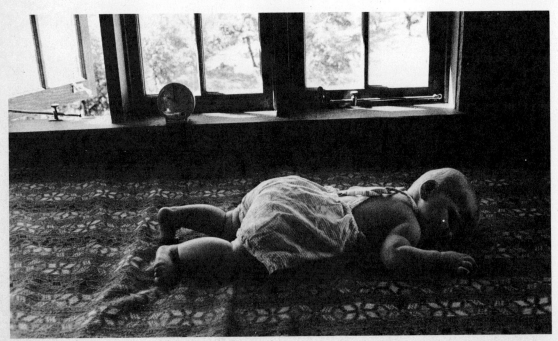

Photo by David Powers/Jeroboam

future personality of the individual. It should be noted that these tasks are never completely resolved, but are worked out further during successive stages. Again, we would emphasize the dynamic nature of personality, with the ever-present possibility for improvement (substitution of more appropriate or effective responses). Erikson has formulated each stage in terms of psychological contrasts that represent the two extremes of successful and unsuccessful task resolution (personality development). The actual outcome in an individual is always somewhere between the two polar extremes for each of the eight developmental tasks.

Early Infancy

This period is the first year or year-and-a-half following birth. The lifelong importance of early childhood environment and experiences would be difficult to overstate. Right from birth, many of the basic human needs are strongly felt. The needs for food, love, and security are overwhelmingly strong and demanding at this time. Deprivation during the first few years, whether physical (such as diet) or emotional, will likely have effects spanning one's entire life.

Studies have shown that an infant is capable of learning new responses from the first few days following birth. The experiences of the first year are very significant. For example, babies who receive plenty of sensory stimulus in the form of holding and other loving attention show more rapid mental (and often physical) development than babies who are deprived of such stimuli.

Since the child is so totally dependent on others at this time, Erikson rates its emotional health in terms of either *trust* or *mistrust*. Trust (sound emotional health in the infant) results from affection and adequate gratification of the infant's needs. Mistrust (developmental failure) results from inadequate need fulfillment— neglect, isolation, deprivation of love, too early or harsh weaning, or physical abuse. For many, this is the first step toward a lifetime of isolation and inability to develop intimacy with others. Intimacy is based on mutual trust and can never develop in an atmosphere of mistrust.

Later Infancy

This period lasts from about the first to the third year of age. Much of one's lifelong self-concept, gender identity, and sexual orientation is formed during this period. In addition to the more basic needs—love, security, and the physiological needs—the need for self-esteem is strongly felt during this period. In fact, Erikson rates developmental success at this age in terms of the child's self-image. Successful development is seen as a sense of *autonomy*. While still recognizing its dependence on its parents, the child feels itself to be an independent person and will often exert its independence. Developmental failure at this age is characterized by feelings of inadequacy, doubts about one's individuality, and a desire to hide one's inadequacies (a sense of shame). Development of basic skills like walking and talking is unusually slow. Many of these same characteristics carry over into our adult lives. Those of us who believe in ourselves tend to be much more successful in anything we try than are those of us who doubt our abilities. Again, the development of intimacy may be blocked by shame and the desire to hide imagined inadequacies.

Parents can make an important contribution to their child's lifelong emotional health by building his or her self-esteem at this time. A feeling of individuality, ability, and value gained at this age may stick with the child for life.

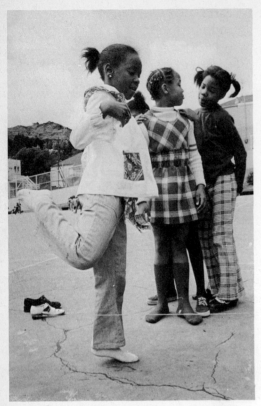

Photo by Suzanne Arms/Jeroboam

Early Childhood This is the period a child goes through between the ages of four and five. In addition to the previously mentioned needs, the need to know and to understand becomes pressing at this time. For many children of this age, the most commonly used word is *why*. Children at this age thrive on an abundance of sensory input. Erikson sees emotional health at this age as characterized by either *initiative* or *guilt*. The child who is developing well has a lively imagination, vigorously tests the limits of reality, imitates adults, and anticipates adult roles. In contrast, developmental failure is characterized by guilt over goals contemplated and acts initiated. This guilt results in an inhibition of normal activity. The child lacks spontaneity and is jealous, posses-

sive, suspicious, evasive, and has difficulty in assuming a social role. Once again, we see that these symptoms of developmental failure carry over in some adults. These unfortunate people gain little pleasure from life because anything that they might do to produce pleasure will also produce guilt. Their relationships with other people tend to be mutually unrewarding and difficult.

Middle Childhood This period lasts from about six to eleven years of age. During this prepubertal stage, most children exhibit fairly stable personality traits. There is seldom a sudden upheaval of established patterns, but rather a gradual evolution of more mature responses. Erikson sees the basic inner conflict at this time as being between *industry* and feelings of *inferiority*. Again, the need for a sense of self-esteem seems dominant in the successful development of children of this age.

The child who is developing successfully holds a positive self-image as someone who has value and is capable of doing worthwhile things. Such a child has a sense of duty and accomplishment, functions up to his or her capability in school, relates well with other children and adults, undertakes and successfully completes tasks at home and at school, and can clearly distinguish fantasy from reality.

Children who are held back by their feelings of inferiority tend to have poor work habits because they have little expectation of success. Their attitude may be "What's the use? Why try? I'm going to fail anyway." They may expend little effort at school work and contribute little to the chores of their home.

An important contributing factor in the development of feelings of inferiority in many children is that they are seldom if ever complimented on things they have done or told that they are "OK." Instead, they only hear negative things about themselves. They are constantly reminded of the "bad" things they have done or the "good" things they have failed to do. Many parents could make a great contribution to the lifelong happiness of their children if they would merely emphasize their positive values and minimize their shortcomings.

School failures can often be traced to prejudice, preconceived notions, stereotyped thinking, and self-fulfilling prophecies. For example, teachers' expectations for a child are sometimes influenced by such factors as the child's sex, ethnic group, appearance, or the opinions of previous teachers. If a teacher expects little from a child, the child will quickly become aware of this feeling and the expectation of failure will be incorporated into the child's self-image. Once a person of any age adopts a self-image of incompetence in any area, his or her failure in that area is pretty well assured—it is a self-fulfilling prophecy. Teachers, parents, and anyone interacting with children can, by taking a positive view of the potential of each child, contribute to a self-image that will lead to success, not failure.

Adolescence In most societies, adolescence (the period between puberty and full maturity) is recognized as a period of special difficulty in adjustment, a critical period in the individual's development. This should not appear surprising if we consider the special stresses to which the adolescent is typically subjected, in comparison to people at most other age levels. Problems of adjustment are minimal during periods when a fairly well-stabilized individual is confronted with environmental demands that are for the most part familiar, and for which appropriate and need-satisfying responses have already been well developed. Neither condition characterizes adolescence in our culture. (Other similar periods of stress are created by entering or leaving school, divorce, career adjustments such as changing occupations or retirement, the death of a spouse, and declining health.)

The onset of puberty brings with it a host of physiological changes, including increases in hormone levels and changes in body structure and function. These changes present special adjustment problems in themselves, but also challenge the individual's basic sense of self, one's identity. In adolescence, one's previous concept of self and sense of continuity is challenged by the rapidity of body growth and the entirely new addition of sexual maturity, with its multitude of physical and

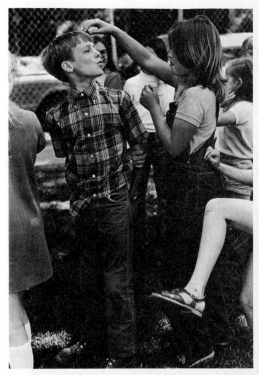

Photo by Linda Montano/Jeroboam

emotional changes. Thus, Erikson sees the success of the development of the adolescent in terms of *identity* versus *role confusion* or *diffusion*.

Adolescents who have an adequately developed sense of identity are characterized by a feeling of self-assurance—a definite sense of who they are, where they are, and in what direction they are moving. They are certain of their gender identity and their sexual orientation. They have been able to integrate their varied partial identifications, such as their identification with each of their parents or other significant adults, their sexual identifications, their intellectual and emotional endowment, and their social roles into a single identity. The consequence of this integrative process is a sense of rightness about who they are and what they are doing. Another result of this integration is a well-defined sense of values.

Identity diffusion (poor self-integration or role confusion) occurs when people cannot adequately integrate their varied identifications. As a result, they may be unable to make definite choices of career, roles, values, or sexual objects. There may be a sense of total confusion—identity confusion, role confusion, authority confusion, value confusion, and even time confusion. All of this uncertainty leads to self-consciousness, anxiety, depression, and a sense of alienation or loneliness.

Many adolescents are forced by these feelings into inadequate and ultimately self-defeating defense mechanisms. Some lean heavily upon alcohol or other drugs as coping devices. Some get caught up in compulsive or irresponsible sexuality. Some seek shelter in a premature marriage. Some withdraw into themselves. In some of the most tragic and severe cases, suicide seems the only way out.

Adolescents with emotional problems are usually identified first by parents or school authorities. Less often, they come to the attention of police, youth leaders, or the clergy. Unfortunately, many adolescent problems are not identified at all until the individuals are having serious emotional problems as adults. Persons outside the home who feel that an adolescent has serious problems may take the matter up with the parents. In many instances, parents are reluctant to take any action unless they are firmly convinced of the need for evaluation and treatment. Perhaps they fear that the problems of their child will be seen by others as a poor reflection of the job that they themselves have done as parents. This, of course, is not necessarily the case, and the problems of adolescents should be treated promptly before more serious trouble results. A therapist should be chosen who has specific training and experience in working with this age group. Various individual and group therapy methods are used with adolescents.

Adulthood Erikson divides adulthood into three stages, each with its own characteristic developmental task. These stages are early adulthood, from about ages 18 to 25; middle adulthood; and late adulthood, which roughly corresponds to the retirement years.

Early Adulthood If the more basic human needs are being more or less adequately fulfilled, the full range of Maslow's higher needs should be manifest by this time. With adequate need fulfillment, the young adult should now be in a position to make a full commitment of him- or herself to others. In fact, Erikson judges the success of one's development at this age on the basis of *intimacy* versus *isolation*.

Some of the characteristics of satisfactory personality development include the ability to establish intimacy, as discussed

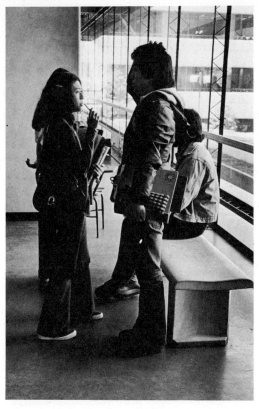

Photo by David Powers/Jeroboam

in the preceding chapter; the ability to work productively; and adequate sexual adjustment. All of these traits have the prerequisite of an adequate sense of personal worth or self-esteem. Lacking this feeling, many people avoid the development of intimacy or exhibit various "personality problems" that work against them, especially in their relations with other people. Sexual dysfunction is quite common among these people, often simply because they lack confidence in their sexual ability. There may be a feeling of "something missing" in sexual relationships. That missing element is intimacy.

As a substitute for intimacy, many people resort to "game playing" in their interpersonal relationships. A "false front" is presented to others, so every rela-

tionship involves a certain element of deception or dishonesty. People who fail to develop intimacy often experience the failure of one or more marriages during their early adult years. They may be unable to establish the kind of mature relationship necessary to provide mutual need fulfillment over a longer period of time.

People experiencing problems of this type need to explore (perhaps with a therapist) the true nature of their relationships with others and the true content of what they are verbally or nonverbally expressing to others. People are often quite amazed to learn how they "come across" to others.

Middle Adulthood In the middle years of life, successful development is characterized by having one's needs adequately fulfilled so that one can help others in the fulfillment of their needs. Erikson uses the terms *generativity* (productivity) as contrasted to *stagnation* for the possible development of the middle adult. Others have applied the phrase *generosity* as contrasted to *self-absorption*.

Successful emotional development in the middle years is characterized by productivity and creativity for one's self and for others. If one has children, they are the source of pride and pleasure. The life of the middle adult should be rich with new experiences and the individual should gain satisfaction in establishing and guiding the next generation.

Poor personality development in the middle adult might be characterized by stagnation and/or self-absorption. Such people might be self-centered, self-indulgent, threatened by new ideas or experiences ("in a rut"), less productive than they could be, and perhaps even forced into premature invalidism by psychogenic or psychosomatic disorders (either term means a physical condition that is caused or aggravated by the state of the mind). Highly self-centered people tend to dwell upon every minor ache or pain to such an extent that a slight pain that most people would ignore seems so serious that it is disabling. No amount of physical treatment can cure such a problem, but appropriate psychotherapy can be rapidly effective in treating psychosomatic disorders.

Late Adulthood The way in which younger people look ahead to maturity and the way in which mature people experience it reveals much of the success of their personality development. Emotionally healthy younger people, while perhaps not eager to grow older, accept the aging process as part of life and try to make the most of every phase of their lives.

Erikson sees the emotional health of the elderly in terms of *integrity*, as contrasted to *despair*. Emotional integrity includes a love and appreciation of the spirit of humanity that goes beyond the love of the self. It is an acceptance of the continuity of past, present, and future. Most importantly, it is an acceptance of the life one has lived as having been valid and worthwhile. People holding such views do not find their mature years clouded by a morbid fear of death.

Conversely, the lack of this integrity is characterized by despair, fear of death; the feeling that one's life has been wasted, that the things one has done are not worthwhile; and the feeling that given another chance, one's life would be lived differently, but that it is now too late to start anew, to try out alternate roads to integrity. It is a feeling of despair and disgust with oneself and with humanity in general, a feeling that there is no meaning in human existence. It is a striking study in contrasts to compare the inner peace and happiness of a well-adjusted elderly person to the bitterness and depression of someone in a state of despair. Later sections of this chapter will explore in more detail the psychological factors in aging and death.

The College Years The so-called college age group in reality includes a broad spectrum of the population ranging from those in late adolescence to an increasing number of people of more advanced ages. The majority of college students, though, are in their late adolescence or early adulthood and are subject to the common problems that Erikson associates with those age groups: identity problems and isolation.

In colleges that provide adequate mental health services, about 10 percent of the students seek such help each year, either voluntarily or by referral. Since the majority of colleges do not have adequate mental health services, many students are left to try to work out their problems on their own or to seek help elsewhere. Most of the problems of college students are easily treated—only 2 percent of students seeking help are hospitalized. However, of the 40 percent of all students who leave college before completing their studies, it has been estimated that half do so for reasons of emotional health.

In the following paragraphs we will briefly examine some of the types of problems experienced by college students:

Identity Formation versus Identity Diffusion During the college years, various identities and activities may be tried, such as various types of love affairs, living arrangements, and organizational affiliations. If a student lacks integrative ability (as discussed in the section on adolescence), if identifications are too ambivalent, or if the pressures from the college environment are too severe, diffusion occurs.

Independence versus Dependence

Separation from the family—either the physical separation for someone going away to college or the removal from one value system to another that occurs for any college student—requires either the strengthening of an established system of values and behavior or the acceptance of an identification with a new system. A student must learn to trust and respect both the person he or she currently is and the person with new knowledge and values that he or she will become.

If the need to be dependent is too great or if accepting new values or developing a new identity seems to imply the rejection of greatly needed parents, separation anxiety or depression may result. Such feelings may lead to compulsive behavior patterns such as compulsive sexuality, compulsive use of substances (food, alcohol, or other drugs), compulsive activity, or the inability to concentrate on studies.

Intimacy versus Isolation

College students must learn to establish new relationships at a level of intimacy probably not experienced before. This requires a strong sense of self-esteem and identity so that one may be emotionally close to another person or accept a new idea without fear of losing one's identity. For someone lacking this confidence, the prospect of an intimate relationship produces anxiety, perhaps a very intense anxiety. But the failure to establish intimacy leads to feelings of isolation, rejection, and loneliness.

Sexual Decisions

Despite a general liberalization in sexual attitudes and practices, decisions on sexual behavior remain a source of anxiety and emotional conflict for many students. Many students come from families where nonmarital sexual activity is still sternly limited. Aside from the elements of identity, dependency, and intimacy that influence the sexual behavior of most students, these students face possible internal conflicts and guilt feelings if they are sexually active. But they also may experience feelings of being strange, lonely, or unaccepted if they are not sexually involved. Problems of this sort are best avoided by having a value system of one's own, not imposed by parents or friends, and with which one can be comfortable at both the intellectual and the emotional or "gut" level.

Problems of the New Student

The student entering college may encounter for the first time a wide variety of values and attitudes that conflict with those of his or her family. The conflict may be interpreted by the student as one of his or her individuality versus family loyalty. The pursuit of individuality, which is natural, may produce guilt feelings about rejecting and devaluing his or her own family.

The transition of a student from high school to college is often assumed by parents to mean the acceptance of adult responsibilities—financial and otherwise—and not all college freshmen are prepared or willing to give up their dependent status. They may feel that their family has abandoned them. At the same time, the parents may not be tolerant of the new values and ideas that the student brings home. The student who lives with parents and commutes to school is in a particularly difficult position as he or she may have to function at two conflicting levels in two quite different environments.

A common problem among college freshmen is the depression brought about by the first failures to maintain the level of grades received in high school. A student who was outstanding in high school may find him- or herself competing in college with many others of equal ability. A student in this position must rebuild the basis of his or her identity and self-esteem before feelings of inadequacy take hold and make success in college impossible.

Unhealthy family relationships may manifest themselves when a student leaves home to attend college. Previously suppressed negative feelings about parents may enter the consciousness, causing guilt and anxiety. If a student has been an ego-extension of one parent, separation from that parent may create anxiety or guilt at having "abandoned" that parent. If the parents of a student divorce soon after his or her entering college, there may be a feeling of responsibility for the breakup of the family. On the other hand, if the parents get along better after the student leaves home, which often does happen, the student may feel rejected because of the apparent ease with which his or her absence is tolerated.

Transferring Students   A transfer from one college to another may be based on a real need such as a change of career choice, financial problems, marriage, or divorce. On the other hand, many students with social or academic problems try to solve these problems by meaningless transfers from one college to another. Students who find their problems transferring right along with them should recognize that these problems are their own personal difficulties and should seek appropriate counsel in resolving them.

Problems of Academic Performance
Poor grades or anxiety over grades are among the most common college problems. For a few students, the problem may be one of basic intellectual deficiency, or unrealistic goals. For these students, the answer may be a reduced course load or perhaps a change to a more realistic goal. More commonly, students have the basic ability to achieve their goals but have difficulty in channeling their efforts to that

end. They may sit at their desks for hours with little to show for their time because they are unable to direct their thoughts to the task before them. Identifying the source of the distractions and dealing with the underlying problems, perhaps with the aid of a therapist, is the only way to break such a study block. The problem may involve social adjustment to college life, dependency conflicts, sexual problems, or even an unconscious effort to fail as revenge against parents or others. Or feelings of guilt or inadequacy may make a student feel unworthy of success so the unconscious mind acts to insure lack of success. Insight-oriented therapy can often be quite successful in dealing with any of these problems.

The Alienation Syndrome   Some students react to the college environment with attitudes of apathy, boredom, lack of involvement or commitment, and general unhappiness. This has been called the *alienation syndrome*. This syndrome is often related to the intellectual or conscious rejection of an individual's value system while emotionally or unconsciously holding on to the same value system. Or a student may reject his or her existing value system without formulating an adequate replacement for it. There may also be elements of repressed guilt if the system being rejected is that of the individual's parents or former religion.

Rejection Reactions   Some students (actually, people in general) suffer extreme reactions in situations that they perceive as rejection. A careless comment, a broken friendship, a bad grade, or a critical remark from someone can produce a hysterical reaction—panic, crying, impulsive acts, or even suicidal thoughts or actions. This type of reaction usually indicates an underlying lack of self-esteem. Great significance is placed on the opinions of others because the individual holds such a low opinion of him- or herself. People experiencing problems related to low self-esteem should seek out things they can do well and concentrate on such ego-boosting activities.

Fear of Leaving School During their last year of college, many students face decisions regarding career, further education, relocation, marriage, and general life-style. If college has served as a prolongation of a comfortable state of dependency, the prospect of graduation can arouse intense inner conflicts. The need to make important decisions plus the threatened loss of security may lead to reactions ranging from minor anxiety to true psychotic episodes. These factors also give rise to the "professional student," who in his or her senior year decides to change majors or who prolongs graduate study almost indefinitely in order to avoid leaving the sheltered environment of the college. Students experiencing this problem should explore (perhaps with a therapist) the emotional functions college has served and their attitudes toward the future.

Aging   Almost without exception, we hope and indeed expect to live as long as possible. Thanks to the contributions of science and modern medicine, we can now look forward to some seventy years of life. Length of life, however, too often becomes dissociated from quality of life and when basic human needs can no longer be met, the prospect of living countless more years does not have the same appeal as it did during youth.

While the most critical social problems concerning aging involve those persons who are in the retirement age bracket, the aging process takes a considerable emotional toll upon many younger persons who have passed some imaginary youth boundary. Our culture is geared toward adoration of youth, its physical perfection, and its hope in its ability to solve old problems with new ideas. In every way we are encouraged to grow up with a self-concept that does not include the inevitable changes that occur throughout life. We tend to conceal from everyone, including ourselves, that we are unable to halt the deterioration of physical function.

There exists a tremendous need to establish more realistic attitudes toward the later stages of life. Until we can come to grips with some of the problems involved in growing old and until we make a commitment toward solving them, we are devaluating these "golden" years, and can only look forward to as dismal a future as is presently experienced by vast numbers of aged people in this nation.

No one age represents all the positive aspects of a fulfilling life. Every age has its own special qualities and we should try to emphasize the positive rather than the negative aspects of each. For instance, in childhood there is freedom of time but there is little freedom of choice. In youth there is self-determination, physical stamina, and adaptability. On the other hand, lack of experience results in many mistakes, and the pressure of competition is fierce during this period. The middle years often represent the period of greatest productivity but there is also an awareness that others are ready and able to replace you, that it is too late to start on another path of endeavor, or that the children are grown and parental usefulness is being threatened. The material rewards of many years of work are most apparent here but these are often overshadowed by changes in physical appearance, doubts about one's real success, doubts about sexual attractiveness, and the realization that there may be no higher level of achievement or challenge to be reached. While there may be no real basis for these fears, they are so common that we refer to them as the *middle age crisis*.

Retirement, which may have been looked forward to during youth as a time when one is finally free to pursue his or her fondest interests, too often turns out to be the beginning of many years of discontent, and rapid decline in capacities. Unless the retiree has been fortunate enough to have had an income substantial enough to save faithfully for the coming years, it is unlikely that Social Security and fixed pension monies will be sufficient to tide him or her through the remaining twenty to thirty years. As the costs of living continue to rise, fixed incomes become less significant in terms of maintaining one's customary standard of living. Travel and hobbies that were anticipated may be either too expensive or they may not satisfactorily fill up the hours once devoted to employment or family. It is obvious that young people need to be taught to prepare themselves for a meaningful retirement in order that they can remain in a position of emotional and financial stability. It is necessary to encourage the young to establish goals early in life so that satisfying objectives can be accomplished that are in accord with plans for life after retirement. The hardest part is trying to get younger people oriented to the reality that they too will grow old.

Even the well-to-do people who purchase homes in retirement communities that apparently offer everything an older person would want out of life may find less happiness than expected. Such communities tend to cut their inhabitants off from contact with the world outside. Many older people miss the mixture of generations and often find the whole scene very depressing. A feeling of loss of usefulness is a common complaint of retirement community members.

With advancing age, the incidence of illness and chronic disease increases rapidly. Perhaps it is so painful to confront this reality because we are afraid to look closely at what we fear may be our own fate. Old people, especially those who are also ill, are often regarded by their families as useless burdens. When they can no longer care for themselves, they are rarely invited to stay with family, but rather are shipped off to homes for the aged or convalescent hospitals. Adjustment to new surroundings, new people, and strange ways is difficult for these elderly people, and they are saddened by the separation from family, friends, and familiar surroundings. The quality of care in such homes varies to both extremes. However, even the best facility lacks the comfort that could be provided by the mere presence of a loved person. Unfortunately, the quality of care in many places is grossly inadequate. Even basic nutrition may be ignored and many patients literally die of gradual starvation and general neglect. For lack of resources, understanding, or alternatives, these homes continue to provide a sanctuary for substantial numbers of aged citizens. Loneliness, combined with lack of interest or purpose, encourages even those who are still potentially productive to retreat from life. Often they die a social death long before bodily systems cease functioning.

Of course, growing old should and can be a wonderful period of life. It can be a time of savoring past experiences and looking forward to still more new ones. Growing old can be a time of continued curiosity and learning, even though physical functions are beginning to fail. It can be a time of sharing one's wisdom with younger people, while having the wisdom to understand youths' limited capacity to accept what they hear. Children especially love to hear old people talk about the way things were and what it was like in the "old days." This is something that many youngsters will never be fortunate enough to hear. In short, our older people are a source of wisdom that in our youth-worshipping culture has remained largely untapped. The young must try to become acquainted with this alienated segment of society and attempt to improve the plight of the aged as well as to prepare society to receive themselves when they reach their own "golden" years.

Death and Dying

No part of our existence is more unconsciously denied than the reality of our own death. While rationally we know that death is an inescapable counterpoint to life, somehow we manage to push aside death-related thoughts, thereby creating an illusion of immortality. It is nearly impossible to picture our own death and when we do, it is in a sort of play fashion, backed with the security of being in control of our thoughts. The majority of people express a desire to die suddenly and painlessly, during sleep. Death and violence are frequently associated with each other and anticipated suffering arouses great fear.

People have always exhibited a fear of death, much of which is attributable to its being an unknown encounter. This fear, however, is a composite of many fears— fear of loss of self, loss of feelings, loss of thoughts, permanent earthly separation, and fear of pain and suffering. It also includes emotions such as anger or jealousy toward those who will remain and who may erase even the memory of our existence. Despite our resistance to death, it is certain to affect each of our lives. The more fully we can come to face our attitudes toward dying, the less helpless we will feel in crises related to death, and the easier it will be to communicate with those who are dying and their survivors. Psychiatrists

think that our unresolved feelings toward death affect our daily living and are reflected in the way we drive, eat, work, sleep, and even in our commitment to love.

Dr. Robert Kavanaugh, a leading authority on the subject of death, believes that life can be lived more fully once we have come to terms with our true feelings about death. He suggests a reflective journey back through our lives, focusing on those experiences that have helped form our death-related attitudes. It is also good to reflect on other people's death fears, examining the emotions they evoke in ourselves. When there is an occasion to visit a dying person or to be in contact with persons who have recently encountered death, do not make excuses to stay away or be otherwise uninvolved. Being comfortable around reminders of death is not easy,

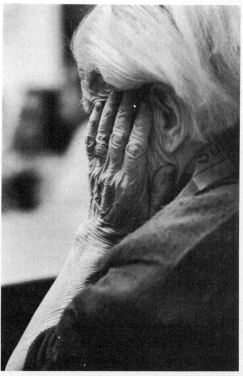

Photo © Sepp Seitz/Magnum

but if we are ever to reach a healthful attitude toward death, it is necessary to dispel our feelings of helplessness.

Our whole culture is based on denial of death and attempts to disguise whatever cannot be denied. First of all, death has almost totally shifted from the home to the impersonal surroundings of the hospital. This shift, to a large extent, has removed its association with other basic facts of life. Even the hospitals in which we die are not adequately set up to serve terminal patients. Death is often seen as an insult to the hospital function of healing and prolonging life. The time of death has become less and less definitive, and can be best described as the time when the decision to discontinue care is made. Funeral directors disguise death with euphemisms, and clergy hide behind standard words of comfort that are doled out in precise amounts. Only people with true and lifelong religious orientation derive the real comforting solace of religion. Expressions of sympathy come largely in the mail in the form of condolence cards. Grievers are only allowed to mourn and display evidence of their loss for certain periods of time. Criticism results when mourning is either too long or too short, irrespective of the circumstances surrounding the death. There are few if any American traditions left that can be identified with death. Wakes are an infrequent occurrence, there are few celebrations on the anniversary of a death, and traditional mourning apparel is out of style. These traditions formerly provided considerable emotional support to the living.

Within the last twenty years or so, there has been a dramatic increase in the number of terminally ill persons who have perhaps several years to live before finally succumbing to the disease from which they suffer. While medicine can still not effect cures for many diseases, it is often able to offer palliative treatment, which gives pa-

tients a substantially longer time in which to prepare for their death. There are very few patients anymore who are not made aware of their diagnosis. Although it may not be accepted initially, when the mind is ready and able to accept it, adjustment to the situation can be made.

While the physical needs of the terminally ill are being met, it is obvious that emotionally they and their families need special help. As patients struggle toward accepting their impending death, they find people are reluctant to listen to fears they need to vent, and they find it difficult to obtain permission to die. In any event, the plight of such persons has had much to do with stimulating interest in the dying process. People like Drs. Kavanaugh and Elisabeth Kübler–Ross have devoted much time to helping the dying and studying how we can best handle this part of life. Their efforts have resulted in a wealth of knowledge, giving us new insights into death.

Dying a peaceful death can be helped by the presence of a special confidant who lends support and encouragement. Such a person will help the dying break off ties to all except that which is part of the self. It is very important for dying people to receive permission to die from those who are closest to them. Once such permission has been given, they will slowly let go of all persons and worldly possessions held dear until everything except their own person has been relinquished.

People who die in peace are often noted as having had a smile on their face. This is associated with their having successfully gone through certain stages of coping mechanisms that lead to the state of acceptance. The first stage is *denial and isolation*. This occurs following the initial awareness of impending death. It is the stage when the person goes from "Not me!" to "Why me?" This is a very trying time for all those involved with the dying person, as anger is displaced indiscriminately. After the anger subsides, the person may try to *bargain* or make deals for a longer period of life. Many of such bargains are made with God, and are commonly promises associated with guilt feelings. The next stage is *depression*, involving sadness about leaving family behind, loss of job, inability to see children grow up, and perhaps leaving behind many bills or much unfinished business. Another part of the depression concerns mourning one's own impending death. This is a vital emotional adjustment in preparing for final separation. The last stage is *acceptance*, and during this stage the person will have already mourned the loss of self, other people, and all earthly possessions. It is not a state of happiness, but one that is nearly void of feelings. Hope is usually held on to until the very end, and only wavers when signs of death are imminent. It is important to know that these stages are not mutually exclusive of one another. They often coexist and can also be repeated. The amount of time it takes for a person to progress through these stages is enormously variable and depends heavily on how much time is actually left. It is possible for an individual to go through all stages and reach the state of acceptance within a matter of days, or it may take many months.

After death has occurred, the survivors experience a deep sense of loss, and a feeling of sadness penetrates their very beings. Dr. Kavanaugh has found certain distinct phases in the bereaved's grieving process. They include shock, disorganization, volatile emotions, guilt, loneliness, relief, and reestablishment. For those who have been expecting death to occur, the period of grief is not as long. However, even when apparently all mourning is finished, there is frequently a resurgence of grief. Grief can be so intense that the body can become seriously ill, or mental stress may culminate in psychiatric disorders. The bereaved usually receive some comfort and help from others, but most support is suspended after the funeral has ended. The need for caring friends who will listen and understand may go on for a matter of months. Mourning is not complete until the bereaved have made an adjustment to living without the one they have lost.

Children are often left out of the mourning experience. However, such attempts to protect children from the grief and finality of death can lead to confusion and the establishment of strange perceptions about death. Frequently, children feel they have had something to do with causing a person to die and feel unnecessary guilt. Children should be aware of the reality of death and even when there are no deaths involving family members, many occasions arise that can be used to approach the subject of death. Such occasions arise, for instance, when a loved pet dies, when a leading national figure dies, or when children bring up the topic themselves. When death does occur in the family, children should be included in discussions that relate to impending death, as well as the discussions and events that follow death. The truth should always be told, within the limits of the child's comprehension. It is never good to tell a child that a dead person is only going away temporarily, such as "on a long trip." Given the opportunity, children adapt to crises and unpleasant realities as well as adults do. Often a child will ask for further explanations or clarification of ideas previously discussed about death. This is common, and usually all that is needed is a reaffirmation that his or her ideas are correct.

Prolonging Life How long should life be prolonged with drugs or the use of machines? Is there any dignity in the artificial maintenance of life when there is no possible hope of recovery? Should it be legal to perform mercy killings when a dying patient requests such a service? Is it the responsibility of the medical profession to lengthen the dying process by any means available despite the person's desire to have all extraordinary life-supporting measures stopped? These are but a few of the questions being raised in response to our advanced and complicated methods of prolonging life.

Euthanasia, which means "good death," is often confused with *mercy killing.* Mercy killing refers to the unnatural interruption of life, such as giving an intentional overdose of a drug in order to end suffering. Euthanasia, on the other hand, is allowing persons to die their own natural deaths without the use of artificial means to sustain life, such as intravenous feedings, respirators, dialysis, and so forth. Persons who are kept functioning only with the aid of machines and who have no chance of ever getting better, either physically or mentally, are not truly benefiting from such heroic efforts.

It is difficult to legislate about what actions are appropriate and those that are not, as regards maintenance of life. Who wants to take the responsibility for playing Supreme Being? Each case has to be looked at and treated independently according to circumstances. The dying person's needs have to be respected as much as possible; however, under the stress of illness and pain, sometimes he or she is not able to make wise decisions.

The Euthanasia Educational Council publishes a form called *"A Living Will"* (see sample copy). This document is a legal request to be allowed to die a natural death in the event there is no reasonable chance of recovery from physical or mental disability.

A Living Will.

Reprinted with permission from the Euthanasia Education Council, 250 West 57th Street, New York, N.Y. 10019. Copies may be obtained by writing to this address.

TO MY FAMILY, MY PHYSICIAN, MY LAWYER, MY CLERGYMAN
TO ANY MEDICAL FACILITY IN WHOSE CARE I HAPPEN TO BE
TO ANY INDIVIDUAL WHO MAY BECOME RESPONSIBLE FOR MY HEALTH, WELFARE OR AFFAIRS

Death is as much a reality as birth, growth, maturity and old age—it is the one certainty of life. If the time comes when I, _____ can no longer take part in decisions for my own future, let this statement stand as an expression of my wishes, while I am still of sound mind.

If the situation should arise in which there is no reasonable expectation of my recovery from physical or mental disability, I request that I be allowed to die and not be kept alive by artificial means or "heroic measures". I do not fear death itself as much as the indignities of deterioration, dependence and hopeless pain. I, therefore, ask that medication be mercifully administered to me to alleviate suffering even though this may hasten the moment of death.

This request is made after careful consideration. I hope you who care for me will feel morally bound to follow its mandate. I recognize that this appears to place a heavy responsibility upon you, but it is with the intention of relieving you of such responsibility and of placing it upon myself in accordance with my strong convictions, that this statement is made.

Signed_____

Date _____

Witness_____

Witness_____

Copies of this request have been given to _____
_____
_____
_____

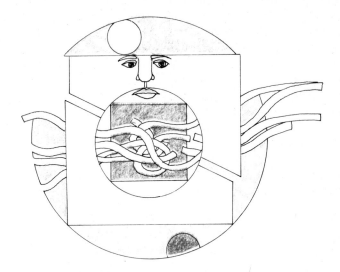

3

EMOTIONAL PROBLEMS

With the increasing complexity of life, extended life expectancies, and the tendency toward greater mobility and social isolation has come a growing challenge for the maintenance of our emotional health. To answer this challenge requires that the individual be aware of and concerned with the positive steps toward maintaining personal emotional health. The challenge to our society is, first of all, to create a social and physical environment that is favorable to good emotional health, and secondly, to provide adequate facilities for the treatment of the many cases of minor and major emotional problems that occur in a complex culture such as our own.

The extent of emotional problems in the United States is high. There are no exact figures available, only estimates, and these vary considerably depending on the way in which emotional illness is defined. According to the concepts we will follow in this chapter, everyone can be considered emotionally disturbed at some time. Of course, there are many degrees of emotional disturbance, but what we are concerned with here is the number of people that have emotional problems serious enough to interfere with normal living patterns.

It is estimated that about one in every ten persons in the United States suffers from a serious emotional disturbance at some time. This estimate means that about 10 percent of the people we know will at some time need professional help with their emotional problems; or that we, ourselves, have one in ten chances of being seriously disturbed at some time.

The Scope of the Problem

The high incidence of these problems places a heavy burden on the resources of our country. For example, every year over one million people are hospitalized in mental hospitals or psychiatric wards of general hospitals for treatment of emotional disorders. On any given day, more than half of all the hospital beds in the country are occupied by mental patients. The cost in terms of dollars and human suffering is staggering.

Since 1900 the rate of hospitalization for emotional problems has more than doubled. This increase is only partly the result of the greater stresses of modern life. Other important causes of this reported increase include a growing public awareness of the problems of emotional health, a higher percentage of the population living in large cities (where stress is greater), a growing population of elderly persons (who may suffer from senility, anxiety, or depression), and a great increase in the facilities available for treating emotional disorders.

Although the rate of hospitalization for emotional disturbance in the United States is one of the highest in the world, this does not necessarily mean that there is a higher incidence of emotional illness here than in other countries. This country has more facilities than any other country for treating emotional illness, and greater effort is made here to help the disturbed. In some countries, little or nothing is done to combat emotional illness.

Although the number of persons entering hospitals for emotional problems has increased, the number of patients requiring lengthy and full-time treatment has dropped considerably. For the great majority of patients now being treated, it has become more a matter of *when* they will be released rather than, as in former times, whether release would be possible. This more effective therapy is a result of new methods of treatment, which will be discussed later in this chapter.

A lingering problem is the *labeling* of psychiatric patients. There remains, in the minds of many people, an unjustified fear of and prejudice against people who have been hospitalized at some time for treatment of emotional problems. The media (newspapers, TV) contribute to this fear through their frequent use of the phrase "ex-mental patient" for a criminal or other person whose hospitalization may have been many years earlier and for a disorder totally unrelated to events now considered newsworthy, such as political candidacy. Many of the people who fear the "ex-mental patient" have been equally in need of treatment at some time for their own problems, but failed to seek treatment. Also, the stigma falls mainly on the poor, as they may have to turn to a public mental hospital for treatment that a more affluent person would obtain through office visits to a psychiatrist or clinical psychologist, who can more easily maintain professional privacy for the patient.

Common Emotional Problems

Several types of emotional problems are extremely common in everyday life. Anyone might expect to experience one or more of these problems from time to time. If they are mild in degree and short in duration, then they really are no cause for alarm. If, however, they are persistent or are at times severe enough to interfere with one's normal functioning—happiness, productivity, or relationships with others—then they definitely warrant some form of therapy.

Anxiety Everyone feels anxiety at times. It is a normal response to threats directed towards one's body, possessions, loved ones, way of life, or value system. The distinction between fear and anxiety is that fear is the response to a realistic danger while anxiety is a response to a vague, obscure, or imagined danger. Some anxiety is normal during any extreme effort or during any period when one's life situation is rapidly or drastically changing and continuous adaptation is required. In fact, moderate anxiety helps stimulate one to useful action and may play an important role in beneficial change and personality growth. In contrast, excessive anxiety not only makes a person unhappy, but detracts from any useful action. Severe, disorganizing anxiety is usually called *panic*.

The experience of anxiety is subjective—it is described differently by different people. But its essential feature is the unpleasant anticipation of some kind of misfortune, danger, or doom. It is accompanied by tenseness, restlessness, and the feeling that something must be done to avoid disaster. Since the source of the anxiety is often vague, the "something" that must be done is also vague and thus nothing constructive is or can be done. Persistent anxiety leads to a feeling of helplessness and the fear of collapse.

There are many physical symptoms of anxiety as well. Some common indicators of anxiety are excessive sweating, muscle tension, especially in the back of the neck, sighing, rapid breathing and/or pulse, digestive symptoms such as indigestion, loss of appetite, diarrhea, or "butterflies" in the stomach, frequent urination, and sexual dysfunctions.

Severe, disabling anxiety should receive immediate treatment, which usually involves psychotherapy to get at the basic source of the anxiety and/or tranquilizers to provide more immediate relief of its unpleasant symptoms.

Depression It can certainly be said that this is a depressing era, considering worldwide conflict and hardship, national political and economic problems, and the individual realities of crime, unemployment, and inflation. It is not surprising that vast numbers of people are suffering from depression. What may be surprising is that even in the best of times, many of these people would still be depressed. For depression, like anxiety, often has no real external cause, but arises entirely within the individual.

Also like anxiety, the degree of depression may range from mild to disablingly serious. Mild depression usually results in a loss of pleasurable interest in life. Spontaneity is gone. Everything one does requires greater effort than before, and provides less satisfaction. One does not feel physically ill, but neither does one feel particularly well ("the blahs"). Fatigue is excessive and much time may be spent sleeping. A person with mild depression such as this still goes to work or school, meets most obligations, and appears normal, but there is no joy in life.

More severe depression may involve deep despondency, a feeling of physical illness, or both. The person feels gloomy, helpless, hopeless, and worthless. Insomnia (sleeplessness) is common; many lonely hours are spent in deep despair in the late evenings or early mornings. Loss of appetite and weight loss are characteristic as is a loss of sexual interest or ability. The most serious consequence of deep depression is that it frequently leads to suicide.

There are two schools of thought regarding the causes of depression and it is entirely possible that both are valid, with each being involved in some cases. On the one hand is the theory that most depression has physiological (biochemical) causes and that any psychological factors are secondary in importance. In support of this position are cited certain detectable differences in body chemistry in depressed people, the hereditary tendency toward certain types of depression, and the frequent occurrence of severe depression in the absence of any apparent psychological cause.

On the other hand are those who relate most depression to a basic lack of self-esteem. There is a great dependency on others for ego-support and approval. But highly dependent people are always vulnerable to disappointment. Since such people need a great deal of support from others, they can rarely get enough. Because needs are often unfulfilled, these people have feelings of frustration and anger. Since the expression of this anger would drive away those on whom they are so dependent, the anger is held in and self-directed. The result is a further decline in self-esteem and subsequent feelings of hopelessness, guilt, and depression.

As in anxiety, treatment usually revolves around psychotherapy and drugs. In deep depression, suicide prevention must always be part of the plan of treatment.

Emptiness Many people today complain of a rather vague feeling in their lives that they often call a sense of emptiness. Not only are they unsure of what they want out of life, but they also do not even have a clear idea of what they feel. They do express painful feelings of powerlessness and lack of direction, often resulting in a great difficulty in making decisions. They know what others—parents, spouses, employers, professors, and society—expect of them, but not what they themselves want. They may satisfy all of these other people, but still feel the overwhelming emptiness. Some typical cases include people who spend their days in boring, routine, assembly-line work and who find little additional fulfillment in their leisure activities. It must be stressed, though, that people in all types of careers, including many who are quite successful by most standards, are subject to emptiness. They do their job and do it well, but there is no satisfaction. The feeling of emptiness is also commonly expressed by many women in traditional housewife roles who feel little identity of their own other than "his wife" and "their mother." Unemployed or underemployed people of both sexes commonly experience similar feelings.

The problem of emptiness usually has as its basis the failure to find self-actualization. There is a need (perhaps even through therapy of some kind) to gain a fuller understanding and acceptance of one's own intrinsic nature—needs, interests, feelings, abilities—and to progress toward self-actualization, the fulfillment of these needs and abilities. There must be a "sorting-out" process in which one's own needs and abilities are identified among the multitude of values and expectations imposed by the various "others."

Loneliness Another common feeling of modern people is loneliness. Though certainly not a new problem, it is increasing in both incidence and severity. A few of the many causes of this increased loneliness are industrialization, with many jobs lacking human contact; increased reliance on impersonal electronic media for entertainment; increased mobility, with many people moving away from friends and relatives; and increasing lifespan, with many older people limited in their social contacts through poor health, small incomes, and social isolation. Among the results of loneliness are emotional problems, alcoholism and other drug dependencies, and many suicides.

The feelings of emptiness and loneliness often go together. Many people today express feelings of being lonely even in the presence of other people, including, perhaps, their own family. The reason for the close association between loneliness and emptiness is that when people do not know what they want or what they feel, they depend on others for their sense of direction in life. But when the goals imposed by others fail to produce that sense of direction, the result is a feeling of having been failed by the others and of being "alone in a crowd." (This, of course, does not apply to people who are lonely because their life situation deprives them of needed social contact, such as many elderly people.) Another common factor in loneliness is the inability to establish intimacy—to form close relationships with people. Many people, for the reasons of ego-defense, keep everyone "at arm's length," forming only the most superficial kinds of relationships.

When loneliness is caused by individual personality traits, it is obviously going to be resolved only through changing those traits. But the loneliness of many people today results from factors beyond their control. Our society could and should do much more to provide opportunities for social contact for the many people to whom circumstances such as age, poverty, or physical handicaps deny adequate social contact.

Emotional Dysorganization

The traditional approach to a discussion of emotional disturbance has been to describe various abnormal behavior patterns and give them definite labels and diagnoses. Unfortunately, these labels mainly describe the way in which the person is acting at the time, and they have little to do with the basic cause of the problem or the most effective approach to its treatment. They are only descriptions of signs and symptoms.

We have chosen to depart from tradition and instead present some of the ideas of Dr. Karl Menninger, one of the founders of the Menninger Clinic in Topeka, Kansas. This clinic is one of the most outstanding psychiatric hospitals in the United States, and Dr. Menninger is recognized as one of the country's leading psychiatrists. In his book *The Vital Balance*, (Viking Press, 1967), Dr. Menninger proposes doing away with much of the labeling of emotional problems and placing emotional problems into a range of severity that extends from relative emotional normalcy to a state of complete emotional collapse.

Dr. Menninger has coined the word *dysorganization* to describe the difficult or painful experiences a person must undergo in trying to cope with life situations. The prefix *dys-* means "painful" or "difficult." Dysorganization does not mean the same as *disorganization*, which is a common term meaning a lack of organization or a state of disarrangement. In dysorganization, the process of organization is difficult and painful, but there *is* organization.

According to Menninger's concept, the degree of emotional illness is in proportion to the amount of dysorganization present. There is, of course, a continuous range of degrees of dysorganization. Menninger divides this range into five levels or steps of increasingly severe emotional disorder. Although these five levels are convenient for purposes of description, it should be stressed that they represent selected steps from a continuum and that there may be other levels of emotional dysorganization that lie between them.

First Level of Dysorganization The first level of dysorganization is what we commonly call "nervousness," a condition we all feel at times. This means that we are experiencing slightly more than the usual amount of difficulty in coping with a situation and feel an increased amount of tension as a result. An increase in such feelings as fear, anxiety, frustration, and anger must be dealt with. It takes more than the usual amount of effort to keep these internal tensions under control.

The nervous person often becomes unusually sensitive to surrounding events and may hear small mysterious noises at night or notice the slightest change in the appearance of something. This alertness is one of the responses to stress that the body makes in preparation for emergency action. Our entire perception is sharpened; the senses of sight, hearing, and smell become keener.

Since the body is alert, a nervous person may have difficulty sleeping at night or may awaken at the slightest noise.

Other first-level symptoms include touchiness, tearfulness, irritability, nervous laughter, moodiness, or depression. Restless behavior is common, such as walking the floor, biting fingernails, chewing pencils, twirling hair, cracking knuckles, or drumming with the fingers.

At this level, the person is often worried and spends an excessive amount of time thinking about some topic of concern. Or the mind may wander into a daydream so as to avoid reality, thus preventing effective thought or action.

Psychosomatic disorders are common among people at the first level. Itching skin, upset stomachs, headaches, and various vague pains can be examples of these disorders.

The symptoms of the first level are a response to stress. Anyone who is placed under enough stress will show some of the symptoms of nervousness on the first level of dysorganization. For this reason Dr. Menninger states that everyone is emotionally dysorganized at times, for everyone reaches the first level at times. But when the unusual stress is gone, most people return to a level of optimum adjustment.

Other people are more limited in their ability to cope with stresses. These people chronically function at the first level, even when they are subject only to normal stresses. If these people are subjected to more than the usual amount of stress, or if they are no longer able to control behavior with the first-level devices, they must develop other self-maintenance devices. These new devices lead to the more serious second level of dysorganization.

Second Level of Dysorganization The symptoms of the second level are somewhat more serious than those of the first level. They may cause a definite detachment of a person from his or her environment. The second-level person is less realistic than the first-level person. The coping process becomes definitely unpleasant and emotionally painful. The individual is unhappy and feels a sense of failure, uselessness, or depression. Other people are seen as either indifferent or as definitely antagonistic, though they may actually be trying to help. Control over words and actions is reduced. One says things one does not really want to say and does things one really would rather not do. Tolerance for frustration is very low.

The second-level coping devices may be used temporarily by a usually normal person placed under great stress, or these devices may become a permanent part of the personality. One is still able to function in society, but these coping methods greatly reduce the pleasure received from life and also make one a difficult person with whom to associate. Although Menninger suggests that such terms be abandoned as obsolete, the common name for a person who lives at the second level is *neurotic*.

Let us now consider some of the common symptoms of the second level of dysorganization. These are all ways in which the person tries to keep unacceptable impulses (like hostility or guilt) under restraint. These may also be used normally, but not to this degree.

Withdrawal A person may unconsciously withdraw from contact with the world temporarily by fainting, developing amnesia (loss of memory), refusing to see or hear certain things, or developing *phobias*. Phobias are excessive and often crippling fears of objects or situations, such as high places, closed rooms, insects, cats, thunder, or darkness.

Self-punishment Some people have repressed such intense hostilities toward other people, groups, or situations that they take their hostilities out on themselves. This type of self-punishment is usually quiet and subtle. It often takes the form of an accidental injury or a psychosomatic disease.

Compensating Acts—Rituals Not all ritual should be taken as indicating emotional conflict. For example, there is nothing particularly unhealthy about the ritual of getting up at the same time every morning, showering, combing hair, and dressing for school. These actions are a means to an end. A ritual indicates a problem when it becomes an end in itself, when the mere act of doing it becomes a kind of release. For example, a student might sharpen a pencil many times while taking a test, not because the pencil point was dull, but because sharpening the pencil relieved some of the anxiety about the test.

Compensating Acts—Obsessional Thinking This is thinking that takes the place of action. Much time is spent in thinking the same thoughts. As such thinking becomes more intense, effective action and productivity decrease. Although this kind of thinking does indicate an emotional problem, it may be of value when a person merely thinks about dangerous aggressive action rather than actually taking such action. Too often, however, obsessional thinking takes the place of needed beneficial action.

Compensating Acts—Compulsions These are irresistible desires or drives to perform acts that seem unreasonable and unnecessary to other people. Compulsive cleanliness is a common example. Some people are so concerned with the cleanliness of their homes that the normal use of the house or apartment becomes impossible. Compulsive overeating is another example. Some compulsions can lead to serious trouble. Compulsive stealing (kleptomania) and setting fires (pyromania) may be motivated by an unconscious desire to be caught and punished.

Personality Deformities Probably the most common second-level symptoms, personality deformities are tendencies to adopt an emergency ego-defense device as a permanent part of one's personality. Many kinds of eccentricities, perversities, dependencies, and unpopular personality traits can be acquired as a chronic maladjustment to the stresses of normal life.

A person may become infantile (helpless) or narcissistic (extremely egocentric); develop into a bully, a braggart, a worrier, or a liar; or become dependent on alcohol or other drugs. These people are often emotionally immature and use these drugs to escape from reality. If they had not turned to alcohol or other drugs, they would probably have made use of one or more of the other second-level defense mechanisms.

Hypochondria Another common characteristic of the second level is hypochondria—an exaggerated anxiety and concern about one's own health. The hypochondriac imagines illness or else makes a big issue over very minor disorders. The psychosomatic disorders and hypochondria are processes the person uses to avoid stressful situations. Illness can be an escape mechanism, a means of avoiding responsibilities. Many people go through life with a series of vague illnesses. These people are never really sick, but they are never well enough to assume normal responsibilities. If a doctor is able to cure one illness in such a person, the person replaces that illness with another one. Many more people use illness as a means of avoiding unpleasant situations. Consider the student who develops a sudden headache or upset stomach when an examination, a speech, or a term paper is due. These ailments are very real at the time to those experiencing them.

Third Level of Dysorganization This level is characterized by the display of aggressive impulses. The person operating on the third level expresses open and direct aggression to people and things. Often the individual who commits an aggressive act is showing that all or nearly all of his or her restricting control has been lost.

In general, such an individual may be described as having the following traits:

1. Aggressive impulses are no longer concealed.
2. No regard is shown for laws and social customs and little attention is paid to conscience.
3. Judgment, consciousness, and perception may be reduced during the aggressive act.
4. Little or no remorse or guilt is felt or displayed after the act of aggression.
5. After the aggressive act, emotional tension is relieved.

As in the case of the first two levels of dysorganization, a person may drop to the third level for a short time while under great stress and then return to a healthier level of adjustment when the stress is gone, or may remain at the third level, adopting repeated aggression as a way of life.

Even when a person reaches the third level only temporarily and briefly, the results may be spectacular. This person may commit murder or assault, or may become violent toward property, leaving a place in shambles. Suicide attempts sometimes occur at this level when the aggression is self-directed. The person who often reaches the third level definitely needs treatment, as a threat is presented to society and to the individual as well.

Fourth Level of Dysorganization
The fourth level represents serious emotional disturbance. The conscious thought processes are greatly disrupted. Because of loss of contact with reality, interpretation of the outside world is badly distorted. Emotional reactions and behavior are inappropriate, exaggerated, and unpredictable. Behavior may be bizarre. Effective productivity, at home, school, or on the job, is lost. Sometimes behavior seems scarcely human.

This is the condition that in the past has been called *lunacy* or *insanity*. A more acceptable word for this fourth level today is *psychosis*. A psychotic person is one who suffers from a serious emotional disorder.

Some psychotic behavior patterns have been described as distinct kinds of emotional illness, but Menninger believes that we should consider these patterns merely as different symptoms of the same general disturbance. The fourth level of dysorganization often takes one of the following forms:

1. *Extreme Depression.* Depressed people may feel overwhelmingly sad, guilty, hopeless, or despondent. They may feel inadequate, incompetent, unworthy, or just no good. There is often a slowdown of physical body functions. Everyone feels depressed at times; only in its extreme forms is depression psychotic.
2. *Extreme Anxiety.* This person shows a great overflowing of poorly controlled energy, talks rapidly, constantly, and incoherently, and may indulge in much bizarre activity, such as walking in a circle day after day or repeatedly stacking and restacking the same objects. As with depression, anxiety is only considered to be psychotic in its most extreme forms.
3. *Excess concern with self.* People may become mute and totally withdrawn into themselves. They may have delusions of their own importance, constantly telling people that they are God, Jesus Christ, the President of the United States, or some other important figure.
4. *Persecution complex (paranoia).* These people may imagine that someone or some group is plotting to get them in some way and may become very suspicious, resentful, and defensive. Someone in this state of mind can be quite dangerous.

Fifth Level of Dysorganization The fifth level represents the greatest extreme of emotional dysorganization. The will to live is gone. All that is left is a self-destructive determination to end life, or to settle for minimal existence.

This extremely disturbed person either commits suicide or becomes like a human vegetable, refusing to eat, drink, or make any contact with reality. Force-feeding may be necessary in order to prevent starvation.

The earnest suicide attempts of the fifth-level person are quite different from the half-hearted suicide displays of people at the previous levels. In the exhibition suicide, the person is consciously or unconsciously hoping and planning for a last-minute rescue. This type includes the person who stands on a rooftop or at an open window while a crowd gathers and the fire department is called. It also includes the person who takes a few sleeping pills and immediately calls for help. These display efforts at suicide stem from various motivations. In general, however, these attempts should be interpreted as a desperate cry for help. The person who makes such an effort should have some professional psychiatric help, as it has been found that such persons often make repeated suicide attempts. The next time they might succeed.

Suicide Suicide is the tenth leading cause of death in the United States today. The "official" annual suicide rate is about 12 per 100,000 population and over 24,000 deaths are recorded as suicides each year. The actual suicide rate is probably closer to double the official rate as many suicides are disguised as accidents or natural deaths to avoid loss of insurance money or stigmatization of survivors.

No group or class of people is free of suicide. Every person is a potential suicide; and almost everyone at some time during his or her life gives some consideration to the possibility of suicide. However, the risk of suicide does relate to certain individual characteristics.

The most significant pattern in the incidence of suicide is the increase with advancing age. Suicide is rare among those under 14 years of age. The rate rises sharply in adolescence and sharply again among college students, for whom suicide is second only to accidents as a cause of death. Several factors are commonly associated with college suicides, the most frequent of which is academic failure. Failure brings not only the disappointment and disapproval of parents, but a shattering of personal self-confidence as well. The second leading cause of college suicide is the end of a love affair. When romance ends, there is more than just disappointment; there is the tumultuous feeling of being rejected and abandoned, the complete loss of self-esteem. College suicides often involve the reserved, introverted, or shy students who, lacking social contacts, tend to internalize their problems. Despite the alarming college suicide rate, many colleges offer little or no on-campus therapy for emotional problems.

The suicide rate rises again in middle age when the male realizes that his career goals have not been attained and are in fact now unattainable. The middle-aged woman may turn to suicide in reaction to menopause, if she feels "finished" as a woman, or upon the departure from home of her children, after which she may no longer feel useful and needed.

Finally, the suicide rate reaches its peak among the elderly, who today suffer from a host of emotionally crippling influences. Our society now emphasizes youth and young ideas. After a forced retirement at age 65, many people feel useless, lonely, bored, and frustrated. In addition, they may suffer great financial insecurity, physical pain from chronic ailments, or may have terminal illnesses. For persons over age 85, the suicide rate is 26 per 100,000.

For the United States in general, the suicide rate among men is greater than among women, though on the West Coast there are more female suicides than male.

Nationally, women attempt suicide at least five times as frequently as men, though because of the method used women are often saved before death occurs. Men are more inclined to use a violent and swift means, such as firearms. On the other hand, women tend to take pills, leaving a considerably longer period of time during which medical intervention can be sought. For "successful" suicides, the percentage of male and female are 70 and 30, respectively. Among college students, males are twice as likely to commit suicide as females.

In recent years the suicide rate for women has risen sharply, while the rate for men has remained fairly static. This increase has been attributed to various causes. Possibly part of the increase is related to increasing opportunities and expectations for women. The opportunity to succeed in a career is also the opportunity to fail. It has been suggested that women are now committing suicide for reasons that were once typical of males, such as despondency over unfulfilled career goals.

The bored housewife is still the greatest potential suicide. A woman who spends her days at home in the traditional role of "wife and mother" may see herself as a failure. Suicide attempts by such women are often extreme and urgent pleas for someone to recognize how alienated and isolated they feel and how little of their potential is being used. There may be conflicts between her desires to succeed in the traditional role of homemaker and in a career as well. There is undoubtedly increasing marital dissatisfaction, as evidenced by the rapidly climbing divorce rate.

In general, suicide is less frequent among married persons, with the notable exception of those under 24 years of age in whom the rate is much higher than in single persons. In single people over 24 and in divorced people of any age, the rate is higher than among married people over 24. The rate among young widows (under 35) is quite high.

Racially, suicide is more than twice as prevalent among whites as blacks. Among young American Indians, however, the suicide rate is at an epidemic level.

There is a direct relationship between suicide and social status—the higher one stands on the social scale, the more susceptible he or she becomes to suicide. The rate is high among doctors, dentists, lawyers, business executives, and similar professionals. Among physicians in general, the rate is 33 per 100,000 (compared with 12 per 100,000 for the general public); among psychiatrists it is reported as between 60 and 70 per 100,000 in various surveys.

Suicide rates even relate to the time of year, soaring in the spring and during holiday periods, especially Christmas. Depression resulting from loneliness and business and social failures may become unbearably painful during the supposedly "happy" times of the year.

Theories on the Causes of Suicide Many psychological theories have been proposed to explain suicide, ranging from the Freudian to the behavioral. Most authorities agree that suicide may have a variety of motivations and that in a particular case there is rarely a single precipitating cause of suicide and that several causes are usually operative in an additive way. All of the following psychological factors are possible motives for suicide: severe depression in which life seems an unbearable burden; psychosis in which suicide is a response to hallucinations or delusions (this sometimes happens in LSD flashbacks); suicide for spite, in which the motive is to hurt the survivors (such as parents, a spouse, or a lover); poor impulse

control, leading to suicide following some minor frustration; identification with celebrities or relatives that have committed suicide; and chronic or terminal illness.

Serious losses (or threats of loss) play a major role in the psychodynamics of suicide. These include loss of health, loved ones, money, earning power, job, pride, beauty, status, friends, children, and independence.

Social isolation is a common factor in those who resort to suicide. The more intimately one is involved with others, the less likely one is to consider suicide. Unfortunately, the severe depression that commonly precedes suicide is likely to lead to social alienation and isolation, further increasing the chance of suicide. Suicide may be considered the final outcome of a progressive failure of adaptation, with isolation and alienation from the usual network of human relationships that support us all and give meaning to our lives.

Danger Signs of Impending Suicide It is not true that people who threaten to commit suicide never do so. Most people who attempt suicide actually give warnings, vocal or nonvocal, beforehand. Potential suicides can usually be recognized before they act. Knowledge of the danger signs can save a life. Any of the following indicates a definite risk of suicide (adapted from Phillip Solomon and Vernon D. Patch, *Handbook of Psychiatry*, 1975):

1. *Previous attempts.* Over half of those who successfully commit suicide have a history of a previous attempt.
2. *Previous psychosis.* A history of psychiatric disturbance indicates the possibility of a recurrence.
3. *Suicide note.*
4. *Violent method.* The more violent and painful the method chosen, the

more serious the intent.

5. *Presence of chronic disease.*

6. *Recent surgery or childbirth.* The birth of a baby leads to severe post-partum depression in some women.

7. *Alcoholism or drug dependence.* Drug or alcohol dependence indicates a person who needs to escape. The permanent escape of suicide is often appealing to such a person. Also, while actually under the influence of drugs or alcohol, the ability to resist the suicide impulse is weakened.

8. *Hypochondriasis.* Constant physical complaints often indicate underlying depression.

9. *Advancing age.*

10. *Homosexuality.* The suicide rate among homosexuals is high.

11. *Social isolation.* Indicates severe depression.

12. *Chronic maladjustment.*

13. *Bankrupt resources.* A person without money, job, or friends may see little to live for.

14. *No obvious secondary gains.* Many suicide threats are really attempts to manipulate others. For example, people often use the suicide threat to keep a dying marriage or love affair going. When there is no such motive and the threat is truly self-directed, the chance of suicide is much greater.

15. *Signs of grave risk:*
   a. *The wish to die.* Repeated statements by a person that he or she would be better off dead indicate very high suicide risk.
   b. *Presence of psychosis.* The psychotic person who is suspicious, fearful, or hears voices should be regarded as potentially suicidal.
   c. *Depression* is the most common cause of suicide. Any of the following symptoms indicates severe risk:
   (1) Guilt.
   (2) Feelings of worthlessness and despondency.
   (3) Intense wish for punishment.
   (4) Withdrawal and hopelessness.
   (5) Extreme agitation and anxiety.
   (6) Loss of the four appetites—food, sex, sleep, and activity.
   (7) Sudden well-being in a previously depressed person may reflect the feeling of relief at having made the decision to die.

Prevention of Suicide Most suicidal people are not fully intent on dying. Though their wish to die may be extremely strong, there is almost always an underlying wish to live. But suicidal people do not wish to live as they are living, for this is seen as being the same or even worse than death. Thus, the crucial element that makes suicide prevention possible is *ambivalence.* Even as suicidal impulses become almost overwhelming, the ebbing wish to live is a root of energy that can be tapped for suicide prevention.

The role of the layperson in the suicide crisis is much the same as in any first-aid situation. It is to preserve life until professional help can be attained—it is not to play "doctor." In many cities there are 24-hour telephone services staffed by mental health professionals or volunteers specially trained in crisis intervention. If such a service is available, one's first efforts should be in aiding or encouraging the suicidal person to call for help. If a crisis intervention service is not available, or if the suicidal person will not cooperate in calling such a service, the person must be kept from committing suicide until other professional help can be attained.

The first step in suicide intervention is to establish a relationship with the suicidal person and maintain contact. As an opening line, the National Save-A-Life League suggests asking, "Are you thinking of killing yourself?'' Communication in crisis intervention must be open and direct. One must remain calm and convey attitudes of helpfulness, hopefulness, and genuine concern, building upon the suicidal person's ambivalence about dying, convincing the person that he or she really does want to live. One must encourage the person to relate everything possible about the problems or troubles and show the person that, with help, these problems can be solved.

Everyone has some strengths. The severely depressed person often loses sight of his or her own strengths or the ability to use them. In talking to a suicidal person, one should keep emphasizing strengths so as to decrease feelings of helplessness and hopelessness.

As soon as the immediate crisis of threatened suicide seems to have abated, the person should be encouraged to seek competent professional help. *Suicidal impulses recur*, and it is dangerous to assume that there will not be further suicide attempts. As many friends or relatives as possible should be involved in the emotional support of the person, because the chance of suicide is reduced through social interaction and increased through alienation.

Recognizing the Severely Disturbed

With today's high incidence of emotional problems, there are few of us who do not occasionally encounter a severely disturbed person. Such a person may be a close relative, a neighbor, or a stranger encountered in a public place. In any case, it is important to be able to recognize the individual as disturbed and to know how to handle such a person. A person suffering from severe emotional disturbance will generally exhibit one or more observable symptoms.

Changes in Behavior Pattern A normally quiet person may become suddenly very belligerent or overtalkative. Or conversely, the happy, outgoing person may become quiet and moody. Any sudden and radical change in a person's normal mood or behavior may indicate emotional conflict. What is important here is a change in the general pattern of behavior extending over a long period of time, not just a passing reaction to some stress or irritant.

Loss of Touch with Reality Emotionally disturbed people usually (some authorities say always) suffer some degree of loss of contact with reality, ranging from slight to total. They may be unable to recall who they are, where they are, why they are there, the day or date, or similar information. Or they may withdraw totally from reality to the extent that they are completely unaware of their environment.

Amnesia Temporary or permanent memory loss is a common symptom of mental disturbance. One of the mind's defense mechanisms is to repress those memories that are too painful for the conscious mind to bear. Loss of memory is also characteristic of the senile elderly person, often as a result of reduced blood supply to the brain due to atherosclerosis.

Delusions A delusion is a distorted belief or idea. Emotionally disturbed persons often harbor beliefs (called *delusions of grandeur*) that they are famous scientists or surgeons, prosperous executives, secret agents, or even God. Much harm may be done to themselves or to others when they act upon such delusions. Even more dangerous are delusions of persecution in which family members, neighbors, members of racial or religious groups, or just a vague ''they'' are believed to be plotting against the person. People suffering from such delusions of persecution may be dangerous, as they may suddenly react to these beliefs by attacking those who they feel are "after" them.

One-sided Conversations In the folk lore of emotional disorders one of the sure signs is "talking to yourself." Actually, we all talk to ourselves from time to time. But a person carrying on an animated conversation to himself or herself in a public place is very likely disturbed.

Hallucinations Severely disturbed persons very commonly suffer hallucinations of one or more of the senses. They hear voices; they see, smell, taste, and feel imaginary things. Though such hallucinations may seem absurd to others, they are very real to those suffering from them, even to the point that they are acted upon, with serious or even fatal results. A frequent problem today is "flashback" hallucination following the use of hallucinogenic drugs, especially LSD and mescaline. Such flashbacks may occur many months after the last drug usage and may be severe enough to produce violent actions directed toward the hallucinating individual or others.

Dealing with the Severely Disturbed

With increasing incidences of emotional disturbance, drug abuse, stressful situations, and increasing population density, the "psychiatric emergency" is becoming more commonplace. This may be defined as a situation in a public or private place in which an individual's behavior becomes dangerous to that person or others and for which prompt and decisive action must be taken. In dealing with a severely disturbed person, the immediate regard is for the safety of everyone concerned. In addition, the ability of the patient to recover and the speed of recovery often depend on the handling received during the acute emergency phase of his or her illness.

The handling of the psychiatric emergency should be thought of as first aid and the basic rules of first aid applied. The prime rule is to recognize your own limitations as an untrained person. To attempt to play psychiatrist is to risk physical injury, lawsuit, and further deterioration of the condition of the disturbed person. Thus, the best course of action is to immediately call for assistance. A physician, even though not a psychiatrist, can often help calm the disturbed individual. Most police officers have both training and experience in handling disturbed persons, and are generally more readily available than physicians. While waiting for assistance, keep cool and calm and take only such action as is absolutely necessary to prevent someone from being hurt. Such action should involve a minimum of physical force or harsh words and should include efforts to reassure the disturbed person that you are a friend and are trying to protect and help the person. If physical restraint becomes necessary, use only as much force as is absolutely necessary.

Types of Treatment

Fortunately, the methods and facilities for the treatment of emotional problems have been greatly improved during recent years. The person who becomes emotionally disturbed today, regardless of the level of dysorganization reached, stands an excellent chance of recovery if he or she receives the benefit of modern methods of treatment and if this treatment is begun promptly. Most patients today begin to show improvement very quickly. If they are hospitalized, they usually return home in only a few weeks, to continue treatment on an outpatient basis.

We shall consider some of the methods of treatment in use today, the different types of personnel working with the disturbed person, and the types of facilities that are now available for the treatment of emotional problems. Many different forms of treatment for emotional disorders have been used at one time or another in the past. Some have been abandoned as newer methods developed and others have been reduced in importance. Of those methods that remain today, some are administered in a hospital and others are used in outpatient clinics. These forms of treatment may be grouped into several main categories.

Psychoanalysis

Psychoanalysis is a system of therapy dating back to Freud in which great importance is attached to the role of the subconscious mind causing emotional conflict. Psychoanalysis attempts to explore the unconscious mind through a long series of sessions in which the patient freely relates anything that happens to come to mind. The therapist, called an analyst, interprets what the patient says, trying to help the patient recognize the subconscious feelings that have led to problems.

Psychoanalysis has been of value to some patients with minor emotional conflicts, but is of little value for major mental disturbances. Also, this type of treatment for even a minor emotional problem may extend over several years of great expense to the patient. It is obvious that factors of effectiveness, time, and expense restrict the use of classical psychoanalysis to a rather limited clientele of only mildly disturbed patients.

Other Individual Psychotherapies

Psychotherapy involves a dialogue between the patient and a specially qualified person. This therapy should result in the patient's having a better self-understanding and learning ways to handle affairs more effectively. The patient should learn to replace ineffective or undesirable coping devices with more appropriate methods. Psychotherapy is usually administered by a psychiatrist, psychoanalyst, or a clinical psychologist. (The distinctions among these types of therapists will be discussed later.) Psychotherapy is commonly given in outpatient clinics, offices, hospitals, and schools, and is of importance today for all levels of emotional problems, from the most minor to the most severe. Those with minor problems may need only a few sessions, but serious cases may need months or years of continued treatment.

Reality Therapy

An interesting (though not universally accepted) concept of emotional conflict is presented by William Glasser, a psychiatrist, in his book *Reality Therapy* (Harper & Row, 1965). His belief is that everyone who is emotionally disturbed suffers from the same basic inadequacy—the inability to fulfill his or her basic human needs. The severity of the symptoms reflects the degree to which the individual is unable to fulfill his or her needs, and whatever the symptom, it disappears when the person's needs are successfully fulfilled.

Glasser sees another common characteristic among all his patients—they all deny the reality of the world around them. His concept of reality therapy is to lead patients toward reality through helping them find effective ways of fulfilling their needs.

According to Glasser, the two needs most often unfulfilled are the need to be loved and to love and the need for self-esteem. We all have these needs, but we vary in our ability to fulfill them. Central to the fulfillment of either need is involvement with other people—at the very least, one person, but hopefully many more than one. For good emotional health we must, at all times in our lives, have at least one person who cares about us and for whom we care ourselves. If we do not have this essential person, we will be unable to fulfill our basic needs. One characteristic is essential in the other person—they must be able to fulfill their own needs and thus be in touch with reality. In other words, they must be in good emotional health. Of course, it is common for two people to mutually fulfill their needs and thus maintain their emotional health through their involvement with each other. Glasser sees the role of the psychiatrist or psychologist as providing someone for temporary involvement until the patient learns to fulfill needs through involvement with others.

Another basic concept in reality therapy is *responsibility*, which Glasser defines as the ability to fulfill one's needs in a way that does not deprive others of the ability to fulfill their needs. This equation of emotional health with responsibility interjects a moral tone into reality therapy that is absent from conventional therapy. Conventional therapists generally consider deviant behavior to be a product of emotional illness, and the patient should not be held morally responsible because he or she is considered helpless to do anything about it. Glasser feels that in their effort to avoid the issue of morality, many conventional therapists accept behavior that does not lead to need fulfillment and that the irresponsibility of many patients is the cause of their emotional disturbance, not its excusable result. Glasser claims particular success in the treatment of delinquent adolescents with his emphasis on responsibility.

Another departure from conventional therapy is that reality therapy does not probe into the patient's past life in a search for deep psychological roots for problems. The emphasis is, rather, on teaching the patient better ways to fulfill needs within the confines of reality and responsibility. The past is discussed only enough to show the patient how and why his or her behavior has failed to fulfill needs in a responsible manner.

It must be emphasized that reality therapy, like all other current theories on emotional disorder, is not universally accepted by all therapists, but is favored by some therapists for some patients.

Primal Therapy Primal therapy, introduced by Arthur Janov, is a comprehensive, clinical system of therapy that forces a patient to relive core (primal) experiences, such as those moments in infancy and childhood when the patient found reality too painful to endure and took refuge in the comfortable half-world of neurosis. In primal theory, neurosis is interpreted as the synthesis of two selves (systems) in conflict. The unreal self or system tries to suppress the real one, but because real human needs cannot be eradicated, the conflict is unending. Trying to find satisfaction, these needs become altered by the unreal self so that they can be satisfied only symbolically. The real needs, which produce anxiety because they are not fulfilled, must be suppressed so that the person is not overcome with emotional pain. For example, compulsive overeating or dependence on alcohol or other drugs is seen as satisfying an unreal system of needs, with the patient's real needs having been displaced. The real needs can no longer be fulfilled because they are not even felt. People often stuff themselves with food in order not to feel their emptiness. To them, food unconsciously symbolizes love. A real need has been displaced by an unreal need. Similarly, alcohol, other drugs, or material possessions such as expensive clothes or cars may be used to ease the tension of unrecognized real needs. But they never fill the void.

In primal therapy, as childhood denials are reexperienced, there is usually the release by the patient of a blood-chilling primal scream as the patient's neurotic defense system is broken down. Since it involves such a total stripping away of defenses, primal therapy is dangerous when practiced by inadequately trained persons.

Fight-or-Flight An approach to emotional problems that is now rapidly gaining advocates, but that is as old as animal life itself, is called *fight-or-flight*. It is based on how animals deal with a threat. There is no time for indecision. An instant choice is made whether to fight the intruder or run for safety. There is no other alternative.

In everyday human life, fight means eliminating or overcoming an obstacle through directly attacking the problem. Flight means cutting ourselves free of the obstacle in order to function as individuals and regain our feelings of independence and self-esteem. Problems arise because, unlike other animals, we are often emotionally involved, become confused, lose objectivity, and fail to make any decision. Further, the decision is complicated by often-conflicting moral codes, social demands and expectations, and our own basic needs. For example, our culture holds much disapproval for the "quitter" and encourages people who are involved in unhappy situations to "stick it out," creating guilt for those who choose flight but continued unhappiness for those who do try to stick it out. If we suffer from a difficult partnership, a painful involvement, an unhappy marriage, or a strangling, dependency-laden friendship, then cutting the tie (flight) becomes a matter of survival in the long run, disturbing as such action may be in the short run.

Often our moral codes make us forget that our first obligation is to ourselves. This may sound selfish, yet true charity can evolve only after we first fulfill our own basic needs. Otherwise we just continue to bribe our way through life with acts that superficially appear to be generous, but that are really selfish and intended to fulfill our own needs. Needless and endless suffering serves no purpose. Contrary to popular belief, suffering does not necessarily make a person a better human being. Constructive action does. Compassion does. Love does.

Unlike other animals, people often make a third choice—inaction. Instead of fight or flight, there is indecision, the failure to do anything. For example, many unhappily married people fail to fight (attack the problem) or take flight (divorce) but merely remain in a bitter situation year after year, gradually dehumanizing both partners. Indecision is fed by conflict between basic individual needs and an overly harsh conscience, by anxiety, guilt, pity, and doubt in the wisdom of one's own judgment. It has a paralyzing effect and perpetuates weakness and insecurity. There is a loss of self-esteem and a growing sense of failure or of wasting one's life.

In fight-or-flight therapy, as in assertiveness training, the emphasis is on action. In dealing with a problem, one must do something specific. Try anything, but do not just sit back waiting to be told what to do.

Milieu Therapy Severe emotional disorders generally require a period of hospitalization. The recovery process is greatly aided if the hospital is organized as a therapeutic community. Thus, *milieu therapy* refers to the conscious use of the social setting or environment in the treatment of psychiatric patients. It is concerned with physical environment, atmosphere within the psychiatric setting, attitudes, interaction among staff and patients, interaction among patients, and social organization. It adds use of the social system to individual therapy. In milieu therapy, the patient becomes an active participant instead of a passive recipient of treatment. One's strengths are emphasized together with those areas in which one needs help. One is recognized as part of a community that has a culture of its own.

The doctors, nurses, and other members of the therapeutic team generally work in street clothes, rather than in uniforms, which tend to create communication barriers and detract from the therapeutic environment. Since staff members act as role models for patients, it is accepted as part of milieu therapy that the appearance of the staff influences the patients. An attractive, vitally alive staff carries much nonverbal impact.

In milieu therapy, the environment is modified to facilitate more effective patterns of interaction. Social interaction is an important part of the treatment of the psychiatric patient. A well-organized milieu program includes provisions for patients and staff to make decisions on matters concerning themselves through the medium of community and small group meetings. Group therapy and patient-centered activities that are planned and carried out by patients are essential to a complete program. Work therapy or vocational rehabilitation is also an integral part of milieu therapy.

Group Therapy Group therapy, in its many forms, involves processes that occur in structured and protected groups and are calculated to cause rapid improvement in personality and behavior of individual members through controlled group interactions. Group psychotherapy was introduced into the United States in 1905 by Joseph Pratt, a Boston internist, to bolster the morale of his tuberculosis patients.

Group therapy is, to a large degree, based on the same theoretical principles as individual psychotherapy. However, it has additional dimensions and is often useful for problems not adequately met by individual therapy. Traditionally, group therapy has been conducted by psychiatrists, psychologists, and social workers. In response to the growing demand for it, many nurses, clergymen, educators, other professionals, and even laypeople have become involved as leaders of group therapy sessions.

The criteria for success in group therapy are essentially the same as for individual therapy, such as relief from emotional distress, insight, enhanced personal dignity, and improved behavior and social relations. Individual therapy is sometimes preferable in achieving insight, but group therapy provides a better opportunity to "see ourselves as other see us."

The success of group therapy depends largely on the skill and degree of involvement of the therapist and the proper selection of patients. Therapists who consider group therapy to be an inferior form of psychotherapy tend to prescribe it for their least promising patients; if the results are then poor, the prejudice is reinforced.

While the lower cost of group therapy is one obvious advantage over individual therapy, it is not the only advantage, nor the most important one. Group therapy, for example, offers a remedy for the social isolation often resulting from the technological aspects of modern life. The group can multiply the effects of therapy by bringing many minds and viewpoints to bear upon each patient's individual problems. Group therapy offers the further advantage of providing each member with a "safe" human-relations laboratory. Within the protection of the group, each patient has the opportunity to test various ways of relating to others and to discover how others respond. The patients' dignity is enhanced when they act as givers as well as receivers of help. Truly valuable insights and interpretations are often given by one patient to another. In an atmosphere of mutual help, the patient also becomes a therapist.

There are many human conditions for which group therapy is often more useful than individual therapy. Among these are shy and lonely people, whose very reluctance to enter group therapy is an indication that they could profit from it; patients who become too dependent on an individual therapist; patients trying to overcome phobias; patients who feel antagonism and fear toward parental and authority figures and thus withhold their true feelings from an individual therapist; patients who have had unsatisfactory relations with siblings or who have been raised without brothers or sisters; adolescents with confused sexual identification; patients with difficulty in getting along with others (those who demand much and give little, or have other ways of alienating people) are likely to show their characteristic behavior in the group and to be made aware of it by the others; patients with problems seen as shameful or unusual (such as bed-wetters, alcoholics, drug abusers, or obese persons) can be of great emotional support to one another; and married couples who, in couples groups, find that the problems they had considered unique to their marriage are often present in other marriages as well.

The many forms of group therapy can be broadly classified as evocative, directive, or didactic. Evocative methods of group therapy are those that encourage spontaneous expression of feelings by patients in an atmosphere of acceptance and of effort toward understanding those feelings. In group therapy the evocative leader promotes mutual interaction among patients in preference to exchanges between patient and therapist. The leader avoids authoritarianism. The leader does not demand that patients express the "right" attitude; they are encouraged to feel free to express their *real* attitudes. In evocative groups, the patients and leader generally sit in a circle. Thus, the therapist is not placed in any special position that would make him or her the focal point of the group's attention. Most group therapy today is of the evocative approach. Some specific forms include activity therapy, group psychoanalysis, T-groups (training groups), encounter groups, transactional analysis, sensitivity groups, and psychodrama.

Directive group therapy methods are those in which the leader asserts authority, especially as an expert on proper attitudes and conduct. Advice and commands may be given. In directive groups the leader stands or sits in a special position, to become the focal point of the group's attention. Some examples of directive therapy include organized religion (the leader being the cleric in the pulpit), Alcoholics Anonymous, and Synanon.

Didactic group methods aim at educating patients, often with factual knowledge about their problems and their treatment. The distinction between didactic and directive therapy is that the didactic approach seeks to educate, whereas the directive approach seeks to indoctrinate. Typical of didactic therapy are classes and seminars for institutionalized patients with psychoses, sex deviations, and other problems that respond poorly to less structured approaches. Through understanding the nature, causes, and treatments of their conditions, the patients' fear and hostility toward treatment are diminished and they are motivated to cooperate with other forms of therapy.

T-Groups, Encounter Groups, and Sensitivity Groups T-groups are training groups that first came into use as a method of training psychiatrists and other mental health professionals, especially those interested in becoming group therapists. T-groups are not therapy groups—their participants are presumed to be well rather than ill. The T-group differs from the therapy group in that it is concerned with conscious or preconscious behavior rather than unconscious motivation. The participants learn human relations, communications, and leadership skills. They learn about the dynamics of their own behavior and that of others by being in the group under the guidance of a "trainer."

The objectives of training include self-insight, better understanding of other persons and awareness of one's impact upon them, better understanding of group processes and increased skill in achievement of group effectiveness, increased recognition of the characteristics of social systems, and greater awareness of the dynamics of change.

A T-group is typically composed of 12 to 15 persons who work together on an intensive schedule of perhaps 6 hours a day for 2 weeks or in marathon sessions that continue uninterrupted for 48 hours. If the group is to be successful in meeting its goals, the following conditions should be met: (1) each individual must share his or her thoughts and feelings; (2) a continuously operating feedback system must reflect the relevancy of each individual's behavior; (3) a group atmosphere of trust is necessary for persons to be able to reveal their thoughts and feelings; (4) each person needs enough knowledge of psychological theory to understand his or her own experience; and (5) each participant must have the opportunity to try new behavior patterns following the sessions. Unless these new learnings can be applied, they will soon be forgotten. Thus the critical steps in the T-group process are presentation of feelings, feedback from others regarding those feelings, and experimentation with new behavior patterns.

The T-group method has been extended from mental health professionals to business executives, clergymen, medical students, and others whose work demands special ability in dealing with people. Recently, some T-groups have developed a new function as a social movement for overcoming alienation or emotional distance between people in general. Such groups are also called *sensitivity groups* or *encounter groups* and participation is not limited to special professional or occupational groups.

Transactional Analysis Transactional analysis focuses on the hidden meanings in interpersonal communications and is a useful tool in group therapy. It was popularized by Eric Berne in 1964 through his bestselling *Games People Play* (Grove Press). He called each unit of communication a *transaction*. When two or more people encounter each other, sooner or later one of them will speak or in some other way acknowledge the presence of the others. This first communication is called the *transactional stimulus*. Another person will then say or do something in response to this stimulus, and that is called the *transactional response*. Transactional analysis is concerned with diagnosing the real psychological motivations behind the transactional stimulus and response. This approach is especially useful for groups of married couples, in whom it may reveal the playing of verbal and nonverbal games. Berne's "games" are repetitive, neurotic interactions with hidden meanings. Among the commonly played games described by Berne are "See what you made me do," "If it weren't for you," and "Look how hard I've tried."

Life Positions Thomas A. Harris introduced the concept of life positions in his book *I'm OK–You're OK* (Harper & Row, 1969). Basically, your life position is how you feel about yourself and other people. According to Harris, each of us adopts a life position rather early in life, based on our childhood experiences. Once an emotional position is confirmed, a person will tend to cling to it throughout life. Yet Harris believes it possible for a person, through self-understanding, to move from one life position to another. There are four possible life positions:

1. *I'm not OK–You're OK.* This is probably the most common life position. It has its origin during early childhood. It grows out of a feeling of being small and helpless in comparison to parents who are large and powerful and who can either give or withhold comforting "strokes." It is fed by a feeling of parental disapproval of what seem to the child to be normal, natural urges. The child is constantly scolded for "misbehavior" and thus loses self-confidence. At the same time, the child is awed by the "all-knowing" parents. The child arrives at a self-estimation of *not OK* and an *OK* estimation of its parents.

   Adults still holding this position have a strong need for recognition and approval ("strokes") from others. Some, finding it too painful to be around "OK" people, withdraw emotionally or seek out companions with whom they can identify as also being "not OK." Some are convinced that they are inherently inadequate and live out a self-fulfilling prophecy, proving to themselves that they indeed are inadequate. (The concept of cognitive dissonance does not allow them to enjoy success when their self-concept is that they are inadequate.)

   Seeking strokes, many people readily comply with the demands of others. Willing and eager, they constantly seek the approval of others. Yet their *not OK* side keeps reminding them of their inadequacy, so that no matter how hard they try, they still feel *not OK.* They may even unconsciously do something to block success when it appears imminent, again to avoid the anxiety produced by cognitive dissonance.

2. *I'm not OK–You're not OK.* This position may be adopted when children see their parents as having failed them— perhaps through inadequate attention or overly strict discipline. People who assume this view usually develop some form of emotional withdrawal. It is easy for such a person to give up, lose hope, and simply exist through a joyless life.

3. *I'm OK–You're not OK.* This view of life may develop in a child who was truly deprived of love and attention (stroking) and is especially prevalent among people who as children were battered—physically abused by their parents. In their isolation between beatings, some battered children find comfort within themselves. The comfort they find in just being left alone stands in such contrast to the pain of their beatings that they conclude that they are OK, but other people are *not OK.* Their survival almost requires such a position. This view of life and history of childhood abuse are shared by many *sociopathic* persons—those who care little about the rights or feelings of others. The feeling of being OK while everyone else is *not OK* may carry itself to the point of justifying any action— robbery, murder, rape—without any feelings of guilt or personal responsibility.

4. *I'm OK–You're OK.* Usually by the second or third year of life a child has arrived at one of the first three positions. All children begin with the first position, but some shift to the second or third.

   Many adults are captives of one of the first two positions, a few of the third. People who feel *not OK* often feed their egos at the expense of others. They bully others, laugh at the mistakes of others, and often put people down in their efforts to bolster their own self-esteem. Material symbols of success—houses, cars, and so forth—assume a great importance to these people.

The move into the fourth and most desirable position of *I'm OK–You're OK* requires a conscious effort. First, you must understand your childhood reasons for being in one of the first three positions. Then you must convince yourself of your own personal worth—that you are *OK*. This must be done intentionally and it takes time. It is done by finding activities in which you can succeed and collecting a series of successes. Doing so, you gradually feel more secure in your ability to succeed and this feeling contributes to further success. It comes down to the old story that failure breeds failure and success breeds success. In order to attain or maintain a feeling of *I'm OK*, you must learn to ignore the inevitable put-downs by other people, knowing that the reason some people must put others down is their own feeling of being *not OK*. It is not easy to learn to feel OK, but it is possible.

Behavior Therapy Behavior therapy is the application to human beings of techniques derived from experiments with animal behavior. The behavior therapies differ in several important respects from traditional psychotherapy procedures. Perhaps the most important difference is that the behavior therapist works directly toward modifying objectionable behavior, rather than attempting to identify the "underlying unconscious disease process" that most psychotherapists (and all psychoanalysts) believe to be the cause of symptoms.

For this reason the behavior therapist does not deal with the unconscious, ego structures, or defense mechanisms, and does not employ insight as a prime treat-ment means. Behavior therapy is mainly used for patients with rather specific behavioral difficulties, rather than for those whose problems are more diverse.

The rationale of behavior therapy is that the undesirable behavior patterns were learned in the first place and, with proper training techniques, can be unlearned (behaviorists use the term *extinguished*). Extinction may involve either weakening the undesirable responses or learning new responses that are incompatible with the ones being extinguished.

There are several major types of behavior therapy. The *classical conditioning therapies* make use of unlearned, constitutional reflex behavior to modify or eliminate unwanted behavior. One of the major classical techniques is *counterconditioning*, in which new, more desirable responses are conditioned to the same stimuli that produce the undesirable responses. Varieties of counterconditioning include *aversion therapy*, in which the undesirable behavior response is accompanied by a nausea-producing drug, mild electric shock, or similar unpleasant experience; *reciprocal inhibition*, in which the patient is taught a response, such as relaxation, that is incompatible with the unwanted response to a given stimulus; and *desensitization*, in which the patient, under "safe" conditions, faces anxiety or fear-arousing stimuli in gradually increasing degrees, so that other responses can be conditioned to them. This is particularly effective in treating phobias of many kinds.

Another type of behavior therapy is *operant conditioning*, in which the undesirable behavior is modified by the appropriate use of positive and negative reinforcers. (A reinforcer is a stimulus or event that changes the rate of a behavior when it follows that behavior.) In operant conditioning, positive reinforcers, such as food or desired objects or privileges, are used to reward desirable behavior; while negative reinforcers, such as pain, verbal reprimand, or the loss of desired objects or privileges, are used to "punish" undesirable behavior. By combining positive and negative reinforcement, a behavior therapist can do much to eliminate undesirable behavior and encourage suitable behavior patterns. This, of course, is basically how most parents raise their children.

Operant conditioning can be effective with relatively large groups of people in social situations. Entire wards in mental hospitals, for example, can be placed under a "token economy" in which coinlike tokens are given (and taken away) as reinforcement for certain behaviors. The hospital thereby becomes more like the world outside, and patients are led to interact with other people in useful ways. The tokens earned may be "spent" for such desired items as food, privacy, minor luxuries, or even leave from the hospital. The token economy can be an important part of milieu therapy, discussed earlier.

Behavior therapy has had a mixed reception among mental health professionals. Behavioral psychologists are highly in favor of it for almost every manner of mental disorder, while other psychologists and many psychiatrists remain unconvinced of its value. The true value of behavior therapy probably lies somewhere between these extremes of acceptance or rejection. As previously mentioned, it is best suited for the treatment of rather specific behavioral problems. It is of less value for most severe psychotic disorders and most general personality disorders.

The greatest success of behavior therapy has been in treating such problems as phobias, severe anxiety, obsessional thinking, sexual disorders of many kinds, overeating, gambling, and other compulsive behaviors. Drug dependence and alcoholism have also been treated, though with somewhat less success. Patients who have spent many years locked in the back wards of mental hospitals because they lack elementary social skills and competencies are often able to leave such wards following behavior modification procedures that teach them the rudiments of social skills. While they are not all able to leave the hospital, many actually do, and many more are able to spend their days in happier circumstances in less restrictive wards.

The advantages of behavior therapy, in cases for which it is suited, include: (1) it often works; (2) it may be administered by such nonprofessional therapists as psychiatric aides, parents, and school teachers, after only a few hours of training; (3) the procedures are clear-cut, unambiguous, and consistent: results may be achieved in a short period of time, often just a few weeks; and (4) it is rare for a new behavioral problem to appear in the place of the old one.

Drug Therapy (Chemotherapy) The development of new drugs has had an important influence on the treatment of emotional illness in recent years; they have become a primary means of treating the seriously disturbed patient. The use of these drugs has reduced the time needed for improvement and recovery and has actually lowered the population of many mental hospitals.

The many drugs available fall into several basic groups. Among these are the tranquilizers, which are used to calm anxiety; the sedatives, which combat overactivity and insomnia as well as anxiety; the antidepressants, which help raise the mood of severely depressed patients; and antipsychotics, used to reduce or temporarily remove such symptoms as hallucinations.

Drugs are sometimes used as the primary treatment in cases of mild anxiety or mild depression. But in more serious cases, drugs are used in connection with psychotherapy. Often, the function of the drugs is to make the patient accessible for psychotherapy. Before these drugs were available, many patients were too agitated or too withdrawn to be reached by psychotherapy.

The old-time psychiatric hospital ward, with some patients wildly agitated and others mute and withdrawn, is fortunately becoming a thing of the past through the use of modern drugs. The drugs are not curing the patients, but they are making them calm and rational enough to participate in psychotherapy. After release from the hospital, many patients continue on drugs, and possibly psychotherapy, for varying periods of time.

Today, perhaps 90 percent of all cases of emotional disorder, including major and minor forms, are treated with psychotherapy, drugs, or a combination of the two. Although the use of other forms of treatment thus has become secondary, we will briefly describe two of them.

Shock Therapy Prior to the advent of tranquilizers and antidepressant drugs, shock therapy was often used in the treatment of mental illnesses. The most important of several kinds of shock therapy, called *electroconvulsive therapy* (ECT) is still being used, but with greater discretion than in years past. Another type of shock therapy, in which insulin is injected, is rarely used because of the many dangers associated with its use.

Electroconvulsive therapy was introduced by Cerletti and Bini in 1937. Originally, electrodes were merely attached to opposite sides of the patient's forehead and a current of electricity was sent through the head. In traditional ECT, the patients lose consciousness immediately, followed by convulsions much like epileptic seizures. Over the years, many improvements have been made in the technique, such as administering premedication to sedate the patient. A drug (Anectine) is usually given to block transmission of impulses from motor nerves to skeletal muscles, thus reducing the convulsive spasms associated with shock therapy. Before the use of this drug, it was not uncommon for individuals to sustain sprains or even fractures.

It is now possible to stimulate specific parts of the brain and thereby produce effects other than convulsions. For example, ECT can be used to treat severe drug intoxication such as barbiturate coma resulting from an accidental overdose or an attempted suicide.

ECT is not, however, indicated in the treatment of all mental disorders and its use should be restricted to carefully selected patients. Because of indiscriminate, and sometimes punitive, use, ECT has been the subject of much controversy and thus more stringent controls of its use have come about. If used and administered properly, this procedure is painless and involves little physical risk to the patient. When used to treat severely depressed or manic (agitated) patients, the results may be strikingly favorable. While symptoms such as over-excitement or stupor are significantly reduced, the basic illness does not disappear. However, with the elimination of these symptoms, patients are more accessible and receptive to psychotherapy.

After receiving ECT, patients usually experience a mild confusion or loss of memory, but these effects rarely persist for more than a few weeks or perhaps months after the last treatment.

State hospitals for the mentally ill once relied on ECT as an important part of their therapeutic programs. However, with the availability of drugs that produce similar results, such treatment is seldom used in these institutions anymore. Also, because of the more rigid criteria in selecting appropriate patients, the time and paperwork involved make it impractical. Private hospitals still conduct ECT therapy but it usually requires the consultation and approval of two or more psychiatrists.

Lobotomy Rarely necessary today, lobotomy is the surgical severing of the nerve tracts that connect the frontal lobes of the brain to the thalamus. The frontal lobes are centers for fear and anxiety. Today the same results produced by a lobotomy can almost always be achieved through drugs.

Types of Specialists Many patients today are treated by a specially trained group of people, rather than by one individual. This group is sometimes called the *psychiatric team*. In addition to physicians and nurses, it may include psychologists, occupational therapists, social workers, and others who are concerned with specialized problems. Let us consider several members of this team:

Psychiatrist. A psychiatrist is a physician (M.D.) who has had additional specialized training in treating mental illness and has been licensed by the American Board of Psychiatry and Neurology. The psychiatrist may use any method of treatment, whether individual, group, drug, or shock therapy.

Psychoanalyst. A psychoanalyst is a psychiatrist who has had additional specialized training in psychoanalytic methodology and has fulfilled the requirements for membership in a psychoanalytic association. Most analysts use some variation of Freudian theory.

Clinical psychologist. The clinical psychologist does not go through medical school, but instead does postgraduate study in psychology and usually holds the degree of doctor of philosophy (Ph.D.) or master of arts (M.A.). Clinical psychologists give psychological tests, make diagnoses, and engage in psychotherapy. They often work in association with a psychiatrist.

Psychiatric social worker. Psychiatric social workers take two years of postgraduate study and hold a master's degree in social work, with training in psychology. They make contact with relatives, friends, employers, and others connected with the patient. They assist them in making any changes in the environment of the patient that seem necessary for the patient's recovery.

Psychiatric registered nurse. The psychiatric nurse is a registered nurse who has had special training and experience with the mentally ill. He or she may supervise a hospital ward and administer treatments under the supervision of a psychiatrist, as well as assisting in therapy.

Mental health aide or assistant. The aide or assistant, referred to as a *psychiatric technician* in several states, is charged with the actual physical care and custody of the hospitalized patient. The aide or technician is a paramedical staff person who has received on-the-job training. A few colleges now offer training programs for psychiatric technicians. Aides are important because of the great amount of time they spend with the patient and the personal influence they may have over the patient. A good relationship between the aide and the patient can greatly speed the recovery process.

Types of Facilities A wide variety of treatment facilities are available for people experiencing major or minor emotional problems. Many people fail to receive needed treatment only because they or their friends or relatives are not aware of the facilities available to them. Treatment is often available at little or no cost to people who cannot otherwise afford help.

Outpatient Clinics   Many patients with minor to moderately severe emotional illness can be treated today while they are still living at home. Psychotherapy sessions usually play an important part in such treatment. The psychiatrist or psychologist administering this care may be either in private practice, supported entirely by patient fees, or in a community clinic, supported by government or charity. Often these community clinics have a sliding scale of fees, determined by the ability of the patient to pay.

Outpatient clinics are also very important in providing care for the patient who has had short-term hospitalization during the acute stage of an emotional illness and is completing recovery at home. Such follow-up treatment can greatly reduce the chances of needing to return to the hospital.

Psychiatric Sections of General Hospitals   There is a growing trend for general hospitals to build or reserve certain sections specifically for the treatment of emotional disorders. These provide the patient with psychiatric treatment in a hospital setting without requiring travel far from home. They also help reduce the social stigma of emotional illness by treating it in the same context as any other disorder.

State Mental Hospitals   In the past, emotional problems often required prolonged hospitalization because no effective methods of treatment were available. Some patients received only custodial care, that is, they were given humane shelter, but no specific treatment. Since hospitalization was so prolonged, the respon-

sibility for its cost was usually assumed by the state government. The main purpose of such hospitals was to confine the ill where they could not bother anyone.

Most states are now applying the newer approaches to the treatment of emotional problems, with results often comparable to those obtained in private hospitals. It has been shown that if a state is willing to spend the money to provide intensive care for newly admitted, acutely ill patients, money will be saved in the long run. Given this intensive care, many patients can leave the hospital in a short time. Without such care, the same patients may require hospitalization at state expense for years, and perhaps even for life. The states that recognize this principle have actually been able to reduce the population of their state mental hospitals during a period in which the population of the country has risen and the incidence of emotional problems has climbed.

Private Mental Hospitals   In recent years, increasing numbers of privately owned hospitals for the exclusive treatment of mental or emotional problems have opened. Some treat all kinds of mental problems, while others are restricted to such groups as adolescents, elderly persons, or alcoholics.

Comprehensive Community Mental Health Centers   Unfortunately, there is still an enormous gap between the best that could be done and what is actually being done for the emotionally disturbed. In many communities, facilities for treating emotional problems are nonexistent. Where available, such services are often priced beyond the reach of all but the most fortunate. Treatment for emotional problems is often specifically excluded from payment by health-insurance policies.

In order to stimulate the development of

comprehensive community mental health centers, the federal government has made available financial aid to centers that meet certain standards of qualification. The following ten criteria describe the comprehensive community mental health center:

1. Inpatient services.
2. Outpatient services.
3. Partial hospitalization services such as day care, night care, and weekend care.
4. Emergency services available at all times.
5. Consultation and education services available to community agencies and professional personnel.
6. Diagnostic services.
7. Rehabilitative services, including vocational and educational programs.
8. Precare and aftercare services in the community, including foster-home placement, home visiting, and halfway houses.
9. Training.
10. Research and evaluation.

To date, the number of such comprehensive centers in the United States remains limited and they are especially scarce outside major metropolitan areas. But these criteria are an excellent yardstick by which a community can evaluate its own mental health facilities. While it is generally impossible for a small community to provide all these services, it is often feasible for several neighboring communities to collectively develop an excellent comprehensive mental health center. Adequate mental health facilities often can be established in a community through the efforts of concerned citizens, working in cooperation with interested professional personnel.

FOR FURTHER READING

Aguilera, Donna C., and Messick, Janice M. *Crisis Intervention*, 2nd ed. Saint Louis: C. V. Mosby Company, 1974. A comprehensive overview of crisis intervention from its historical development to its utilization.

Alberti, Robert E., and Emmons, Michael L. *Your Perfect Right*, 2nd ed. San Luis Obispo, Calif.: Impact, 1974. A Guide to building self-esteem through assertive behavior.

Berne, Eric. *Games People Play*. New York: Grove Press, 1964. Describes the significance of specific patterns of interpersonal communication.

Caprio, Frank, and Leighton, Francis. *How to Avoid a Nervous Breakdown*. New York: Hawthorn, 1969. Emphasizes the point that individuals must maintain a strong self-image in order to control the harmful effects of stress.

Goble, Frank. *The Third Force*. New York: Grossman Publishers, 1970. Describes the psychology of Abraham Maslow.

Harris, Thomas. *I'm OK–You're OK: A Practical Guide to Transactional Analysis*. New York: Harper & Row, 1971. Written for the lay person; engagingly describes the insights and advantages of transactional analysis methods.

James, Muriel, and Jongeward, Dorothy. *Born to Win*. Menlo Park, Calif.: Addison–Wesley, 1971. Applies transactional analysis theory to everyday life.

Janov, Arthur. *The Primal Scream*. New York: Dell Publishing, 1970. An explanation of the author's primal therapy system, through which the patient's primal (early) experiences are relived, in order to avoid symptoms of neurosis.

Linder, Robert. *The Fifty-Minute Hour*. New York: Bantam Books, 1971. A collection of true psychoanalytic tales.

Maslow, Abraham. *Motivation and Personality*, 2nd ed. New York: Harper & Row, 1970. Classic presentation of basic human emotional needs.
_____. *The Farther Reaches of Human Nature*. New York: The Viking Press, 1971. Expands Maslow's observations of personality.

Mayeroff, Milton. *On Caring*. New York: Harper & Row, 1971. A noted philosopher explores the meaning and importance of caring.

Rogers, Carl. *Carl Rogers on Encounter Groups*. New York: Harper & Row, 1970. A comprehensive and sensitive analysis of the encounter group—its implications for psychotherapy, its methods and procedures.

Schaefer, Halmuth H., and Martin, Patrick L. *Behavioral Therapy*, 2nd ed. New York: McGraw–Hill, 1975. A look at behavioral therapy as a valuable means of facilitating human adjustment.

Selye, Hans. *The Stress of Life*. New York: McGraw–Hill, 1956. Explains Selye's widely accepted theory of the General Adaptation Syndrome.

Smith, Manuel J. *When I Say No I Feel Guilty*. New York: Dial Press, 1975. Excellent book on how to cope using the skills of systematic assertive therapy.

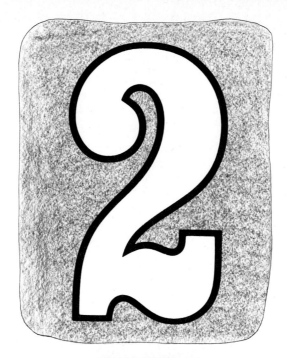

DRUGS, ALCOHOL, AND TOBACCO

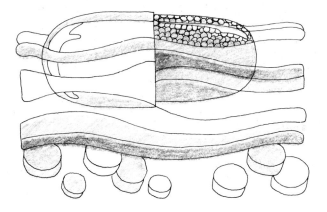

4

DRUGS: USE AND ABUSE

Drugs are a basic part of our cultural concept of good health. Primarily, drugs are used to treat diseases. Yet drugs can be, and are being, misused and abused to a point where they adversely affect health. Alcohol is used in a variety of social situations, but its abuse can lead to alcoholism. The habitual use of tobacco is pleasurable for many people, yet the resulting cancers and heart diseases are major causes of death.

If you were asked to define the word *drug*, you might simply say that a drug is any substance used in treating a disease. However, a more complete definition would be: any substance, other than food, *that alters the body or its functions.* Today the word *drug* is a loaded term. In common usage, it now has two connotations—one positive, reflecting the crucial role of the natural (obtained from a natural source such as a plant) and synthetic (produced in a chemical laboratory) substances used in medicine, and one negative, relating to self-destructive and socially destructive patterns of abuse. Many of society's problems with drugs develop at the point where society has to deal with an *individual's behavior* caused by substances that have little or no medical value, or where the nonmedical behavior modification interferes with therapeutic (disease-treating) uses. The problem of drug control is further complicated by the fact that some drugs play dual roles. For example, barbiturates and narcotics are considered beneficial when used as sleeping pills and painkillers, but destructive when used as downers, or depressants.

Drug Use — Methods and Medicine

The medical and non-medical use of drugs dates back thousands of years. At first, drugs were used by early societies as part of religious healing ceremonies. In most of these societies, however, more reliance was placed on prayers, incantations, and charms than on the particular drug used. Eventually, the powers of certain drugs became highly guarded secrets known only to the individuals who governed their use.

It was not until the latter half of the nineteenth century that scientists began to perform experiments to discover precisely what chemicals were contained in drugs and what effect individual drugs might have in alleviating pain or curing disease. Before that, prescribing drugs was a hit-or-miss affair. Physicians and quacks often ascribed wonderful curative properties to "patent medicines" that were worthless or harmful.

In the past thirty years, new drugs have revolutionized the practice of medicine. Since the development of sulfa drugs and antibiotics in the 1930s, hundreds of new drugs have been introduced, many of them capable of reversing the course of serious disease and saving lives.

Because of the development of these "wonder" drugs and the ready acceptance of them by the medical profession, many people have built up unrealistic expectations about what drugs can do for them. The people of the United States are, in general, drug users. In our zealous search for miraculous cures, we too often decide for ourselves what prescription drugs and what dosages we need instead of leaving this difficult and delicate decision where it belongs—in the hands of trained physicians. The authors of this book feel that it is necessary for everyone to learn something about how drugs work. We hope that the more each of us knows about drugs, the more cautious we will be regarding self-diagnosis, self-treatment, and the misuse of drugs.

Medical Use of Drugs

Present knowledge of the chemical structure of drugs often enables scientists to predict what a drug will do and what the results of its actions will be. Drugs are administered to an individual for a specific purpose: to cure a disease or alleviate the pain or discomfort of an illness or injury. Any drug that is powerful enough to be effective has the potential to produce some adverse reactions, which are not always predictable. These actions can be classified as either side effects or untoward effects. A side effect of a drug is any action or effect other than the one for which it is administered. Side effects are not necessarily harmful to the individual. Morphine is usually given to relieve pain, not for its ability to constrict the pupil of the eye. This constriction is a side effect. An untoward effect is a reaction regarded as harmful to an individual. The untoward effects of morphine—nausea, vomiting, constipation, and addiction—are obviously undesirable and harmful.

Doctors are usually conservative about dosage size when prescribing drugs because of the possible untoward effects. A responsible physician is often reluctant to prescribe new drugs that have not been widely used and thoroughly tested, partly because of the risk of undesirable consequences.

People who visit a physician, seeking relief from an illness, sometimes respond with impatience and resentment when the doctor does not give them a prescription for drugs. But a doctor will not prescribe a medication until the condition being treated is known, and the process of making a diagnosis may take time. If a doctor too quickly prescribes drugs that temporarily relieve the symptoms of the illness, the drugs may interfere with diagnosis and may endanger the patient's health.

In addition, it is important to remember that most Americans are symptom-oriented. This may be a direct consequence of the standard methods of advertising medicines; television, radio, and magazine advertisements are designed to gear our attention toward symptoms, not underlying causes of illness or pain. Thus, many people seek immediate relief of symptoms and want their doctor's assistance in doing so. But if a doctor prescribes a drug that eliminates symptoms, most patients do not feel the same urgency to continue with diagnosis and treatment—the phases of medical attention that are really most important in terms of the individual's long-range health.

Drug Administration and Actions

As the next figure shows, drugs can be introduced into the body in various ways. Some drugs (penicillin, for example) can be taken orally in the form of capsules or can be injected. Other drugs, such as insulin, which is used in the treatment of diabetes, cannot be exposed to the digestive system's chemical action. It must be injected into the body.

After being taken into the body, drugs are distributed by the bloodstream to the many organs, tissues, and cells. The action or effect of a drug may be on the surface of cells, within the cell, or in the body fluids surrounding the cells. In most cases, the action takes place within the individual cells of the body and has either a direct or indirect effect on the central nervous system. Drugs enter the cells in the same way that water and other nutrients do, through the membranes of the cell. Many drugs include molecular parts similar to those found in the cell's normal "diet," and this permits the drugs to participate in a few stages of the cell's normal chemical processes. Ultimately, of course, the differences between the drug and the normal chemical will be detected by the systems of the cell. But by this time the drug's work has been done. The cellular processes are no longer normal; the cells, the organs, and the interrelated body systems have been altered—the drug has taken effect.

Definitions of the Problem

Most drugs that have come to the attention of society have legitimate and useful places in the treatment of disease and alleviation of pain and discomfort. This is the "proper" use of drugs. Theoretically, any drug can be abused; that is, used for purposes other than those intended by a physician. Drug abuse is defined as the self- administration of drugs in excessive or otherwise inappropriate dosages, which results in damage to an individual and/or society. Despite the usefulness of this definition, the term is still a difficult one to define completely and adequately. The

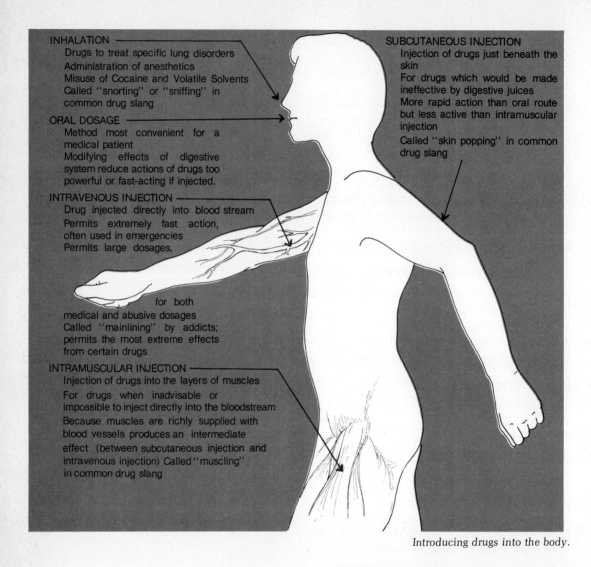

INHALATION
    Drugs to treat specific lung disorders
    Administration of anesthetics
    Misuse of Cocaine and Volatile Solvents
    Called "snorting" or "sniffing" in
    common drug slang

ORAL DOSAGE
    Method most convenient for a
    medical patient
    Modifying effects of digestive
    system reduce actions of drugs too
    powerful or fast-acting if injected.

INTRAVENOUS INJECTION
    Drug injected directly into blood stream
    Permits extremely fast action,
    often used in emergencies
    Permits large dosages,
                        for both
    medical and abusive dosages
    Called "mainlining" by addicts;
    permits the most extreme effects
    from certain drugs

INTRAMUSCULAR INJECTION
    Injection of drugs into the layers of muscles
    For drugs when inadvisable or
    impossible to inject directly into the bloodstream
    Because muscles are richly supplied with
    blood vessels produces an intermediate
    effect (between subcutaneous injection and
    intravenous injection) Called "muscling"
    in common drug slang

SUBCUTANEOUS INJECTION
    Injection of drugs just beneath the
    skin
    For drugs which would be made
    ineffective by digestive juices
    More rapid action than oral route
    but less active than intramuscular
    injection
    Called "skin popping" in common
    drug slang

Introducing drugs into the body.

spectrum of responsibility—from individual to social—frequently clouds important scientific and medical debates about drugs. Attitudes towards drug abuse have also taken on political significance, again adding to the scientific confusion.

Habituating or Addicting?   In the past, certain commonly abused drugs were said to be *habituating* or *addicting*. The expla-

nations of these terms most often quoted today are those of the Expert Committee on Addiction-Producing Drugs of the World Health Organization. These definitions are given in the following table. But the terms *addict*, *user*, or *habitual user* can be ambiguous. In common usage, these words are defined in terms of the drug involved. For example, the addict has been described as someone who is dependent on the physically addicting drugs such as opium and its derivatives, synthetic narcotics, barbiturates, alcohol, and solvents. The user has been described as one who has an habituation to cocaine, amphetamines, marijuana, LSD, or other hallucinogenic drugs.

Dependency

The terms *addict* and *habitual user* have become obsolete because they fail to serve all situations and conditions—the needs of science, medicine, law, and society. Medically, a physician must know if a person is addicted (physically dependent on) a specific drug, in order to direct proper treatment. Whether a drug is addicting or habituating makes no difference to the law or to legal control of a drug. But society will not accept addiction, while it will accept the periodic, recreational, or "weekend" use of a drug. The behavioral problems of addiction are treatable emotional problems of an individual. The physically addicting properties of a drug have no significance in determining whether or not there are social and legal problems associated with a specific drug.

The terms *habituating* and *addicting* are now being replaced by *psychological dependence, drug dependence, substance dependence,* or *dependency*. With the repeated use of any *substance* (food, tobacco, aspirin, alcohol, narcotics, and so on) some individuals develop a *dependence on the substance*. The exact definition of this dependence varies with the type of substance being abused (narcotic, food, tobacco, sedative, hallucinogen); the social acceptability (degrees of acceptability of tobacco, alcohol, and heroin); and the individual reasons (social or emotional) for dependence on the substance.

Large amounts of food are consumed by individuals dependent on food as an emotional stabilizer. Large amounts of mild pain relievers (analgesics) with aspirin or aspirinlike ingredients are consumed

Definitions of Addiction and Habituation

Drug Addiction is:	Drug Habituation is:
a state of periodic or chronic intoxication produced by the repeated consumption of a drug (natural or synthetic) that produces in the individual—	a condition resulting from the repeated consumption of a drug that produces in the individual—
1. an overpowering desire or need (compulsion) to continue taking the drug and to obtain it by any means	1. a desire (but not a compulsion) to continue taking the drug for the sense of improved well-being or effect it produces
2. a tendency to increase the dose (tolerance)	2. little or no tendency to increase the dose (little or no tolerance)
3. both psychic (psychological) and physical dependence on the effects of the drug and hence presence of abstinence syndrome (withdrawal illness)	3. some degree of psychic dependence on the effect of the drug, but absence of physical dependence and hence of abstinence syndrome
4. a detrimental effect on the individual and on society	4. detrimental effects, if any, primarily on the individual

every day. Tranquilizers, sedatives, and hypnotics are the most widely prescribed and consumed drugs in the United States and the world. Many people believe they cannot get up, do their work, keep their nerves quiet, or go to sleep unless they have a drug to help them. There is sound medical basis for the temporary use of these drugs by some, and the permanent use by a few. But in general this is a form of "socially acceptable" drug dependence.

Problem Drugs The drugs, whether socially acceptable or not, that cause problems for society are those that cause death (tobacco in particular), or marked personality changes and abnormal social behavior. Such drugs may be alternately described as *mood modifying* (substances that modify moods and change behavior), *psychoactive* (substances that alter mood, perception, or consciousness), *psychotropic* ("mind-changing" substances), or *psychotoxic* ("mind-poisoning" substances). The most accurate term is *psychoactive*. Most psychoactive substances are abused because they cause euphoria (an extreme or exaggerated sense of pleasure or well-being), hallucinations (perceptions of objects with no relation to objective reality), or recognizable changes in personality or behavior. Psychoactive substances that are considered dangerous and unacceptable to society when used in excessive amounts include narcotics, solvents, hypnotics, sedatives (including alcohol), tranquilizers, forms of cannabis, hallucinogens, cocaine, and amphetamines.

Depressants and Stimulants In general, psychoactive substances act in or on cells to increase or decrease cellular activity of nerve centers and their conducting pathways (nerves and nerve tracts). *Depressant* substances have the ability to temporarily depress cellular, and consequently, body functions. Such drug-induced depression of the central nervous system is frequently characterized by a lack of interest in surroundings, inability to focus attention on a subject, and a lack of motivation to move or talk. The pulse and respiration become slower than usual, and as the depression deepens, the ability to use senses, such as touch, vision, hearing, smell, and taste, diminishes progressively. Psychological and motor activities decrease. Reflexes become sluggish and finally disappear. Depressant drugs are often quite accurately called *downers*. They literally slow down the cellular activity of an individual's nervous system. If a strong depressant is used, or if abusively large doses are consumed, depression progresses to drowsiness, stupor, unconsciousness, sleep, coma, and death.

A central nervous system *stimulant* is a drug that temporarily increases cellular processes, which causes an increase in body or nerve activity. Stimulant drugs quickly produce a dramatic effect, but their medical usefulness is limited because of the complexity of their actions and the nature of their side effects. Such side effects may include hallucinations, euphoria, anxiety, extreme nervousness, and tremors.

Because the milder stimulant and depressant drugs do not seem to produce the clear-cut physical dependence and are mood modifying, many users never progress beyond these relatively mild drugs. Individuals are able to control the effects they desire at a particular time. "Social drinking" of alcoholic beverages is an example of this kind of drug control. Others who start on the milder drugs progress to stronger ones because they enjoy the slight differences of effects. And some users, seeking a more pleasurable reaction, eventually become unable to control their drug use.

As already mentioned, each of the psychoactive substances either stimulates or depresses cellular functions. Caffeine, for instance, stimulates the nerve cells, while a barbiturate depresses them. Because of the complexity of the body's functions, drug action is often complex. At times, this makes it extremely difficult to place a group of drugs on a progressive continuum chart. Also, the complexity of a drug's actions often leads to apparent paradoxes. For example, alcohol is a depressant and depresses nerve functions. If this is so, why do people seem stimulated by a small-to-moderate amount of alcohol? The answer is that the brain contains a group of cells whose function is inhibition. These cells normally keep an individual from responding irresponsibly to every passing impulse. These inhibitory cells are more sensitive to alcohol and similar drugs (sedatives, hypnotics, and solvents) than the other brain cells. As the alcohol concentration in the blood begins to rise, the inhibitory cells are depressed and cease to function properly; many impulses, ideas, and actions that would otherwise be suppressed are acted out by the individual. Therefore, moderate amounts of alcohol, a depressant drug, can cause excitation by depressing a cellular inhibitory function.

Tolerance The repeated use of most psychoactive drugs, such as the narcotics, can produce biochemical and physiological changes that cause the user to keep increasing the dosage to maintain the same mood-modifying effect desired. At this point, a drug user is said to have developed a tolerance for the drug. *Tolerance* is an acquired reaction to a drug that necessitates an increase in dosage to maintain a given action or effect. As tolerance increases and more of the drug is used, body cells are gradually exposed to greater and greater quantities of it.

For a period of time, the body will adjust to these slowly increasing dosages of a drug. However, it is always possible that a user will take a larger dose than the body can tolerate (an overdose), leading to extreme illness or death.

If you are to deal with the psychoactive drugs, or understand individuals who use them, it is wise to learn something about the mind-altering or psychotropic effects of some of the more commonly abused drugs.

Psychoactive Substances

Today much research on drugs is concerned with how drugs alter states of mind. Researchers are attempting to discover how certain chemical substances work in modifying people's moods, personality, and behavior.

Such studies are especially necessary in view of the widespread use and abuse of psychoactive drugs. In the United States, over 20 million people use sleeping pills, over 10 million use amphetamines, and more than 50 million use tranquilizers. This includes those who have medical approval for their use of drugs as well as estimated "amateur" users. By considering the sheer number of users, we can see that the medical, psychological, sociological, philosophical, and legal aspects of drug use and abuse are extremely important.

The abnormal social behavior of some drug abusers, moreover, causes other problems. One of these involves the issue of personal responsibility during times of drug-induced behavioral changes, which may be called "times out." During such an interval, a person might do things that represent a complete departure from normal rationality and morality.

The degrees of depression and stimulation of drugs affecting the central nervous system are independent actions. The figure showing the continuum of drug effects and responses was suggested and formulated by Dr. Robert W. Earle of the University of California at Irvine.

The continuum of drug effects reaches to overstimulation and death at one extreme, and to depression and death at the other. The neutral area of this continuum is the range of stimulation and depression an individual encounters normally. Often drugs in different groups have similar actions. For example, narcotics are used to relieve pain but they may also, as a side effect, induce sleepiness. Barbiturates are used for their ability to induce sleep but they do not have the ability to relieve pain. Thus, the sleep-producing effects of these two depressants, narcotics and barbiturates, overlap on the continuum chart. In fact, many of the drugs that affect the central nervous system have similar actions.

As we progress along the chart from the neutral area outward, we can locate the specific points where the effects of drugs overlap. These points show where the continuum moves from the major effective area of one group of drugs into the area of another more powerful group of drugs. The weaker drugs are nearer the center, while the most powerful drugs are at the two extremes.

If dosages are increased, any of the drug groups listed may produce the complete range of effects of stimulation or depression. This overstimulation or extreme depression is the effect the drug abuser is seeking. Consequently, dosages used by drug abusers are far in excess of the dosages normally used in medical practice. The complete range of effects produced by increased dosages is represented in the next figure.

The drug continua in these two figures serve to point out the fact that the extreme effects of many different drugs are actually very similar. For example, any of the stimulants will produce hallucinations if

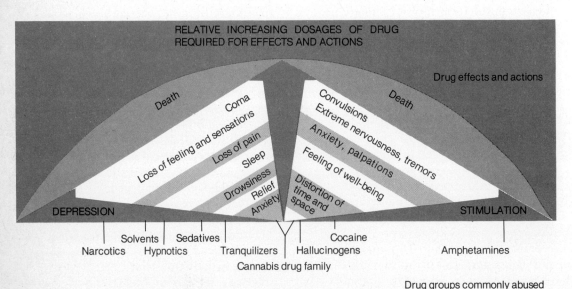

This graph shows the relationship of increased dosages to the continuum of drug effects. As the dose of drugs is increased, the effects progress along a continuum of effects until a lethal dosage is taken.

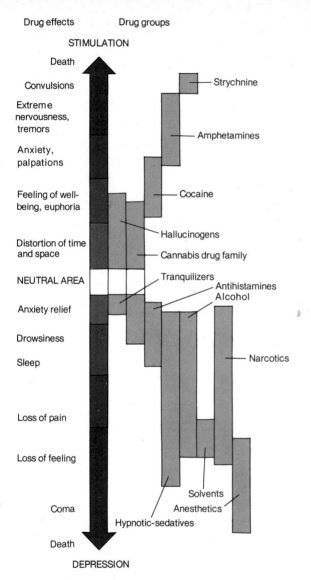

Drug effects   Drug groups

STIMULATION

Death

Convulsions — Strychnine

Extreme nervousness, tremors

Anxiety, palpations — Amphetamines

Feeling of well-being, euphoria — Cocaine

Distortion of time and space — Hallucinogens

— Cannabis drug family

NEUTRAL AREA — Tranquilizers

— Antihistamines
Alcohol

Anxiety relief

Drowsiness

Sleep — Narcotics

Loss of pain

Loss of feeling

Solvents
Coma   Anesthetics

Hypnotic-sedatives

Death

DEPRESSION

This illustration shows the continuum of drug effects and actions, as well as overlapping effects of drug groups.

the dosage is large enough. This is why many individuals, while usually preferring one drug over another, will abuse any available psychoactive drug. As the specific actions of a drug become more familiar and less spectacular, the individual may experiment with new ways to use the drug. A user often combines drugs of the same type, or of different types (poly-drug use) to produce a more intense effect. Examples of common combinations of drugs are alcohol and marijuana, alcohol and methadone, and methadone and heroin. Or, a user progresses from taking the drug orally, to injecting it under the skin, to injecting it directly into a vein. Some drug abusers are not satisfied with experiences from one drug at one consistent dosage, and often progress toward the extremes of the continuum.

The more commonly abused drugs, such as marijuana, barbiturates, and alcohol, are close to the center of the chart because of their mild effects when used in small dosages. The popularity of these drugs lies in the ability of the user to control the amount and, consequently, the relative effect of the drug. Many users of these drugs, particularly if they are not generally excitable or emotional, are contented with low dosages. On the other hand, highly emotional users or users seeking a specific "kick" are likely to increase the dosage and obtain a more intense effect. However, this ability to control drugs is offset with some drugs when tolerance (increasing cellular resistance to the usual drug effects) of the drug develops, or when usage reaches addictive levels. Then, regardless of the individual's desire or emotional state, a small but increasing dose is regularly required to keep the individual from entering withdrawal. This increasing level must be reached daily to keep the individual functioning at approximately the same level. Or, with the tolerance-producing nonaddicting drugs, the individual must either increase the amount he is using to produce the desired effects or move up the continuum to a stronger drug. Thus, he finds himself locked into a pattern of constantly increasing dosage amounts with the drugs that are tolerance-producing or addictive.

Controlled Substances: Uses and Effects

Drugs	Schedule*	Often Prescribed Brand Names	Medical Uses	Dependence Potential: Physical	Psychological
Narcotics					
Opium	II	Dover's Powder, Paregoric	Analgesic, antidiarrheal	High	High
Morphine	II	Morphine	Analgesic	High	High
Codeine	II III V	Codeine	Analgesic, antitussive	Moderate	Moderate
Heroin	I	None	None	High	High
Meperidine (Pethidine)	II	Demerol, Pethadol	Analgesic	High	High
Methadone	II	Dolophine, Methadone, Methadose	Analgesic, heroin substitute	High	High
Other Narcotics	I II III V	Dilaudid, Leritine, Numorphan, Percodan	Analgesic, antidiarrheal, antitussive	High	High
Depressants					
Chloral Hydrate	IV	Noctec, Somnos	Hypnotic	Moderate	Moderate
Barbiturates	II III IV	Amytal, Butisol, Nembutal, Phenobarbital, Seconal, Tuinal	Anesthetic, anti-convulsant, sedation, sleep	High	High
Glutethimide	III	Doriden	Sedation, sleep	High	High
Methaqualone	II	Optimil, Parest, Quaalude, Somnafac, Sopor	Sedation, sleep	High	High
Meprobamate	IV	Equanil, Meprospan, Miltown Kesso-Bamate, SK-Bamate	Anti-anxiety, muscle relaxant, sedation	Moderate	Moderate
Other Depressants	III IV	Dormate, Noludar, Placidyl, Valmid	Anti-anxiety, sedation, sleep	Possible	Possible
Stimulants					
Cocaine†	II	Cocaine	Local anesthetic	Possible	High
Amphetamines	II III	Benzedrine, Biphetamine, Desoxyn, Dexedrine	Hyperkinesis, narcolepsy, weight control	Possible	High
Phenmetrazine	II	Preludin	Weight control	Possible	High
Methylphenidate	II	Ritalin	Hyperkinesis	Possible	High
Other Stimulants	III IV	Bacarate, Cylert, Didrex, Ionamin, Plegine, Pondimin, Pre-Sate, Sanorex, Voranil	Weight control	Possible	Possible
Hallucinogens					
LSD	I	None	None	None	Degree unknown
Mescaline	I	None	None	None	Degree unknown
Psilocybin-Psilocyn	I	None	None	None	Degree unknown
MDA	I	None	None	None	Degree unknown
PCP‡	III	Sernylan	Veterinary anesthetic	None	Degree unknown
Other Hallucinogens	I	None	None	None	Degree unknown
Cannabis					
Marihuana	I	None	None	Degree unknown	Moderate
Hashish					
Hashish Oil					

*Scheduling classifications vary for individual drugs since controlled substances are often marketed in combination with other medicinal ingredients.

†Designated a narcotic under the controlled Substances Act.
‡Designated a depressant under the Controlled Substances Act.

Tolerance	Duration of Effects (in hours)	Usual Methods of Administration	Possible Effects	Effects of Overdose	Withdrawal Syndrome
Yes	3 to 6	Oral, smoked	Euphoria, drowsiness, respiratory depression, constricted pupils, nausea	Slow and shallow breathing, clammy skin, convulsions, coma, possible death	Watery eyes, runny nose, yawning, loss of appetite, irritability, tremors, panic, chills and sweating, cramps, nausea
Yes	3 to 6	Injected, smoked			
Yes	3 to 6	Oral, injected			
Yes	3 to 6	Injected, sniffed			
Yes	3 to 6	Oral, injected			
Yes	12 to 24	Oral, injected			
Yes	3 to 6	Oral, injected			
Probable	5 to 8	Oral	Slurred speech, disorientation, drunken behavior without odor of alcohol	Shallow respiration, cold and clammy skin, dilated pupils, weak and rapid pulse, coma, possible death	Anxiety, insomnia, tremors, delirium, convulsions, possible death
Yes	1 to 16	Oral, injected			
Yes	4 to 8	Oral			
Yes	4 to 8	Oral			
Yes	4 to 8	Oral			
Yes	4 to 8	Oral			
Yes	2	Injected, sniffed	Increased alertness, excitation, euphoria, dilated pupils, increased pulse rate and blood pressure, insomnia, loss of appetite	Agitation, increase in body temperature, hallucinations, convulsions, possible death	Apathy, long periods of sleep, irritability, depression, disorientation
Yes	2 to 4	Oral, injected			
Yes	2 to 4	Oral			
Yes	2 to 4	Oral			
Yes	2 to 4	Oral			
Yes	Variable	Oral	Illusions and hallucinations (with exception of MDA); poor perception of time and distance	Longer, more intense "trip" episodes, psychosis, possible death	Withdrawal syndrome not reported
Yes	Variable	Oral, injected			
Yes	Variable	Oral			
Yes	Variable	Oral, injected, sniffed			
Yes	Variable	Oral, injected, smoked			
Yes	Variable	Oral, injected, sniffed			
Yes	2 to 4	Oral, smoked	Euphoria, relaxed inhibitions, increased appetite, disoriented behavior	Fatigue, paranoia, possible psychosis	Insomnia, hyperactivity, and decreased appetite reported in a limited number of individuals

Narcotics Narcotics include opiates (opium and its derivatives) and synthetic narcotics (drugs chemically similar to opiates, but produced in a laboratory). Narcotics work by depressing specific parts of the body's central nervous system. Depending on which cells and areas of the brain are depressed, and to what extent, narcotics produce *analgesia* (relief of pain), their first and foremost medical use. A number of side effects often result from narcotics. These effects include sedation (freeing the mind of anxiety, relaxing the muscles, and calming the body), hypnosis (induction of sleep), and euphoria.

Narcotics are used in medicine primarily for their analgesic effect—that is, their ability to relieve pain. Administered in controlled dosages, they cause insensitivity to pain without producing loss of consciousness or even excessive drowsiness. Doctors generally use anesthetics or members of the hypnotic–sedative group when they want to anesthetize patients for operations. They never use narcotics alone for this purpose, because narcotics used in dosages large enough to produce sleep or stupor could depress the respiratory center sufficiently to cause death.

A physician administering a narcotic usually gives a subcutaneous injection. This method produces too slow an action for most addicts, who prefer to have an intravenous injection. Because of the more rapid distribution throughout the body, an intravenous injection or "mainline" gives the desired effect immediately.

Some narcotics users start out by taking the drug orally. They will switch to injections when they learn—usually by associating with other users—that injections are more efficient. Less of the drug is then needed to obtain the effect wanted. Also, the drug acts faster and its effect is more prolonged.

An individual abusing narcotics may develop a physical dependence on the drug. Tolerance to narcotics develops very quickly. When a person whose body has developed a tolerance is cut off from a supply of drugs, he or she develops a condition called *withdrawal illness* (in this case, *narcotic–solvent-type abstinence syndrome*).

Withdrawals are caused by the drug-tolerant cells trying to return to a nondrug, normal condition. The intensity and nature of withdrawal illness varies with the type and strength of narcotic abused. Methadone produces a very mild withdrawal when compared to opium and its derivatives (such as morphine and heroin). The latter produce withdrawals marked by irritability, depression, extreme nervousness, pain in the abdomen, and nausea—all to a severe degree. After withdrawal, if the person abstains from using narcotics, the body will readjust to a predrug normal condition and lose the tolerance that has developed. Now even a relatively small dose of a narcotic can constitute an overdose and cause death. Because of the relatively weak preparations of narcotics sold in the United States, many individuals use them intermittently for years without ever becoming addicted.

The following are the major narcotics abused throughout the world.

Opium Opium is the juice obtained from cutting the unripe capsule of the oriental poppy *(Papaver somniferum)*. This drug is generally smoked in an opium pipe or eaten. Because it is difficult to obtain, American drug abusers seldom use opium today, but there is a great abuse of its derivatives, morphine, heroin, and codeine, which are the most important narcotic substances obtainable from opium.

Morphine The major derivative of chemically refined opium is morphine. Morphine is the best analgesic available. It may be pure white, light brown, or off-white in color and comes in many forms: cubes, capsules, tablets, powder, or liquid solution.

Very little morphine is sold on the streets. Rather, morphine is used when heroin is not available and is usually stolen from doctors' offices or pharmacies. Morphine is also often obtained by forging prescription forms that have been stolen from physicians.

Heroin Heroin is produced from morphine. During this process the total amount of the drug is reduced in volume, which facilitates smuggling. This makes the heroin more potent per ounce than the morphine that went into the process. In studies carried out in England by Dr. J. H. Willis, nondrug users and drug users were unable to tell whether they were being given morphine or heroin. Heroin is able to enter the central nervous system more easily than morphine. Consequently, heroin seems to be a more potent drug. Pure heroin is a grayish-brown powder. Because of its strength and the economics of illegal drug traffic, heroin is diluted or adulterated ("stepped on" or "cut") many times before it is sold on the street. Usually heroin is cut with milk sugar (lactose), mannite (a substance derived from the ash tree and used as a mild laxative), procaine (a local anesthetic used by dentists), or quinine. Very often unsafe chemicals such as strychnine, LSD, phencyclidine (PCP, or Peace Pill, a horse tranquilizer), and amphetamines, are used to adulterate the heroin, because they will intensify the "kick." Street heroin ends up as a white, off-white, or brown ("Mexican" heroin) powder, usually containing no more than 1 to 4 percent pure heroin.

The main reason why laws controlling heroin have been unsuccessful is the tremendous amount of money made each year by the illegal sale of heroin in the United States. Heroin is a billion-dollar product on the streets. It passes through five or six levels of distribution before reaching the user. For example, one kilogram (2.2 pounds) of heroin can be purchased for $5,000 to $10,000 by someone who has a "connection" with the individuals preparing the heroin from morphine. This "importer" will have the heroin brought into the United States, have it diluted, and then sell it to a "wholesaler" for $18,000 to $20,000. The wholesaler dilutes it again, divides it into plastic bags containing about an ounce of cut heroin, and sells these to local "dealers" for about $700 a bag. The wholesaler obtains about $32,000 for his bags. The dealer dilutes it again and divides it into smaller portions called "pieces," "street ounces," or "vig ounces" (vig is a term used to describe the high interest charged by loan sharks). The street ounce is folded into squares of glassine paper ("papers"), put into clear or colored capsules ("caps"), or, most often, put into balloons folded to about the size of a fingertip (it is easier to transport and hide this way) and sold to the street "pusher." The dealer obtains about $70,000 for the batch. The pusher will now sell to the individual user at the street price, after cutting it again or removing some for personal use. This practice varies from time to time or from city to city. On the street the original one kilo of heroin can return $225,000. This single kilogram of heroin has produced $215,000 in profit.

Some individuals can use heroin off and on, on a nonregular basis, for years without becoming addicted. These individuals are called "joy poppers" or "chippies." Persons who use heroin regularly become addicted faster than users of any other narcotic. The body's tolerance to heroin builds up very rapidly. Thus, an addict requires increasingly larger doses to get the desired effect and to prevent entering withdrawal. (See the graph showing the results of an experiment in drug tolerance.)

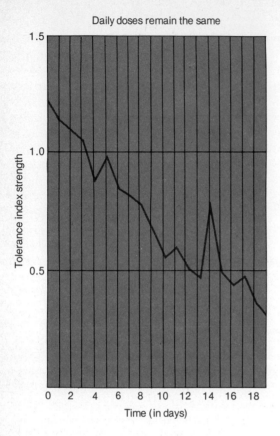

Daily doses remain the same

Tolerance index strength

1.5

1.0

0.5

0 2 4 6 8 10 12 14 16 18

Time (in days)

At the National Institute of Mental Health Addiction Research Center in Lexington, Kentucky, a group of individuals were given an equivalent dose of heroin every day for 19 days. The euphoric effects were measured each day during the 19 days and graphed as the Tolerance Line. The effects of the standard dose decreased, and by the 19th day were almost nonexistent—even though the same chemically measured amount of heroin was given on day 19 as on day 1. Heroin users respond to the development of tolerance by progressively increasing their dosages of heroin.

Adapted from W.R. Martin and H.F. Fraser, "A Comparative Study of Physiological and Subjective Effects of Heroin and Morphine Administered Intravenously in Postaddicts," Journal of Pharmacology and Experimental Therapeutics, 1961, p. 397. Copyright © 1961 by Williams and Wilkins Co., Baltimore, Maryland.

Codeine Codeine is a relatively mild narcotic. The pure product is a white crystal powder, which is sometimes taken in tablets for pain relief in combination with other ingredients (one such tablet is labeled "Empirin with Codeine"). Codeine is also widely used as an ingredient in liquid cough medicines.

Narcotics addicts sometimes resort to the use of codeine when deprived of their supply of stronger drugs, but codeine is not widely abused because it is too mild to give a "hard" narcotic user the high wanted. Still, codeine, especially that found in some cough medicines, is often abused by young people when they can obtain it. It is an addictive drug, particularly when used frequently in large amounts.

Synthetic Narcotics The synthetic narcotics differ from the opium derivatives and their compounds in that they are made synthetically in the chemical laboratory—not from opium, but from coal tar or petroleum products. Some of the more common synthetic compounds are marketed under the names Darvon, Percodan, Demerol, Perco-barb, Methadone, and Nalline. Their chemical properties resemble those of various opium derivatives; their narcotic effect (and addictive potential) varies. But all narcotics, including synthetic ones, are addictive.

Nonnarcotic Analgesic Substances
These substances are not psychoactive and do not produce drastic mood or behavior changes. Consequently, they are not in-

cluded on the chart showing the continuum of drug actions. Nonnarcotic analgesics are used medically to reduce mild pain and to lower fever. In some instances they are also used as very mild sedatives or anti-inflammatory agents. In this category are drugs that contain aspirin (the popular name for acetylsalicylic acid), phenacetin (acetophenetidin), and Tylenol (acetaminophen).

Volatile Solvents   The practice of inhaling vapors of volatile chemicals, chemicals that evaporate readily at room temperature, is also a major concern of society. The solvents in plastic or model-airplane cement are volatile chemicals and are often inhaled for their mood-modifying effects. These effects are primarily feelings of pleasantness, cheerfulness, euphoria, and excitement—feelings that closely simulate the early stages of alcohol excitement. As a person inhales more, he begins to appear "drunk," exhibiting disorientation and speaking in a slurred manner. Such behavior may continue for 30 to 45 minutes, followed by drowsiness, stupor, or unconsciousness. Unconsciousness may last for as long as an hour. If the person has inhaled too much glue vapor, or if exposure to the vapors has been prolonged, the person may die.

Several toxic solvents are used in the manufacture of airplane cements. Common to many brands are isoamyl acetate and ethyl acetate. Other toxic solvents used in many products include benzene, toluene, and carbon tetrachloride. High concentrations of these solvents may be found in cleaning fluids, paints, and paint thinners. Also, the hydrocarbons in gasoline (such as butane, hexane, and pentane) may cause solvent intoxication when inhaled. Prolonged inhalation of the fumes of any of these fluids may cause death. Labels on many types of solvents and gasoline include the warning "Use only in a well-ventilated, open area."

Tolerance to solvents develops rapidly, and the user soon must inhale the vapors from the contents of several tubes of cement to experience the effects desired.

The toxic effects of solvents have been carefully observed. They include irritation of the mucous membranes, the skin, and the respiratory tract; alternate excitation and depression of the central nervous system; cellular injury in the heart, liver, and kidneys; alteration of bone marrow activity, which results in anemia (reduction in red blood cells), and leucopenia (reduction in platelets in the blood). There have also been reports of brain tissue deterioration, acute liver damage, and death from kidney failure.

In their quest to find volatile chemicals that have mood-modifying effects, some young people have tried to "sniff" anything that is in a pressurized can—from hair spray to the Freon gas used in refrigerators. Most of these spray cans either displace the oxygen in the air or coat the lungs with resins when "sniffed" in a closed area and have caused the deaths of hundreds of young people.

Hypnotic-Sedative Drugs   Each drug in this group has the ability to depress the central nervous system into a condition resembling sleep. The difference between a hypnotic and a sedative is one of degree of depression. A hypnotic drug, given in a moderate or even a small dose, will produce sleep soon after it is given. Such reduced dosages of sedative drugs, even when administered several times a day, will calm a person without producing sleep. With increasing dosages, all of the drugs in this group produce a continuum of effects from tranquilization to sedation (the allaying of excitement), to the loss of psychomotor efficiency, to sleep, and then to coma and death.

For thousands of years the only hypnotic drugs known were alcohol, opium (actually now classified as a narcotic), and belladonna (a drug extracted from *Atropa belladonna,* or "deadly nightshade," a plant found in Europe and Asia).

Alcohol and Alcohol Derivatives

The oldest hypnotic-sedative drug used in medicine is alcohol. Derivatives of alcohol have been used as hypnotics and sedatives for many years. The first alcohol derivative was *chloral hydrate,* developed in 1869; next was paraldehyde, introduced in 1882.

Occasionally these drugs are used to control patients who are hospitalized with delirium tremens, withdrawal illness, and convulsions. But their use decreases yearly, and they have been replaced largely by the barbiturates.

Barbiturates The barbiturates were first used in the United States as hypnotic-sedatives in the form of barbitol, developed in 1903. Since that time, many new barbiturate compounds have been produced and put on the market. Doctors prescribe them mainly to help patients sleep. On the illegal market, barbiturates are known as "sleeping pills," "goofballs," "reds" (because of the usual capsule color), "downers," or "stumblers."

Barbiturates produce a surprisingly variable effect in the brain and nervous system of the person who uses them. After taking these drugs, many users undergo a variable period of hyperactivity and excitement. Then, as the drug depresses their central nervous system, they become relaxed, euphoric, and sleepy. But a user may take a dose of barbiturates at bedtime and discover that they have no sedative or hypnotic effect at all because the period of hyperactivity and excitement has lasted throughout the night and no sedative or hypnotic effect ever took place. For some users, certain barbiturates produce a "truth serum" effect in which long-forgotten events are remembered. With abusive dosages, drastic and sudden mood changes may occur. Users are often described as friendly one minute, and mean the next, much as with another sedative drug—alcohol (see chapter 6).

Barbiturates are addictive drugs when abused. Tolerance develops quickly and physical dependence eventually develops when large abusive dosages are used over a prolonged period of time. Barbiturates are usually taken orally ("dropped"): however, users can dissolve the compound and inject it with a hypodermic needle, but it is very destructive to tissue when injected. Sometimes the capsules are dropped in combination with a stimulant such as Benzedrine, Dexedrine, or Methedrine. This combination overcomes the depressing effects of the barbiturates and extends the excitement and euphoria. The use of a stimulant drug to antagonize the depressant effect of a barbiturate is extremely dangerous. The cardio-circulatory system cannot take drastic "ups" and "downs" which may end in a *stroke* or *heart attack.*

A very risky practice indulged in by some persons who abuse barbiturates is combining them with alcohol. Because the barbiturates interfere with the body's normal disposal of alcohol through the liver, the two drugs taken together have a total depressant effect far greater than the sum of their individual effects. Often, an overdose of either drug is taken unknowingly; the person is "too drunk" or "too doped up" to realize what he or she is doing. Because of this confused state, it is difficult to tell whether a fatal drug overdose was suicide or accidental. The use of alcohol and barbiturates in combination, even in small amounts, is extremely dangerous and often results in death.

Since both are hypnotic-sedative drugs,

the effects of barbiturates and alcohol are very similar. A small amount of barbiturates makes the user feel relaxed, sociable, and good-humored, but less alert than normally. After taking more of the drug, the user becomes sluggish, gloomy, and quarrelsome. The tongue becomes "thick," and the user gradually falls into a deep sleep. If a large amount of the drug has been taken, especially in combination with alcohol, the deep sleep may progress into a coma. At this point, only prompt medical attention can save the person's life. Such attention has saved the lives of people who showed no sign of life after lapsing into a barbiturate-induced coma.

The effects of barbiturates and alcohol are similar, but barbiturates are by far the more potentially lethal drug. An excess of alcohol may be vomited up, but barbiturates are seldom vomited up. Intead, all of the drug taken into the stomach will be absorbed unless the stomach is pumped. On the other hand, a large amount of alcohol consumed at one time (such as a fifth of whiskey), if unvomited and retained by the stomach, car cause almost instantaneous death.

The chronic user of barbiturates, who takes the drug for either its exciting and euphoric effects or to sleep at night, eventually finds that the dosage must be increased in order for the drug to be effective and to keep from going into withdrawal. Without a regular, daily dose, an addicted individual will experience *alcohol-barbiturate abstinence syndrome*. This includes hallucinations, mild-to-severe *delirium tremens*, and convulsive seizures that resemble *grand mal* epileptic convulsions. Often these are severe enough to cause death. Alcohol-barbiturate withdrawal is far more serious than narcotic-solvent withdrawal. A physician treating someone in barbiturate withdrawal must know the name of the drug (or combination of drugs) the individual was using.

Sedative Anestheticlike Drugs These substances are highly psychoactive and produce an extremely wide range of actions, many of which are similar to the barbiturates. Often, they depress the central nervous system as much as an anesthetic would. Because of their marked, varying effects, it is difficult to place them into standard depressant categories. Thus, the authors have not attempted to place the varied group of individual drugs on the continuum of drug actions.

The most commonly abused of this group is Methaqualone. Heavy, continued use of Methaqualone produces tolerance and physical dependence. Abrupt withdrawal produces severe alcohol-barbiturate abstinence syndrome.

In street use, Methaqualone is claimed to be an aphrodisiac or "love-enhancing" drug. This is because the sedation causes users to feel relaxed, friendly, receptive, and uninhibited. But in reality it actually lowers the ability to perform sexually. In the United States, it is marketed as Quaalude, Sopor, Parest, Optimil, and Somnafax; in England, combined with an antihistamine, it is called Mandrax. Street names are derived from brand names: "Quallude," "Quas," "Quads," "Luding," "Sopors," "Soapers," or "Mandrakes."

Other psychoactive substances in this group that have been abused, when locally available, include: Noludar (Methyprylon), Ethchlorvynol (Placidyl), and Glutethimide (Doriden or "ciba"). All produce physical dependence (addiction); are potent hypnotic-sedative depressants; and are extremely dangerous—especially when taken with alcoholic beverages. All have been totally misused.

Tranquilizers Tranquilizing drugs prevent or relieve uncomfortable emotional feelings. They relieve tension and apprehension and promote a state of calm and relaxation. Dramatic effects in calming violent, overactive, psychotic individuals take place.

In the early 1950s, the term *minor tranquilizers* was introduced to distinguish the ones that reduce anxiety, tension, and agitation from the *major tranquilizers*, which are used in the control of violent, overactive psychotics (mental patients).

Major Tranquilizers   These drugs do not cure mental illnesses, but they are extremely important in making mental patients easier to manage and control. These drugs are true mood-modifiers. They modify the moods and alleviate many of the symptoms of mental-illness. Major tranquilizers are in reality "antipsychotic" drugs, reversing the processes of mental illness in specific groups of individuals. They are not abused to any extent because of their mild actions in all but this one group.

Minor Tranquilizers   These drugs are the most widely used prescription drugs in the United States. At present, there are more minor tranquilizers sold than sleeping pills, amphetamines, and narcotics put together.

Meprobamate, synthesized in 1950, was the first minor tranquilizer. Today, under its own name, and the trade names Miltown, Equanil, Kesso-Bamate, Meprospan, and SK-Damate, over 250 tons are sold each year. Other frequently used minor tranquilizers are Librium or Librax (chlordiazepoxide), and Valium or Diazepam. Medically, these drugs are used to relieve tension, anxiety, behavioral excitement, and insomnia, as well as during acute periods of depression (as after the death of someone close, divorce, and so on).

After repeated use, tolerance develops and dosages must be increased to obtain desired results. But no tolerance to a potentially lethal dosage (amount needed to kill) develops. Care must therefore be taken because only a limited quantity of these drugs can be taken safely. There is heavy nonmedical abuse of tranquilizers. Alcoholics use them along with sedatives to prolong intoxication. Narcotics addicts often take large quantities to increase their kick. Librium and Valium have been shown to cause physical dependence when taken in large dosages over periods longer than six months. Also, withdrawal is very similar to that from barbiturates and alcohol (convulsions, abdominal and muscular cramps, vomiting, and sweating). Most of the others are believed to lead to dependence. However, it is difficult to substantiate physical dependence among users of minor tranquilizers because of a large number of variables: differences in individual psychology, emotional disposition, and the time of day the drug is used. Abuse by the general public is becoming so wide-spread that the American Medical Association has warned doctors about overprescribing and allowing prolonged unsupervised use. As of July 1, 1975, the Drug Enforcement Administration moved minor tranquilizers from a Class IV to a Class III controlled drug in the federal Controlled Substances Act (see chapter 5).

The Cannabis Drug Family   Tetrahydrocannabinol (THC) is the psychoactive substance obtained from the common hemp plant (*Cannabis sativa*), grown throughout the world. The plant is grown extensively in Jamaica, Mexico, Columbia, Africa, India, and the Middle East. Most botanists consider all hemp plants to belong to a single species with many varieties. The leaves and flowering tops of the plant contain an amber-colored resin, a mixture of many chemicals, one of which is tetrahydrocannabinol (THC). The potency of the intoxicating drugs produced from the Cannabis plant varies widely, depending on which plant variety, which

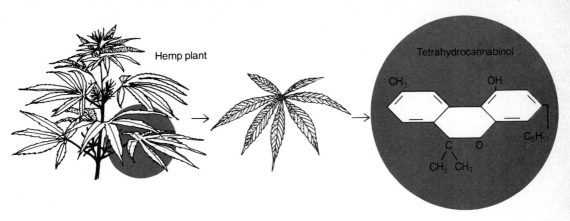

Hemp plant

Tetrahydrocannabinol

Most drugs produced by plants can be obtained only through some form of extraction technique. Marijuana plants are picked and processed. The potency depends on the available concentration of the active agent, tetrahydrocannabinol (THC).

part (stems, roots, and seeds do not contain tetrahydrocannabinol), method of preparation, and storage used.

This drug family, more than any other, cannot be described accurately without specifying dosage levels. *Marijuana*, a popular name for the plant itself, is the drug prepared by drying the leaves and flowering tops of the plant to make a tobaccolike material. Marijuana as used in the United States is probably the weakest preparation of the plant used in the world. Plants grown in the United States and northern Mexico are low in THC, containing between 0.2 and 2.0 percent. Marijuana from southern Mexico, often called "Acapulco Gold," and from southeast Asia (called "Vietnam Green"), may contain between 2 to 4 percent THC. "Panama Red" grown around the Canal Zone and surrounding islands, including Jamaica, may have a THC content of 4 to 8 percent. *Ganja*, a preparation containing only flowering tops and the small leaves or bracts, may contain 8 percent or more THC if it comes from the Jamaican area. The most potent preparation of cannabis is *charas* (prepared mainly in India) or *hashish*. Charas is the pure tetrahydrocan-

nabinol resin obtained from the dried flowers of *Cannabis indica* (a specific variety of cannabis). Hashish, as the term is used correctly, is a powdered and sifted form of charas. It is a chalky brown or black substance. Hash generally contains 12 to 20 percent THC.

Marijuana has been illegally imported into the United States for decades. In 1974, marijuana sales in the United States were estimated to be over five billion dollars. Hashish or "hash" and "hash oil" extracts are being illegally imported and sold in the United States. The most potent extract of THC is delta-9-tetrahydrocannabinol, delta-9-THC. Another form, delta-3-tetrahydrocannabinol (delta-3-THC) has been produced synthetically. It was found to be far less potent than the naturally occurring mixture of tetrahydrocannabinols, but most users do not know this, and they try to buy pure THC on the street. THC is difficult to manufacture and costs at least $50.00 per dose to manufacture. Consequently, the white powder "THC" being sold on the street for about $2.50 a capsule is not actually THC. When tested, the street THC has been found to be a combination of substitute psychoactive substances (methamphetamine, mescaline, LSD, or some cocaine). Most often the material is PCP (phencyclidine, a "horse" sedative, or anesthetic, often called the "peace pill"). PCP is very dangerous and will be discussed further on in this section. None of the liquid forms of THC is pure and often what is sold as liquid THC is a broad mixture of unknown chemicals that could be very dangerous.

The different forms of cannabinol can be used in many ways. While marijuana and hashish are usually smoked, they are also baked into foods or added to drinks. Taken in large, strong doses, the cannabis drug family bears many similarities to the hallucinogenic drugs, such as LSD. This is why, for the last few years, it has been classified as an *hallucinogenic drug* and will continue to be classified as such by many experts. The effects from a low dose or "social" use of marijuana are quite different and tend to approximate mild intoxication with some reactions similar to those produced by alcohol. Because of these

findings, and recent research on and reports of the effects of cannabinol drugs (*National Institute on Drug Abuse* report to Congress in 1974, *Eastland Report* to Congress in 1974, and Vera D. Rubius' *Ganja in Jamaica,* published by Mouton in the Hague, Netherlands, 1975), the authors feel it should be given a classification distinct from all other drug families. The cannabis drug family has been placed across the "neutral area" of the drug continuum because of its wide range of actions and effects depending on the form of the drug used (marijuana to hashish), the amount used at one time, and the many "variables" (such as emotional state, "set," "setting," personality, and social factors) that affect the individual's response to tetrahydrocannabinol. Depending on these factors cannabis intoxication can be similar to either hallucinogens (stimulants) or sedatives, such as alcohol (depressants).

The mood-modifying effects of cannabinol derivatives can only be described in terms of some important variables, of

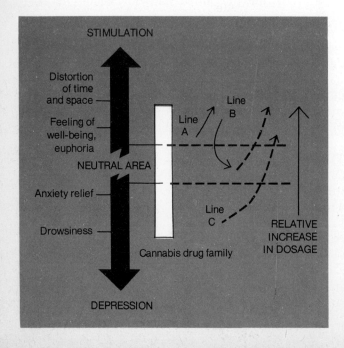

This continuum of drug effects and actions shows the diverse effects when consuming cannabis drugs. The three lines (A, B, and C) account for the varied reactions to cannabis drugs because of potency, "set," "setting," and amount consumed at one time. (A) Line A represents the direct stimulation experienced when using potent forms of cannabis (such as hashish) or consuming a large number of marijuana cigarettes at one time. (B) Line B follows the apparent depression and relaxation produced by 2 or 3 (social dosage) cigarettes when consumed by an individual who is already stimulated, excited (set), or is in a stimulating setting (rock music, strobe lights, etc). Broken section of line B shows the stimulation which occurs as the individual consumes more than a social dosage. (C) Line C represents the direct stimulation any amount of cannabis will produce in an individual who is relaxed, depressed, or in a relaxed setting while consuming the drug.

which dosage is the most important. As shown in the preceding graph (line A), if an individual uses a potent form (such as hashish) or consumes a large amount (a number of marijuana cigarettes) the physical and emotional effects will continue to go toward the stimulant end of the continuum of drug actions. If a lower dosage is consumed (part of a cigarette to one or two cigarettes), often termed a "social dose," or "recreational dose," the reactions of the individual are more closely tied to the emotional and social variables present. As shown in the graph by line B, if the individual is stimulated, or in a stimulating environment (music, colored lights), the reaction will be a slight depression causing him to relax and enjoy the situation. But continuing to consume the drug at this time will cause the emotional reactions of the individual to progress up the continuum of drug actions toward the stimulating effects of the increased dosage (hallucinations, feelings of depersonalization). Also, as shown by line C, if the individual is depressed at the beginning of the evening, there will be feelings of stimulation with any intake of marijuana. This ability to control an individual's emotional reactions to his environment, the ability to change moods only slightly, are the major reasons marijuana is used in a social or recreational context.

Hashish Individuals using potent extracts from cannabis plants experience distortions of auditory and visual perception, hallucinations, and a sense of depersonalization similar to that occurring with the use of LSD. Tolerance does develop when high dosages are used over prolonged periods, but there is no cross-tolerance (tolerance to one drug group affecting the effectiveness of another drug group) with any of the hallucinogenic drugs such as LSD or mescaline. The effects of even large dosages of hashish are milder and more easily controlled than with hallucinogens. The differing "trips" or "highs" of the two classes of drugs are readily distinguishable by users; hashish users, even at high dosages, lack the major anxiety, panic, and stress reactions found in hallucinogen users. Since most hashish is actually powdered or liquid, the method of use becomes important. Smoking and inhalation cause rapid absorption into the bloodstream, but a certain amount is lost into the air and does not reach the lungs. Oral ingestion diminishes the effects of the drug, but prolongs its actions. Hashish capsules "dropped" and absorbed through the intestinal tract may cause a trip to last as long as 6 to 8 hours.

Marijuana Marijuana is usually rolled into cigarettes and smoked. It cannot be confused with tobacco, being green rather than brown and having a different (alfalfa or tealike) smell. These cigarettes, "joints," burn hotter than do cigarettes made of tobacco, and the burning tip is brighter. Also, the lighted tip of a marijuana cigarette will go out easily unless an effort is made to keep it lit.

A number of variable factors exert an important influence upon an individual's feelings and state of consciousness while using marijuana. The amount consumed is the most important variable. As with most psychoactive drugs, the larger the dose, the greater the physical and mental effects and the longer the effects will last. The effects of the usual low "social" dosage, a moderate dosage, and a high dosage will be explained.

As mentioned previously, the *method of use* is important. Important variables in the individual's response to marijuana are the emotional environment ("set") and physical environment or "setting" in which the experience takes place. The emotional environment—personality, life-style, philosophy, past drug experiences, mood at the time of drug use, and expectations of drug effects—is very important in determining the type and degree of response an individual will experience from a social dosage. These factors and the social setting—alone, with friends, at a party, or at a large event (such as a rock concert)—greatly account for the belief of marijuana users that they are experiencing a "high" even when using a nonmarijuana substance (called a placebo) presented as marijuana. Tolerance is also important in low-dosage marijuana usage. There is little evidence that a tolerance develops, although it has been shown that with time and repeated consumption, the original level of satisfaction (or high) may last for a shorter period of time. The phenomenon of reverse tolerance has been observed; that is, the individual requires smaller doses to achieve the same high. Perhaps such reverse tolerance is related to one's *set*, especially the expectations of drug effects, and is actually the result of learning to get high and learning to recognize the more subtle mood changes taking place at low dosages.

A person's reactions to marijuana are highly individualistic, and probably the closest analogy is the experience of daydreaming or the parade of passing thoughts, ideas, or feelings just prior to falling asleep. These effects are not constant and tend to be cyclic, periodically increasing and decreasing in intensity. At low *social doses*, the marijuana user experiences an increased sense of wellbeing, some early restlessness and hilarity, followed by a dreamy, carefree relaxation (see line B on chart). Sensory perception is altered. There is an expansion and exaggeration of time and space relationships, cracks may look like rivers, and brief incidents may seem to take hours. The senses are heightened, intensifying smells, tastes, sounds, and sights. There are very subtle changes in thought formation and expression that often seem unusual to the un-

knowing observer. The individual finishes the experience, comes down feeling hungry, especially for sweets, often called "the munchies." To an unknowing observer, a person under the influence of this dosage of marijuana would not appear noticeably different from normal.

At moderate dosages, the physical and emotional reactions are intensified, but the intoxication of the individual would still be scarcely noticeable to an observer. At these higher levels of use, an individual may experience rapidly changing emotions, changing sensory reactions, lapses of attentiveness, altered thought formation, fragmented thoughts and sentences, flights of ideas, impaired short-term memory, inability to associate ideas and physical senses, and an altered sense of self-identity. Some perceive an internal feeling of great insight.

At very high dosages, the marijuana experience closely resembles the "psychotomimetic" (or psychosis-mimicking) reactions of the hallucinogenic drugs (such as LSD). These include distortions of body image, loss of personal identity (depersonalization), sensory and mental illusions, fantasies, and hallucinations. Nearly all individuals who continue to use cannabis after experiencing these effects describe them as pleasurable. However, consistently unpleasant reactions may discourage further use.

When high dosages of cannabis (marijuana or hashish) are used over a long period, *compulsive cannabis use* can develop. The compulsive, chronic use of cannabis is the same as the compulsive, chronic use of any psychoactive drug. The individual has a preoccupation, and an abnormal desire for the effects of the drug being abused. An individual may recognize the beginnings of a *compulsive use pattern* and a preoccupation with marijuana (or hashish) by experiencing vague feelings that something is wrong and that they are functioning at a reduced level of efficiency. This is called "dropping out" or "dropping down." Individuals feel a loss of desire to work, to compete, to face challenges. Interests and major concerns become centered around marijuana. They may drop out of school, leave work, or ignore personal hygiene. The results of this reduced efficiency has been termed the "amotivational syndrome."

Controlled research studies to expand the available knowledge concerning marijuana are currently in progress. As time passes, additional information will become available to provide a more complete picture of the implications of cannabis use at various dosages and patterns of use.

Hallucinogenic Compounds Hallucinogens are drugs that create vivid distortions of the senses without greatly disturbing the individual's consciousness. Such distortions (hallucinations) may cause persons to see, hear, or smell things that are not really there. Or, they may view the world much differently from the way it really is (or from the way they usually view it). Persons who abuse the hallucinogens may share with individuals who are mentally ill a tendency to experience hallucinations when they do not want to or when they are no longer under the influence of a drug. This is why some hallucinogens have been termed psychotomimetic (psychosis-mimicking) or psychotogenic (psychosis-producing) drugs. Such drugs, some authorities feel, are capable of temporarily turning a normal person into a psychotic. Users have often been hospitalized to prevent them from doing harm to themselves or others during what seems to be such a temporary psychosis.

During recent years, psychiatrists have been increasingly interested in hallucinogenic drugs. Some have taken doses of these compounds themselves in order to experience something of what their severely ill psychiatric patients must feel. Other researchers, influenced by colleagues who have defined these hallucinogenic drugs as "psychedelic," "mind-realizing," or "mind-expanding," have tried using them in an attempt to gain insight into their own minds. These drugs have also been given to alcoholics and other emotionally disturbed patients as part of therapeutic treatment. The results of these experiments have been contradictory, and in general they have not borne out the expectations of the investigators.

A large number of people acquire these drugs illegally and take them without medical supervision, sometimes while participating in group experiences. Occasionally a severe psychotic reaction or a prolonged delirious reaction follows the use of hallucinogens. Psychiatrists report that they are frequently called upon to give emergency help to persons who are suffering "bad trips" ("bummers") from these drugs. For its own protection, society has become involved in legislation against the abuse of all psychotogenic compounds.

Mescaline Mescaline is named after the Mescalero Apaches, who developed a cult that involved using the drug in religious rituals. Mescaline is found in the small buttonlike cactus plant called *peyote*. This plant grows naturally in the watershed of the Rio Grande. Indian tribes in the southwestern United States chew the cactus in order to experience hallucinatory states as part of religious ceremonies. Considerable controversy developed several years ago over whether the United States government should, or should not, permit such drug use. At present, the government feels that the constitutionally defined right of freedom of religion would be withheld if these Indians were forbidden use of peyote in religious ceremonies.

The buttonlike peyote plants are usually dried and then chewed. Sometimes they are boiled in water to make a broth. The effect of mescaline involves hallucinations and euphoria lasting for a period of between 8 hours and 2 days. These hallucinations may include the appearance of fantastic geometric patterns, distortions in the sense of time and space, and feelings of depersonalization.

Peyote itself is by no means convenient to use, a fact that limits its illicit use among persons who seek psychedelic experiences. The texture of the buttons is extremely unpleasant, and the juice from them is sickening. Persons who use peyote, even Indians experienced in its use, can expect to vomit several times while taking the drug. Besides an upset stomach, peyote causes sweating, elevated blood pressure, increased pulse rates, and muscle twitching. Pure mescaline, which is extracted from peyote buttons, is available on the illegal market in capsule form. The caps, of course, are much easier to take, although some users experience slight nausea at the beginning of their trip. Neither mescaline caps nor peyote buttons are physically addictive.

LSD LSD, commonly referred to by users as "acid," is a tasteless, colorless, and odorless drug derived from lysergic acid diethylamide. The primary danger in taking LSD is that it may cause temporary psychosis, accompanied by a wide range of behavioral disturbances. Some users experience panic or depression, while others feel euphoria and a sense of great mental clarity or comprehension. Visual hallucinations are commonly experienced.

An LSD trip lasts 8 to 16 hours. Afterward, users who have enjoyed their trip may describe a feeling of having been reborn, of having seen the world for the first time. This feeling is often accompanied by a sense of deep affection for others, particularly those who were present and participating in the trip.

LSD is the most potent of the hallucinogens. Doses of LSD are measured in micrograms; an average dose can be anywhere from 150 to 250 micrograms. This means that there are about 300,000 trips in one ounce of LSD. A user taking much larger doses may experience delirium and convulsions. After any dose, "flashbacks" may occur; that is, the psychotic effects of the drug may recur from time to time a year or more after the trip. In recent years the individual street use of LSD has decreased tremendously. But the use of LSD is as prevalent as in the past. It is now being used in ritualistic groups, "cults," or associated with "mystic" experiences. In these situations, the individual is prepared for the experience, and the group is supportive while on the trip, reducing the number of bad trips and tragic experiences that were associated with LSD in the past.

LSD dilates the pupils of the eyes, raises the blood pressure, stimulates the brain's sensory centers, and blocks off its inhibiting mechanisms. It intensifies hearing, increases the ability to differentiate among textures, and may produce a tingling sensation and numbness of the hands and feet. Subjects often report crossovers of sensation; for example, they may seem to hear colors or smell the scent of music (an experience known as *synesthesia*).

A user of LSD may experience minor physical discomfort, including nausea and abdominal pain. The possibility of much more serious, long-term effects of LSD has been reported, such as deformities among children born to women who took LSD while pregnant.

Cocaine Cocaine is extracted from the flowering branches of a shrub or small tree, the coca plant (*Erythroxylon coca*), which grows to heights of 12 or 15 feet and is found in Peru and Bolivia. Medically, cocaine is used as a local anesthetic to relieve or prevent pain at a particular area of the body. When applied to the surface of the skin, or injected subcutaneously, it blocks transmission of pain and touch sensations rapidly and completely. Because of its dangerous side effects cocaine has been replaced by synthetic local anesthetics such as: procaine (novocaine), lidocaine (Xylocaine), Butacaine (Butyn), and benzocaine (ethyl aminobenzoate).

This is the only depressant effect of cocaine—when it is used as a local anethetic. Its general effect on the body is to stimulate, alter mood and behavior, and induce excitement. Cocaine is the most powerful natural stimulant known. Neither physical tolerance nor other tolerance develops, but cocaine produces a very strong psychological dependence.

Cocaine, or "coke," is processed into an odorless, white, fluffy, fine crystalline powder, often referred to as "snow" because of its appearance. It is sold in the same types of containers as heroin. Cocaine is called the rich man's drug because of its high price. It currently sells for $50 to $60 per gram or about $1,600 per ounce. Because it is so profitable, cocaine is often cut with the other local anesthetics such as procaine, lidocaine, and benzocaine.

Cocaine users usually sniff the drug into their nostrils. A few users take the drug by hypodermic injection. Sniffing is the more popular method but it is highly destructive to the tissues lining the nose and respiratory tract because the drug is absorbed slowly through the membranes of the nose. When sniffed, its effects last longer and are less violent than when it is injected. Advanced narcotic addicts may mix cocaine and heroin together. This combined injection is called a "speedball."

Cocaine can cause death by two distinct routes. In some people, a relatively small dose can cause complete circulatory collapse and instant death from heart failure. There is no way to tell which individuals will react in this manner. The other route is indicated by the increased dosage on the chart showing the continuum of drug effects. As the dosage is increased the euphoria, laughter, restlessness, and excitement are replaced by anxiety, depression, headache, confusion, dizziness, fainting, and death by respiratory failure. These signs of an overdose in any individual require immediate medical care.

Unclassified Stimulant Drugs These are varying groups of drugs that act on the central nervous system as stimulants or hallucinogens; in some cases they also possess depressant, tranquilizing, and anesthetic qualities. Some of these drugs are naturally occurring, while most are synthetics (with new ones being produced every year).

The most widely abused of this group is phencyclidine (or Sernyl), which has been variously called PCP, "hog," "angel dust," or "the peace pill." It was first produced in the 1950s and is medically used as an animal tranquilizer, sedative, and anesthetic. Its effects are related to the dosage taken. PCP is chemically related to depressants, but at abuse dosages an individual experiences hallucinations and feelings of apathy and isolation. When used by someone who normally feels apathetic and socially or emotionally isolated, PCP can precipitate a psychotic problem. Because of the wide range of psychoactive effects, PCP has been sold on the illegal market as nearly every psychoactive drug abused (LSD, hashish, THC, and so on). PCP is never prescribed for humans because the range between an effective dosage and a lethal dosage is too narrow.

Psilocybin and Psilocyn are hallucinogens obtained from certain mushrooms grown primarily in Mexico. DOM (or STP) is one of a series of psychoactive substances that produce the effects of amphetamines while also producing hallucinations. DMT (or DET) is found in seeds of certain plants. In the West Indies and South America, the pulverized seeds have been used for centuries to produce "a state of mind enabling man to communicate with God." MDA and MMDA are between hallucinogens and amphetamines. They produce serenity and an exaggerated sense of wellbeing. Premoline (Cylert), in abusive dosages, produce a wide range of stimulant effects. Preludin (Phenmetrazine) is used in place of amphetamines as an appetite suppressant, but it produces a wide range of effects characteristic of amphetamines. Jimson weed (*Datura stramonium*) or Jamestown weed is actually a group of plants, found worldwide, that contain a number of psychoactive substances capable of producing a wide range of stimulant effects.

Amphetamines Included in the stimulant group are a large number of drugs that mimic the actions of adrenalin. In general, the physical reactions they produce are an increase in heart rate, a constriction of certain blood vessels, an increase in the breathing rate, an increase in perspiration, and a cottonlike dryness of the mouth. These side reactions are always combined with the primary actions of amphetamines on the brain—an increase in bodily activity and an elevation of mood. Feelings and behavior aroused by amphetamines include increased confidence, euphoria, fearlessness, talkativeness, impulsive behavior, loss of appetite, and a decrease of fatigue.

In 1970, the Food and Drug Administration (Drug Enforcement Administration) limited the legal use of amphetamines to three types of conditions: narcolepsy, hyperkinetic behavior (as observed in hyperactive children), and short-term weight-reducing programs.

Narcolepsy is a very rare disorder in which an individual has sudden, uncontrollable desires for sleep, often as many as a hundred times a day. Amphetamines block these patterns and keep the individual awake.

Hyperkinetic or *hyperactive* children have an unusually short attention span, are unable to sit still, and in spite of normal or superior intelligence are frequently underachievers in school. Amphetamines have the paradoxical effect in such children of acting as a tranquilizer, increasing attention span, and decreasing hyperactive behavior. Considerable controversy has been focused on drug treatment for hyperactivity. Methylphenidate (Ritalin) is similar to amphetamines but less potent. It has also been used in the treatment of hyperkinesis (and narcolepsy) and many feel it is superior to amphetamines because of its lower potency. In recent studies, *caffeine* has been found to be as effective as amphetamines (and Ritalin) in treating hyperkinesis. The symptoms of some hyperactive children have been relieved by keeping them from eating foods that contain artificial sweeteners and flavorings (see chapter 8).

Amphetamines have been used for years for appetite control because they suppress hunger. There are two dangers in prolonged use of amphetamines for weight control. First, tolerance to the appetite suppressant characteristics of the drug develops very quickly. Even moderate dosages lose their ability to control appetite within 4 to 6 weeks. Second, overeating is a behavior problem, just like drug abuse, and is primarily controlled by psychological factors, not by the physiology of the body. Consequently, amphetamines reinforce the dependent behavior of the individual, simply transferring it from food to the drug.

The amphetamines used for weight reduction are the most widely abused. Dexedrine and Benzedrine are prescribed for this purpose and on the illegal market they are known as "bennies," "dexies," "pep pills," or "whites" (because Benzedrine is often sold as a white tablet) or as "uppers" or "leapers" because of the mood elevation (see illustration). Several drug companies, without showing substantial evidence, make claims that their particular compound suppresses the appetite without causing central nervous system stimulation. No amphetamine or amphetaminelike compound has only one of these two effects on the body. Consequently, the usual circumstance is that while users lose weight, they also lose sleep.

Many individuals occasionally take small dosages of amphetamines orally to reduce fatigue, elevate mood, and produce prolonged wakefulness while doing an unpleasant task, to help recover from an alcoholic hangover, or just to "get high."

Actually, most chronic (compulsive) pep-pill users use a desire for weight loss as an excuse for taking these drugs and as a means for obtaining the drugs. These individuals obtain amphetamine pills from doctors for weight control, but take them 3 or 4 times a day in excess of the prescribed dose, for the stimulation and euphoria produced by the drug. These people develop a strong psychological dependence on the pills and feel that they cannot get along without them. If an individual stops taking daily amphetamines, withdrawal depression occurs. Renewed pill use stops the depression. Consequently, the drug dependence becomes very difficult to break, and many individuals increase their daily intake of amphetamines and begin to take sleeping pills (barbiturates) or alcohol

to relieve the insomnia that develops. This "upper–downer" cycle is especially dangerous because it greatly increases the probability of overdose.

There are several ways in which these drugs can cause physical damage when they are used over long periods of time. The mechanism in the liver that activates amphetamines is destroyed or impaired quite quickly. Therefore, users have to increase dosage levels continually to maintain the desired effectiveness. Prolonged use of increasing dosages causes long periods of sleep loss and mood and behavior changes, which may develop into a severe mental disorder or psychosis. The people suffering from this mental illness are usually characterized by extreme activity for long periods of time, feelings of superiority, bizarre forms of suspiciousness, hallucinations, and excitement—all to an exaggerated degree. Those that suddenly stop using amphetamines (often because these drugs have stopped being effective) usually go through a rather prolonged period of lethargy, depression, nightmares, and restlessness.

Young people particularly are abusing amphetamines for the mood-modifying qualities of these drugs. They frequently mix these drugs with either alcohol or barbiturates. Such abuse is extremely dangerous. It can cause death or lead to impulsive acts of poor judgment and to accidents. Especially abused is the amphetamine compound Methedrine (methamphetamine hydrochloride), commonly called "speed" or "meth." Some people swallow Methedrine pills, but the majority inject the compound into a muscle ("skin pop") or vein ("mainline") to get a quick euphoric flash or rush. With continued injections, they will stay awake for days and eat very little, until their bodies become completely exhausted ("strung out"). Then the worst part of a speed cycle be-

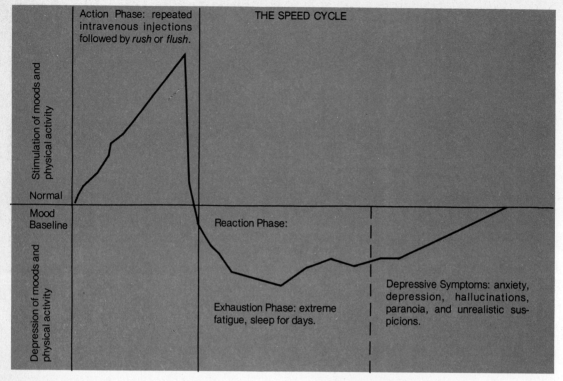

Action Phase: repeated intravenous injections followed by *rush* or *flush*.

THE SPEED CYCLE

Stimulation of moods and physical activity

Normal

Mood Baseline

Depression of moods and physical activity

Reaction Phase:

Exhaustion Phase: extreme fatigue, sleep for days.

Depressive Symptoms: anxiety, depression, hallucinations, paranoia, and unrealistic suspicions.

The Speed Cycle

Adapted from David E. Smith, "The Characteristics of Dependence in High-done Methamphetamine Abuse," International Journal of the Addictions, 4 (September, 1969): 453–459.

gins, the withdrawal from the drug, or "crashing." Heavy users stop their injections, slip between coma and sleep for days, then awaken and start their injections again. David E. Smith described these symptoms as the "speed cycle" in terms of an "action-reaction" sequence, as shown in the following diagram. During the "action phase" the hyperactive individual continues to shoot methamphetamine many times a day to stay "high." In time, the "speed freak" becomes physically exhausted because the extreme stimulation has kept this person from sleeping or eating for days. Following this action period, the individual slips into prolonged depression, which may last for days or weeks. During this "depression-reaction phase," the individual exhibits five adverse psychological reactions.

1. Exhaustion syndrome—intense feelings of fatigue. The individual may sleep continuously for 1 or 2 days.
2. Anxiety reactions. Individual becomes fearful and has unrealistic concerns about his or her physical well-being (hypochondria).
3. Amphetamine psychosis. Individual misinterprets the actions of others, hallucinates, and becomes unrealistically suspicious (paranoia).
4. Prolonged depression.
5. Prolonged hallucinations. Individual continues to hallucinate long after the drug has been completely metabolized.

Many do not consider amphetamines as addicting because they do not produce a classical withdrawal syndrome. This distinction results from a disagreement over the definition of addiction, physiological dependency, and withdrawal, not over the actual physical symptoms exhibited by the individual. During amphetamine withdrawal, the individual exhibits extreme apathy, decreased physical activity, and sleep disturbances that can last for weeks or months. Suicides have occurred during amphetamine withdrawal, so people should be under medical supervision during this time.

A great danger from amphetamines is the effect they have on automobile drivers. When a number of pills are taken at one time, or if they are used for a long period of time without rest or sleep, they may produce hallucinations or delirium. Users may feel that someone or something in another automobile is pursuing them. Or, they may black out suddenly while driving at high speeds. These effects are so dangerous that many states have made it a felony offense to drive while under the influence of amphetamines.

Beyond the chemistry and physiology of drug use is an extensive body of laws, attitudes, procedures, and treatments—as our society attempts to maintain some policy and method of dealing with these substances. This social aspect of drug abuse is explored in the next chapter.

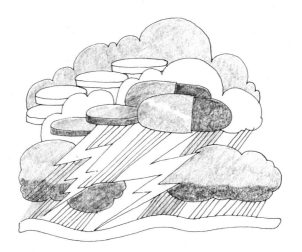

5

THE PROBLEMS OF DRUG ABUSE

Most Americans use drugs. The "drug problem" is actually a problem of the abuse of drugs relating to the amount of mood-modifying drug being used by an individual and the circumstances surrounding the drug use.

The difference between the use and the abuse of mood-modifying substances lies in the degree and patterns of usage. The reasons for taking mood-modifying drugs are complex. Basically an individual wants to change the pace of life, moods and feelings; to reduce anxiety, tensions and boredom; to increase physical activity; to facilitate social interactions; or just "to have fun."

Classifying the Problem

The term *mood-modifying* describes the behavioral effects of psychoactive substances and is not a chemical or medical classification. Not everyone who comes into contact with psychoactive drugs will follow the same predictable pattern of behavior. But all people who try psychoactive drugs belong to one or another of the categories outlined in the following figure. Some may only experiment with such substances because of social influences (peer pressures), curiosity about the reported pleasant effects, or because of short-range emotional problems. Such individuals should be termed "drug experimenters," as they stop using such drugs after their experimentation. Their continued action is unrelated to serious drug abuse because they have already made their decision not to abuse drugs. Unfortunately, often they have been arrested during their experimentation and may carry a criminal record of this experiment for the rest of their lives.

Individuals who experiment and continue to use psychoactive substances find they desire the gratification, mood-modifying effects, or accompanying social environment drugs give them. This is a form of psychological dependence. These people use such substances infrequently, yet consistently, which is usually more than once a month but less than several times a week. (Individuals who use alcohol in this manner are called "social drinkers.") Many use marijuana in relatively low dosages and a similar pattern of use, which is called a *social* or *recreational* use of marijuana. These individuals should be termed *occasional* or *intermittent users.*

Use of psychoactive drugs daily or at least several times a week, extending over a long period of time constitutes "regular," or "moderate" to "heavy" substance abuse. A cigarette smoker who smokes between eight cigarettes and a pack a day (twenty cigarettes) is a regular user. A user of two packs a day is a heavy smoker.

Categories of Drug Use

Experimenters — Experiment with drugs, often not more than three times. Half will never use illegal drugs again. Have only a minor place in discussion of drug abuse. A single incident may indicate hidden emotional problems. One single experiment can lead to a conviction for drug possession.

Occasional Users — Enjoy the social, personal, and emotional gratification the mood-modifying drugs give. Very socially conscious. Use current "in" substance. "Social drinkers," "social" or "recreational" users. Have no serious problem with drugs.

Regular Users — Use drugs regularly, one or more times a week. Part of the drug subculture. Greatest defenders of personal right to use drugs. Striding fine line between controlled use of drugs, heavy use of drugs, and compulsive, uncontrollable abuse of drugs. Dividing line between drug *use* and drug *abuse.*

Compulsive Abusers — Abuse drugs compulsively. Associated with abnormal personality and emotional illness. Use drugs as the only means of coping with stresses of society. Under influence of drugs, personality shifts, social behavior, and modified moods are very dramatic. Representative of the most serious kinds of drug problems.

People who use tranquilizers just to insulate them from their environment, or amphetamines for the extra energy they produce, or a drink of alcoholic beverage to relax or "slow down" every evening are included in this category.

Often regular drug users experiment with a wide variety of drugs and are "poly-drug users" or use the "in" drug currently in fashion. They function within their society, but drugs are a major focus of their lives. Drugs, for them, are not just an intermittent assist in the pursuit of a happy life but a part of a more general "turned-on" ideology and membership in a lifestyle or counterculture.

Regular users of mood-modifying drugs are called "heads," "pot-heads," "coke heads," "acid heads," or "weekend drunks," depending on the specific drug used. Often these users are the greatest defenders of the personal right to use drugs. They seldom have had bad experiences with drugs and have closed minds concerning factual information about drugs because of *street experimentation*. The person who says, "I know because I have been there," is in a dangerous phase of regular drug abuse.

The most dangerous aspect of regular drug use is the danger of lapsing into a *personality deficiency* and inability to control one's substance use that may restrict a user's ability to deal constructively with life. The self destructive dependence of a smoker on cigarettes is a good example. Increased dependence on psychoactive drugs eventually will lead to compulsive drug abuse, very heavy drug use, addiction, or alcoholism—all of which are different names for a single basic problem.

Compulsive abuse (addiction, alcoholism) of mood-modifying substances is always associated with an abnormal personality. Whether this behavioral distortion is the cause or the result of the drug abuse is not known. The abnormal social behavior and modification of moods in such individuals is more of a problem to society than is the drug abuse itself, the responsibility for which lies solely with the individual.

In all cases of repeated drug abuse, the person who misuses such drugs chooses to do so, but is unable to control this use. Once started, this abuse will lead to psychological dependence, in response to personality, or to drug addiction (physiological dependence), according to the physical properties and physiological effects of the drug involved, On the other hand, the person who does not find a pleasurable experience in drug abuse, or whose only reason for experimenting was strong social pressure, will probably not continue to abuse drugs. The personality does not lack, or seek, what the drug has to offer and therefore tends to reject it.

There must be recognition of the various patterns of drug abuse if our society is to reach a humane, just, and successful method of dealing with the serious problems posed by drugs.

Drug Abuse Behavior The taking of psychoactive drugs (legal or illegal) is a type of behavior, and follows the same rules and principles as those of any other human behavior. Behavior patterns persist when they either increase the individual's pleasure or reduce discomfort. People are not just choosing *any* drug; they want substances that give them a pleasurable experience.

Drug use can be an important coping mechanism. In humans, adaptation to the environment is much more complicated than in simpler animals. We have the ability to reason and make decisions based upon learned behavior, and physiological and emotional needs. Why do we do the things we do? Why do we feel the way we do? The answers to these questions come largely from our understanding of how basic human needs are fulfilled and how the frustrations of unfilled needs are met.

Basic Human Needs and Drug Abuse

The most basic human needs are the *physiological needs* (food, water, sleep, and sexual satisfaction). Drug abusers substitute the substance being abused for many physiological needs. They may consume only the food and water needed to remain alive. Drug abusers often suffer from insomnia. And the decrease in sexual drive in drug abusers and alcoholics is well documented.

Curiosity or the need to know and understand is often the major reason for first drug experimentations (especially among young people). Often, the knowledge of drugs these individuals possess is *street knowledge*, while others have had organized drug education. Ironically, these classes may produce the curiosity to experiment with drugs.

The need for comradeship and belonging is very important to all of us. People feel a strong need for friends, companionship, and acceptance by a group. Group acceptance through drug taking may cause an individual to progress from experimentation to being an occasional, regular, or compulsive member of a drug-oriented group. Drug use is a means of establishing and reinforcing *self-esteem*. The desire to be accepted as an "adult" confers status. Many young people also use drugs as a means of annoying and upsetting their parents and as a token rejection of accepted social and moral standards.

Personality and *emotional maturity* can be divided into three areas: (1) personal pleasure and gratification, (2) mature, appropriate behavior, (3) ideals for self-image and personal judgment of right and wrong. Maturity acts as a regulator between the need for pleasure and satisfaction and the demands of conscience (personal evaluation of acceptable behavior). An individual matures as he or she learns to respond to emotional, social, and environmental pressures while still attaining satisfaction and pleasure.

Aggression or dominant behavior is seen by many authorities as a childish means of obtaining pleasure. Young children enjoy being aggressive. In maturity, aggression can be expressed in both harmful and beneficial ways. Drug abuse is often a self-inflicted form of aggression.

Mature people learn to balance social and personal responsibility with the drive for pleasure for its own sake. Many regular and all compulsive drug abusers cannot control their behavior adequately and operate at a "child role" level of maturity, a significant aspect of mental illness.

Drugs, especially depressant drugs such as alcohol and heroin, are abused as a coping mechanism by individuals who are frustrated and unfulfilled in their basic emotional needs. Their drug use is directly related to the "rage of impatience" when helpless and powerless to change the social and economic forces which shape their lives. And, when all opportunities for reinforcement of self-esteem and self-satisfaction have been removed by poverty and social degradation, the occasional user turns to drugs either to block out these feelings or to provide experiences that make the everyday tension and stress seem insignificant. The ability to tolerate emotional tension and stress varies considerably among individuals. When frustrations exceed a person's ability to cope, they either must be relieved or the individual suffers extreme consequences.

The emotionally ill experience an abnormal amount of tension and show it through nervous, exaggerated, or irrational behavior. The occasional drug taker who starts to become a regular drug user is establishing a pathological pattern of drug use. These individuals, when not under the influence of drugs, become increasingly alert (hyperalert). Sounds are exaggerated, lights seem more intense, and perception is keener. As the illness progresses, they look for possible dangers, and display restlessness (often walking or driving aimlessly). There is increased touchiness, tearfulness, irritability, nervous laughter, moodiness, or depression.

During prolonged periods between drug taking (when "straight" or "on the wagon"), these individuals may appear to be normal and may function acceptably within society. But, under stress, they readily turn to drugs. Changes in personality are often apparent. This is why drug abuse is termed a *personality deformity* or *personality disorder*.

Before an individual ever comes into contact with drugs, he or she has an attitude either for or against drug use. This attitude generally corresponds to that of family, friends, social group, neighborhood, community, or city. Where the use of drugs is discouraged, both the availability and the abuse is low. Equally crucial to the person's continued use of drugs after experimentation is the reaction of the social group to the initial drug experience; approval or disapproval, reward or punishment, praise or ridicule. However, even a person with a mature personality needs strong social pressures and guidance to reverse the course of drug abuse after the establishment of drug dependence.

Selection of a specific drug (heroin, marijuana, alcohol) is generally dictated by factors such as availability, practices of friends, and social environment. Individuals tend to have drug experiences related to their own basic emotional needs. Drug users who never progress beyond social, occasional use may suffer physical discomfort (hangover, withdrawal, shakes, and so on) but they are able to control their emotional reaction to drugs. Psychological processes can override physical drug effects. Emotional factors become more important in drug abuse and social and physical factors less important as use becomes heavier and more compulsive. For example, depressant drugs remove an individual from stresses and anxieties of society. Heroin does this very quickly; alcohol does this slowly, but for a longer period of time. Hallucinogenic drugs and cocaine can compensate for a lack of "peak" or "high" experiences, can help control emotions, or can help someone deal with the frustrations leading to aggression. Amphetamines help increase output of physical energy.

There is no single reason for abusing drugs, no single pattern of abuse, and no inevitable outcome. Many individuals are able to use psychoactive drugs without harm to themselves or society. Others are susceptible to factors that are responsible not only for chronic abuse but also for relapses. People desperately trying to stop abusing drugs must progressively fulfill their emotional and social needs in order to resume control of their lives.

Drug Abuse Treatment

All drug abuse treatment programs are ultimately based on the motivation of the individual. By placing final responsibility and hope for "cure" on the will of the individual, we have also implied that the alteration of certain external factors will not be sufficient to reverse the tragic patterns of abuse that have occurred in recent decades.

The Goals of Treatment As might be expected, the usual point at which the drug abuser and society as a whole first really meet is at the time that the user runs up against the law. Enforcement of the drug laws temporarily takes the user out of his environment, and, for the period of his jail sentence, forces him to do without drugs. Also, another beneficial effect of a jail sentence is that, for the moment, the innocent (the "forgotten person" in our laws) is protected from the compulsive drug user.

But emphasis solely on punitive confinement has never successfully helped any significant number of drug abusers. "Drunkards" have been jailed for centuries. Opium eating was once a serious problem in the United States, but it was the elimination of the supply from China, rather than the early narcotics laws, which reduced its incidence. Heroin addiction is demonstrably a consequence of factors that do not seem to be affected by short-term detention.

Compared with the other possible modes of control—social, legal, and so on—self-control is the only one that can ultimately be relied upon for treatment. The environment or *setting* and the emotional *set* of the individual must be changed if he is to live a life free of drug abuse. Development of *an individual's self-control* and changing the *setting* and *set* are the aims of most drug treatment programs. Punishment alone does not work.

Treatment Laws and Facilities There are two kinds of agencies available for treatment of drug abuse: private and public. The private programs mainly emphasize treatment through family members or peers. Individuals lacking the personal self-control to stay within the framework of a private program, and who would leave it against medical advice, are placed within the legal controls of public programs. However, too often we commit people to public treatment programs out of anger and vindictiveness rather than humane concern. This is certainly emphasized by the penalties for drug possession. The predominant method of dealing with drug abuse has been to place abusers in jail. Following their release, they gener-

ally resume abusing drugs. We still do not have effective methods of treatment for this kind of drug abuser.

The federal Narcotics Addict Rehabilitation Act of 1966 guides states and local communities in the treatment of drug abusers. Many states have also passed legislation supplementing and defining the procedures of this act. In California, there is the Mental Health Act of 1969 (the Lanterman–Petris–Short Law), which defines in detail the conditions that permit voluntary and involuntary hospitalization for drug abuse. Under the federal statute, eligible individuals charged with a drug crime may be told by a judge that the criminal charge will be "held in abeyance" if they submit to a medical examination to determine whether they are an addict and could be rehabilitated through treatment. The drug offender has 5 days in which to make a decision. If treatment is elected, he or she is then retained in a hospital for not more than 60 days for examination purposes. If found to be a suitable candidate for treatment, the drug abuser is placed in a state hospital through a civil commitment procedure.

The civil commitment is a legal mechanism used in place of a criminal commitment. This procedure ensures control over drug abusers during rehabilitation—first in a hospital or drug treatment institution, later in a halfway house, and still later in the community under the close supervision of a probation or parole officer. The significant step in this procedure is that the drug abuser does not establish a criminal record when seeking treatment and help.

Drug abusers are limited to a 2-year maximum confinement, unless the judge renews the procedure at a later date. If, after release to the community, they resume using drugs they may be returned for further treatment or the criminal proceedings may be started again. Should he or she be found guilty, any time served in the treatment program will be counted toward the time to be served under the criminal sentence.

If someone has been convicted of a non-violent crime, and a judge believes the criminal offender is an addict or in danger of becoming an addict, the judge may order the offender to be examined and then committed to a treatment program for an indeterminate period of time. This period may not be more than 10 years but must be more than 6 months. The offender then may be released under the supervision of a probation officer. This is a criminal commitment procedure and (differing from state to state) may result in a criminal record.

In 1972 the Drug Abuse Office and Treatment Act was signed. This law allocated over $1.1 billion to help control and treat drug abuse. During the same year, the Special Action Office for Drug Abuse Prevention (SAODAP) was established by the federal government to see that these, and future funds, are spent according to federal guidelines. This agency was established to help with short-term and long-term planning and coordination of drug abuse treatment programs at the local and state levels.

In 1973, the federal government established the Alcohol, Drug Abuse, and Mental Health Administration (ADAMHA). This agency oversees the National Institute of Alcohol Abuse and Alcoholism (NIAAA) and the National Institute of Drug Abuse (NIDA). One of the significant outcomes of these agencies is the recognition of alcoholism as a drug abuse program and treating it as such. These agencies help states to develop training programs and to construct, staff, and operate drug treatment facilities. The support has helped the states expand their programs and facilities to meet their increasing needs.

Modes of Drug Abuse Treatment

Most drug users (experimenters and occasional users), given adequate supervision, will eventually give up the use of illegal drugs after a period of drug-free living, if only to avoid an involuntary return to an institution.

Medical authorities find that the compulsive drug user is emotionally disturbed and often physically ill from the toxic effect of the drug being abused. He or she may need emergency treatment for the physical effects of the drug and psychological help, often continuing throughout life, to keep from going back to drug abuse when leaving the hospital. Drug abuse therapy must be aimed at the psychological and sociological problems of the individual abusing drugs and his or her family. Many drug abusers (including alcoholics) would prefer not to stop using drugs, but to return to controlled, moderate drug use or drinking. But most authorities are convinced that at the present time, the return to controlled drug use is often an unrealistic or most often an impossible goal. Very few compulsive drug users including alcoholics have been able to return to controlled drug use. Such individuals must also be wary of their use of prescription and certain over-the-counter drugs for medicinal purposes. Many of these drugs have properties, similar to the drugs they were abusing, that could cause the drug abuse problem to recur.

No single method of treatment has been developed that has significantly reduced the complex problem of drug abuse to a treatable problem. All treatment programs tend to reduce compulsive drug abuse, addiction, and alcoholism to the level of an individual problem. Thus, all treatment programs should be available to all individuals. If someone is not progressing with one type of treatment, another type is tried until a treatment program appropriate to the individual is found. This is called a multimodality treatment program and many professionals feel it is essential to the control of drug abuse. The 1973 National Committee on Marijuana and Drug Abuse therefore recommended a community multimodality approach to drug abuse. More flexibility of treatment and of our definitions of successful treatment are needed. Any person who can be a productive member of society, while using a drug (or a level of drugs) acceptable to society, would be considered "cured." The goal of a "cured drug user" (completely free of all drugs) is simply not a reliable prospect. A great deal more research will be necessary in order for our society to maintain any level of cure and rehabilitation. The damage done by drug abuse is so powerful and so widespread that the only practical long-range complete solution is prevention.

Drug treatment programs can only succeed when they deal with the basic fact that the compulsive user or addict has no ability to combat the ordinary stresses in life. Such a user has relied for months, or perhaps years, on the external solace provided by drugs. A cure of this dependency must help redirect attitudes toward personal weaknesses.

Emergency Therapy When an individual under the influence of drugs comes to the attention of a hospital staff or a private physician, it is usually in an emergency situation. Some doctors in high drug-abuse areas may see thousands of drug users every year.

The first information needed by the physician is the name of the drug or combination of drugs the individual is using, in order to prescribe appropriate treatment. This is often difficult to determine because the user may be unconscious, semicoherent, disoriented, frightened, unreliable, and may often behave as an acute

psychotic. Reassurance in a quiet and "cool" environment will often produce an accurate story of what happened and simplify this phase of treatment. Friends, the contents of the user's pockets, and the surrounding conditions under which the adverse reactions occurred may help the doctor in his evaluation. During this acute phase of treatment, a well-established rapport between the physician and the patient can be a valuable tool.

During this "talk-down" phase, little more than acceptance and reassurance is necessary. If definite signs of toxic complications occur, the physician will treat them as they appear, regardless of what the patient has told him or her.

A very important complicating factor in this procedure is the fear of legal incrimination. In addition to emotional and physical distress, the patient will probably fear the introduction of the police into the situation. He or she will try to cover up potential evidence, will become wary of the doctor's questions, and may well have difficulty distinguishing medical from legal personnel.

Most drug prosecutions are based on evidence of possession (even for one's own personal use) of an illegal drug. If the police obtain such evidence at the time the patient was brought to a health facility, the fears are simply too late. But they will not pursue the search into the examining room. A doctor is not a law enforcement official. The doctor's goal is to help the patient come out of what was probably an extremely disturbing and dangerous experience. And the physician needs the patient's greatest possible cooperation in order to succeed.

Drug Detoxification When treating a victim of addicting drugs, a doctor has a complicated task. Abrupt withdrawal, the so-called "cold turkey," is painful and can be fatal. Gradual withdrawal is usually done in a hospital. The American Medical Association suggests that a physician should not normally try to attempt withdrawal unless the individual is in a hospital.

During narcotics withdrawal, the drug abuser will suffer nausea, watery eyes, muscle spasms in the stomach and legs, and hot and cold flashes. The drug methadone may be substituted for any major opiate drug. This is called *methadone detoxification*. It tends to block the euphoric effects of an opiate and relieves the craving for other narcotics.

In barbiturate withdrawal, grand mal epileptic-type convulsions and delirium tremens may occur. Here, the drug pentobarbital can be used as a substitute drug during detoxification withdrawal. Abrupt withdrawal from barbiturates is extremely dangerous and often ends in death from respiratory failure because the drug has depressed the respiratory center in the brain until the person's breathing stops. Alcohol, another hypnotic-sedative drug, and many other substances greatly increase the chances of overdose and death when taken with barbiturates. Consequently, a physician must know both the quantity and nature of the barbiturates used before the patient can be effectively treated.

Narcotic Antagonists The first "chemical treatment" approach to drug abuse was the use of narcotic antagonists—drugs chemically and structurally so like narcotics that they apparently are able to "occupy" the sites of narcotic action in the brain and thus are able to block the action of a narcotic. Antagonists, when given to a person physically dependent on a narcotic (usually heroin), will bring on withdrawal symptoms rather than prevent them. Even if the individual has taken only one or two doses of the narcotic within the last week, there are recognizable changes (such as in pupil size) that take place. The changes in pupil size have been used for years in the Nalline tests for narcotics use. From the withdrawal symptoms and the pupil changes, a physician can tell if an individual is currently taking narcotics. There are four currently recognized narcotic antagonists: nalorphine (Nalline), levallorphan (Lorphan), naloxone (Narcan), and cyclazocine.

Of the four antagonists, naloxone and cyclazocine show promise as therapeutic agents. These drugs, when taken prior to a shot of heroin, block the euphoric effects of the heroin. While someone is taking several daily dosages of cyclazocine, they will not feel the effects of a narcotic nor will they become addicted to it. Thus, during a treatment program, antagonists may provide a means of "unlearning" drug-abusing behavior. With these drugs people may keep from becoming physically addicted, making it possible for them to continue working and participating in a rehabilitation program. To be effective, these drugs must be part of a broad program of psychological and social rehabilitation.

Maintenance Therapy (Narcotic Substitutes) Because of the short-acting ups and downs of psychoactive drugs such as heroin, a regular and compulsive drug abuser thinks about drugs and obtaining drugs all the time. The first step in treatment is to eliminate the need for psychoactive drugs and establish normal social functioning, perhaps by giving the individual a daily "maintenance" dose of a drug that allows the person to go to school, work, and be an active member of society. Methadone acetylmethadol (CAAM), Darvon-N, also sold as PN (propoxyphene napsylate), and a combination of methadone and naloxone (a narcotic antagonist) called Methenex are synthetic narcotics that can relieve a person's physical need for other narcotics without producing drastic mood modifications.

Individuals on a methadone maintenance program are given one oral dose daily. The effects of acetylmethadol last long, and a patient using it needs a dose only 2 or 3 times a week. Darvon-N seems to have two advantages over methadone: (1) less chance of causing death in overdoses, and (2) much less physical dependence. One of Darvon-N's disadvantages is that it is less potent than methadone. Methenex is used to interrupt the diversion of methadone into illegal channels. Methenex is taken orally; this way, the methadone part satisfies the narcotic needs of the addict, while the naloxone has no effect. But if Methenex is injected the naloxone blocks the narcotic effect and causes withdrawals.

With maintenance drugs, some users have been able to stay off psychoactive drugs and rejoin the general society through a combination of programs including psychotherapy and rehabilitation education. A number of nonaddicting drugs have been tried, with varying degrees of success.

In 1965, Drs. Vincent Dole and Marie Nyswander of Rockefeller Institute in New York City developed the first systematic methadone maintenance program. This program is based on a slightly different use of methadone. The patient is given a quantity of the drug on a daily basis, thus having the opportunity to live a fairly normal life. Unlike the narcotics addict who is relying solely on illegal opiates, the individual being treated with methadone need not focus an entire existence on obtaining drugs. Methadone thus offers the user a more immediate, responsible view of self and society.

By 1972, 25,000 heroin addicts were enrolled into methadone programs. This prompted the Food and Drug Administration to release more methadone for expanded use. However, poor administration and control put much of this methadone on the streets for illegal abuse. Methadone does not produce euphoria when taken orally, but it does produce euphoria and mood modification when injected. On the street capsules of methadone are known as "dollies" (after a trade name for methadone, Dolophine).

In 1973, the Methadone Control Act established rigid control over the distribution of methadone to try to slow the illegal traffic. Control has not been successful; abuse of methadone remains a major problem. In 1973, Dr. Dominick DiMaio, Acting Chief Medical Examiner of New York City, listed 924 narcotics-related deaths. Of these deaths, 181 were directly caused by methadone overdose, while 98 were directly due to heroin. Both methadone and heroin were found in 145 of these dead users. Also, Dr. Robert Newman, director of the city's methadone program, noted that only 10 of the 181 methadone deaths were enrolled in methadone clinics. Since then, the abuse of methadone has continued to increase.

Originally methadone maintenance programs were to run for a specific length of time. Within this time (say, two years), the individual was to be "cured" of drug abuse. Many physicians, politicians, and others feel that the use of methadone is based upon a morally and ethically imperfect scheme of substituting one addictive drug (methadone) for another (heroin).

As mentioned earlier, such a "cure" is an unrealistic goal. However, with proper support programs, maintenance does offer some help. For example, the patient must take the drug day after day, year after year, just as a diabetic must continue to take insulin. Both situations are unfortunate, but they do serve to remind the individual that this is a unique problem that requires ongoing treatment and concern. A continuing treatment program is the basis of all successful drug treatment programs (for example, A.A. and Teen Challenge).

Therapeutic Communities Another distinct approach involves the establishment of complex social systems, houses, homes, or communities that are directed almost exclusively by ex-addicts. These are called *therapeutic communities*. Such organizations as Synanon (California), Daytop House, Phoenix House and Odyssey House (New York), Gateway House (Illinois), and the federally sponsored Tacoma Narcotics Center (Washington) are some of the better known therapeutic communities. Individuals are not required to remain at these centers continuously, and are free to leave permanently at any time. However, in order to remain at the center, they must participate in the center's programs and must conform to the strict community rules.

Therapeutic communities are designed to provide care through three mechanisms: (1) encounter group therapy, (2) a highly structured community organization, and (3) a reward–punishment system based on simple behavioral psychology. The key to the therapeutic process is the group encounter, usually called the "Synanon game," "attack therapy," or the "verbal street fight." The second phase consists of a complete behavioral dissection through the encounter therapy and scaled program of house jobs, starting with dishwashing or garbage control, and progressing to ordering supplies and leading group therapy sessions (this phase can last for years).

These communities are designed to develop and reinforce standard middle-class norms of behavior and attitudes. Theoretically, the community tries to make the individual goal-oriented—willing to work hard and sacrifice in order to obtain eventual security and success. Men and women's roles are carefully defined and sexual behavior is subject to the censure and influences the individual would encounter outside the community (homosexual relationships are prohibited;

heterosexual relationships are permitted only after an extended period of time in the community).

More black and brown individuals and groups criticize this type of program because of the personality and identity destruction that goes on in encounter therapy. These people feel that they have been stripped of their identity by white society long enough and that the reconstruction of black and brown identity should be a valid concern of these programs. Also, most of the programs are conducted exclusively in English, so that the Spanish-speaking person is at a disadvantage. The middle-class norms do not take into consideration the poverty backgrounds of most black and brown addicts. Therefore, new programs, such as *The Community Thing* in New York City, based upon positive racial identification and self-help, have been started and seem to be successful.

There are two distinct approaches and goals within therapeutic communities. The first is illustrated by Synanon in Santa Monica, California. In the past, reentry into society was the desired last stage of all successful therapeutic community treatment programs. But Synanon found that very few of its residents ever achieved full-time life outside the structure of the community. A common criticism is that therapeutic communities do not make people independent. Synanon provides a life that is better than life "outside." This encourages addiction to community life rather than to drugs. Synanon believes that a dependent user can never be cured if he or she lives in the outside world. Experience now indicates that many addicts require the permanent support of a therapeutic community in order to prevent the resumption of their drug-taking behavior. This also seems to be the case with alcoholics; they must continue their association with Alcoholics Anonymous. Narcotics addicts must remain on methadone maintenance. In the beginning, there was very little emphasis on education within the communities because it interfered with the therapeutic process. In recent years, with entire families becoming permanent residents, therapeutic communities have become strongly education-oriented. Synanon operates its own elementary and secondary schools and encourages colleges and universities to hold classes in its facilities. And now Synanon is establishing "Synanon City," which will provide lifelong residency.

The second approach to therapeutic communities is illustrated by Daytop Village, on Staten Island, New York. Daytop Village uses group sessions (encounter groups called "copout sessions" or "probe sessions") and has apparently provided a successful forum for the black and brown individuals in the group. But Daytop Village feels that the ex-user can go into the outside world and be able to live without lifetime support. They design their programs so that the individual lives in the community for six months to a year.

Local Community Programs Almost every community has a peer-organized and peer-run temporary treatment and help program. Over the years, these have evolved into programs that help people with all kinds of medical and behavioral problems. "Hot lines" now handle drug problems, sex problems (rape, abortion, and so on), and offer suicide prevention care. The drug-related problems range from identification of street drugs to promoting emergency help for drug overdoses.

Some peer-group programs have developed into established centers where trained volunteers and professionals are available to help individuals with any behavioral or medical problem. These may be peer-staffed "rap centers," paraprofessional and professionally staffed "crisis intervention centers," or medically equipped and staffed "free clinics." Other centers are residential ("crash pads"), where individuals can live while trying to stay off drugs or working out a behavioral problem.

Experimental Programs Many experimental treatment programs are being used throughout the United States. Some physicians feel that dependent drug users and alcoholics suffer from specific physiological deficiencies. Some users are being treated by salt detoxification. In this process, different mineral salts are given during and after withdrawal to correct chronic metabolic imbalances believed to be present. Others are being treated with large doses of vitamins on the same theory. This treatment is called *megavitamin therapy*.

Many programs designed to cause the individual to relax physically and emotionally are being tried. These include medications such as tranquilizers, hypnosis, biofeedback, and acupuncture. Hypnosis is used to take the individual back to pre-drug-using years to isolate the behavioral patterns that led to the drug-taking behavior. Biofeedback is a technique in which an individual is taught to control physiological activities that influence or control moods, attention levels, and a wide variety of emotional sensations. With extensive training and discipline, an individual may be able to achieve desired moods and emotional sensations without drugs. Transcendental meditation and "turning on" without drugs seek the same results as biofeedback.

Acupuncture has been used successfully to reduce pain and completely block withdrawal symptoms. Treatments are given three or four times a day, which makes it impossible to use acupuncture over long periods of time. However, a variation on traditional acupuncture seems to help individuals over longer periods. A *surgical staple* is implanted in the ear of the addict and when he or she feels the signs of withdrawal, he or she massages the staple and it relieves the symptoms for a short period of time. This staple technique is also being used successfully in helping individuals to lose weight.

The Return to Society

After an individual has been treated for drug abuse and returns to society he or she faces many personal problems, which may be social, legal, economic, and medical. Often, with drug problems, the offender and the victim are the same person and the social pressures that encourage the drug abuse in the first place are still present in this environment when the patient returns to it.

If there are facilities available to provide for a gradual reentry into society, or if the drug abuser has not established a criminal record (civil commitment rather than criminal conviction) because of drugs, there is a much better chance of adjustment. Short visits home should be made at first; then a halfway house, work camp, parish house, or a day–night hospital may help after the person leaves the therapeutic community. Any of these settings is potentially useful in providing the abuser with social, therapeutic, educational, and vocational services. These give controlled contacts with the community.

But all too often, treated drug abusers leave the hospital (or more often, the jail) and are literally "dumped back on the street." Consequently, it is a very short time before they are again abusing drugs and are back or beyond where they were when treatment was initiated.

Obviously, the trend is away from purely punitive measures and toward rehabilitation and treatment. There is no doubt that rehabilitation and planned prevention hold much greater promise for both the individual and society than does punitive confinement.

A person who has been rescued from a possible life of drug abuse has saved society a good deal more than the cost of the future treatment. The more our nation's policy makers become convinced that the cost of ambitious, well-planned, humane programs is money well spent, the more progress we can expect to witness.

Control and Enforcement

Control of drug use in the United States has had a mixed and confused history, and few guidelines are clearly revealed. Prohibition of alcoholic beverages during the 1920s has generally been considered an overwhelming failure. It most probably did not discourage drinking (in fact, quite the contrary), nor did it produce a generation of nondrinkers. Yet, control-by-prescription laws of certain other drugs has certainly determined that these substances will not be routinely abused on a wide scale. A person cannot simply walk into a drug store and purchase morphine without a prescription. A five-year-old child cannot purchase even aspirin. Surely the legal requirement that certain substances be dispensed only upon the approval and under the direction of a physician has affected most people's attitudes toward drugs.

One of the most interesting aspects of the problem is the current argument centered on the decriminalization of marijuana. Reflected against the history of drug control in our country, this debate highlights some interesting points. The pressure for decriminalization of marijuana is hardly universal and the change of status of this substance, in all states, is certainly not a foregone conclusion at this time. But some recurring themes can be found in the arguments of the decriminalization proponents. Mainly, the analogies to the prohibition of alcohol demand some attention.

Proponents of legalization have insisted that prohibition during the 1920s did not work and that the restrictions on the cultivation, sale, use, and possession of marijuana are not working either. Marijuana does little to the body that alcohol does not do, according to these same arguments, and yet society has hypocritically banned one and permitted the other. A driver "stoned" on grass is a potential danger on the highways, but the major cause of serious automobile accidents in the United States is alcohol. To those who say that we need more information and more time to understand the effects of marijuana—before we can confidently legalize it—proponents respond that we know little about certain major aspects of alcohol use. The nature of the damage alcohol does to the metabolism, the causes of alcoholism, and the cure for a hangover are still relative mysteries, yet alcohol is permitted a controlled but important place in our society.

The major conclusion to be drawn from the present marijuana argument is that our society has the most difficulty in developing useful policies toward those substances that occupy a middle ground in the public consciousness. Alcohol, tobacco, and marijuana have attained such an undefined position primarily because their effects are not readily predictable, and their use does not necessarily interfere with normal functioning in our society.

As Prohibition went headlong against the attitudes of many Americans and thus failed, so has the outlawing of marijuana use come into conflict with the viewpoints and life-style of a generation.

Our society is seeking sound solutions to the basic causes of drug abuse. It pre-sently relies on a certain body of laws to protect itself. Laws can be preventive measures, but the current controls now available are not meeting present needs. Some type of control is needed for the treatment of drug abuse. This may be legal, social, or self-control, but it must be present. More control than is necessary becomes punishment, but less control than is necessary is useless. Up until the middle 1960s the major laws were established to control illegal possession, manufacture, and sale of drugs rather than their abuse. Treatment programs were left out completely. As described earlier, during the middle 1960s laws were established that governed research into the effects and actions of drugs that permitted greater flexibility in the treatment and control of drug abuse and the rehabilitation of drug abusers. This trend separated treatment laws from those governing the possession and sale of drugs.

Federal Drug Control Laws The federal government's control of the sale and possession of drugs is based on laws that have been enacted over the last sixty years. In tracing the history of these laws, we will be recapitulating the record of drug abuse in this country.

During the 1800s, narcotics were taken as constituents of patent medicines and curealls. This use increased greatly with the invention of the hypodermic needle and syringe just before the Civil War. Doctors actually encouraged their patients to buy this equipment and to use narcotics on a "do-it-yourself" basis. The "miracle medicines," "elixirs," and "tonics," which contained large amounts of narcotics—usually opium preparations—were easy to obtain and were reputed to be cures for everything.

By the end of the Civil War, thousands of soldiers had received injections of narcotics to relieve their suffering from wounds and sickness. Many became addicted to these drugs. A much greater percentage of the population was addicted at this time than is today. Then, with the growth of advertising and the promotion of patent medicines containing narcotics, great numbers of people took such medicines and became addicted to them. Some, having discovered the fact that these medicines contained opium, bought and used "straight" opium. Narcotic abuse climbed steeply even after 1914, when the first effective drug-control laws were enacted. There was very little actual reduction in the abuse of narcotics until the Federal Bureau of Narcotics was established in 1930 to enforce the earlier narcotics laws and apprehend violators. The name of this agency has since been changed to the Drug Enforcement Administration (DEA).

The first federal measure seeking control over drugs was enacted by Congress on February 9, 1906. The federal Pure Food and Drug Act prohibited the importation of opium, its preparations, and its derivatives, except for medicinal purposes. A second law was enacted December 17, 1914, the Harrison Narcotic Act, which further restricted the importation, manufacture, sale, and dispensing of opiates. It required the keeping of accurate records and inventories of narcotics and made the possession of narcotics a criminal (felony) offense. It established the legal definition of a narcotic as *any drug that produces sleep or stupor and relieves pain*. Certain specific drugs were legally labeled narcotics regardless of their medical nature. Opium, its derivatives, coca leaves and their derivatives (such as cocaine), marijuana, peyote (mescaline), and any synthetic drug that produces sleep or stupor and relieves pain was declared a "habit-forming narcotic drug."

The Harrison Act required physicians to dispense opiates only "in the course of their professional practice" for bona fide medical purposes. It limited the selling of narcotics to licensed druggists and only after they received a lawful written prescription issued by a qualified medical or dental practitioner.

The next federal statute, approved in 1922, was an extensive revision of the Harrison Act. It is known as the Narcotics Drugs Import and Export Act. This revision and subsequent minor revisions are considered the official position of the federal government with regard to the legal and illegal possession, importation, manufacture, and exportation of narcotics. It authorizes the importation of specific quantities of crude opium and coca leaves needed to provide for the medical and legitimate scientific needs of the United States. It prohibits the importation of any form of narcotic drugs, except the prescribed limited quantities of crude opium and coca leaves. It specifically prohibits the importation of opium for smoking or for the manufacture of heroin. This law made it illegal to possess heroin in any form in the United States.

Another principal federal statute controlling narcotics was approved in 1942; it is known as the Opium Poppy Control Act. This act was passed when World War II cut off the supply of opium to the United States from Asia. The law requires that a license be issued by the federal government for the cultivation of the opium poppy in the United States. The issuance of this license is conditioned by a determination of the necessity of supplying the medical and scientific needs of the country. The development of synthetic narcotics has minimized the likelihood that a scarcity will occur.

From 1951 to 1956 intensive studies were conducted by congressional committees on the rising narcotic problem among young people in the United States. These committees recommended that heavier penalties be imposed as a more effective deterrent to narcotic traffic and abuse. Consequently in 1956 Congress passed the Narcotics Control Act, which set forth a range of stringent, mandatory minimum sentences and fines for violation of federal narcotics laws.

The law known as the Marijuana Tax Act was patterned after the Harrison Act and was enacted in 1937. This act later became part of the Internal Revenue Code and is really a tax law, rather than a narcotics control law. The statute requires the registration and payment of a tax by all persons who import, manufacture, produce, compound, sell, deal in, dispense, prescribe, administer, or give away marijuana. This catalog of possible illegal actions is interesting for two reasons. First, like other drug-control laws there is no functional reference to the use of the prescribed drug. Second, the law, by specifying a wide range of actions, seeks to cover all aspects of the drug abuse with the same legal umbrella.

The need for more stringent controls over the manufacture, distribution, and illegal abuse of the dangerous drugs became a point of focus in the early 1960s. In 1965, the Drug Abuse Control Amendments to the 1938 federal Food, Drug, and Cosmetic Act were enacted by Congress. This law applies not only to barbiturates and amphetamines, but it established the current definition of a dangerous drug. Under the 1965 amendments all wholesalers, jobbers, and manufacturers of dangerous drugs are required to register annually with the Food and Drug Administration and keep records of sales of these drugs. Pharmacists, hospitals, researchers, and doctors who regularly dispense and charge for the controlled drugs must maintain records that are available for inspection by the Food and Drug Administration. Prohibitions include refilling a prescription more than five times or later than six months after the prescription is originally written, and require the registration of drug firms that manufacture, process or sell controlled drugs.

In 1970 a new schedule of federal drug penalties was established (Comprehensive Drug Abuse Prevention and Control Act). This law established five classes of drugs whose illegal manufacture, distribution, possession for use, possession for sale, and sale are controlled by the federal government. The following table is an outline of these five classes. Also, the law does away with the term *dangerous drugs* by defining drugs as either *narcotics* or *nonnarcotics*.

Both narcotics and nonnarcotics are placed in Schedule I when they have a high potential for abuse because of their mood-modifying effects, and are not currently used in medicine in the United States. These drugs may be used in approved research projects, but may not be possessed for any other purposes.

Schedule II substances (narcotic and nonnarcotic) have the same potential for abuse as Schedule I drugs. Abuse of these substances will lead to severe psychological or physical dependence. Schedule II drugs are currently being used in medical practice. The controls, fines, and penalties for illegal manufacture, distribution and possession of both Class I and II substances are essentially the same.

Substances placed in Schedule III are considered to have a potential for abuse that is lower than Schedule I and II substances. These drugs are used in medical practice and are considered to produce moderate or low physical dependence or high psychological dependence. The penalties for illegal trafficking, distribution, and sale of Schedule III drugs are less severe than for Schedule I and II drugs but more severe than for Schedule IV or V drugs.

Schedule IV and V drugs have the lowest potential for abuse, the lowest penalties, and the least controls. The major difference between Schedule IV and V drugs is that Schedule IV drugs require a prescription from a physician, while most of the Schedule V drugs are sold over the counter.

As shown by the table on penalties for violations of the federal drug laws, there are major differences in the prescription requirements of the different schedules. Also, the penalties for trafficking (sale or

Schedules and Penalties for Violation of the Comprehensive Drug Abuse Prevention and Control Act of 1970

Drug Schedule	Potential for Abuse	Dispensing Controls	Example of Substances in Each Schedule	Maximum Penalties for Illegal Trafficking	Maximum Penalties for Personal Possession
I	High	Research use only	Nonmedical opium derivatives, cannabis, hallucinogens.	Narcotics: first offense—4 to 15 years; $25,000 fine. Second offense and subsequent offenses—6 to 30 years; $50,000 fine. Nonnarcotics: First offense—2 to 5 years; $15,000 fine. Second and subsequent offenses—4 to 10 years; $30,000 fine.	First offense—up to 1 year (probation possible); $5,000 fine. Second offense—up to 2 years; $10,000 fine.
II	High	Written prescription. No refills.	Medically used narcotics and injected amphetamines.		
III	Moderate to low	Written or oral prescription. With MD's authorization, refills up to 5 times in 6 months.	Mild narcotics, noninjected amphetamines, methadone, barbiturates, and minor tranquilizers.	First offense—2 to 5 years; $15,000 fine. Second and subsequent offenses—4 to 10 years; $20,000 fine.	
IV	Low	Written or oral prescription. With MD's authorization, refills up to 5 times in 6 months.	Mild sedatives, hypnotics, narcotics, and some stimulants.	First offense—1 to 3 years; $10,000 fine. Second and subsequent offenses—2 to 6 years; $20,000 fine.	
V	Low	Over-the-counter. Prescription by oral order by MD.	Restricted over-the-counter drugs. Low percentage mixtures of narcotics, sedatives, and amphetamines.	First offense—up to 1 year; $5,000 fine. Second and subsequent offenses—up to 2 years; $10,000 fine.	

NOTE: Schedule and penalties may be changed by the U.S. Attorney General at any time.

possession for sale) are different for different classes but the possession for one's own use of any controlled substance in any schedule is always a misdemeanor on the first offense, punishable by one year in jail, and up to a $5,000 fine. For a first offense, an individual user twenty-one years of age who is convicted of possession may be placed on probation, and if he or she successfully completes the probation, the official arrest, trial, and conviction can be erased from the record.

The director of the Drug Enforcement Administration (DEA), under the direction of the attorney general, decides which schedule a new drug belongs in on the basis of its "potential for abuse." This is also the procedure for moving drugs from one schedule to another.

In 1973 the Heroin Trafficking Act was signed into law. It increased the penalties for traffickers in heroin and made it much more difficult for traffickers to obtain bail for such offenses.

State Drug Control Laws State laws dealing with drugs are highly variable. In 1932 a model uniform state narcotics law, patterned after the Harrison Narcotics Act, was submitted to several states. Since that time most states have enacted laws similar to this act. It also became the basis of the laws controlling the nonnarcotic or dangerous drugs. Some states enacted legislation with even heavier penalties. For example, in 1955 Ohio provided a twenty-five-year minimum penalty for the unlawful sale of narcotics. In 1973, New York State passed the most severe drug control penalties of any state. This law provides penalties of up to life in prison for possession and sale of narcotics. Some convictions, such as for the sale of an ounce or more of heroin, carries a mandatory life sentence. Also, an arrest for possession of marijuana carries a mandatory referral to a drug treatment clinic.

Other states reduced some of their penalties during the same period. All fifty states and the District of Columbia have reduced the penalty for first-offense marijuana possession from a felony to a misdemeanor. Six states, led by Oregon in 1973, have "decriminalized" their laws concerning individual possession of small amounts of marijuana for personal use. Oregon's law basically states that persons found in possession of up to one ounce of marijuana can be charged with a *violation*, which is similar to a parking ticket. They face a fine of not more than $100. Transportation and possession of more than an ounce, and sale or cultivation of marijuana remain a felony with a maximum penalty of up to ten years in prison. Maine, Alaska, California, and others have since followed Oregon in decriminalizing simple possession of marijuana.

Since 1970, many states have followed the example of the federal government and established five classes for narcotics and dangerous drugs, bringing their laws into conformity with the federal Comprehensive Drug Abuse Prevention and Control Act.

In Conclusion   Medical, educational, and legal experts have struggled for years to develop a simple, clear model of substance abuse and its treatment and cure. The complexities of the social and personal factors—compounded with the chemical and medical aspects—have prevented simple solutions to this dramatically serious problem.

The past several decades have shown that the drug problem does not fade away—it only changes form, severity, and location. Hopefully, new research and fundamental changes in attitudes will reduce the serious effects of drug abuse in the future.

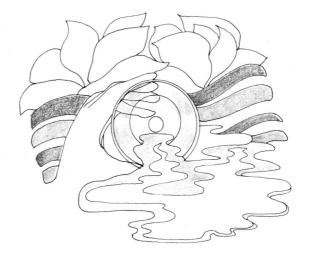

6

ALCOHOL: A LEGAL MOOD—MODIFYING DRUG

At a time when there is great public interest in the mood-modifying drugs, which have become substantially identified with the "youth culture" in our country, it is important and useful to remember that the most prevalent and potentially dangerous mood-modifying drug consumed in the Western world is alcohol. Yet alcohol occupies a very distinct place in our society—its use, manufacture, advertisement, and sale are major parts of our environment.

There are many aspects of the alcohol use situation. Most Americans find alcohol a pleasant and generally enjoyable part of dinner parties, social gatherings, celebrations, and so on. Unlike most of the hallucinogens and opiates, the use of alcohol in our society is not *necessarily* questioned or condemned; nor is it illegal. It becomes a legal or social problem for individuals and society only under specific conditions—driving while under the influence of alcohol, public intoxication, the tragic personal consequences of alcohol abuse (excessive drinking, problem drinking, and alcoholism).

The effects of alcohol are part of a complex web—some are definitely caused by problems of body chemistry (and thus may be inherited); some are caused by social control and responsibility; and often these effects are complicated by severe psychological problems. Abuse of alcohol is a behavioral problem with physiological implications and as such is comparable to the abuse of the drugs discussed previously. It is also difficult to predict all the effects of alcohol directly, or to understand how it affects each individual.

Ironically, because of the generally freer attitudes toward alcohol use, we are able to see and understand more of its harmful results. With the possible exception of heroin addiction, we know more about the damage done by alcohol than we know about any other drug mentioned so far.

Yet, at the same time, millions of people derive great enjoyment from the delightful alcohol products available without ever seriously threatening the well-being of themselves or society. The reasons for the differences between these two groups are not all clear, but in this chapter, we will consider those facts known to science and medicine.

Alcoholic Beverages

Alcohol is a sedative (See chapter 4) and is the most widely used and abused psychoactive sedative in the United States. Because of

Source and Alcoholic Content of Alcoholic Beverages

Beverage	Source	Distilled	Percent of Alcohol By Volume
Beer	Malted barley	No	4–6
Ale	Malted barley	No	6–8
Wine	Grape juice	No	12–21
Whiskey	Malted grains	Yes	40–50
Brandy	Grape juice	Yes	40–50
Rum	Molasses	Yes	40–50
Vodka	Various sources	Yes	40–50
Gin	Various sources	Yes	40–50

legal availability, the average person has a much greater chance of becoming physically dependent on alcohol than on any other psychoactive substance.

Among the many varieties of alcohol is *methyl alcohol*, commonly called "wood alcohol," which is used in many commercial products, such as antifreezes and fuels. *It must never be consumed*, since even small amounts can cause blindness and death.

A second common type of alcohol—also poisonous—is isopropyl alcohol. While it is usually called "rubbing alcohol," it is also used as a disinfectant and a solvent.

The only kind of alcohol that can be consumed safely in alcoholic drinks is *ethyl alcohol*, or *grain alcohol*. Denatured alcohol is ethyl alcohol to which poisonous chemicals have been added to prevent human use. The removal of these poisons requires complex laboratory procedures, so there is no household way to make denatured alcohol safe for drinking. Ethyl alcohol is produced from various forms of starches and sugars. Each type of carbohydrate produces a particular type of alcoholic beverage. Beer, for example, is made from fermented malted (sprouted) barley. Wine is fermented grape juice. The hard liquors are made from the distilled products of the fermentation of various grains and other plants. Because distillation greatly concentrates the alcoholic percentage of a beverage, the distilled liquors are much stronger than beer or wine and are often made into highballs, that is, diluted with water or soft drinks. The table on alcoholic content shows the percentage, distillation processing, and source of the alcohol in various common beverages.

The alcoholic content of distilled beverages is expressed as the "proof," a figure that is exactly double the alcoholic percentage. Thus 86 proof whiskey is 43 percent alcohol. The alcoholic content of wine is usually expressed directly as a percentage.

In addition to alcohol and water, alcoholic beverages contain mainly flavoring and coloring agents. They have almost no food value except calories. As shown in the following table, there are no vitamins, minerals, fats, proteins, or usable carbohydrates in most alcoholic beverages. The one exception is beer, and the amounts available are nutritionally insignificant.

Calories, however, are abundant in all alcoholic beverages. Most of the caloric value of alcoholic beverages is derived from the alcohol itself. These are "empty calories" because they must be changed into fat and then back into body sugar before they can be used—this provides nothing towards good nutrition, but displaces potentially nutritious foods from the diet. Alcohol provides just calories and nothing else.

Thus, alcohol can be described as a mood-altering drug with a significant caloric value. As a food, alcohol can be consumed with meals and will go a long way towards providing one's daily calorie requirement. But as a drug, alcohol can have serious effects on the normal functioning of the mind and body.

Alcohol is a mood-modifying substance and can temporarily produce a state of euphoria and an apparent stimulation. This, undoubtedly, is the basis of its attraction. The stimulant effect of alcohol is an illusory one, however. Actually, alcohol is

Nutritional Values of Alcoholic Beverages

Food Nutrient	Type of Beverage and Quantity		
	Beer (12 ounces)	Whiskey (2 ounces)	Wine (8 ounces)
Calories	171.0	140.0	275.0
Calories from alcohol	114.0	140.0	240.0
Protein (grams)	2.0	0.0	0.0
Fat (grams)	0.0	0.0	0.0
Carbohydrate (grams)	12.0	0.0	8.5
Thiamine (milligrams)	0.1	0.0	0.0
Nicotinic acid (milligrams)	0.75	0.0	0.0
Riboflavin (milligrams)	10.0	0.0	0.0
Ascorbic acid (milligrams)	0.0	0.0	0.0
Folic acid (milligrams)	0.0	0.0	0.0

a *depressant*; it slows down the functions of the brain and central nervous system. The first part of the brain to "go" is the center that controls judgment and inhibitions. Thus, paradoxically, alcohol stimulates drinkers for a brief period by depressing the restraining factors of their personalities. They become talkative, happy, and assume they are being witty and charming. Frequently, the stimulation will cause people to say and do things they would, if sober, prefer were left unsaid and undone.

The best quantitative measure of what is happening as a normal healthy person drinks is the blood-alcohol concentration. After a drink, alcohol shows up in the bloodstream very quickly. At first, in small amounts, alcohol is absorbed into the blood through the lining of the stomach, but this process slows and then stops just as quickly. The presence of food in the stomach impedes absorption; this is the reason many people prefer a light snack at cocktail parties—it helps modify the effects of the alcohol. Unlike the stomach, the intestinal lining absorbs alcohol rapidly, regardless of the amount of alcohol or the presence of food. Consequently, moderate and high blood-alcohol concentrations are controlled by the emptying time of the stomach. Anything that increases the emptying time of the stomach reduces the blood-alcohol concentration by spreading its absorption over a long period of time. Carbon dioxide (CO_2) is one such factor; it speeds up the passage of alcohol into the intestines. A carbonated mixer with a whiskey drink is more potent than a whiskey-and-water highball. Dissolved CO_2 is what gives champagne its extra kick.

The table on blood-alcohol levels shows the relationship between body size, number of drinks, and resultant blood-alcohol concentration. Body size is a factor because the larger the bloodstream into which the alcohol passes, the more dilute it will be. Blood-alcohol concentration levels are the basis of drunk driving determinations in almost all states. The appearance and demeanor of a suspected drunk driver has no bearing on whether he can be found guilty of driving while intoxicated. Alcohol is believed to be a contributing factor in 25 to 50 percent of all fatal traffic accidents. Although alcohol is not officially listed as the actual cause in many of these cases, it is believed that many accidents blamed on "high speed" or "failure to negotiate a curve" are actually caused by excessive drinking. Research has shown that alcohol starts to be a factor in accidents at blood levels as low as 0.03 percent.

Because all the voluntary muscles are under the control of the brain and nervous system, muscle control is impaired at all blood-alcohol levels. This results in a loss of coordination and a lengthened reaction time, and, of course, these changes are especially detrimental to automobile drivers. Some people feel that their driving ability is improved by small amounts of alcohol, but the truth is that alcohol only makes these people *think* they are driving better. Drinking drivers seldom realize how much their driving ability has deteriorated, because the same effects on the brain that cause them to be dangerous drivers also make them unaware of how poor their driving has become.

At low blood-alcohol levels, the main effect on driving is a reduction in the level of judgment and care used. Most people can still drive straight enough, but they may take chances they might otherwise not risk. With higher blood-alcohol levels, there are the additional factors of poor vision and slowed muscular reactions. As the drinker takes in more alcohol, more primitive or lower parts of the brain are de-

Blood-Alcohol Levels (Percent Alcohol in Blood)

Body Weight	Drinks[a]											
	1	2	3	4	5	6	7	8	9	10	11	12
100 lb	0.038	0.075	0.113	0.150	0.188	0.225	0.263	0.300	0.338	0.375	0.413	0.450
120 lb	0.031	0.063	0.094	0.125	0.156	0.188	0.219	0.250	0.281	0.313	0.344	0.375
140 lb	0.027	0.054	0.080	0.107	0.134	0.161	0.188	0.214	0.241	0.268	0.295	0.321
160 lb	0.023	0.047	0.070	0.094	0.117	0.141	0.164	0.188	0.211	0.234	0.258	0.281
180 lb	0.021	0.042	0.063	0.083	0.104	0.125	0.146	0.167	0.188	0.208	0.229	0.250
200 lb	0.019	0.038	0.056	0.075	0.094	0.113	0.131	0.150	0.169	0.188	0.206	0.225
220 lb	0.017	0.034	0.051	0.068	0.085	0.102	0.119	0.136	0.153	0.170	0.188	0.205
240 lb	0.016	0.031	0.047	0.063	0.078	0.094	0.109	0.125	0.141	0.156	0.172	0.188

Under 0.05	0.05 to 0.10	0.10 to 0.15	Over 0.15
Driving is not seriously impaired[b]	Driving becomes increasingly dangerous	Driving is dangerous	Driving is *very* dangerous
	0.08 legally drunk in Utah	Legally drunk in many states	Legally drunk in any state

[a]One drink equals 1 oz of 100-proof liquor or 12 oz of beer.
[b]There is substantial evidence from recent studies that drivers below the age of twenty-five may experience serious impairment of their driving skills even if their blood alcohol level is below 0.05 percent. Also, studies show that some persons with a blood alcohol level below 0.05 percent are involved in accidents. Figures in the table are "average" figures based on the "average" person under "average" conditions. Individual differences—both physiological and psychological—must be considered.

Taken from: The New Jersey Department of Law and Public Safety, Division of Motor Vehicles, Trenton, New Jersey.

pressed progressively. If extremely high levels of alcohol are in the blood, the primitive reflex centers that control breathing and other body functions may be depressed to the point that the person dies. Such high blood-alcohol levels are seldom reached through normal drinking, however, because a person usually vomits or becomes unconscious first. Nevertheless, a fatal dose of alcohol could be consumed if a person very rapidly drank a large quantity of distilled liquor.

Sight is the first sense affected by alcohol. Although small amounts of alcohol increase a person's sensitivity to light, he or she is less able to distinguish between two different intensities of light, and focusing becomes more difficult. Increasing amounts of alcohol cause a great loss of vision. Hearing is affected less than sight, but is still significantly impaired at higher blood-alcohol levels.

Alcohol interferes with both the storage and retrieval of information. When a person is under the influence of alcohol, the ability to learn and to recall past events and information is decreased. Problem-solving ability is also greatly diminished.

Even simple puzzles and arithmetic problems may be difficult or impossible for the intoxicated person to solve.

Another serious aspect of alcohol use is the chemistry of the hangover. There is considerable evidence that hangovers are due to three factors. First, the buildup of acetaldehyde causes toxic reactions in the brain. Second, part of the hangover is caused by the overactivity that is characteristic of an individual who is drinking. And third, the nausea of a hangover (or during drinking itself) is apparently caused by *congeners* (chemicals other than alcohol), which determine many of the characteristics of alcoholic beverages. Vodka, which is almost pure alcohol, is low in congeners. Bourbon whiskey, on the other hand, is high in congeners and apparently produces more nauseous hangovers than vodka. Alcohol speeds up excretion of water through the kidneys, thus causing the intense thirst usually associated with hangovers. The alcohol-induced changes in kidney function can also include a shift of water from inside the body's cells to the intracellular fluids. Over a long period of time, this shift of body water can cause the bloated look common to heavy drinkers and alcoholics.

The steady, heavy drinker and the alcoholic (a distinction we will discuss in a later section) show additional, and in some cases different, effects of drinking from those mentioned here.

For example, alcohol frequently damages the stomach of the heavy drinker. High concentrations of alcohol are definitely irritating to the stomach lining and may lead to chronic gastritis. The irritating effect of alcohol on the stomach lining is also the reason that persons who drink too much may vomit. Vomiting is a reflex action that relieves the stomach of irritating substances.

Probably the most serious organic damage caused by alcohol abuse is to the liver.

The liver is the primary chemical organ of the body. Almost 90 percent of the ethyl alcohol taken into the body is metabolized by the liver and converted into a material known as *acetaldehyde*. This chemical is toxic to many organs of the body. The acetaldehyde is then converted into carbon dioxide and water, which can then be exhaled and excreted. The liver is the basic mediator of the chemical processes that remove the alcohol from the body. The ability of the liver to handle this process determines the speed at which a person will "sober up." Generally, the conversion process can handle one drink per hour. During a 4-hour party, drinking at the rate of one drink per hour will probably not cause excessive intoxication.

Every individual has a rate at which he or she can oxidize alcohol. This rate varies among different people, but it cannot really be affected by such factors as drinking black coffee or walking in cold night air. Only time can sober up an individual.

Evidence indicates that for a long period of time, during the progression of alcoholism, prolonged drinking of more alcohol than the liver can comfortably metabolize (about a quart a day) leads to the development of a supplemental system for alcohol metabolism in the liver. Under these circumstances, the ability of the liver to metabolize alcohol may double. But this tolerance is reversed later (due to liver cell death), greatly reducing the liver's ability to metabolize alcohol.

Liver ailments are especially common among alcoholics. One such ailment is fat deposition in the liver, which is a measure of the degree of malnutrition present in the individual. Abnormal liver tests often show alcoholic hepatitis, a result of liver cell death. The lesion produced by alcoholic hepatitis is fatal to about one in ten patients or it may heal as cirrhosis (occurring in one of two cases), a hardening of the liver. Cirrhosis is six times as common among alcoholics as among the general population. Death from cirrhosis of the liver has risen to the point that in large urban areas, such as New York and Los Angeles, it is one of the major causes of death between the ages of twenty-five and forty-five. In 1974, at the University of Southern California Medical Center, cirrhosis of the liver was the number one cause of death between twenty-five and forty-five years of age. In New York, cirrhosis ranks third as a cause of death between the ages of twenty-five and sixty-five. Most of these individuals were alcoholics.

The predictability of many of the unpleasant side effects of excessive drinking is usually instrumental in helping people control their use of alcohol. After a few years of alcohol use, most people do learn how much alcohol is "enough" for mild, pleasant stimulation; how certain drinks affect their ability to function sensibly and responsibly; and what combination of beverages might be harmful or unpleasant to them.

Alcoholism as Drug Abuse

Alcoholism is probably America's number one "hidden" health problem. Behind the public attitudes and condemnation, alcoholism does extensive damage to individuals, families, and to society as a whole. The alcoholic has difficulty holding a job, continuing an education, and maintaining a stable family life. An important factor in bringing a formerly hidden disease out into the open is the potential for cure. To many people, the available treatment methods seem nebulous and difficult to understand. There is no one method, no one drug, that can provide a cure. Since it appears to people that there is little to gain from open discussion of the problem, many people will choose to avoid dealing with the problem of alcoholism.

What Is Alcoholism? There is no clear-cut, widely accepted definition of the word *alcoholism*. Some people would suggest so simple a definition as "an alcoholic is someone who drinks too much." But what is "too much" drinking? With alcohol, as with any mood-modifying substance, there are levels of use. The *moderate drinker* is an occasional user who enjoys the social, personal, and emotional gratification of alcohol and who enjoys the company of individuals surrounding the "social" use of the drug. A *heavy drinker* is a regular user who, for at least a year, drinks daily and has six or more drinks on one occasion at least twice a month, or has six or more drinks at least once a week for over a year—but who shows no personal or physical problem related to alcohol consumption. A *problem drinker* is a heavy drinker with alcohol-related problems, but not enough such problems to be classified as an alcoholic.

An *alcoholic* is a heavy drinker who has alcohol-related problems in at least three of the following four areas:
1. Marital problems, or social dispproval of drinking by spouse, friends, or parents.
2. Job trouble, traffic arrests, or other police trouble.
3. Frequent "blackouts," tremors, or other physical symptoms of severe alcohol toxicity and physical dependence.
4. Loss of control (inability to control amount of alcohol consumed at one time), and morning drinking.

The most widely accepted definition of alcoholism is that of the American Medical Association and the World Health Organization: *An alcoholic is a person whose drinking interferes with a major aspect of life on a continuing basis.*

The National Council on Alcoholism, a voluntary health organization, and Alcoholics Anonymous distribute twenty questions that were originally used by

Johns Hopkins University Hospital (Baltimore, Maryland), as a test to see if someone is an alcoholic:

1. Do you lose time from school or work due to drinking?
2. Is drinking making your life at home unhappy?
3. Do you drink because you are shy with other people?
4. Is drinking affecting your reputation?
5. Have you often felt sorry after drinking?
6. Are you in financial difficulties as a result of drinking?
7. Do you turn to lower companions and an inferior environment when drinking?
8. Does your drinking make you careless of you or your family's welfare?
9. Has your ambition decreased since you started drinking?
10. Do you feel you "really need a drink" at a definite time daily?
11. Do you want a drink the morning after drinking?
12. Does your drinking cause you to have difficulty in sleeping?
13. Has your efficiency decreased since you started drinking?
14. Is drinking jeopardizing your education, job, or business?
15. Do you drink to escape from worries or trouble?
16. Do you drink alone?
17. Have you ever had a complete loss of memory while drinking?
18. Has your physician ever treated you for drinking?
19. Do you drink to build up your self-confidence?
20. Have you ever been to a hospital or institution because of drinking?

If a person answered yes to any one of the questions, he or she may be an alcoholic, or in danger of becoming an alcoholic. If answering yes to any two of the questions; the individual is probably an alcoholic. If he or she answered yes to three or more, he or she is definitely an alcoholic.

Alcoholism Despite years of research efforts at a cost of millions of dollars, the causes of alcoholism are still not definitely known. Many theories have been presented, some of which are backed by extensive scientific evidence, while some are pure speculation. It has not been clearly determined whether alcoholism is caused by physical factors, psychological factors, or a combination of the two. Each theory has strong supporters. There is certainly reason to believe that personality problems are a facet of alcoholism. Yet there is also evidence that some people simply respond differently to alcohol. This variability is probably related to some metabolic problem such as the lack of an enzyme that prohibits the normal processing and removal of alcohol from the liver. Possibly, some factor in brain action is also involved in alcoholism. All authorities today do agree that alcoholism should be thought of as a disease, regardless of its cause, and that the alcoholic should be treated as an ill person, rather than condemned as a sinner or a good-for-nothing. Public acceptance of other drug abusers as "ill" individuals is taking a longer period of time.

Certain personality traits are commonly found among alcoholics. The alcoholic typically has a low sense of personal worth, and therefore feels insecure and isolated from other people. These feelings cause emotional pain, and drink helps wipe out this pain. These feelings are also found among drug abusers and overeaters.

When drinking does become associated with family problems, it is of prime importance to determine whether the drinking is the cause of the family problems or a symptom of a deeper personal emotional problem. In the past, alcohol was automatically held responsible for family poverty, divorce, child neglect, juvenile delinquency, and most other family problems. Today alcoholism is often recognized as being one of several complex emotional problems. However, a vicious circle often develops in which personal and family problems lead to excess drinking, which leads to further family problems, which leads to the eventual destruction of the family unit.

The police spend much of their time and effort in handling problems associated with the abuse of alcohol. Many of these cases involve relatively minor offenses, such as drunkenness in a public place, being drunk and disorderly, or "vagrancy." But others have become involved in much more serious offenses, such as felonious traffic violations, assault, and murder. For example, in half of all murders in the United States, either the killer or the victim, or both, had been drinking at the time of the crime.

Stages of Alcoholism In trying to deal with the consequences of alcohol abuse, society has been forced to rely on the consistent patterns and few predictable sides of the problem—in the absence of definite knowledge of causes and cures.

No one ever decides to become an alcoholic. Almost every new drinker assumes that he or she will always be able to handle liquor—and this assumption is almost always right. But there is no way to predict which drinker will be the one who does develop the disease of alcoholism. The great majority of those becoming alcoholics do not even realize what is happening to them until it is too late to stop.

Fortunately, there are ways in which a person can observe signs of developing alcoholism. Recognition of the incipient problem requires both knowledge of the

warning signals and the honesty to admit the seriousness of what is happening. There is often only one remedy—to stop drinking—and it requires a good deal of strength and determination to seek out this one cure.

As they become dependent on alcohol, many people learn to appreciate and rely on the feelings of relief from tensions and escape from reality that alcohol can provide. The first step toward alcoholism occurs when a person starts to drink specifically for these effects. About one-fifth of all drinkers can be classified as *occasional*

Photo © Leonard Freed/Magnum

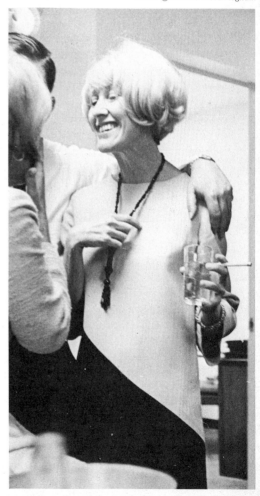

escape drinkers. These people are not yet alcoholics, but they should be aware of the possible development of the condition. In those who are progressing toward alcoholism, escape drinking becomes more and more frequent. It may quickly develop into a pattern of heavy drinking every night or every weekend.

Another pattern of developing alcoholism that should not be ignored is the "binge" pattern. The binge, or periodic, drinker may go for weeks or months without drinking any alcohol, but then goes on a drinking spree that lasts for days or even weeks. The periodic drinker may be just as much an alcoholic as the regular drinker. He or she is even more likely to lose a job, because of the habit of staying drunk for days at a time.

An *alcoholic blackout* is a period of temporary amnesia. It should not be confused with passing out, which involves unconsciousness. Anyone who drinks too much will pass out. He or she will then be unconscious or asleep. Passing out is not a sign of alcoholism; it merely indicates the drinker's own poor judgment or lack of experience with alcohol—or, of course, a desire to reach a state of temporary oblivion.

A blackout is something else entirely. It may occur after the drinker has taken just a few drinks. The drinker remains conscious and appears fully aware of what is going on. He or she may appear normal to others, and may seem fully capable of walking, talking, driving, dancing, and drinking as usual.

But after finishing drinking, the drinker who has had a blackout will have no memory of what took place while drinking. He or she will remember neither the major events nor the minor details. The memory will have "blacked out" everything that happened after the first few drinks. A blackout usually lasts for several hours.

During a binge, however, it may last for several days.

Anyone who has had such a blackout either *is* an alcoholic or is very nearly so. Blackouts usually occur after several months or years of drinking, but some alcoholics report that they experienced blackouts from the very beginning of their drinking.

The most important symptom of alcoholism is *loss of control*. This means that the alcoholic cannot stop at a reasonable number of drinks, but must continue until drunk or sick. Depending on the drinking pattern of the individual, such drinking will continue for hours, days, or even weeks. Loss of control does not mean that the alcoholic cannot choose whether or not to drink on a certain day. But if the alcoholic does take a single drink, he or she cannot really determine when to stop.

Alcoholism is a progressive disease. Every case of alcoholism develops at its own speed. Some alcoholics reach an advanced state in just a few months. Others take many years to reach a pattern of problem drinking.

The alcoholic has several defense mechanisms that partially deal with the guilt resulting from his or her drinking problem. He or she may appear extremely jovial, but the remorse felt will show itself in crying jags and serious periods of depression.

Most alcoholics have problems with employment and finances. Intoxication on the job is usually grounds for dismissal from any position. Once a person has been fired for drinking, it becomes very difficult to find another job. In the face of such seeming failure to earn a living, the alcoholic may go on spending sprees, making extravagant investments and purchases. As self-esteem sinks lower, he or she tries to establish social position by buying drinks for total strangers.

The female alcoholic generally reaches the extreme stages of the syndrome faster than a man. In previous years, a woman with a drinking problem could hide her illness in the home. But like many aspects of alcoholism, the problem among women is now subject to more examination and treatment. Boredom, dissatisfaction with a life bound to the home, and marital difficulties are frequently cited as causes of alcoholism among women.

Many of alcoholism's effects on marriage are the results of the financial strains just described. Money problems always place a strain on marriage, but when these problems are the direct result of the excessive drinking of one spouse, the other spouse is likely to be highly resentful.

Other problems in the alcoholic's marriage result from the family's loss of companionship and, in some cases, the abuse of family members while the alcoholic is under the effects of alcohol.

The alcoholic's family tends to become socially isolated. Members no longer bring friends home because they fear embarrassment by the alcoholic's actions. This fear is an especially painful problem for children who can never be free of the fear that an alcoholic parent may be at home and intoxicated at any time of the day or evening.

Another problem in the alcoholic's marriage is jealousy. This is one of the many cause-and-effect dilemmas of alcoholism. Some alcoholics give a spouse's infidelity as a reason for their drinking problem, while others recognize that the drinking problem has ruined the marriage and driven a spouse into an extramarital relationship.

The alcoholic often suffers a loss of sexual drive. As the sexual relationship in the marriage deteriorates and intercourse becomes less frequent, the alcoholic tends to blame the deterioration on anything but the real cause—alcohol-induced reduction of sexual drive. Very often, the alcoholic's spouse is then accused of having extramarital love affairs. And it is this suspicion and jealousy that can lead to the eventual end of the marriage.

True Alcohol Addiction The basis of the physical addiction in alcoholism seems to be an altered metabolism that is alcohol-induced and that produces chemicals in the body similar to those produced in opiate addicts. Alcoholism and drug addiction are similar processes, the major differences are the length of time and the dosage required for development of physical dependence. In 1970, the Expert Committee on Alcohol and Alcoholism of the World Health Organization stated: that recent evidence makes it appear that there is more resemblance between the responses of the withdrawal from alcohol and from opiates than was previously realized . . . when serious symptoms follow the withdrawal of alcohol they persist almost as long as do those following the withdrawal of opiates. Consequently, the World Health Organization now defines physical dependence as either *narcotic-solvent abstinence-syndrome type addiction* or *alcohol-barbiturate abstinence-syndrome type addiction*.

When a physically dependent alcoholic is suddenly withdrawn from alcohol, extreme hypersensitivity to all external stimuli usually appears within a week after the alcohol blood levels return to normal. Such hypersensitivity in its most extreme form (delirium tremens or convulsions) is *alcohol-barbiturate abstinence syndrome* and requires emergency medical treatment. This is caused by a return of function to previously anesthetized neurons, aggravated by prolonged magnesium and potassium deficiency. Many physicians believe that magnesium deficiency is responsible for the alcohol-withdrawal syndrome and often treat it with magnesium compounds.

After several attacks of delirium tremens, a very serious condition called "wet brain" may develop. This is a chronic or long-term condition, seldom curable, and often fatal. The alcoholic's thought processes are completely disrupted. All functions of his nervous system are impaired. The alcoholic who reaches this stage will either die or spend the rest of his or her life in an institution.

Treatment of Alcoholism Most chronic alcoholics do not voluntarily stop drinking. Even if an alcoholic could stop, he or she would risk serious or even fatal withdrawal symptoms. An alcoholic must, therefore, have intensive medical treatment during the sobering-up ("drying-out") period. He or she may require hospitalization during this time. Such drugs as minor tranquilizers, insulin, thiamine, magnesium compounds, and caffeine may be used in the treatment. Once alcoholics have passed through the more serious physical parts of the withdrawal period, many therapists feel that alcoholics must never take another drink and generally should seek continuing treatment the rest of their lives.

Some therapists are using the phrase "uncontrolled drinker" in place of "problem drinker" and "alcoholic." Uncontrolled drinkers are individuals who refuse to stop drinking regardless of the environmental and personal consequences. These individuals are unable to control their emotional impulses or direct their energies towards appropriate tasks. Behind this reluctance to stop drinking are the following factors:

1. An inadequate ability to deal with internal distress and emotional organization.
2. A lack of alternatives to drinking as a coping mechanism.
3. An inability of their lives to fulfill their *basic human needs* and produce "peak" experiences (periods of extreme pleasure).
4. An inability to feel "themselves" as a result of the anesthetic effects of alcohol.
5. The illusion that they are "happy drunks" most of the time.
6. A deep fear that they will not be able to stop drinking despite their efforts.

These therapists feel there are three different types of uncontrolled drinkers. First, there is the person whose alcohol (or poly-drug) use is seriously interfering with life, but who does not accept that drinking is the reason for his or her problems. Second is the person who acknowledges that alcohol is a problem and freely admits that they have to stop drinking, and want to stop, but think that they cannot. Third is the most difficult and frustrating type of uncontrolled drinker—the person who admits that alcohol is creating health, family, employment, or legal problems, but who enjoys drinking, receives pleasure from it and does not want to stop. Their personalities are very complex, and often the following pressures or threats are the only means of stopping all drinking:

1. A mandate from a physician that the person will not live long if he or she continues to drink.
2. An ultimatum by a spouse or family that they will leave the alcoholic or kick him or her out of the house.
3. An ultimatum that the alcoholic will lose his or her job.
4. The legal suspension of a driving license, or jail.

This type of uncontrolled drinker has been manipulated and coerced into treatment to change behavior that the drinker really does not want to change. If this person will accept complete abstinence from alcohol and other mood-modifying drugs, classical types of treatment *may* work. But most often this insistence upon abstinence as the only possible treatment may be unrealistic. Some therapists feel this person can be brought into a "controlled drinking schedule" (meaning a specific amount of alcohol, at a specific time, under specific social conditions) through an *awareness process*, where the drinker and therapist agree upon a "contract" between them.

The other two types of uncontrolled drinkers are not fully aware of how much he or she is currently drinking. They have been told they are drinking too much but are not fully aware of what this really means. In these cases the awareness process is to make them aware of their drinking behavior and responsible for changing it.

The first step is to have them review their drinking habits and establish the quality, quantity, circumstances, and financial cost of their drinking behavior. The second step is to have the person keep an accurate record of each day's drinking—quality, quantity, circumstances, and the cost. The drinker is then asked to evaluate the financial and personal costs of his or her drinking behavior. This process develops an awareness of the drinking behavior, and records the costs and motivations for drinking. The third step consists of a study of the structure and function of the drinking behavior. What aspect of the drinking does the individual like, what part does he or she get something from? what part is not liked? and what are the negative effects? The fourth step consists of detailing the "solutions" that alcohol is providing the individual and some mutually acceptable alternatives. The fifth step is the development of alternatives to the real problems faced, such as handling anger, anxiety, and awkwardness. Finally, the individual becomes fully aware of the extent of his or her use and abuse of alcohol. The cessation of the use of alcohol as a means of coping lets the individual use his or her own resources. When the person reaches this step of awareness, he or she begins to change from a focus on drinking to an awareness of themselves, other people, and the world. Such individual awareness is the unstated but understood goal of most psychoactive drug abuse treatment.

Psychotherapy   Since alcoholism is at least partly the result of emotional illness, it is understandable that one approach to its treatment is psychotherapy. The success of psychotherapy depends greatly on the amount of understanding the therapist has of the personality of an alcoholic. It is very difficult for someone who has never been an alcoholic to understand what it means to be one. Group psychotherapy is becoming increasingly important, because alcoholics really do understand each other. This approach has some similarity to that of Alcoholics Anonymous.

Aversion Therapy   This type of therapy involves the use of drugs, or other methods that make a person sick if he drinks alcohol. These can be administered in two ways. One is by a daily dosage of a drug such as Antabuse (Disulfiram), which causes unpleasant bodily reactions if any alcohol—even a small amount—is consumed. Breathing becomes difficult, the heart pounds, and nausea and vomiting occur. As long as a person is taking Antabuse, he or she is not likely to drink. This drug is sometimes taken for months or years. For Antabuse to be successful, the patient must want to stop drinking; otherwise he or she will simply stop taking the drug.

Another type of aversion therapy that sometimes works is to give alcoholics a drink of alcohol along with a drug that makes them sick. After several of these treatments, they may develop a conditioned reflex so that alcohol alone makes them sick.

The problem with either type of aversion therapy is that severe psychotic symptoms may occur if the alcoholic is suddenly deprived of the escape. Most alcoholics have become dependent on alcohol as an escape from life; if no effective psychotherapy is given or if it cannot provide replacement, they may undergo severe emotional stress and disintegration.

Alcoholics Anonymous   One of the most successful approaches to the treatment of alcoholism has been that of Alcoholics Anonymous (commonly called A.A.). It is believed that A.A. has the greatest recovery rate—75 percent of those who *want* to stop drinking—of all methods of treatment for alcoholism.

Alcoholics Anonymous is an organization whose only purpose is to help its members stay sober. Today, almost every city has regularly meeting A.A. groups ranging in size from a handful of members to over a hundred. A large city might have groups meeting every night of the week. There are even special groups for teen-age alcoholics and for spouses and children of alcoholics.

The approach taken by A.A. is that of group therapy. Like the "dope fiends" of Synanon groups, which to some extent are patterned after A.A. meetings, alcoholics often find a deep personal, emotional, and spiritual experience through close association and conversation with others who have shared the experience of addiction. An evening's program usually consists of several members telling informally how miserable their lives were during their drinking years and how they have changed since joining A.A. New members often find that these admitted alcoholics have had experiences similar to theirs. They can identify with the older member, who "speaks their language." As they tell of their past experiences, the older members are helped too. The stories serve as a constant reminder of the unhappiness of their periods of drinking and help to prevent a return to drinking.

Alcoholics Anonymous does not claim to cure the alcoholic; rather it feels it helps him or her stop drinking and regain sobriety. A.A. emphasizes that an alcoholic is always an alcoholic, even when not drinking; if one starts drinking again, he or she would still drink in an alcoholic manner. For this reason, members always begin their personal stories by stating "I am an alcoholic."

There are many cases where members of A.A. decided, after years of sobriety, to try a return to social drinking. These attempts are never successful. Alcoholics Anonymous can only help those who have a strong desire to stop drinking forever and are *aware* that their drinking behavior is the basis of their personal, social, or economic problems.

The Making of an Alcoholic

As we have seen, there are no clear definitions of problem drinking and alcoholism—both are forms of compulsive drug abuse. But there are about 10 million Americans whose drinking has created some problem for themselves or their families, employer, or the police *within the last year*.

Many psychologists feel that serving a child a colorful nonalcoholic drink made of ginger ale and maraschino cherry juice (a "Shirley Temple"), which simulates the appearance of an adult alcoholic cocktail, is the first step. Serving children such a drink encourages them to adopt an adult habit in order to gain adult approval. Many alcoholics report learning, at an early age, that alcohol is a symbol of fun. Children should be taught that alcohol is not a harmless social beverage, but a dangerous drug. Also, in recent years, parents have seemed relatively unconcerned about their children's drinking habits. They are panic stricken when their child uses marijuana, but merely send a drunk youngster to bed quietly. This inconsistent behavior is caused by the abundance of scare information concerning marijuana and the legal and social disapproval of marijuana. Actually, many teen-agers use both marijuana and alcohol.

The use of alcohol by young people has been accelerated by the inexpensive "pop" wines. These wines help make the transition from soda pop to alcohol very easy. The alcohol is disguised with sweet fruit flavors and most young people treat them as just an adult soft drink. Actually, this "kid stuff" contains 9 percent alcohol; more than twice as much as beer. With the pop-wine phase behind them, they go on to distilled alcoholic drinks. The following table sets forth some effects of alcoholic beverages.

Young people are often multiple or poly-drug users. Many experts feel this situation occurs because of the social acceptance of psychoactive drugs other than alcohol, such as marijuana. Also, the widespread misuse of methadone treatment programs has changed the pattern of abuse of alcohol and other drugs. Some narcotic addicts now turn to alcohol as an alternative, legally available drug. Sedatives, stimulants, and minor tranquilizers are being mixed with alcohol—into "cocktails." Such poly-drug use has greatly increased overdose deaths and complicated withdrawal syndromes that often are not recognized until it is too late to save the patient.

Most teen-agers who begin to drink do so at home under parental supervision and approval. Much of this drinking occurs on holidays or as part of family and social occasions. Whether and how much a person drinks are strongly associated with sex, age, ethnic background, religious affiliation, education, socioeconomic status, occupation, area of residence, and degree of urbanization.

The highest proportion of heavy drinkers among men occurs between the ages of eighteen to twenty and thirty-five to thirty-nine. Women between the ages of twenty-one and twenty-nine are more likely to be heavy drinkers. The largest number of drinkers (in the range from social through alcoholics) is found in the younger age groups (to twenty-four years). Larger numbers of abstainers are found among older persons. Problem drinkers and alcoholics tend to be infrequent among ethnic groups whose drinking habits are well integrated with the rest of their culture. Irish-Americans demonstrate a higher rate of problem drinking than other American groups of the same social class. Conservative religious groups show the lowest percentage of drinkers of any group. Those who attend church often are more likely to be infrequent drinkers.

Some Effects of Alcoholic Beverages

Amount of Alcoholic Beverage Consumed		Concentration of Alcohol found in the Blood (in %)	Effects		Time required for alcohol to be oxidized (hours)
1	highball (1½ oz. whiskey)	0.03	Slight changes in feelings		2
1	cocktail (1½ oz. whiskey)				
3½	oz. fortified wine				
5½	oz. wine or pop wine				
2	bottles beer (24 oz.)				
2	highballs	0.06 (0.08— Legally drunk in Utah)		Feelings of warmth, emotional relaxation, slight decrease in fine skills. Less concern with minor irritations and social restraints.	4
2	cocktails				
7	oz. fortified wine		Increasing effects with variation of individuals and within the same individual at different times.		
11	oz. wine or pop wine				
4	bottles beer				
3	highballs	0.09 (0.10— Legally drunk in many states)		Emotional buoyancy, exaggerated emotions and behavior. Person talkative, noisy or morose.	6
3	cocktails				
10½	oz. fortified wine				
15½	oz. (1 pt.) wine or pop wine				
6	bottles beer				
4	highballs	0.12		Impairment of fine coordination, clumsiness. Slight to moderate unsteadiness in standing or walking. Loss of peripheral vision.	8
4	cocktails				
14	oz. fortified wine				
22	oz. wine or pop wine				
8	bottles beer (3 qts.)				
5	highballs	0.15 (Legally drunk in all states)	Intoxication, unmistakable abnormality of body and mental control.		10
5	cocktails				
17½	oz. fortified wine				
27½	oz. wine or pop wine				
½	pint whiskey				

NOTE: Based upon individual of "average" size (150 pounds). See table entitled Blood-Alcohol Levels (Percent Alcohol in Blood) to see effects on individuals of varying weights.

Amount of education is strongly related to whether a person drinks and to the quantity consumed. The highest proportion of abstainers is found among persons with less than an eighth-grade education. The proportion of heavy drinkers increases fairly steadily with educational level until reaching the college graduate. There is a slight decrease in heavy drinkers among persons with postgraduate degrees. Moderate and heavy drinkers increase as social class rises. Farm owners have the lowest proportion of drinkers, whereas professional men and businessmen have the highest proportion of heavy drinkers, while female service workers have the highest proportion of heavy female drinkers. Alcohol consumption varies considerably by geographic region. There are more drinkers in New England, the Middle Atlantic states, and the Pacific Coast than elsewhere in the country.

The Proper Use of Alcoholic Beverages

There are some people who argue that any consumption of alcoholic beverages is improper. But the majority of Americans find no medical, moral, legal, or religious reason for not making moderate use of alcoholic beverages. We shall therefore offer some suggestions that may help a person avoid drinking problems.

Even those people who fully approve of drinking and themselves drink regularly usually disapprove of certain types of drinking behavior, for example, drunken driving or such antisocial behavior as physical or verbal violence. Almost all those who approve of drinking do feel that there are times and places where drinking is not appropriate. Any time when a person needs his or her fullest mental facilities, such as when driving, flying or operating machinery, is obviously a poor time to drink. For many employers, drinking or being drunk on the job is grounds for immediate dismissal. It is very poor policy to drink for courage, for example, in preparation for a job interview or sales conference. This is using alcohol as a crutch and is a step in the direction of alcoholism.

There is, of course, no set answer for the question of how much to drink. While drinking is acceptable in American society, getting drunk is definitely frowned upon. The person who drinks is expected to drink in moderation, without serious impairment of physical or mental functions.

The social drinker learns to drink slowly and to pace his drinking so that he does not build up a high blood-alcohol level.

If a person who can oxidize the alcohol from one drink each hour spaces four drinks over the span of a four-hour party, he or she will not reach an excessively high blood-alcohol level.

The host or hostess of a party at which drinks are served should feel a certain responsibility for the amount of alcohol the guests drink. They must ask themselves how they would feel if someone was involved in a fatal accident after leaving their home. There should be nonalcoholic drinks available for those who prefer them, and the person who prefers not to drink should not be pressured or ridiculed. No pressure should be put on any guest to drink more than he or she really wants. If guests want to stop at one drink, they should be allowed to. During the last hour or so of a party, coffee should be served. This serves several purposes. Coffee does not counteract alcohol, but the caffeine may help overcome the drowsiness that can be as much a cause of accidents as intoxication. The time spent drinking coffee serves as a "sobering-up" period, as well. Finally, the serving of coffee is accepted by most guests as a signal that the party is about over so the host or hostess can bring a party to a close when they wish to. Anyone who is obviously in no condition to drive home should be strongly encouraged to stay overnight, take a taxi, share a ride, or *anything* other than drive.

In Conclusion The last few pages have summarized a substantial portion of what science can contribute on the subject of alcohol use. A large part of the task of developing sensible and enjoyable attitudes toward alcohol thus rests on the individual. Undoubtedly, the people who really enjoy alcohol the most are those who use it properly.

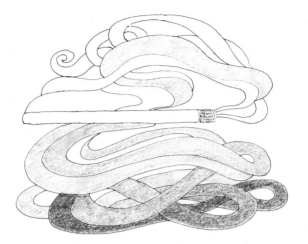

7

THE EFFECTS OF TOBACCO

In 1972, U.S. Surgeon General Jesse L. Steinfeld stated that "cigarette smoking is deadly." His statement officially acknowledged that tobacco smoking is probably the most wide-spread and dangerous drug usage in the United States. More people smoke, and show the harmful effects, than is the case with any of the substances mentioned previously. To challenge the smoking habit is to challenge a habit of nearly 48 million Americans; however, this habit has not always been so widespread. Cigarette consumption in the United States has generally been subject to certain predictable factors. For example, the greatest increases in smoking have occurred during wars. As shown by the graph on cigarette consumption, a brisk rise began in 1915. World War II produced another jump; the rise between 1942 and 1946 (the actual war years) was extremely sharp.

The main reason for this periodic increase is that during a time of national crisis the population in general experiences increased tension. Facts that might ordinarily go unquestioned, moreover, such as the impressive evidence that smoking is harmful, no longer seem important when the whole nation is under such stress. Another reason for this increase during wartime is that young service personnel are introduced to smoking as a tension reliever and morale booster. Many of today's habitual smokers were first introduced to cigarettes with the gift packages donated by charities and cigarette companies during the war. Only in recent years have military hospital administrators stopped the practice of gift cartons being given to ill or convalescing service personnel. Many cigarette companies have long encouraged the development of the smoking habit by giving away cigarettes through their "representatives" on college campuses.

Certain government actions have substantially changed this picture. In 1970, Congress passed the Public Health Cigarette Smoking Act, which prohibited the broadcasting of cigarette commercials on TV or radio after January 2, 1971. Cigarette advertising has had two purposes. First, it helps develop brand loyalties, and emphasizes the differences between basically similar tobacco products. This goal is accomplished by the creation of an image for the product and for the type of people who choose a particular brand. Secondly, cigarette advertising encourages young people to take up smoking in the first place, and this is the reason the government has sought to control cigarette advertising.

The cigarette advertising industry is immense and powerful. Through 1970 and into 1971, the cigarette companies strengthened their campaigns in the printed media. Estimated newspaper ads

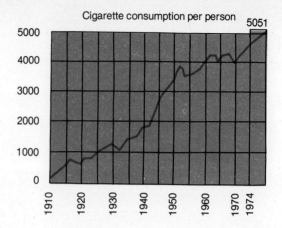

A profile of the growth of cigarette consumption in the United States between 1910 and 1974. These figures include nonsmokers and smokers 15 years old and over.

Compiled from United States Department of Agriculture, Economic Research Service Publications.

rose during this time from $16 million in 1969 to between $50 and $75 million; magazine advertising rose from $10 million to about $40 million; and billboards went from $2 million to $6 million. In 1970, anticigarette campaigns of the United States Public Health Service National Clearinghouse on Smoking and Health spent about $500,000. The American Cancer Society spent some $700,000 in its efforts, and other voluntary health agencies and public service groups were only able to spend an additional $500,000. Consequently, only about $1,700,000 could be spent to counteract a campaign of between $96 and $121 million spent to promote cigarette smoking.

The tobacco industry circumvented the federal control of TV advertising by introducing the little cigar in 1972 and 1973. These are the size of cigarettes and have the advantage of not being labeled as being as much of a health hazard as cigarettes are. Also, their access to TV and radio advertising is uncontrolled. TV advertising is presenting these cigars the same way it presented cigarettes in the past—as part of a life-style most young people find attractive and exciting, full of beautiful people, enjoyable activities, and interesting places. Physical appeal, success in business, and other positive attributes are consistently associated, by advertising, with a particular brand and with smoking in general.

Furthermore, at the same time the government was launching its antismoking campaign, it continued a multimillion dollar tobacco subsidy program. The U.S. Department of Agriculture (USDA) provides the tobacco industry with free grading and inspection of its products (a service paid for by the producers of all food products such as fruits and vegetables), which is estimated to cost us (as taxpayers) about $2.9 million a year. Former Surgeon General Luther Terry urged an end to tobacco industry supports, saying "the expenditure of 73.2 million dollars of taxpayers' funds in the support of the tobacco industry is inconceivable in the face of known health facts" (American Society Fact Sheet: New York, 1972).

The Extent of Smoking

The use of tobacco by Americans has increased tremendously since the turn of the century. In 1900 the consumption rate was less than 50 cigarettes per year per person (both smokers and nonsmokers, 18 years of age and over). By 1930 this had risen to 1,389 cigarettes consumed per person per year, and then to 4,345 in 1963 (when this continual increase ended). Internal Revenue Service statistics on cigarette sales taxes show that in late 1967 and early 1968 there began a drop in per-person consumption of cigarettes. According to figures published by the National Clearinghouse for Smoking and Health, 33.8 percent of men smoking in 1966 had quit by 1970 and 25.4 percent of the women smoking in 1966 had quit during that same period. This trend reversed and smoking started to rise in 1971 (3,960 cigarettes consumed per person), during the first year of the television cigarette commercial ban. Contributing to this rise is the increase in smoking by women and teen-agers promoted by aggressive advertising in magazines. The consumption rose through 1974 (5,051 cigarettes per person) and has continued to rise since then. During the 1970s the percentage of women in the United States who smoke has increased until over 30 percent now smoke.

Who Has Stopped While 25 percent of male smokers who stopped stayed off cigarettes, only 11 percent of females have continued to stay away from cigarettes. Also, during this period individuals in the 14- to 18-year-old range have increased along the same lines as the women. If this trend continues through the 1970s the heaviest smoking population will be the 25- to 34-year-olds, especially females (50.6 percent of males and 38.6 percent of females).

Despite public information campaigns on the subject, too few smokers realize the degree and extent of damage to their bodies associated with cigarette smoking. Early morning hacking and smoker's cough are so common that millions of Americans consider these "normal," rather than signals that warn of damage to the body. Each day in the United States, 2,060 people die of heart attacks, 220 of lung cancer, and 150 from other cigarette-related diseases. Minor ailments directly related to smoking compete with the common cold as major causes of time lost from work and school.

It is very disturbing that the greatest number of smoking women (38.6 percent) is in the age group 25 to 44, which include the critical childbearing years (25 to 34). Women who smoke during pregnancy affect two lives—mother and child. They also have more spontaneous abortions, stillbirths, and premature babies than do nonsmokers.

Rights of the Nonsmoker

Studies have shown that exposure of anyone to a "smoking environment" causes measurable effects in their body. These include increased heart rate, blood pressure, and amount of carbon dioxide in the blood. Other possible effects individuals may feel include eye and nose irritation, headache, sore throat, cough, hoarseness, nausea, and dizziness. Because of the uncomfortable feelings of nonsmokers, air carriers have agreed to set aside nonsmoking areas. The American Medical Association has asked member doctors to keep people from smoking in their waiting rooms. In 1971 the Interstate Commerce Commission issued a regulation requiring separate seating on all interstate buses for smokers and nonsmokers. Since this time hotels have set aside nonsmoking floors. States and cities have outlawed smoking in public buildings and on public transportation. And many restaurants also have nonsmoking areas.

Smoking in the presence of a nonsmoker should be considered "an act of aggression." Cigarette smokers in a crowded, ill-ventilated room or automobile can raise the level of carbon monoxide to a point dangerous to one's health. Experiments show that in a small room a smoker can raise the level of carbon monoxide to 50 parts per million. At this level, after an hour and a half, a nonsmoker can have trouble discriminating time intervals and visual and auditory cues. The right of smokers to enjoy their habit is frequently cited in opposition to antismoking regulations. However, the rights of nonsmokers to a clean, smoke-free environment must also be recognized. Nonsmokers definitely should feel free to discourage smoking in their presence, especially in their homes.

The Smoking Habit

As early as 1967 the World Conference on Smoking and Health concluded that the individuals who exhibit a continuing need to smoke show a dependence that is similar to all other major forms of drug dependence. The evidence seems to indicate that there are two basic groups of dependent smokers. In one group the dependence is more psychosocial and giving up smoking is relatively easy, involving little physical discomfort. The other group of smokers seems to be physically dependent on tobacco. In this case the dependence is harder to eliminate, and withdrawal symptoms are definitely present. Because of the large number of deaths linked directly to cigarettes, smoking is the most dangerous form of drug abuse in the United States today.

Substances in Tobacco Smoke Of all the substances known to be present in tobacco smoke, only nicotine has effects that could produce the dependence associated with smoking. This statement is based on established scientific facts concerning the properties of nicotine, the descriptions of symptoms given by those who smoke (or try to stop smoking), and comparisons made with other drug abuses.

Forming the Smoking Habit A person's first experiences with smoking tobacco are usually tied to psychological and social pressures. A person with this extent of dependence falls into the psychosocial category, and can smoke or not at will. As a result, this smoker may have periods of smoking and abstention throughout his or her lifetime. The smoking periods will be in response to peer, social, or psychological pressures. But the continued use of tobacco is encouraged, reinforced, and then made habitual by the dependence-producing effects of nicotine. The effect of tobacco on the smoker seems to be that of a stimulant and can be followed by depression, depending on the person's real or imagined reaction to smoking. But whatever the particular reaction, nicotine-free tobacco, or cigarettes made from other plant materials (such as lettuce), do not satisfy smokers.

As mentioned earlier, the years from the early teens to the early twenties are the years in which a majority of people begin to develop the habits and social patterns that will cause them to start to smoke or to become smokers later. Two factors help explain why young people begin smoking: (1) the desire to imitate those around them, and (2) the wish for adult status. In many cases there is a relationship between smoking and a need for status among friends and peer groups, an increase of self-assurance, and a desire to feel or appear more mature. Psychiatrists see smoking behavior as an accelerated striving for social status in the sense that the beginning smoker is often trying to show an adultlike need for personal and social standing.

A strong relationship has been found to exist between parents' and youngsters' smoking habits. Apparently, parents' smoking habits influence the age at which children take up smoking more than it influences whether the children will be smokers or nonsmokers. Consequently, many authorities believe that the most effective way to cut down smoking among young people is to decrease smoking among their parents.

It should also be noted that many studies reveal that the health damage is greater among individuals who start cigarette smoking early in life than among those who start later. Also, the ability of an individual to stop smoking whenever desired is clearly related to how long he or she has been smoking.

There have been a few scientific studies of the personal and social reasons for smoking. Evidence suggests that early smoking is linked with self-esteem and status-seeking in ambitious young people. The pattern or style of living an individual seeks within the family, community, and peer group seems to have a strong influence on smoking behavior. A permissive cultural climate (one in which smoking is

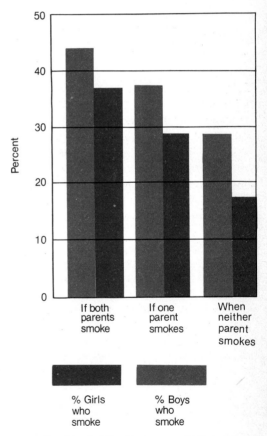

Smoking habits of teenagers and their parents. A large majority of teen-age smokers come from homes where one or both parents smoke.

Taken from American Cancer Society, Profile 1970.

readily permitted) results in an increase of smoking among young people, especially among those who tend to conform to the society's liberal standards.

Although no "smoker personality" has been shown to exist, certain common personality traits have been reported among smokers. Smokers tend to be extroverted (outgoing) people who place a strong emphasis on immediate pleasure. Because smokers often take a large part in various social activities, they are placed in situations that reinforce their smoking habits. They are also more open to suggestions from social influences and friends.

Generally, it seems that different personality types tend to establish specific smoking habits. The pipe and cigar smokers often look for sedation in smoking. The cigarette smoker more often wants stimulation. Consequently, very few cigarette smokers can change to pipes or cigars and be as satisfied as they were with cigarettes.

Stress seems to be conducive to smoking, as it is to so many other habits. Tense or challenging situations contribute to the beginning of the smoking habit, its continuation, and to the number of cigarettes a person smokes. Increased experiences of stress among young people, together with social situations favorable to smoking, may set off experiments with smoking. Later, tense or strained situations tend to reinforce or strengthen the habit. By the time a smoker has developed the habit, he or she may respond to even the slightest tension by reaching for a cigarette.

Intelligence does not seem to be a factor in whether or not individuals take up smoking. But evidence indicates that smokers tend to achieve less in schoolwork than nonsmokers. The reason for this tendency is extremely hard to determine. It is unlikely that smoking, in itself, is responsible for unsatisfactory schoolwork. But it is possible that whatever causes an individual to smoke may also reduce interest in school—for example, the increased social activity that smokers seek at this age. Smoking may also be a reaction to failure or frustrations.

Tobacco—A Dangerous Drug?

Tobacco is not legally classified as a dangerous drug, for the most part because it does not cause the drastic mood modifications or behavior changes found among those who abuse the more potent drugs. However, smokers do exhibit mood modifications when without cigarettes. These are not dangerous enough to society to warrant legal controls of the severity of those used against heroin. But tobacco should be classifed as a "socially acceptable" mood-modifying psychoactive drug. Also, although the immediate effects of tobacco are mild, the overall, long-range physical effects are drastic because of the continuing physical damage to the body and health of the individual—enough, in fact, to classify its use as drug abuse.

The Effects of Smoking

Tobacco contains more than a hundred known chemical compounds, including nicotine. Some of the substances found in tobacco remain in the ashes of a burned cigarette; others are greatly changed during the burning process. Moreover, additional compounds are produced during combustion, and it is some of these materials that are of great concern to scientists and physicians. The composition of the cigarette smoke that enters the human body has been the primary aim of most analytical studies.

Cancer-Causing Substances

Nicotine and at least fifteen other compounds found in cigarette smoke are known to be carcinogens—cancer-causing substances. In addition to those known carcinogens, cigarette smoke also yields substances that have not yet been tested to

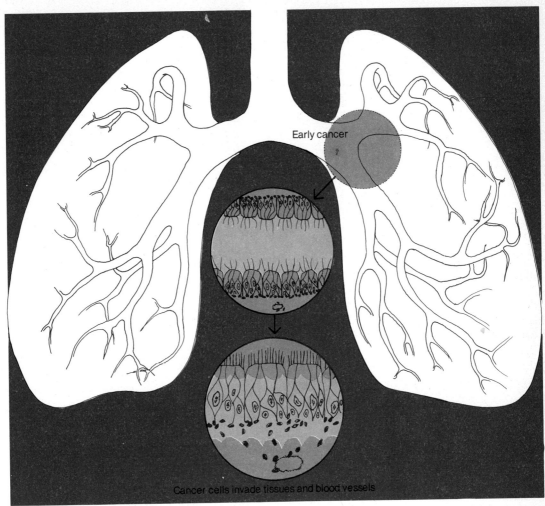

Early cancer

Cancer cells invade tissues and blood vessels

The respiratory system. The bronchial tube begins at the windpipe (trachea), then divides into two tubes (bronchial tubes). The deeper a cigarette smoker inhales, the further along the bronchial tree the smoke moves. Dotted lines represent the bronchial tubes as they pass behind the heart. This is where changes leading to cancer are most likely to occur. The surface of the bronchial tubes contain cilia which propel irritating substances out of the lungs. In response to the smoke, the cilia gradually disappear altogether, thus depriving the tubes of this protective mechanism.

determine their cancer-causing properties. Also present are hydrocarbons— chemicals closely related to the chemicals in gasoline. As explained earlier in the section on solvents, the long-term effects of hydrocarbon inhalation may also cause death.

When a person inhales cigarette smoke, the smoke passes down the trachea (windpipe) to the bronchial tubes and into the lungs. The drawing of the lungs shows that each bronchial tube is wider at each fork. The air or smoke slows down as it enters this region of greater width and deposits particles it may contain. This process is much the same as that of a river that deposits its sediment in the form of a delta where the river broadens into a lake or ocean. The exposure of the bronchial tubes to the particles (including carcinogens) contained in cigarette smoke is thus greatest at the points where the tube is widest. Autopsies of hundreds of human lungs have shown that it is precisely in these areas of maximum exposure that precancerous changes are most likely to take place—and where lung cancers are most likely to appear.

Smoking also causes damage to the protective mechanisms of the lungs. The lining of the bronchial tubes is normally moist. It is covered with mucus that is produced by cells along the surface of the tubes. Many of the surface cells also contain small whiplike fringes called *cilia*, which, with a back-and-forth waving motion, propel the mucus upward and outward toward the throat. Any irritating or poisonous particles or dust entering the bronchial tubes or lungs are trapped in the mucus and propelled by the cilia out of the lungs and bronchial tubes into the throat. This protective mechanism removes the unwanted and irritating foreign materials from the easily damaged lungs.

Cigarette smoke paralyzes the action of the cilia in the broncial tubes. It also causes changes to occur in the lining of the tubes, so that the cilia eventually disappear altogether. Thus, some relationships between smoking, lung cancer, and many other respiratory conditions, at least in part, are due to the effects of smoke on the cilia rather than to the direct carcinogenic action of the chemicals in the smoke. Furthermore, cigarette smoke is itself an irritant. Heavy smokers can feel this irritation in their throats and very often develop "smoker's cough" after a few years of smoking.

All of the effects of cigarette smoke on the tissues of the body are damaging. The actual role of cigarettes in the production of diseases is great because there is a com-bination of harmful factors. Any one of them could be responsible for damage, but together they are deadly.

The relationship between smoking and health has received a great deal of attention. Research brought to light by the 1964 surgeon general's report *Smoking and Health* has shown definite links between smoking and the occurrence of a variety of diseases, some of which we will discuss. This report and subsequent revision through 1973 (*The Health Consequences of Smoking*) continue to confirm previous findings and suggest additional mechanisms that may cause diseases such as cancer in smokers. Section Two of *Progress Against Cancer 1970* (Research on Chemical Carcinogenesis) reaffirms these findings, establishing more links between smoking and disease. These links have become stronger every year since then.

In fact, such a tremendous body of information had been accumulated as early as 1967 that, in September of that year, a World Conference on Smoking and Health was held in New York. In the opening address, Dr. Luther L. Terry, former surgeon general of the U.S. Public Health Service, set the theme of the conference and summed up the case against cigarettes:

We have come to the end of one era in the smoking and health field. The period of uncertainty is over. While science will continue to probe the reason why, there is no longer any doubt that cigarette smoking is a direct threat to the user's health. . . . There was a time when we spoke of the smoking-and-health "controversy." To my mind, the days of argument are over.

Dr. Terry was the U.S. surgeon general who issued the historic 1964 report.

Evidence has accumulated that explains the processes and chemicals in tobacco smoke that cause the many disease problems associated with smoking. The amounts of carcinogenic chemicals in tobacco are very small; in some cases they are measured in fractions of micrograms. But the normal functioning of the cell is a very delicate process. Constant irritation over long periods of time allows these carcinogens to change normal cells into cancerous cells. The chances of cancer for nonsmokers and smokers, verified by scientific investigations, are described and summarized in the table on expected and actual deaths for cigarette smokers. This table also shows the increased death rates from cancer expected of heavy smokers in any one year.

The most common type of cancer found in smokers is lung cancer; more people die of lung cancer than of any other type of cancer—the majority of them being male smokers. The number of victims has risen sharply during the past thirty years, and lung cancer now exceeds automobile accidents as a significant cause of death.

The first symptoms of lung cancer—a cough, wheeze, or vague chest pain—are so commonplace in smokers that they rarely cause a person to consult a physician and suspect that he or she might have cancer. Thus lung cancer is seldom diagnosed in its early stages. The smoker's familiarity with these symptoms increases the likelihood the disease will continue to its most dangerous stages. Yet lung cancer is the most preventable and one of the most treatable forms of cancer.

The relationship between it and smoking is clearly and irrefutably established. Although lung cancer is not unknown among nonsmokers, it is many times more common among smokers. Cigarette smoking is more likely to result in lung cancer than is cigar or pipe smoking, since an individual is more likely to inhale cigarette smoke than pipe or cigar smoke,

Expected and Actual Deaths for Smokers of Cigarettes

Underlying Cause of Death	Expected Number of Deaths in the General Population	Actual Number of Smokers Dying in General Population	Increased Ratio of Smoker Deaths
Cancer of lung	170.3	1,833	10.8 to 1
Bronchitis and emphysema	89.5	546	6.1 to 1
Cancer of larynx	14.0	75	5.4 to 1
Oral cancer	37.0	152	4.1 to 1
Cancer of esophagus	33.7	113	3.4 to 1
Stomach and duodenal ulcers	105.1	294	2.8 to 1
Other circulatory diseases	254.0	649	2.6 to 1
Cirrhosis of liver	169.2	379	2.2 to 1
Cancer of bladder	111.6	216	1.9 to 1
Coronary artery disease	6,430.7	11,177	1.7 to 1
Other heart diseases	526.0	868	1.7 to 1
Hypertensive heart disease	409.2	631	1.5 to 1
General arteriosclerosis	210.7	310	1.5 to 1
Cancer of kidney	79.0	120	1.5 to 1
All causes of death[a]	15,653.9	26,223	1.7 to 1

NOTE: This table shows the expected and actual deaths for smokers of cigarettes only and the ratios of such deaths to expected deaths in the general public.

[a] Includes all other causes of death as well as those listed above.

Adapted from *The Health Consequences of Smoking*, Washington, D.C.: U.S. Department of Health, Education, and Welfare.

but cigar and pipe smokers are substantially susceptible to lip, tongue, mouth, throat, and larynx (voice box) cancer. These cancers are associated with all forms of tobacco usage (cigarettes, pipes, cigars, and chewing tobacco), but the risk of lip, tongue, and mouth cancers is greater among pipe and cigar smokers than among cigarette smokers.

Smoking does not make these cancers inevitable. They are not even the greatest hazard associated with smoking (heart disease is more common). But the chance of getting lung cancer and the other forms of cancer just mentioned is greatly increased by heavy smoking.

Cardiovascular Diseases from Smoking

Recently, studies of large groups of people have shown that cigarette smokers are more likely to die of certain cardiovascular disorders than nonsmokers. Such diseases of the heart and blood vessels are the most common causes of death in our population. A cause-and-effect association has theoretically been established between cigarette smoking and the incidence of coronary attacks in humans, especially among men between 35 and 55 years of age. The risk of death in male cigarette smokers in relation to nonsmokers is greater in middle age than in old age. Statistics indicate that smokers are often struck down with disease when they should be most active and enjoying life. They also imply that men who stop smoking have a lower death rate from coronary diseases than those who continue to smoke.

Respiratory Diseases from Smoking

Smoking is increasingly linked to the development and progression of respiratory diseases, such as bronchitis and emphysema. Air pollution and respiratory infections as well as smoking cause and aggravate chronic bronchitis and emphysema. Any pollutant, condition, or infectious agent that can cause permanent damage to the respiratory system can be linked with these diseases. However, smoking causes an increased irritation above and beyond the pollutants and irritants commonly encountered.

The American Tobacco Institute

In the past ten years, the cigarette companies, represented by the American Tobacco Institute (ATI), have attempted to present the "other side" of the smoking-cancer debate. The studies on which the surgeon general's 1964 report was based were statistical ones. They included massive evidence of a *statistical correlation* between smoking and cancer. There are also many reports of animal cancers induced by application of cigarette residues to exposed portions of tissue.

But the ATI repeatedly emphasizes that no *human* case of cancer has ever been demonstrably induced by cigarette smoke in the laboratory. The industry insists that the studies simply have not proven that cigarette smoking causes human cancers. The cigarette companies put a good deal of faith in this assumption. They suggest the possibility that both smoking and lung cancer are "caused" by the same third, unknown factor that results in their being linked statistically. And though it seems nonsensical, there is at least the theoretical possibility that cancer causes smoking—this would also yield the same statistics.

At the same time that they protest the government's reliance on the surgeon general's reports of 1964, 1968, 1971, 1972, and 1973, the cigarette companies do see what is in store for them. For example, suits have been brought against the companies by victims or survivors of emphysema, lung cancer, and heart disease. For these and other reasons, there is currently a trend among the cigarette corporations to diversify and minimize their dependence on cigarettes, in anticipation of eventual illegalization of cigarettes and public rejection of smoking. At the same time, they are making a comeback (which may be only temporary) with the little cigars, which are selling in amounts close to cigarettes.

Another extraordinary phenomenon has been the introduction and early success of the 120-mm cigarettes. Starting in early 1975, these "fashionable" new products have met increasing success. This is somewhat difficult to understand, considering the fact that they offer exactly the same *amount* of tobacco as shorter cigarettes. Despite the predictions of cutbacks in the cigarette industry and slumping revenues, the new longer cigarettes were initially promoted with the same investment and fanfare of brands introduced ten and fifteen years ago.

Breaking the Smoking Habit

After an individual has started smoking, there is good evidence that the ability to stop is related to the forces that led to the smoking habit in the first place, the number of cigarettes smoked per day, and the number of years of smoking. An ability to stop smoking has consistently been found to be highest among those who started late in life and whose average cigarette consumption is low.

If a person is unable or unwilling to quit, he should at least try to reduce his consumption of cigarettes as a means of decreasing the harmful effects of smoking. The National Clearinghouse on Smoking and Health (*If You Must Smoke*, Public Service Publication No. 1786, Washington, D.C.: U.S. Government Printing Office, 1968), recommends the following five steps to reduce one's intake of cigarette smoke:

1. *Choose a cigarette with low tar and nicotine.* The U.S. Department of Health, Education, and Welfare publishes a current list of the tar and nicotine contents of cigarettes every 6 months. See how your brand compares and find out how much you can reduce your tar and nicotine intake by switching to another brand. Will such a switch result in your smoking more? Probably not. Most smokers who make such a change either continue to smoke at their previous rate or even smoke less. One possible reason for the lower rate is that nicotine and tar contribute to the taste of a cigarette. Lower tar and nicotine cigarettes will not seem as flavorful to a smoker who is used to high tar and nicotine concentrations. This can result in finding smoking in general less enjoyable.

2. *Don't smoke your cigarette all the way down.* No matter what cigarette you smoke, the most tar and nicotine is found in the last few puffs. The sooner you put your cigarette out, the lower your dose of harmful ingredients. Ths same fact also points up the added risk of the new longer cigarettes. Their extra puffs are really extra perils for you.

3. *Take fewer draws on each cigarette.* With practice, some people find they can substantially cut their actual smoking time without really missing it.

4. *Reduce your inhaling.* Easier said than done? Perhaps. But remember it is the smoke that enters your lungs that does most of the damage. It is this smoke that causes lung cancer and creates the cardiovascular changes that can bring on heart attacks.

5. *Smoke fewer cigarettes per day.* Pick a time of day when you promise yourself not to smoke. It may be before breakfast. Or while driving to school or work. Or after a certain hour each evening. It's always easier to *postpone* a cigarette if you know you will be having one later. Maybe you're a pack-a-

day smoker. Buy cigarettes one pack at a time. Try buying your next pack an hour later each day. It may also help to carry your cigarettes in a different pocket. Or, at work, keep them in a drawer of your desk or in your locker—any place where you aren't able to reach for one automatically. The trick is to change the habits you have developed over the years. Make a habit of asking yourself, "Do I really want *this* cigarette?" before you light up. You may be surprised how many cigarettes you smoke you don't really want.

In August 1968 the newsletter of the National Interagency Council on Smoking and Health reported that one-fourth of all American men and one-fifth of all American women who have ever smoked have quit. But, there are still 48 million smokers in this country. Of this number, an estimated 40 million feel some concern about their continuing smoking habit. Many of these people find it too difficult to overcome the smoking habit.

In the September 1968 issue of *Diseases of the Chest*, Lawrence Stross (M.D., Menninger Clinic, Topeka, Kansas) stated:

In the face of the overwhelming medical evidence about the inevitable dangers and harmful effects of cigarettes, as a psychiatrist I would categorically say that anyone who continues smoking or begins smoking is acting in an irrational way and denying reality. I think cigarette smoking can properly be described as a kind of masochistic perversion in which people get pleasure out of hurting themselves and making themselves sick.

Methods of Breaking the Habit   Thus, for a person to stop smoking he must first stop ignoring the health dangers of smoking and accept his smoking as a personal problem he must conquer. Breaking the habit is now being accomplished in a number of ways, but the most successful methods fall into the following categories: (1) individual medical care provided by physicians or psychologists; (2) self-help programs based on books, magazines, lectures, and pamphlets (such services are available from such organizations as the American Cancer Society, the American Heart Association and others); and (3) withdrawal clinics or "smoker's clinics," often conducted by hospitals or medical and health organizations.

Withdrawal Clinics   Withdrawal clinics, which are quite successful, are actually group therapy sessions in which physicians and health professionals conduct a series of sessions that explain the health hazards of smoking. They often have a psychologist who conducts part of the session to help reinforce the individual and suggest methods of stopping or reducing smoking. The participants are encouraged to explain how well they are doing and to make suggestions to other members of the group. Also, past participants may conduct part of a session with small groups who identify with the problems these individuals had when they stopped smoking.

Once the group has been established there are three goals to accomplish to successfully stop smoking: (1) to assist the individual in building a strong motivation for stopping smoking; (2) to constructively confront the individual's attitudes toward smoking, especially those relating to events and feelings associated with the withdrawal experiences taking place with the group; and (3) to provide support and guidance during and immediately following the period of withdrawal from tobacco.

Drug Therapy   Preparations containing lobeline, a drug with actions similar to those of nicotine, are now sold over the counter at drugstores. The smoker takes such lobeline compounds in decreasing doses once he or she has cut down on the consumption of tobacco. While these drugs claim to help the smoker to break the dependence on nicotine, they do not replace the habit of smoking. Thus the smoker may find, on trying to stop, that new habits replace smoking. To keep the hands busy, he or she may become a "fiddler." To satisfy what has been called "oral need," he or she may overeat or become a nailbiter. But because these habits are seldom as satisfying as smoking, the individual more often than not returns to tobacco.

Advantages of Not Smoking

Little is known of the relationship between not smoking and normal health. The main areas of study have so far been confined to the relationships between smoking and disease. These studies are just beginning to show which body changes in response to cigarettes are transitory and which are permanent.

In a study based on 12 years of experience in conducting smoking withdrawal clinics, Dr. Borje E. V. Elrup, Clinical Associate Professor of Medicine, Cornell Medical Center, New York, has been able to demonstrate the following anatomical and physiological changes in ex-smokers.

Digestive and eating patterns start to change even during withdrawal from cigarettes. Soon after a person stops smoking, intestinal motility decreases—often causing constipation for a short time. The absorption of food is greater, the appetite is better, and both the taste of food and the sense of smell are improved—all contributing to a weight gain.

Patterns of circulation also change. The ex-smoker is less tired. He often arises earlier in the morning and is more alert during the day. Skin circulation improves.

The complexion of the face can be seen to change for the better, even during the process of stopping. Increased circulation helps to slow the pulse rate, reduce blood pressure, and increase heart efficiency— both at rest and after exercise.

Responses from the respiratory tract show a decrease in breathing rate, as well as an increase in maximal breathing capacity, and a better exchange of oxygen between the lungs and the circulatory system. Such respiratory conditions as chronic bronchitis improve and coughing disappears during withdrawal. Emphysema patients are able to breathe more easily and many asthma conditions improve substantially.

The age at which one stops smoking has a lot to do with the benefits. The younger a person is when he stops, the greater the benefits. There have been studies showing increases in death rates for smokers as young as 11 years of age. An individual between 35 and 54 shows a marked decrease in the chances of dying from diseases associated with cigarettes if he stops smoking. However, a person between 55 and 74 shows only a slight decrease in his chances of dying as a result of such diseases.

In Conclusion

Although quitting smoking is seldom easy, the effort required may be handsomely rewarded. For example, a two-pack-a-day smoker will have $365 per year savings (average cost of cigarettes is $.50 per pack). You will have cleaner teeth, will require less professional teeth cleaning work at your dentist, and you will keep your own teeth longer (especially women). You will not run the risk of burned clothing, upholstery, or furniture. Added years of good health and fewer chances of early death are, of course, the most important gains. If you smoke—quit now. If you don't smoke—don't start.

Andrews, Matthew. *Parent's Guide to Drugs*. Garden City, N.Y.: Doubleday & Co., 1972. A reference for parents outlining the range of drug abuse by young people.

Bejerot, Nils. *Addiction: An Artificially Induced Drive*. Springfield, Ill.: C. C. Thomas, 1972. Shows the psychological aspects of drug abuse regardless of the drug being abused.

Bludworth, Edward. *Three Hundred Most Abused Drugs*. Tampa, Fla.: Trend House, 1973. A dictionary of drugs with description of their psychoactive properties.

Brecher, Edward M. *Licit & Illicit Drugs*. Mount Vernon, New York: Consumers Union, 1972. The most complete volume concerning psychoactive drugs in print.

Canadian Government Commission of Inquiry. *The Non-Medical Use of Drugs*. Santa Fe, N.M.: Gannon, William, 1973. A single view of drug abuse.

Fast, Julius. *How to Stop Smoking and Lose Weight*. New York: Newspaper Enterprise Association, 1969. This book offers the most data available on diet and weight control while stopping smoking.

Fort, Joel. *The Pleasure Seekers: The Drug Crisis, Youth & Society*. New York: Grove Press, 1970. A paperback update of the earlier book; written by a pioneer in drug treatment programs. Traces patterns of abuse among young people.

——————————. *Alcohol: Our Biggest Drug Problem*. New York: McGraw–Hill Book Co., 1973. A book for the general public describing alcohol as the major drug problem in the United States.

Jones, Kenneth; Shainberg, Louis; and Byer, Curtis. *Drugs: Substance Abuse*, 2nd ed. San Francisco: Canfield Press, 1975. An overview of the abuse of drugs, alcohol, and tobacco.

——————————. *Drugs and Alcohol*. New York: Harper & Row, Publishers, 1973. A scientific, popularly written report on the sources and effects of drugs and drug abuse.

Linkletter, Art. *Drugs at My Door Step*, New ed. New York: World Book, 1973. Describes the drug problems of his daughter, in the hopes that others will recognize the problem before something tragic happens.

Mauser, Bernard, and Platt, Ellen S. *Smoking: A Behavioral Analysis*. Elmsford, N.Y.: Pergamon Press, 1971. One of the best books written to help individuals to understand smoking and how they may stop smoking.

National Commission on Marihuana and Drug Abuse. *Marihuana: A Signal of Misunderstanding*. Washington, D.C.: U.S. Government Printing Office, 1972. An excellent study on marijuana and its abuse.

Nowlis, Helen. *Drugs on the College Campus*. Garden City, N.Y.: Doubleday & Co., 1968. A classic study containing an excellent section describing the reasons for drug abuse.

Ochner, Alton. *Smoking: Your Choice Between Life & Death*. New York: Simon and Schuster, 1971. Discusses smoking and how to stop.

Petrie, Sidney. *How to Stop Smoking in Three Days.* Monroe, N.Y.: Library Research Associates, 1973. Describes direct method for stopping smoking.

Phillipson, R. *Modern Trends in Drug Dependence and Alcoholism.* New York: Appleton–Century Crofts, 1970. Shows the interdependence of all types of drug dependence.

Royal College of Physicians of London. *Smoking & Health Now.* Philadelphia: J.B. Lippincott Co., 1971. A complete volume on the implications of smoking.

Williams, John B. *Narcotics and Drug Dependence.* Los Angeles: Glencoe Press, 1974. Update of previous books on drugs. Compete coverage in concise sections.

Witters, Weldon L., and Jones–Witters, Patricia. *Drugs & Sex.* New York: Macmillan Co., 1975. Two separate books under one cover. Complete coverage of drugs and drug abuse.

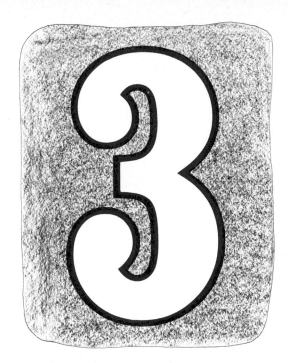

GOOD HEALTH IN THE MARKET PLACE

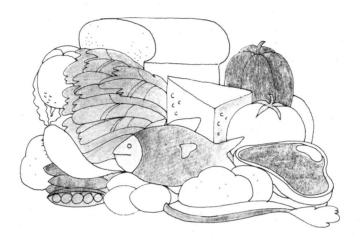

8

NUTRIENTS AND NUTRITION

Food is one of our most basic survival needs. After oxygen and water, food is an immediate requirement for the maintenance of life. A food can be defined as any substance—besides air and medicines—that provides for the body's growth, maintenance, repair, and reproduction. The substances in food that perform these functions are called *nutrients*. Food may be either natural or man-made, may come from plants or animals, and is the source of all nutrients. Nutrients are chemicals that:

1. Provide energy for body activities.
2. Provide materials for growth and maintenance of body tissues.
3. Provide substances that act to regulate body processes.

What Is Food? Although the hundreds of substances we consume as food (hamburgers, steak, salads, ice cream, and so on) show little similarity, the nourishing materials they provide fall into only six chemical classes of nutrients.

Carbohydrates The carbohydrates consist of sugars and starches. For the majority of people in the world today, carbohydrates are the most important source of energy. It is estimated that, of the total calories consumed in the United States, about 40 to 50 percent come from carbohydrates. If the diet is low in carbohydrates, fats or proteins will be converted into glucose (blood sugar) as a source of energy. If there is a surplus of carbohydrates in the diet, the surplus is converted into human fats and stored in the adipose tissues for possible future use. Foods high in carbohydrates include rice, corn, grains (and grain products), potatoes, and all sugar products.

Carbohydrates consist of one or more simple sugar units. The simple sugars are glucose (also known as *dextrose*) and fructose, found in many fruits and honey; and galactose, found in milk. Examples of carbohydrates consisting of two simple sugar units connected together (compound sugars) are sucrose, which is table sugar (cane and beet sugars are identical); maltose, produced by germinating grains; and lactose, found only in milk.

Carbohydrates consisting of long chains of simple sugar units connected together are called *starches*. One starch, cellulose, although present in most of our foods that come from plants, is not converted into energy by humans, because we lack the digestive enzymes necessary for its breakdown. Cellulose is useful, however, in stimulating intestinal activity.

It actually matters little whether carbohydrates are consumed as simple sugars, compound sugars, or starches, since the process of digestion reduces all of them to their simple sugar units before they are absorbed into the blood. The simple sugars other than glucose are further converted by the liver into glucose. Glucose is the only carbohydrate that can be used as a source of energy by the cells of the body. The liver and muscles store some carbohydrates in the form of glycogen (an animal starch), which is then available for rapid conversion into glucose when extra energy is needed.

Fats In addition to being a high calorie source, fats serve as the body's energy storage, form a part of the membranes of cells, act as carriers for the fat-soluble vitamins A, D, E, and K, and provide both insulation and protection for the body.

A fat is made up of one glycerol molecule connected to three fatty-acid molecules. (Through digestion fats are broken down into four components.) The human body is able to produce most of the fatty acids it needs through the conversion of carbohydrates. Fatty acids that the body needs but is unable to produce itself in sufficient amounts are called *essential fatty acids*. These must be obtained from our food. Fortunately, essential fatty acids are widely and abundantly distributed in foods such as meats, whole milk, cheese, nuts, olives, and fish. Such food products as butter, margarine, oils, and shortenings are almost pure fat.

Some fats are designated as "saturated" fats and others as "unsaturated" fats according to the amounts of hydrogen in the molecule—the more hydrogen, the more saturated the fat. Although there has been some suggestion that too high a ratio of saturated fats in the diet can have a direct influence on atherosclerosis (fatty deposits in the bloodstream), this idea is not an established fact. For certain types of conditions, physicians may recommend substituting unsaturated fats for saturated ones, but it appears that normal bodies need both kinds of fats. In an effort to reduce intake of saturated animal fats, some people have used "imitation milk" products. In imitation milk the butterfat is replaced with coconut oil, an unfortunate choice of fats, because it is one of the few fats from plant sources that is highly *saturated*. Thus imitation milk would be a poor choice for someone who was trying to decrease the intake of saturated fats.

Proteins Proteins in the diet are a source of nitrogen, both in its elemental form (uncombined with other chemicals) or in the form of amino acids (simple nitrogen compounds found in nature). There are twenty-three amino acids, some of which cannot be synthesized by the body—the eight essential amino acids must be derived from the proteins consumed in food. The other amino acids can be made from molecular pieces and other substances in the body.

Proteins containing all eight essential amino acids in significant amounts are *complete*. Proteins low in one or more of these amino acids are *incomplete*. Most animal proteins are complete while most plant proteins are incomplete. This is why it may be difficult for a vegetarian to obtain all the essential amino acids. Two incomplete proteins may be used to complement each other, if they are deficient in different amino acids. The combination of a whole grain and a legume (beans, peas, peanuts) serves this purpose and plays an important dietary role in many parts of the world (for example, beans and rice or beans and corn).

From the constituent amino acids, the body makes the enzymes (chemical catalysts), hormones, secretions, and tissues it needs. These are highly complex substances, made possible by the literally millions of possible combinations of amino acids that the body can prepare.

In contrast to fats and carbohydrates, amino acids are not stored in the cells. Thus, a person needs a daily supply of protein in the diet. The table on energy values compares the three basic energy-yielding food groups (carbohydrates, proteins, and fats). These are the only nutrients that can be converted into energy.

Minerals Many mineral elements are found in the body. They may occur as simple compounds or be incorporated into very complex materials. Many of these elements (such as calcium, phosphorus, sodium, potassium, chlorine, magnesium, iron, sulfur, iodine, manganese, cobalt, copper, and zinc) perform essential functions in the body—they make up vital parts of cells, bones, teeth, and the blood. Other mineral elements make up important parts of hormones and secretions.

As is true of all nutrients, there are specific patterns of deficiency and abundance in the distribution of minerals in the American diet. For example, phosphorus deficiency can occur when someone does not eat adequate amounts of fresh green vegetables. Men consume more calcium than women at all age levels, because of their greater total intake of food. Also, food processing can result in high losses of minerals, especially magnesium, phosphorus, and calcium.

Caloric Values of Energy-Yielding Nutrients

Type of nutrient	Kilocalories per Gram	Kilocalories per Pound
Carbohydrates	4	1860
Fats	9	4220
Proteins	4	1860

NOTE: This table assumes a gram or pound of pure substance. Very few foods are pure and release the total number of kilocalories.

Vitamin	Rich Sources	Properties	Function	Deficiency Symptoms	Recommended Dietary Allowance
Fat-soluble vitamins					
Vitamin A	Cheese, green and yellow vegetables, butter, eggs, milk, fish liver oils; carotene in vegetables converted to vitamin A by liver	Lost through oxidation during long cooking in open kettle; overdose possible	Necessary for growth, tooth structure, night vision, healthy skin	Slow growth, poor teeth and gums, night blindness, dry skin and eyes (lack of tears)	1500–5000 I/U, child 4000–8000 I/U, adult
Vitamin D	Beef, butter, eggs, milk, fish liver oils; produced in the skin upon exposure to ultraviolet rays in sunlight; no plant source	One of the most stable vitamins; large doses may cause calcium deposits, poor bone growth in children, congenital defects	Necessary for metabolism of calcium and phosphorus; essential for normal bone and tooth development	Rickets; poor tooth and bone structure; soft bones	400 I/U
Vitamin E	Widely distributed in foods; abundant in vegetable oils and wheat germ	Lost through oxidation during long cooking in open kettle; overdose not known	Not definitely known for humans	Not definitely known for humans	7–9 I/U, child 12–30 I/U, adult male 10–25 I/U, adult female
Vitamin K	Eggs, liver, cabbage, spinach, tomatoes; produced by bacteria of intestine	Destroyed by light and alkali; absorption from intestine into blood depends on normal fat absorption	Necessary for blood clotting	Slow blood clotting: *anemia* (low oxygen-carrying capacity of blood)	Not established. Given to pregnant women and newborn infants, since newborns lack bacteria normally producing adequate supply
Water-soluble vitamins[a]					
Vitamin B₁ (thiamine)	Meat, whole grains, liver, yeast, nuts, eggs, bran, soybeans, potatoes	Usually not destroyed by cooking, but can be destroyed by alkali—May dissolve in cooking water. Not stored in body, daily supply needed.	Necessary for carbohydrate metabolism, normal nerve function; promotes growth	Beriberi; slow growth, poor nerve function, nervousness, fatigue, heart disease	0.7–1.2 milligrams, child 1.0–1.5 milligrams, adult

Vitamin	Good Sources	Stability	Function	Deficiency Symptoms	Recommended Amounts
Vitamin B$_2$ (riboflavin)	Milk, cheese, liver, beef, eggs, fish	Not destroyed by cooking acid foods, unstable to light and alkali	Essential for metabolism in all cells	Fatigue, sore skin and lips, bloodshot eyes, anemia	0.8–1.2 milligrams, child 1.5–1.8 milligrams, adult male 1.1–1.4 milligrams, adult female
Niacin (nicotinic acid)	Bran, eggs, yeast, liver, kidney, fish, whole wheat, potatoes, tomatoes; can be synthesized from amino acid tryptophan	Not destroyed by cooking, but may dissolve extensively in cooking water	Necessary for growth, metabolism, normal skin	Pellagra; sore mouth, skin rash, indigestion, diarrhea, headache, mental disturbances	9–16 milligrams, child 16–20 milligrams, adult male 12–16 milligrams, adult female
Vitamin B$_6$[b] (pyridoxine)	Meat, liver, yeast, whole grains, fish, vegetables	Stable except to light	Functions in amino acid metabolism	Dermatitis, deficiency rare	0.6–1.2 milligrams, child 1.6–2.0 milligrams, adult
Vitamin B$_{12}$ (cyanocobalamin)	Meat, liver, eggs, milk, yeast	Unstable to acid, alkali, light	Necessary for production of red blood cells and growth	Pernicious anemia	1.0–2.0 milligrams, child 3.0 milligrams, adult
Vitamin C[c] (ascorbic acid)	Citrus fruits, tomatoes, potatoes, cabbage, green peppers, broccoli	Least stable of the vitamins; destroyed by heat, alkali, air, dissolves in cooking water	Essential for cellular metabolism, necessary for teeth, gums, bones, blood vessels	Scurvy, poor teeth, weak bones, sore and bleeding gums, easy bruising, poor wound healing	40 milligrams, child 45 milligrams, adult
Folacin (folic acid)	Liver, yeast, leafy vegetables such as asparagus, lettuce and broccoli and whole wheat products	Destroyed by cooking at high temperatures; keep leafy vegetables under refrigeration	Needed for synthesis of DNA and RNA, extremely important during pregnancy	Gastrointestinal disorders, diarrhea, and anemia, can cause anemia during pregnancy and childhood	100–300 micromilligrams, child 400 micromilligrams, adults 800 micromilligrams for pregnant female 600 micromilligrams while breast feeding

[a]Several other water-soluble vitamins are believed essential to human nutrition, but are not as well understood as the above vitamins and their deficiency is less common.

[b]A female using an oral contraceptive pill should increase her intake of vitamin B$_6$ to 2.5 milligrams daily.

[c]There is some controversy over the amount of vitamin C an individual should consume.

Vitamins Vitamins are a group of important compounds that are found in very small proportions in food. They are needed in trace amounts for the proper functioning of the body. Vitamins function along with enzymes to carry out very specific, important chemical reactions in the body. Like enzymes, vitamins act by helping a reaction take place (in some cases, enzymes and vitamins make reactions possible that could not occur in their absence), but vitamins are neither changed nor incorporated into the products of the reaction. Because of this action, vitamins are called *coenzymes*.

Except for vitamins D and K, vitamins cannot be synthesized directly in the body; they must be obtained from the diet. And even though vitamins D and K are synthesized within the body, the chemicals from which they are synthesized still must come from what we eat. Consequently, they also depend on a proper diet. As shown in the vitamins table, whether a vitamin will dissolve in water or in fat (or oil) is important. This can tell you the source of a vitamin, how it is absorbed into the body, and what happens to it inside the body. Water-soluble vitamins are not stored in the body and should be taken in each day. In general, fat-soluble vitamins are stored within body tissues and can cause toxic effects in large overdoses. Excessively high intake of fat-soluble vitamins, such as A and D, especially in infants, whose bodies are small, should be avoided. On the other hand, the absence of fat-soluble vitamins has serious consequences. An entire class of diseases, called *vitamin deficiency diseases* (see vitamins table) , can result from a lack of these vital chemicals in the diet.

A number of vitamins, such as B_6 (pyridoxine), C, and E, have become very controversial in the last few years. Powers have been ascribed to them that many nutritionists feel are unproven, while others insist large amounts of these vitamins are needed for good health. It will take years of continued research to completely substantiate many of the claims made for these vitamins.

Water No material serves the body in as many vital functions as water. The importance of water to the body is so great that the loss of only 10 percent of the body's water can result in an individual's death. The body is over 50 percent water, and many of the tissues of the body (such as blood) are as much as 90 percent water. Digestion, absorption, and the secretion of materials must take place in water. All chemical reactions of metabolism also require water. It provides the moisture in the cells of the lungs that enables the membranes to exchange oxygen and carbon dioxide. It is important in distributing heat uniformly throughout the body. It transports many vital substances throughout the body. And it also serves as a cushion for the brain and spinal cord.

How much water people require each day depends largely on the air temperature around them and the kind of physical activity they are engaged in. Water loss may range from 2½ quarts for a moderately active person to several times that much for a person working vigorously in the hot sun. The loss occurs primarily through the kidneys, lungs, digestive tract, and skin.

This water loss can be replenished by liquids and foods of all kinds. All foods—even dry bread—contain some water. Some water is produced within the body through the metabolic breakdown of stored nutrients. Since there are variables both in water needed and water available from different sources, it is not possible to state the specific amount of water a person should drink each day. In general, a person should drink a little more water than is sufficient to satisfy thirst. The slight excess beyond thirst provides for good kidney health.

Food supplies the nutrients for growth and replacement of worn or damaged cells, as well as for the manufacture of cellular products, such as enzymes and hormones. The overall composition of the body is about 59 percent water, 18 percent protein, 18 percent fat, and 4.3 percent mineral. At any one time there is less than 1 percent carbohydrate in the makeup of the body. These substances that make up the body are not distributed equally in all organs. For example, the percentage of water varies from 90 to 92 percent in blood plasma to 72 to 78 percent in muscle, 45 percent in bone, and only 5 percent in tooth enamel. Proteins are found most abundantly in muscle. Fat tends to concentrate in the adipose (fat) cells under the skin and around the intestines. Carbohydrates are found mainly in the liver, muscles, and blood. As for the minerals, high levels of calcium and phosphorus form part of the bones and teeth, sodium and chlorine are found mainly in the body fluids (blood plasma and lymph), potassium is the main mineral in muscle, iron is essential to red blood cells, and magnesium is general throughout the body. These are the main minerals supplied to the body as food, but many other minerals are essential to the human body in proportionately smaller amounts. These minerals are termed *trace elements,* and they too must be ingested with our food. Other chemicals (vitamins) are needed in very small amounts for various functions of the body to take place.

The Chemistry of Nutrition

All food is not alike. Nor are humans able to synthesize all of those chemicals that they fail to get through eating. Supplying known physiological requirements demands eating a balance of nutrients in kind and amount. A well-fed person is not necessarily a well-nourished person. Balance is the key—balance not only in vitamins and calories, but also in protein, minerals, essential fatty acids, and water.

The quantity of energy released from a given quantity of food is measured in Calories (the capital C designates this unit as equaling one thousand "small" calories). One Calorie is the amount of heat energy required to raise 1 kiloliter (approximately one quart) of water 1 degree centigrade. In nutrition, this large calorie (C) is most often not capitalized and referred to as a *kcal* (kilocalorie).

The energy released from food, though measured in a heat energy unit, is readily converted into those forms of energy needed by the system—electrical energy (for nerve impulses), light energy (as in the glow of a firefly), mechanical energy (for movement of the body and of internal muscles such as the heart), and sound energy.

The human body is an efficient machine, and like any machine, it needs energy to function. The body converts certain types of food into the energy it needs. Such food contains *potential energy,* or energy in a form that can be set into action. The body is able to convert this potential energy into heat, movement, growth, and all the processes that take place in the body. Energy that is being used or is working is termed *kinetic energy.*

The conversion of potential energy into kinetic energy takes place through chemical reactions in every cell of the body. The term *metabolism* refers to the total of all the chemical processes that make up the functions of life. The extent of metabolic functions in the human body can be viewed as existing on two levels. The body requires energy just to stay alive; this energy is used for those processes that sustain the living system—breathing, heartbeat, and glandular secretions. This basal metabolic rate (BMR) is the total energy needed by the body for internal body functioning only. The BMR is a useful measure of the healthy functioning of the body. The basal metabolic rate is most directly under the influence of the thyroid gland, through its secretion of the hormone thyroxin.

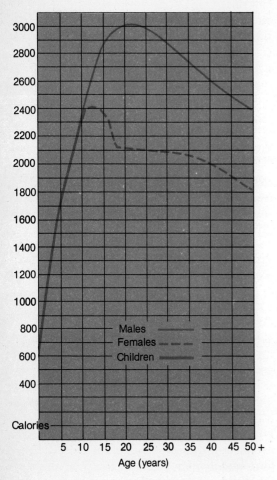

The normal basal metabolic rate at different ages is shown by graphing the caloric needs at different ages.

Adapted from U.S. Department of Agriculture, Recommended Daily Dietary Allowances (Washington, D. C., 1973).

As shown in the graph, the basal metabolic rate (BMR) is highest in childhood and drops gradually throughout life. This requires a gradual decrease in the amount of food a person should eat to avoid excess weight. The average man (late teens to early thirties) needs about 1,600 to 1,800 kcal per day for basal metabolism. Women typically have a lower basal metabolic rate than men and need 1,200 to 1,450 kcal per day.

Determination of your BMR (usually measured while you are awake, but reclining and relaxed) should be added to the number of calories you use by general resting activities throughout the day (sleep, general minimal movements). This sum is an individual's *resting metabolism* (BMR plus calories used while at general rest) and is about 10 percent above the BMR. The RM (resting metabolism) ranges from 0.8 to 1.4 kcal per hour per kilogram (2.2 pounds) of body weight, depending on the amount of fat present or *lean body mass* (LBM), as shown in the following table.

You can also calculate your approximate RM. An average man requires about 1.2 kcal per hour (24 hours per day) for each kilogram (2.2 pounds) of body weight. A 154-pound (70-kilogram) man would need 1.2 times 24 times 70, or 2,016 kcal per 24 hours. The resting metabolism for an average woman (128 pounds or 58 kilograms) is about 1,320 kcal per day or 0.9 times 24 times 58, or 1,320 kcal per 24 hours.

But an individual's energy requirements also include the degree of physical activity he or she engages in during the day. The need for kcal is proportional to the amount of daily exercise and one's RM. If you are an inactive individual, add 30 percent of your resting metabolism; add 50 percent if you engage in light activity; 75 percent for moderate activity; and 100 percent for strenuous physical activity. A brief description of exercise categories is given in

Resting Metabolism According to Body Weight and Composition

Men	Women	% of Body Fat	110	121	132	143	154	165	176
					Weight in Pounds				
					kcal per 24 hours				
Thin		5	1188	1399	1613	1856	2117	2376	2669
Average		10	1128	1333	1555	1778	2033	2304	2573
Plump	Thin	15	1068	1267	1483	1700	1949	2214	2496
Fat	Average	20	1008	1201	1411	1638	1865	2124	2400
	Plump	25	960	1135	1339	1560	1797	2034	2304
	Fat	30	960	1069	1267	1482	1714	1944	2208

Degrees of Physical Activity

Very light (sedentary)	Sitting most of day, studying, talking. About two hours of walking or standing.
Light activity	Typing, teaching, shop work. laboratory work. Some walking throughout the day.
Moderate activity	Walking, housework, gardening, carpentry, light industry. Little sitting throughout day.
Strenuous activity	Unskilled labor, forestry work, skiing, outdoor games, dancing. Very little sitting. Periods of running.
Very strenuous activity	Tennis, swimming, basketball, football, running. Short periods of rest throughout day.

the above table. Calculate your daily energy requirements and see if you are eating too much or exercising too little.

Organic Versus Inorganic

The term *organic* as used by scientists refers to any substance that contains carbon (a chemical element) and that belongs to groups of chemical compounds that are derived from living sources. Those substances that are not from living sources and do not contain carbon are termed *inorganic*.

Health food faddists have a different definition of organic food: any food that is obtained from a living plant or animal and is not chemically treated. The term is also used for those foods grown without pesticides, herbicides, or artificial chemical fertilizers. These are popular, but totally erroneous and unscientific uses of the term *organic*.

Plants and animals contain both organic and inorganic materials or nutrients. Carbohydrates, fats, and proteins are organic nutrients because they all contain carbon. These are also the only nutrients that can be used to supply energy to the body. Vitamins also contain carbon and are therefore organic substances. Minerals are inorganic substances because they are single-chemical elements that do not contain carbon. A nutritious food is one that supplies both the organic nutrients (carbohydrates, fats, proteins, vitamins) and the inorganic nutrients (minerals) for the body.

What's in Your Food?

One of the greatest problems with most foods is their relatively short storage life. In the past, people have used many methods to try and preserve perishable foods—the most common being drying and salting, or adding salt, sugar, or spices.

Additives   There are two ways in which we classify chemicals that are in our food as a result of food-processing technology. *Additives* are substances in foods that are deliberately added to foods for specific reasons. *Residues* are substances that remain in foods as a result of agricultural processes or environmental contamination. By conservative estimates, there are at least ten thousand additives or residues that may wind up in your food.

Convenience foods are made possible by the use of food additives used to improve the appearance, texture, taste, nutritional value, and ability of the food to be packaged and stored. By 1980, over half of the foods sold will contain additives. Currently five pounds of food additives are used for every person in the United States.

Hazards Posed by Additives   Official policy governing the use of additives varies widely. While some countries have strict regulations, the United States has allowed wide proliferation of new additives (preventing adequate evaluation of each new one). Many are loosely accorded "generally recognized as safe" (GRAS) status, on the basis of long-established use without "evidence of harm." Relatively few food additives have been accepted for specific and limited uses on the basis of sound investigation.

It is acceptable for food processors to give food reasonable shelf life, but not to "embalm" food that can no longer be considered fresh.

Some additives are now under suspicion. The antioxidant butylated hydroxytoluene (BHT) is suspected of inhibiting the uptake of oxygen by hemoglobin in the red blood cells. One emulsifier, polyoxyethylene (no longer used in the United States), was found to greatly in-

crease the rate of iron absorption in some animals—leading to too great an absorption of vitamin A.

The most disturbing element in the use of additives is that they are not always fully investigated *before* being used in foods. This is particularly true of substances in use prior to the Food Additives Amendment to the federal Food, Drug, and Cosmetic Act, as well as with those included as GRAS. In some cases, the use of a particular additive, with great food industry resistance, has been discontinued *only* after the fact—after possible physical damage to unwary and trusting consumers.

Before purchasing processed foods, read the ingredients list on the label. The ingredients are listed in descending order of abundance—the first item listed is the most abundant. If there seem to be more chemicals than food, you might consider buying another product. Remember that some of the ingredients with chemical-sounding names, such as ascorbic acid, are actually important vitamins or other nutrients. Some foods, such as ice cream, can still be sold with no ingredients listing, although a multitude of chemicals may be included.

Antioxidants   Some foods, particularly unsaturated fatty-acid-containing foods, tend to oxidize (combine with oxygen). Frozen peaches become brown and unattractive. Some cake mixes become useless unless the shortening in them is kept fresh. Antioxidants are used to minimize these problems.

Acids   Baking powder or cream of tartar (tartaric acid) reacts with baking soda and produces carbon dioxide to leaven bread and cake, making it light. Certain other acids (phosphoric, citric, malic) are used to counteract the excessive sweetness of many soft drinks.

Emulsifiers Emulsifiers break up fats and oils into very small particles. They are used in bakery goods to improve uniformity of texture, fineness, and softness; in ice cream to control particle size (smoother ice cream); in salad dressing to prevent the oil and vinegar from separating.

Artificial Sweeteners Substitute sweeteners (sweet-tasting compounds with no food value) have a long history. Two of the most important are saccharin and cyclamate. These have long been used by diabetics. Saccharin is over 300 times as sweet as table sugar (sucrose), while cyclamates are only about 30 times as sweet as table sugar. Although safe within recommended doses and as used by diabetics, the use of these sweeteners is restricted or prohibited in some countries because they are nonfoods (contain no food value) and are possibly dangerous when consumed in large quantities.

Coloring Agents Coloring agents have been used in food since the early 1900s. Many scientists are questioning the safety of a number of federally certified food-coloring agents, particularly the sodium nitrite used in meats and the "rainbow" of coloring agents made from coal tar used to increase the eye-appeal of beverages, cereals, meats, desserts, fruits, and vegetables.

Sodium nitrite is used as a preservative, flavoring agent, and coloring fixative in hot dogs, bacon, ham, luncheon meats, smoked fish, and related products. It is added to over seven billion pounds of such food products each year to give them the nice pink color everyone expects. The FDA limits the use of nitrites to 200 parts per million in food; this is not toxic. Many food manufacturers have been cited for overstepping these limits up to the range of 3,000 parts per million. At this level, sodium nitrite can be toxic. This is the only material added to food during processing that is known to cause death in humans.

Dyes made from coal tars are going into your food supply at the rate of about four million pounds a year. Coal-tar dyes are complex chemicals that are not found in nature. Many are currently being used that, scientists believe, have never been adequately tested for harmful effects. Over the years, a dozen of the dyes have been banned after it was proven that they caused either cancer, birth defects, long-term mutagenic harm, or serious allergies.

These coloring agents, along with artificial sweeteners, in recent studies by Dr. Ben F. Feingold, chief emeritus of the Department of Allergy at the Kaiser-Permanente Medical Center in San Francisco, have been suggested as the cause of hyperkinetic behavior in at least twenty-five youngsters. When these youngsters were allowed to eat foods containing these materials they showed the classic symptoms of a hyperkinetic condition. While on a diet free of such additives they returned to normal. Dr. Feingold has asked the federal government and the food processing industry to identify more clearly the coloring and sweetening agents used in foods. A listing of dyes (and other additives as well) are not required on so-called *standard food items* such as ice cream, cheese, and butter. On other food products the coloring agents need only be identified as "artificial coloring," or "certified color added."

Chemical Bleaching Years ago, flour was aged, stored, and turned periodically to bleach it white for white bread. Today, chemical bleaching agents are added to whiten bread. The baking industry states that the sole purpose for bleaching is consumer demand for white bread. One or a combination of chemicals may be used to bleach flour. The amount used is stated as "a quantity not more than sufficient for bleaching and/or to produce an aging effect." Bleaching agents include oxides of nitrogen, chlorine, nitrosyl chloride, chlorine dioxide, acetone, peroxides, or azodicarbonamide. A flour treated by these chemicals must be marked "bleached" on the label. The complete actions of many of these are unknown.

Enrichment Chemicals Some chemicals are added to white flour in order to "enrich" it. The food industry insists these chemicals are identical to the vitamins and minerals that have been removed in processing. The problem is that the "enriching" may restore only 25 to 60 percent of the original amount (a net loss). Vitamins and minerals are added to certain food products to replace those that have been lost during processing or to make up for an inherent deficiency in the food. For example, white flour has several vitamins and minerals added to replace those lost in milling, and most milk has vitamin D added because it is normally present in only trace quantities.

Other Additives *Pectin* is a thickening agent that is added to certain fruits in order to give a consistent and desirable thickness to jams and jellies. Wieners, like other sausages, contain *flavoring agents*. Canned shredded coconut contains a *humectant* to keep it moist. Table salt, powdered sugar, and malted milk powder all contain *anticaking* agents. Salt and sugar are still used as preservative and flavoring agents.

Nutrition and Health
Good health is much more than the absence of disease; it is also physical and intellectual vigor, vitality, and freedom from emotional and functional illnesses of all kinds. The level of general public health in the United States has been improving through the years, but consistent health problems do trouble certain segments of our population. Diet, the customary amounts and types of food and drink taken by a person from day to day, and nutrition, the relationship between the needs of our body and the food we consume, are important factors in good health. In fact, to a certain extent, food is the basis of good health. How adequate our diet and nutrition are in contributing to good health may be measured in the following ways.

Nutritional Levels Adequate nutrition is attained when individuals are eating diets that enable them to grow, mature, reproduce, and function in a healthy and normal manner. Insufficient nutrition occurs when the nutritional level and diet are inadequate for an individual to maintain adequate health. It may result from one of two things—undernutrition or malnutrition. The effects of these two may appear separately or together.

Undernutrition This is an insufficiency of calories in the diet, and is usually caused by an insufficient supply of food. When famine strikes, those most severely hit are the very young, the old, and those in the lower socioeconomic groups. It is estimated by the United Nations Food and Agricultural Organization (FAO) that 10 to 15 percent of the world's population is undernourished.

The most obvious symptoms of continued calorie deficiency are the conditions of underweight and starvation. The undernourished body begins to utilize its own fat, protein, and other tissues, causing first a loss of weight and then a stunted growth and development. In serious cases of starvation, the metabolic rate is reduced, the pulse is slowed and weakened, the blood pressure is reduced, muscle tone is decreased, the skin becomes less elastic, mental processes are dulled, and the person is easily fatigued. In cases of extreme starvation the body becomes severely waterlogged, and death commonly occurs from heart failure.

Pregnant women suffering from severe undernourishment may have longer

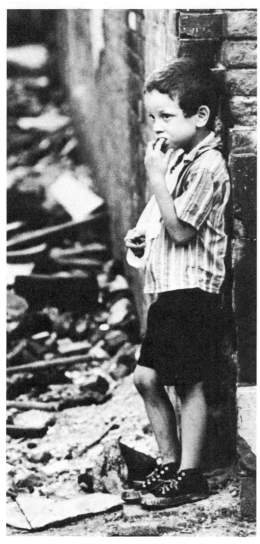

Photo by Eileen Christelow/Jeroboam.

of a child slows down, but then catches up with that of normal children when food is available. There is no permanent effect on eventual size and weight. During periods of chronic undernutrition, however, children show reduced resistance to diseases such as tuberculosis. Their muscular development is weakened, their skeletal development delayed, and permanent bone abnormalities may be produced.

Malnutrition Malnutrition is a type of selective starvation. It is the absence of some of the needed nutrients in the diet and is responsible for the deficiency diseases that affect human beings.

Protein deficiency may result from severe hemorrhaging, extensive burns, severe injuries, or loss of the body fluids. This can cause shock and circulatory collapse. More commonly, protein deficiency occurs when there is an inadequate protein intake or excessive body breakdown of proteins.

Kwashiorkor, a severe protein-deficiency disease, is the most widespread and most serious deficiency disease in the world today. It affects children from the time of their weaning to the sixth year of life. Kwashiorkor is common in southern Mexico, northern South America, tropical Africa, and India—all countries with low agricultural productivity. Recent governmental investigations have revealed evidence of the disease among the very poor in the United States.

Toward the end of a child's first year of life, if its mother's milk fails to supply enough protein and the supplementary foods given to it are largely carbohydrates, the child will suffer a greatly reduced protein intake, causing serious symptoms. The syndrome usually includes severely retarded physical and mental growth, apathy, loss of appetite, tissue swelling, loss of pigmentation, diarrhea, and anemia, as shown in the

periods of labor at childbirth, creating hazards to both child and mother. Since the mother's production of milk is often affected, infant mortality increases sharply. The famines in certain European countries occupied by the Germans during the 1940s caused a reduction in the size of children at birth. There is even some evidence that poor nutrition during pregnancy may increase the incidence of congenital handicaps.

During a temporary famine, the growth

photograph. The word *kwashiorkor*, of Ghanaian origin, means either "red boy" in reference to the change in skin and hair pigmentation among afflicted African blacks, or "displaced child" in reference to the onset of the disease in the elder child when a younger child is nursed by the mother. Before modern medical facilities were available in Africa, the mortality rate there from the disease ranged from 30 to 100 percent. Treatment consists of a diet largely composed of dry skim milk.

The symptoms of kwashiorkor also include the inability to combat such diseases as pneumonia, measles, whooping cough, diarrhea, and tuberculosis.

Vitamin A is necessary for normal bone growth, normal vision, and normal skin. In victims of xerophthalmia, a vitamin A deficiency disease, there is impaired night vision, a breakdown of the layers of the skin, and a tendency for secondary infection to readily occur. Conditions such as these can be avoided by including vitamin A or carotene in the diet.

Because of increased cloud cover, the northern latitudes tend to receive less winter sunshine than do more southerly ones. Within the United States, for example, the percentage of winter sunshine varies from 20 to 40 percent around the Great Lakes area to 70 to 90 percent in the Southwest. The amount of sunshine people receive relates directly to the amount of ultraviolet radiation they absorb and, in turn, determines the amount of vitamin D in their bodies. Ultraviolet light hitting the skin causes the body to produce vitamin D, which is essential to the proper utilization of calcium and phosphorus in the formation of bones and teeth. Fish liver oils (liquid extracts of the vitamin-rich storage tissues of the liver) are useful sources of vitamin D and are frequently given to children, especially in regions and at times when sunshine is insufficient.

Rickets and osteomalacia are vitamin D deficiency diseases typical of cold climates where foods are unavailable that are rich in vitamin D or have it added (such as whole milk). The bones of a child with rickets enlarge at the extremities (the arms and legs) and become so soft that they bend under the weight of the body. The disease has its most serious effects during the first two years of life, when growth of the long bones is most rapid. Osteomalacia, a softening of the bones caused by vitamin D deficiency, occurs chiefly in adults. Although not killers, these two diseases retard and deform, thus reducing one's work capacity and resistance to disease.

Thiamin deficiency (deficiency of vitamin B_1) is associated with diets based primarily on milled rice, which causes the disease beriberi. This deficiency disease is largely restricted to the rice-eating areas of the world, such as Southeast Asia, Venezuela, and Madagascar. In dry beriberi, the lower extremities become weak and unresponsive, seriously restricting walking. In wet beriberi, edema (accumulation of large amounts of fluids in the intercellular tissue spaces of the body) occurs, causing swelling. Cardiac beriberi is associated with heart failure. Infantile beriberi may occur in nursing infants when the mother is deficient in thiamin. All forms of beriberi may be fatal. Infantile beriberi is the leading cause of infant mortality in many developing areas of the world.

Niacin deficiency can cause the nutritional disease called *pellagra*. Prevalent in the temperate zones of the world, it is more severe during the warmer months. It appears to occur where corn is the principal food crop. It is important to realize that the cause of the disease is not the eating of corn, but rather the niacin deficiency patterns that are epidemic in those regions where corn and other starches might be relied upon in place of niacin-rich foods, such as whole grains, organ meats, and eggs.

The history of the discovery of causes of deficiency diseases consistently shows this same type of pattern. A particular food is consumed to the exclusion of another food; any change in diets occurring within that population permits the observation of a comparison between the two. For example, in China, beriberi was most common among the upper classes, the only portion of the population that could afford the expensive process of hulling and husking its rice. The vitamin B_1, held onto the rice grain by the thin hull of the grain, was removed in the rice going to those who could afford the more attractive white rice. The poorer population ate the hull and the grain and so its incidence of the disease was much lower.

This is also true in the case of scurvy. Scurvy is a deficiency disease caused by lack of ascorbic acid (vitamin C). Its incidence was consistently higher among those people who were unable to consume fresh fruits and vegetables—sailors on long voyages and rural populations during the inactive winter. It was so common during English winters that it was given the name "London's disease." Scurvy can cause pain in the joints, hemorrhaging, gum softening, and tooth loss. Inadequate amounts of vitamin C can occur in people of any age or sex, regardless of their general level of health. In fact, during the 1950s a slight outbreak of scurvy's milder symptoms was observed in a wealthy Michigan suburb, probably as a result of skipping breakfast—the one time of the day when most Americans try to get some vitamin C in their diet.

Iodine deficiency can be caused by an insufficient supply in the diet or the inability of the body to use the iodine available. Insufficient amounts of iodine in the body lead to inadequate amounts of thyroxin, a hormone responsible for the rate of metabolism in the body. Thyroxin is manufactured by the thyroid gland in the neck.

An iodine deficiency can cause the thyroid to enlarge in an attempt to produce sufficient thyroxin. This enlargement of the thyroid gland is called *goiter*, a condition more unsightly than serious in its early stages.

Iodine is most commonly found in sea water and in the plants and animals in the ocean. A useful way of assuring a sufficient supply of iodine is to include some fish in one's diet. In inland regions of the United States, the unavailability of fish often led to a serious iodine shortage, but iodized salt has successfully reduced the prevalence of this deficiency in the United States.

Reduction in the number of red blood cells or the amount of hemoglobin in red blood cells is called *anemia*. Since hemoglobin contains iron, an iron deficiency may reduce the hemoglobin concentration and cause an iron-deficiency type of anemia. Eating food rich in iron, such as liver, meat, shellfish, egg yolk, legumes, and dried fruits, can prevent this type of anemia.

Other Nutritional Disorders Many kinds of human disorders arise from faulty nutrition. For example, certain types of high blood pressure (hypertension) can be related to too much salt in the diet. Thus the use of low-salt diets is commonly recommended for those with high blood pressure. The depositing of cholesterol in the inner layer of the arteries relates to the formation of blood clots and blood vessel diseases. An excessive cholesterol level in the blood may be related to the amount and kinds of fats or carbohydrates in the diet. Nutrition plays an important role in such metabolic diseases as gout, diabetes, and obesity. Acne, eczema, dermatitis, and other skin diseases often have nutritional origins. The skin is affected by many nutritional problems—the lack of vitamins A and C, and protein. Well-nourished skin appears better able to resist skin infections. High-quality nutrition also helps to counteract both physical and emotional stresses.

Inadequate amounts of protein in the diets of children have a direct bearing on their intellectual development. Lysine, one of the amino acids, plays an important part in supplying adequate protein, which, according to some authorities, may play a significant role in how the memory operates.

The human body is like any other natural system. It must maintain a balance between the food taken in and the energy expended to operate correctly. A proper amount of nutrients and adequate exercise are needed for optimum health. Often a parent assumes that a child is healthy because there is no standard of what a healthy child should be. For this reason, the following general list of obvious characteristics of the healthy, well-nourished individual is contrasted with the unfit, undernourished or poorly nourished person.

Healthy	Unhealthy
Well developed body	Body may be undersized, or show poor development
Average weight for height	Thin (more than 10 percent underweight) or overweight (fat or flabby)
Muscles firm	Muscles small and flabby or overdeveloped
Skin firm and of a healthy color	Skin loose, sallow, waxy, or off color
Membranes of eyelids and mouth reddish pink	Membranes of eyelids and mouth pale
Eyes clear	Eyes reddened, puffiness, or dark hollows or circles
Full of life	Irritable, overactive, fatigues easily, listless, fails to concentrate
General health excellent	Susceptible to infections, lacks endurance and vigor

The following chapter (Diet and Weight Control) is a guide to the kinds and amounts of nutrients needed while the next chapter (Total Fitness) describes programs of regular energy output needed to help in maintaining healthy individuals.

Food and Affluence

Rapid global population growth continues to increase the demand for food, but, in addition, the rising affluence of nations has become a new factor affecting world food resources.

The FAO recommends a daily minimum of 2,650 calories (kcal) per person, although more than half the world's people today live on less than 2,200 calories per person per day. The diets of the world's poor nations consist primarily of plant foods and cannot be considered balanced diets. Consumed directly, cereal grains provide 52 percent of the world's food. Consumed indirectly, in the form of meat and livestock products, cereal grains provide a sizable share of the remaining 48 percent of the world's food supplies. The problem with consumption of grain through high-protein foods lies in the amount of grain needed to produce meat, milk, and eggs. for example, it takes 7 pounds of grain to produce 1 pound of beef, 4 pounds of grain for 1 pound of pork, and 3 pounds of grain for 1 pound of chicken. In the poor countries of the world, there are about 400 pounds of cereal available per person per year. Nearly all of this must be consumed directly (roughly 1 pound a person per day) to meet minimum energy needs. Little can be spared for conversion into expensive animal protein. As people's incomes rise, their consumption of grain increases, until annual income reaches $500. Then the direct consumption of wheat decreases until it levels off at about 150 pounds consumed annually, in the form of breads, pastries, and breakfast cereals. The total amount of grain consumed indirectly in the form of meat, milk, and eggs continues to grow rapidly as income climbs. In the United States, it is almost 2 tons per person per year.

Yearly consumption of beef in the United States has grown continuously, from 55 pounds per person in 1940 to a high of 192 pounds in 1971. However, in 1972 the per-person consumption of meat in the United States declined to 189 pounds. In 1973, the drop continued to 175 pounds. This may be the result of higher beef prices, or it may be a fundamental shift in eating habits in which more and more individuals prefer to eat vegetables and grains and less meat. If this trend continues, it could help the world food situation by shifting Americans toward a simpler life-style and a more balanced use of vegetables and plant foods.

In other industrial countries, from the United Kingdom, Europe, and Soviet Union to Japan, the consumption of beef has increased until now it more or less approximates the 1940 level in the United States. Increasing personal income in these countries is being used more and more for meat, milk, and eggs.

Hunger in the United States   Despite the highest food-production levels in the world and excellent distribution facilities, not every American is getting enough to eat or adequate amounts of the right foods. A large group of Americans are malnourished for many reasons.

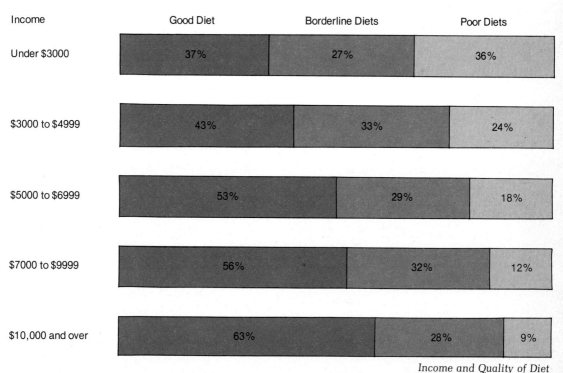

Income and Quality of Diet

Taken from U. S. Department of Agriculture, Agricultural Research Service Bulletin (Washington, D.C.).

1. Many have incomes far below their needs. The average American spends proportionately less on food than almost all other people. But while average Americans spend 20 percent of their income on food, a low-income American family may have to spend more than half of its total income in order to obtain a minimum-cost, adequate diet. Low-income families have a greater tendency to have poor diets than high-income families, because they lack the money to buy the required nutrients, as seen in the following figure.

2. A number of Americans know too little about nutrition to prepare well-balanced meals, even when they have the money to do so. Low-income families do not obtain sufficient nutrients for their money. However, having money does not ensure a proper selection of nutrients, either. Even some families in the high-income brackets still have poor diets.

3. Many people resist altering long-established preferences for foods that are nutritionally deficient. Traditional eating patterns that conform to ethnic and family preferences are frequently difficult to change in the adult years. Many family eating patterns are basically unhealthy, emphasizing fatty and starchy foods while minimizing vitamin content and mineral-rich vegetables and fruits. A person raised in this kind of environment is likely never to develop really sound eating habits.

4. Some people have far more children than their resources enable them to feed adequately. It has been assumed for years that, given equal educational opportunities and environmental advantages, a child will be as bright, imaginative, and productive as other children of the same age. Now it is being suggested that behind the empty-eyed stare of the malnourished child is a mildly retarded to severely retarded child. Severely undernourished children are smaller than average and are found to have 15 to 20 percent fewer brain cells than well-nourished children. Within the United States, high birth rates are usually found among lower-income, less educated, and non-white families. Too often these families are one and the same. Consequently, the cycle of poverty produces children who are physically, culturally, and educationally disadvantaged. These children are unable to make good use of improved educational facilities in order to upgrade their lives. Improving their nutrition could enable these children to get a better education and to take advantage more fully of opportunities to lift themselves out of poverty.

The information and machinery exist for eliminating hunger in the United States. The token efforts of the past have been inadequate and unacceptable responses. Food-distribution programs should provide high-nutrition food, not farm surpluses that cannot sell on the open market. Along with food, there should be educational programs schooling families in nutrition and explaining the rewards of producing fewer children.

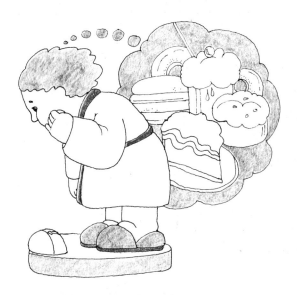

9

DIET AND WEIGHT CONTROL

Every cell of the human body requires certain chemical nutrients in the fluids that surround it. In order to supply these nutrients, the body must break down complex foods into molecules small enough to pass through tissues, enter the bloodstream or lymphatic systems, and be delivered in a usable soluble form to the various body cells. This breaking down of insoluble forms is know as *digestion*. The passage of such substances into the blood or lymph is known as *absorption*.

A Healthy Diet

A healthy diet must meet certain basic requirements. It should provide sufficient amounts of all the nutrients known to be required by good

Recommended Daily Dietary Allowances Designed for the Maintenance of Good Nutrition of Practically All Healthy People in the U.S.A.

Age (Years)	Weight (kg)	Weight (lbs)	Height (in)	Energy (kcal)	Protein (g)	Fat-Soluble Vitamins			Water-Soluble Vitamins							Minerals					
						Vitamin A Activity (IU)	Vitamin D (IU)	Vitamin E Activity (IU)	Ascorbic Acid (mg)	Folacin (mg)	Niacin (mg)	Riboflavin (mg)	Thiamin (mg)	Vitamin B$_6$ (mg)	Vitamin B$_{12}$ (mg)	Calcium (mg)	Phosphorus (mg)	Iodine (mg)	Iron (mg)	Magnesium (mg)	Zinc (mg)
INFANTS																					
0.0–0.5	6	14	24	kg × 117	kg × 2.2	1400	400	4	35	50	5	0.4	0.3	0.3	0.3	360	240	35	10	60	3
0.5–1.0	9	20	28	kg × 108	kg × 2.0	2000	400	5	35	50	8	0.6	0.5	0.4	0.3	540	400	45	15	70	5
CHILDREN																					
1–3	13	28	34	1300	23	2000	400	7	40	100	9	0.8	0.7	0.6	1.0	800	800	60	15	150	10
4–6	20	44	44	1800	30	2500	400	9	40	200	12	1.1	0.9	0.9	1.5	800	800	80	10	200	10
7–10	30	66	54	2400	36	3300	400	10	40	300	16	1.2	1.2	1.2	2.0	800	800	110	10	250	10
MALES																					
11–14	44	97	63	2800	44	5000	400	12	45	400	18	1.5	1.4	1.6	3.0	1200	1200	130	18	350	15
15–18	61	134	69	3000	54	5000	400	15	45	400	20	1.8	1.5	2.0	3.0	1200	1200	150	18	400	15
19–22	67	147	69	3000	54	5000	400	15	45	400	20	1.8	1.5	2.0	3.0	800	800	140	10	350	15
23–50	70	154	69	2700	56	5000	—	15	45	400	18	1.6	1.4	2.0	3.0	800	800	130	10	350	15
51+	70	154	69	2400	56	5000	—	15	45	400	16	1.5	1.2	2.0	3.0	800	800	110	10	350	15
FEMALES																					
11–14	44	97	62	2400	44	4000	400	12	45	400	16	1.3	1.2	1.6	3.0	1200	1200	115	18	300	15
15–18	54	119	65	2100	48	4000	400	12	45	400	14	1.4	1.1	2.0	3.0	1200	1200	115	18	300	15
19–22	58	128	65	2100	46	4000	400	12	45	400	14	1.4	1.1	2.0	3.0	800	800	100	18	300	15
23–50	58	128	65	2000	46	4000	—	12	45	400	13	1.2	1.0	2.0	3.0	800	800	100	18	300	15
51+	58	128	65	1800	46	4000	—	12	45	400	12	1.1	1.0	2.0	3.0	800	800	80	10	300	15
PREGNANT				+300	+30	5000	400	15	60	800	+2	+0.3	+0.3	2.5	4.0	1200	1200	125	18+[a]	450	20
LACTATING				+500	+20	6000	400	15	80	600	+4	+0.5	+0.3	2.5	4.0	1200	1200	150	18	450	25

IU stands for International Unit.
1 kilogram (kg) = 2.2 pounds (lbs)
1 kilogram (kg) = 1,000 grams (g)

1 kilocalorie (kcal) = 1,000 calories
1 gram (g) = 1,000 milligrams (mg)
1 milligram (mg) = 1,000 micrograms (mcg)

Taken from Food and Nutrition Board, National Academy of Science—National Research Council, *Recommended Daily Dietary Allowances*, Revised 1973.

[a] This increased requirement cannot be met by ordinary diets; therefore, the use of supplemental iron is recommended.

NOTE: Slightly abridged.

health. It should provide these substances in amounts that are compatible with the needs of the individual. And it should not provide any nutrient in dangerous excess. (Some nutrients can be stored in the body if excess occurs; other nutrients can be eliminated if more than the basal amount is provided. Other nutrients might be toxic in high concentrations in the body.) A diet should include a variety of textures to maintain good intestinal tone and should provide a sufficient amount of water. There are several guidelines—some developed by research agencies in government and private industry, some provided by educational institutions to help in the teaching of sound nutrition—which can help you select a good diet.

Recommended Dietary Allowances

The following are basic recommendations for the daily amount of food that should be available to everyone. In 1973 and 1974, new food-labeling regulations were issued by the U.S. Food and Drug Administration (FDA). They required that labels on foods packaged within the United States list the proportions of U.S. Recommended Daily Allowances (RDA) of nutrients that one serving contains.

The RDAs are based on statistics gained from studies of large groups of people. Individuals vary in terms of physical structure and biochemical makeup. Since some people need more, some less, than the recommended amounts of certain nutrients, it must not be automatically assumed that certain food practices are poor or that people are malnourished simply because the recommendations are not being completely met. Also, the RDAs are ample enough to provide some margin of safety for each nutrient in order to take care of variations among different individuals. For most people in this country, the recommended allowances can be considered

adequate for maintaining good health and preventing nutritional diseases.

In addition to defining what are sufficient amounts of each nutrient, we should take a look at the matter of excess amounts of certain nutrients in the body. Fat-soluble vitamins can be stored in the body, and can be toxic when taken in excess. The RDAs for such vitamins should be adequate for most individuals. Excess water-soluble vitamins are excreted by the body, but if excess amounts are consumed without enough water to carry them through the kidneys, they can cause permanent kidney damage. Also, excess amounts of fatty and starchy foods produce overweight individuals, while high-protein diets can cause kidney damage. All the nutrients that one consumes should be balanced to promote good health.

The Reference Man and Woman   The reference man for Recommended Dietary Allowances is 22 years old, weighs 147 pounds, and is 5 feet, 8 inches tall. The reference woman is 22 years old, weighs 128 pounds, and is 5 feet, 4 inches tall. The allowances are intended to provide for individual variation among most normal persons living in the United States under the usual environmental stresses. The table presents the Recommended Dietary Allowances as revised in 1973. Diets should be based on a variety of common foods in order to provide other nutrients for which human requirements have not been well defined.

Variations from Reference Individuals
The dietary allowances recommended so far have basically been set up for the average, healthy, active adult male and female at age 22. These allowances would not be considered adequate for other normal life periods, such as infancy (from childbirth

up to 1 year of age), childhood (from 1 to 10), adolescence (from 11 to 18), pregnancy and lactation (the time following childbirth during which the mother is producing her own milk), middle years (from 23 to 55), and after age 61. The recommended diets for these periods are sufficiently different from those recommended for reference individuals that dietary adjustments must be made. Dietary adjustments from the reference person will also be required during times of illness and certain other health problems. Since suggestions for dietary adjustments due to illness should be made by a physician, changes in eating habits during such times will not be included here.

The energy requirement for the reference man is 3,000 Calories per day and for the reference woman, 2,100 Calories. Adjustments in caloric intake must be made for differences in age, body size, and activity.

Adjustment for Age Average energy requirements are low in infancy, increase through childhood, and are high during the late teen years. They then decline progressively with advancing age. In addition to age, the amount of energy required also depends on the person's resting metabolism (RM) and the amount of physical activity engaged in.

Adjustment for Body Size Caloric allowances must be adjusted upward or downward in terms of differences in body size and the amount of body fat an individual carries. Weight–height tables such as shown here provide a convenient guide to desirable body weight. It shows the desirable weight for adults (those 18 and older). Adjustments are indicated on the table for sex, height, and body build. An individual with a smaller-than-average frame would be expected to weigh somewhat less than the weight recommended

Desirable Weights for Adults

Height[a] (feet and inches)	Weight (pounds) Men	Women
5 ft.		109 ±9[b]
5 ft. 2 in.		115 ± 9
5 ft. 4 in.	133 ± 11	122 ± 10
5 ft. 5 in.		128 ±10[c]
5 ft. 6 in.	142 ± 12	129 ± 10
5 ft. 8 in.	151 ± 14	136 ± 10
5 ft. 9 in.	154 ± 14[d]	
5 ft. 10 in.	159 ± 14	144 ± 11
6 ft.	167 ± 15	152 ± 12
6 ft. 2 in.	175 ± 15	
6 ft. 4 in.	182 ± 16	

[a]Heights and weights are taken nude.
[b]Desirable weight for a small-framed woman at this height would be approximately 109 lb. minus 9 lb., or a total of 100 lb.; for an average-framed woman, 109 lb.; for a large-framed woman, 109 lb. plus 9 lb., or a total of 118 lb.
[c]Reference woman
[d]Reference man

for a given height, whereas an individual with a larger-than-average frame would usually weigh more.

Of course, the goal of any reducing program is not to normalize body weight according to a table but to reduce to normal the amount of fat stored in the body. Body fat is stored mainly in specialized cells called *adipose cells*. When filled with fat, adipose cells contain about 85 to 90 percent fat, 2 percent protein, and 10 percent water. When body weight is reduced, the water leaves these cells first, which accounts for the rapid weight loss during the first few days of a weight-reduction diet.

There are a number of ways to measure the extent of body fat. One is to estimate the thickness of folds of skin and fat pinched up in several places on the body (the upper back, abdomen, chest, arms, or legs). If such a skinfold is over an inch thick, an individual should lose weight. Another method of calculating body fat-ness is to take circumference or "envelope" measurements of torso, legs, and arms, especially the circumference of thighs and buttocks. These measurements very easily show whether an individual is overweight.

Although maximum body weight is usually attained by age 20 in the male and by age 18 in the female, people in the United States tend to continue gaining body weight until about 60 years of age. Actuarial studies (the calculation of insurance risks and premiums) indicate that these weight gains are undesirable and that the most favorable health expectation is achieved when the weight normally reached by age 22 is maintained throughout life. This is why the recommended caloric allowances for adults relate to the desirable body weight (or the average weight of individuals of a given sex and height) at age 22 and why the age of the reference man and woman is given as 22. These recommended caloric allowances thus pertain to a desirable body weight throughout life.

Adjustment for Activity   There is no easy way to determine the number of calories used during physical activity. Some suggestions are made in the energy expenditure table in terms of the reference man and woman. Normally, people increase their caloric intake as they increase their activity. But the greatest problem is in reducing caloric intake when a person's activity decreases. An easy way to become overweight is to continue eating approximately the same amounts of food as living becomes easier, because of modern conveniences and less activity.

Calculations of Dietary Needs   There are no definite requirements for carbohydrate intake, and the amount of carbohydrates in the diet can be varied considerably. Carbohydrate-rich foods like sugars and starches provide an economical energy source, furnish some minerals and vitamins, and add flavor (especially as sugar) to foods and beverages. No more than a small supply of carbohydrates needs to be present in the diet if fats and proteins are available.

Nutritionists believe that no more than 25 percent nor less than 10 percent of the food one eats should be fat. Some fat should always be in the diet because the body needs essential fatty acids, and most fat-soluble vitamins, especially A and D, gain entrance to the body through fat-rich foods. Whenever reducing fat intake in a low-fat diet, you should supplement your diet with vitamin A in capsule form.

Adults can adapt to a wide range of protein intake, but the least amount consumed should give a liberal margin over the minimum daily requirements listed in the RDA table. On the other hand, superabundant protein intake provides no advantage and just adds weight. In general, it is unwise to limit the intake of protein over long periods. Each day an individual should eat a minimum of about 0.5 grams of protein per kilogram (2.2 pounds) of body weight to ensure the best nutritional conditions.

It is important that the protein come from a wide variety of sources, with at least 25 to 50 percent of the total from animal or other high-quality protein sources. This should provide about twice the minimal needs for the average child, and allow a reasonable margin for growth.

More calories, proteins, minerals, and vitamins are required during the body's growth period. Development for normal individuals will vary considerably depending on differences in height and weight.

Infants and Adolescents   Dietary needs can be calculated for life periods other than the reference period, which is 19 to 22 years. The following figures graphically show caloric allowances for males and females of average size and activity from ages 1 to 18. Separate charts are required because there are major differences in growth rates between females and males after age 9.

Healthy adolescents show marked variations in food intake, and for this reason these caloric allowances must be interpreted with caution. There also are wide variations in their physical activities. Individuals who are inactive may become obese even when the caloric intake is clearly below the recommended allowances, while those who are extremely active must have larger allowances.

Caloric Needs During Pregnancy If a woman has established good eating habits and is well nourished when she becomes pregnant, she has little cause for concern. She needs only to increase intake of some foods she is accustomed to eating. Her nutritive needs are best met by a simple, wholesome diet, based upon milk (and dairy products), eggs, meat, legumes, whole grains, fruits, and vegetables.

From the first through the fourth month of pregnancy, nutrient needs for the daily growth of the fetus are so small that the mother should eat just what any woman normally could consume to preserve or build up health and vitality. However, nausea during this time may cause a woman to eat smaller meals at shorter intervals. If vomiting is severe or prolonged she should notify her doctor. Vitamin–mineral supplements should be taken only if prescribed by the doctor.

After the fourth month, the National Research Council recommends increased allowances for almost all essential nutrients. These recommendations are shown in the RDA table. By the sixth month, the fetus is gaining about 10 grams of weight daily. About half of the total weight increase of

the fetus occurs in the last two months. Therefore, it is very important that a pregnant woman eat foods unusually rich in all nutrients during this two-month period.

Any caloric increase during pregnancy must be closely observed. An excessive weight gain during pregnancy is undesirable and may lead to complications at delivery. Also, some women may find that this excessive weight gained during pregnancy may never be lost. A normal and desirable weight gain during the forty weeks of pregnancy is 20 to 25 pounds. The expectant mother must greatly curtail

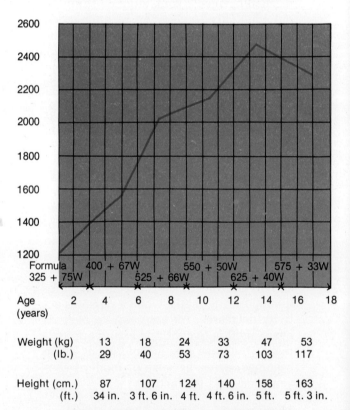

Calorie allowance for females by age and formulas for adjustment by weight. W in formulas is weight in kilograms. To convert formulas for weight in pounds, divide factor by 2.2.

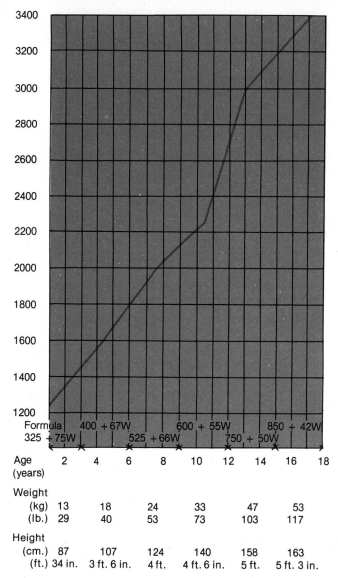

Age (years)	2	4	6	8	10	12	14	16	18

Formula: 400 + 67W   600 + 55W   850 + 42W
325 + 75W   525 + 66W   750 + 50W

Weight						
(kg)	13	18	24	33	47	53
(lb.)	29	40	53	73	103	117

Height						
(cm.)	87	107	124	140	158	163
(ft.)	34 in.	3 ft. 6 in.	4 ft.	4 ft. 6 in.	5 ft.	5 ft. 3 in.

Calorie allowances for males by age and formulas for adjustment by weight. W in formulas is weight in kilograms. To convert formulas for weight in pounds, divide factor by 2.2.

her consumption of sweet, starchy, or fatty foods, concentrating on those foods that yield large amounts of proteins, vitamins, and minerals in proportion to their caloric

value. Only about 11 pounds of this weight is lost at delivery in the form of child, placenta, membranes, and fluids. Some weight is also lost during the next several weeks. Any other excess weight is likely to remain permanently. As a consequence, many women grow heavier with each child, while other women who are active during and after their pregnancies retain slender figures. A woman who wants to control her weight during a pregnancy should increase her physical activity and not cut down on the essential nutrients she is eating.

Teen-age mothers have about 15 percent of all the births in the United States. At the present time, about 40 percent of all brides in the United States are between the ages of 15 and 18 years. Yet studies have shown that in this country, teen-agers are more likely to be undernourished than any other segment of the population, and therefore are poor prospects for a healthy pregnancy.

At birth, a child is already more than nine months old in terms of nutrition and development, and a child's nutrition can be no better than that of the mother. Both for themselves and their children, it is most important that pregnant women eat a balanced diet.

Caloric Needs During Breast-Feeding
The nutritive requirements of nursing mothers are higher than those for pregnant women. As shown in the RDA table, all nutrients need to be increased for the lactating (milk-producing) mother. A woman who has gained an adequate amount of weight (20 to 25 pounds) during pregnancy will have a fat reserve on which to call to help meet her lactational needs. Breast-feeding her infant will help to normalize her weight after a pregnancy.

While breast-feeding, a woman should eat an extra 500 calories per day. She should make sure that at least 85 of these calories, or about 20 grams, are protein. Since milk is very rich in calcium and phosphorus, a breast-feeding mother should increase her intake of milk by one pint to one quart to meet the demands of her child. Vitamin content of the mother's milk is greatly dependent upon her daily intake of vitamins, and this is especially true of the water-soluble vitamins. She should increase her intake of vitamins about 50 percent. Before giving birth, the wise mother will use nutritional information to plan how she is going to meet the increased needs of breast-feeding.

Caloric Needs During Aging One problem common among adults is a failure to realize that their energy requirements decline as they grow older. In order to maintain ideal weight, their caloric intake should be reduced by 5 percent per decade (every ten years) between the ages of 23 and 50, by 8 percent per decade between the ages of 50 and 75, and by 10 percent in the years following age 75.

Such a reduction of caloric intake can prevent obesity as the person becomes older. Obesity can occur simply because the person is accustomed to certain eating habits and continues in spite of increasing age and lowering energy requirements. As people get older, there is a reduction in their rates of basal metabolism (BMR) and in their physical activity. Because the exact degree of reduction in basal metabolism and activity is impossible to predict for each individual, tables such as that showing desirable weight for adults serve only as a reference.

Although total caloric intake should be reduced with advancing age, the body's ability to utilize proteins efficiently decreases as the individual ages, and therefore it is suggested that the protein allowance remain the same for all ages. The same suggestion is made for minerals and vitamins.

In order to cut down the number of calories consumed, there must be a reduction in the intake of such common foods as bread, cereal, fats, and sweets. This reduction is important, since too much caloric intake from these sources will interfere with the proper utilization of proteins. Consequently, the best advice is to cut down on fats and sweets as you grow older.

Diet and Weight Control It is an extraordinary paradox that while much of the world's population is fighting starvation, more than 25 percent of the people in the United States are overweight due to excessive eating. The preoccupation that captivates many people in this country is that of weight control. The magnitude of the problem is shown by the one-quarter to one-half billion dollars a year that Americans pay "fat doctors" to help in overcoming this problem. Such concern is not only a reflection of the importance we attach to proper weight, but also a frank commentary on the failure many people encounter in their attempts to maintain a satisfactory weight.

Appetite and hunger control relate to the ability to control weight. Appetite and hunger are known to be controlled by a small area in the brain called the "appetite center" or *appestat*. It is composed of two sets of nuclei. One determines your perception of hunger and one determines your perception of a satisfied feeling; your willingness to eat is regulated by the comparison between the two. Thus, the appestat works something like a thermostat controlling the temperature of a room.

As to what activates the appestat, there is still some question. It may be the glucose level (blood-sugar level) in the blood, body temperature changes, or the level of amino acids in the blood. But it is known that the appetite center has nerve connections with the cortex of the brain and may also be consciously controlled. This means that emotional factors, as well as chemical ones, appear to control appetite. Worry, tension, frustration, and conflicts in interpersonal relations can influence a person's appetite. Other research has shown that appestats vary in different individuals. Thus a person may inherit a "higher setting" in the appestat than another person and require more food before feeling satisfied. Consequently, we can say that appetite is regulated by emotions, body chemistry, and inheritance. All of these factors influence the ability to control weight. Most of us succeed in accomplishing things we want to acomplish; we do things that interest or motivate us. If we are to maintain a desirable weight we must *want* to. Reasons for losing weight or maintaining a desirable weight that appeal to or motivate people include the following:

1. *A desire to look attractive.* Whether a person likes it or not, he or she must admit that clothing styles are directed toward slender figures. Of course, larger sizes are provided for those who need them, but these are not the fashion ideal. Few people are not influenced by the fashion market. Then again, it's always pleasant to fit into a standard-size theater or lecture-hall seat, or to take no more than our third of the car seat. The overweight person faces such dilemmas daily.

2. *Longer life.* According to studies, a man 45 years of age, of medium height and frame, and weighing 170 pounds, can expect to live 2 to 4 fewer years than a similar man weighing 150 pounds. A man 45 years of age, of medium height and frame, weighing 200 pounds, can expect to live 4 to 6 years fewer than a similar man weighing 150 pounds.

3. *Fewer diseases.* Cardiovascular disease, diabetes, gallbladder disease, cirrhosis of the liver, certain forms of cancer, and arthritis occur more often or can be more serious in overweight people than in those of desirable weight.

4. *Fewer painful conditions.* Overweight is a factor in such common conditions as varicose veins, high blood pressure, gout, pulmonary emphysema, nephritis, and toxemia in pregnancy. It is estimated that for every pound of added fat an additional two-thirds of a mile of blood vessels are required to keep this pound of fat alive.

Excess fat complicates all surgery and increases surgical risks. The same is true in the delivery of a child. It takes extra body effort to carry body weight that is not needed; thus, the overweight person is more often tired. Fat accumulates around internal vital organs (such as the heart and lungs) and tends to crowd them. The overweight person is less agile, has more balancing problems, moves more slowly, and has more physical accidents than a person of normal weight.

Patterns of Obesity Obesity is the medical condition of overweight caused by excess fat on the body frame. It is thought to be due to one of two basic causes. It may be caused by a difference in the ability of the body to utilize food in the same manner as the majority of people (known as *metabolic obesity*). Or obesity can be caused by an inability to regulate food intake, called *regulatory obesity*.

Metabolic obesity depends on the rate at which food is being built up for storage and broken down for use (the rate of metabolism), which varies from person to person. These differences occur in response to specific hormone and enzyme activities in the body. Rate differences may be the result of inherited or developmental differences, or they may be the result of disease in the pituitary gland or the thyroid gland. Such conditions can cause overweight or underweight, but less than 5 percent of all cases can be blamed on the glands.

Regulatory obesity occurs far more often; this is the result of failure on the part of a person to voluntarily control his or her food intake. If such overeating is continued long enough, it may cause basic metabolic changes. Some factors that can affect a person's eating habits and weight include the following:

1. *Family eating and exercise habits.* According to U.S. Department of Health, Education, and Welfare (HEW) statistics, over two-thirds of the parents of obese children are themselves obese. It has not been determined to what extent hereditary factors are responsible for this relationship, but it does seem that nonhereditary factors are also important. The role of the parents as models for eating and exercise habits seems particularly significant. Some individuals come from homes in which parents provide meals that are excessive in calories. Others are accustomed to heavy between-meal eating of soft drinks, candy, ice cream, and pastries. Still others have been accustomed to too little exercise as a result of easily available transportation, too few sports, modern conveniences, and sheer laziness.

2. *Emotional factors.* Some people use food as a comfort, crutch, or compensation for feelings of frustration, unhappiness, or worry. They overeat to counteract domestic troubles, financial problems, family illness, or social upsets.

3. *Poverty.* Some families, because of limited finances, buy cheap foods that tend to be high in carbohydrates or fats, in place of more expensive protein-rich foods.

4. *Uncontrolled snacking and nibbling.* This habit can lead to the consumption of uncounted calories. When such snacking is added to regular meals, it can mean more calories taken in than the body is using, and thus more stored fat. Controlled nibbling is not damaging as long as the nibbling does not interfere with good nutrition and excesses are avoided.

5. *Failure to cut down eating during reduced activity.* It has already been pointed out that as a person becomes less active with age or occupation, he or she requires fewer calories to maintain weight level. If, on the other hand, food intake is not decreased but remains about the same, he or she puts on added weight.

6. *Ignorance.* Some people are frankly ignorant of caloric values of various foods. They tend to confuse the wide differences in the caloric content of favorite foods and drinks (see table).

Regardless of the underlying causes of obesity, the basic problem is simply one of taking in more calories than are needed for one's total activities—basal metabolism, heat loss, work, and exercise. Unused calories from any source are stored in the body as fat; each pound of stored fat is the equivalent of 3,500 calories. All calories taken in are either stored or used, and the more calories that are stored, the greater the degree of obesity.

Reducing Reducing calls for unyielding determination. A person must be prepared to face the rigors of ignoring the sight and smell of appealing food within his reach. This calls for high motivation and willpower.

A person must accept a personal responsibility for a weight problem. It cannot be blamed on family problems, spouse, un-manageable children, lack of friends, or troubles in general. Although admittedly these may affect the obese person, in the end it is that person who has been voluntarily overeating.

A reducing diet is based on the principle that reducing the calorie intake will permit daily caloric needs to exceed the available amount from the diet. In this way, stored body fat can be used up and weight can be reduced.

The Calorie Content in Some Favorite Foods and Drinks

Breakfast	Calories	Drinks	Calories
1 scrambled egg	110	Whole milk, 1 cup	160
2 slices fried bacon	100	Nonfat milk, 1 cup	90
Ham, slice, lean and fat	245	Malted milk, 1 cup	280
1 wheat pancake	60	Cocoa, 1 cup	235
1 waffle	210	Orange juice, frozen, 1 cup diluted	110
Grapefruit, ½ whole	55	Apple juice, 1 cup	120
Cantaloupe, ½ melon	60	Grape juice, canned, 1 cup	165
Corn flakes, 1 oz	110	Yoghurt, 1 cup	120
Oatmeal, 1 cup	130	Cola drink, 1 cup	95
White bread, 1 slice	60	Ginger ale, 1 cup	70
Butter, 1 pat	50	Beer, 1 cup	100
Jam, 1 tablespoon	55		

Lunch or Dinner		Snacks	
Tomato soup, 1 cup	90	Cheddar cheese, 1-inch cube	70
Spaghetti, meat balls and tomato sauce, 1 cup	335	Bologna, 1 slice	85
Pork chop, 1 slice lean	130	Peanut butter, 1 tablespoon	95
Roast beef, 1 slice lean	125	Peanuts, roasted, 1 cup	840
Hamburger, meat only, 3 oz	245	10 potato chips	115
1 frankfurter, cooked	155	Raisins, dried, 1 cup	460
Chicken, ½ breast	155	1 apple	70
Mashed potatoes, buttered, 1 cup	185	1 banana	85
Pizza, 1 section	185	1 orange, navel	60
Cottage cheese, creamed, 1 cup	240	1 peach	35
Custard, 1 cup	285	Watermelon, 1 wedge	115
Angelfood cake, 1 section	110	Popcorn, 1 cup	65
Iced chocolate cake, 1 section	445	2 graham crackers	55
Apple pie, 1 section	345	1 doughnut, cake type	125
Ice cream, 1 cup	285	Candy, milk chocolate, 1 oz.	150
Sherbet, orange, 1 cup	260	Marshmallows, 1 oz.	90
Cornstarch pudding, 1 cup	275	Pretzels, 5 small sticks	20
		1 fig bar	55
		1 cookie, 3-inch	120

Taken from U.S. Department of Agriculture, *Nutritive Value of Foods*, Home and Garden Bulletin No. 72, rev. ed. (Washington, D.C.: U.S. Government Printing Office, 1964.)

Reducing Diets There are many ideas and suggestions about how to lose weight. These range in severity from the "miracle diets" that guarantee to take off 10 pounds in 2 weeks to oils, tablets, seeds, juices, extracts, and high-fat or protein diets. There are also prepared formulas on the market in the form of canned drinks or cookies. Some of these have value, some are worthless, and some are actually dangerous.

Low-carbohydrate diets have been prominent in recent years. While they are known by many names and variations, the basic premise of all of these diets is that if carbohydrates are restricted enough, other calorie sources, even fats and alcohol, may be consumed in unlimited quantities without interfering with weight loss. While such diets have enabled many people to lose weight, at least temporarily, there are strong warnings from many medical authorities regarding the dangers inherent in the extreme low-carbohydrate diet. The AMA Council on Foods and Nutrition has stated: "The council is deeply concerned about any diet that advocates an unlimited intake of saturated fats and cholesterol-rich foods. Individuals responding to such a diet with a rise in blood fats will have an increased risk of coronary artery disease and atherosclerosis, particularly if the diet is maintained over a prolonged period." Another concern is that when carbohydrate intake is very low, fats are broken down to chemicals called *ketones*, creating an acidic condition in the blood. Among the known or suspected effects of extreme low-carbohydrate diets are weakness, faintness, depression of the functions of the central nervous system, kidney and liver damage, and the development of gout (a painful accumulation of uric acid crystals in the body).

1. *See a physician.* A doctor should decide whether it is safe for you to lose

A 1200-Calorie-Per-Day Diet Pattern

Breakfast

Fruit—1 medium serving, fresh, frozen, or canned
Egg—1, poached or boiled
Toast—1 slice with 1 teaspoon butter or margarine

or

Cereal—½ cup with ¼ cup milk, no sugar
Coffee or tea—no cream or sugar

Midmorning Snack

Nonfat milk or buttermilk—1 glass

Luncheon

Meat or cheese—1 3-oz. portion
Vegetable—1 medium serving; may be raw, as a salad such as lettuce and tomato, or cooked; use lemon or vinegar for seasoning rather than butter or salad dressings
Fruit—1 medium serving, fresh or unsweetened canned
Bread—1 slice
Butter or margarine—1 teaspooon or 1 pat
Tea or coffee—no cream or sugar

Midafternoon

Iced tea, lemonade, or a soft drink

Dinner

Bouillon or consommé or vegetable-juice cocktail—1 serving
Meat—1 3-oz. portion
Potato or a substitute for potato—1 small serving of mashed or baked potato, steamed rice, corn, lima beans, or macaroni; or 1 slice bread
Vegetable—1 serving, raw, as a salad, or cooked; one vegetable a day should be a green, leafy one
Butter or margarine—1 teaspoon, for potato
Fruit—1 medium serving, fresh or unsweetened canned
Tea or coffee—no cream or sugar

Evening or Bedtime

Nonfat milk, buttermilk, soft drink, or glass of beer
Crackers or pretzels—2

weight, how much to lose, and how long the reduction should take.

2. *Choose a practical diet.* Under the direction of your physician you should choose a reducing diet that can be followed without undue punishment or undue cost. It should be compatible with eating habits you are accustomed to. It is not necessary to stop eating the foods you cherish, but it will be necessary to regulate the amount of them that you eat. Such regulation is demanded not only for losing pounds, but also for maintaining a desirable weight when it is reached. Once the reducing diet is over and you have lost the unnecessary pounds, you should never return to the old excessive weight. Unless you learn to live on a maintaining diet, all of your agonies of losing weight will have been in vain.

3. *Reduce the calories taken in.* Opinions vary on whether caloric reduction can best be done by limiting carbohydrate intake, fat intake, or protein intake. But whatever the method, there is no doubt that calories do count (even if you refuse to count them). You must watch your foods, particularly the rich ones. Some of these tantalizing and irresistible foods are loaded with calories. Remember that fats have over twice the calories, per unit of weight, of carbohydrates or proteins, so learn what the high-fat foods are and how to cut down on them.

4. *Plan the diet.* One of the most important facts about weight reduction is that the same number of nutrients must be "fitted" into a smaller number of calories. Your reducing plan should include all the basic food groups—meat, milk, vegetables, fruits, grains, minerals, vitamins, and water. Also, your body will still need a daily supply of proteins, minerals, vitamins, and limited calories. A good reducing diet should provide at least 1,200 to 1,800 calories a day. Some commercially prepared, canned reducing formulas supply a minimum of 900 calories per day. These are acceptable when they contain carefully measured supplements of essential vitamins and minerals. The 1,200 calorie-per-day table shows how many combinations of food are available for a well-planned diet.

5. *Know your reducing goal.* You should know how many pounds you intend to lose and how long the reduction should take. Each pound of body fat represents 3,500 calories. To lose 1 pound in 1 week, you must reduce your calorie intake by 3,500 calories over that period of time. "Crash" diets that claim to take off 10 pounds in 2 weeks mean a calorie reduction of 2,500 calories a day, which is more than some people normally eat altogether.

6. *Graph your progress.* Since you gain weight gradually, you should lose it slowly. But, because gradual reducing

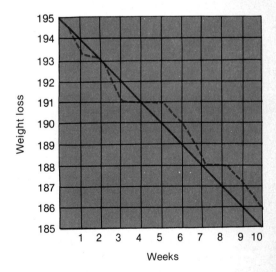

A typical weight-reducing graph. The straight line shows the ideal weight change from steady maintenance of a low-caloric diet plan; the dotted line is the more realistic pattern of expected weight change.

plans can be discouraging, you may lose sight of your goal. Therefore, a good psychological aid is to keep track of progress by setting up a simple graph at the beginning of the program. You should plan to lose 1 or 2 pounds a week, and construct a typical reducing graph similar to the one shown here. In constructing the graph, you should allow as many weeks as there are pounds to lose, draw a straight line from where your beginning weight is to where it should be at the end, weigh in each morning on the bathroom scales, and place a dot on the graph at your weight point for that day. The graph can be a reminder of your progress and keep you determined to succeed.

7. *Exercise regularly.* A reasonable program of regular exercise helps to burn up energy, improves muscle tone, and creates a feeling of well-being, both physically and emotionally. Many people, including certain authorities, have tended to underestimate the role of exercise in weight control and of inactivity as a contributing factor in obesity. But now, many authorities are placing added emphasis on the importance of exercise in addition to diet. Some people rationalize their inactivity, stating that exercise would increase their appetite, canceling its beneficial effects. But this is rarely so. In fact, for most people exercise lets the appestat function more effectively, reducing the amount of "nervous" eating that is often the result of inactivity. Thus exer-

cise may actually decrease the appetite of a sedentary person.

Underweight Whether or not someone should be called underweight should not be determined by weight alone, but on the presence or absence of associated symptoms of malnutrition. It is possible to eat a balanced diet, in moderation, and remain in excellent health even though slender. But symptoms such as lack of endurance, easy fatigue, frequent infections, intermittent diarrhea, or sores on the skin or mucous membranes might indicate a definite problem of undernutrition—there is not enough food intake for normal body function. In severe cases, the results can include deficiency diseases, injury to vital organs (especially heart and kidneys), and even death. Underweight can be caused by emotional state (nervousness, worry, anxiety), diseases, malnutrition (poor selection of foods), hormonal disorders, or unrealistic dieting.

The treatment of underweight is not always just a simple matter of starting to eat more. There should be a physician's consultation to detect the presence of any infectious or glandular disease or other contributing condition. If the problem appears to be purely dietary, emphasis should be on a good balanced diet, adequate in protein and other nutrients. If the problem is an emotional one, as is often the case, efforts should be made to either correct, or learn to cope with, the underlying conditions. Increased exercise may help relieve nervous tension, leading to improved diet.

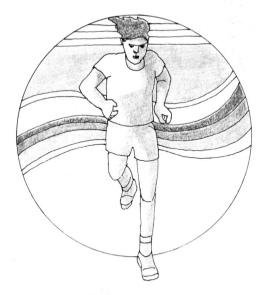

10

TOTAL FITNESS

According to Dr. Roger Bannister (the first person to run a mile in four minutes), *fitness* is one of the most misused words in the English language. It can mean anything from a general, overall joy in living to a specific suitability for particular kinds of mental and physical tasks.

The Measure of Total Fitness

Total fitness implies the ability to function at an optimum level of efficiency in all daily living. This encompasses the whole philosophy of the science of health: intellectual, emotional, and social, as well as physical conditioning. A totally fit individual has the strength, speed, agility, endurance, and social and emotional adjustments appropriate to his or her age. Each of these characteristics involves energy.

All body activities require energy. Very simply, energy is produced by breaking down foods (carbohydrates, fats, and proteins) in the presence of oxygen. The body can store food, but it cannot store oxygen. If the body takes in more food than is needed, it uses what it needs and stores the rest for later. Not so with oxygen. We cannot store oxygen, so we breathe in and out every moment of our lives to keep the supply coming in. If the oxygen supply were suddenly cut off, the oxygen stored in the body would not last more than a few minutes. The brain, the heart, all body tissues would cease to function, and we would die. The oxygen in the air is readily available; as we need it, we breathe it in. The problem is getting enough oxygen to all parts of the body where food is burned.

Most of us produce enough energy to perform ordinary daily activities; that is, to walk, talk, think, or study. However, as the activities become more vigorous, we sooner or later reach our maximum performance or maximum oxygen consumption. A person's maximum oxygen consumption is known as his or her *aerobic capacity*. The range between our minimum oxygen requirements (amount of oxygen used at rest) and our maximum capacity is one factor in the physiological measure of our total fitness. The most totally fit persons have the greatest range of capacity; the least fit, the narrowest range. In some persons, their minimum energy requirements and maximum physical capacity are almost identical. A totally fit individual should have, among other qualities, adequate aerobic capacity and physical strength to engage in daily physical activities, including such sports as tennis, swimming, bicycling, and handball, without producing undue fatigue.

To achieve this level of fitness an indi-

Energy Expenditure Per Hour During Different Types of Activities

Form of Activity	Calories per Hour Man (154 lbs.)	Calories per Hour Woman (128 lbs.)
Sleeping	65	50
Awake lying still	77	71
Sitting at rest	100	98
Standing relaxed	105	85
Dressing and undressing	118	107
Tailoring	135	115
Typewriting rapidly	140	129
"Light" exercise	170	160
Walking slowly (2.6 miles per hour)	200	186
Carpentry, metal-working, industrial painting	240	221
"Active" exercise (brisk walking)	290	272
"Severe" exercise	450	427
Sawing wood	480	441
Swimming	500	457
Running (5.3 miles per hour)	570	533
"Very severe" exercise	600	557
Walking very fast (5.3 miles per hour)	650	637
Walking up stairs	1100	1016

Adapted from A.C. Guyton, *Basic Human Physiology,* 4th. ed. (Philadelphia: W.B. Saunders, 1971).

vidual must participate in a daily fitness program. Programs must be individually tailored to the needs of the person. For example, the term *weight lifting* applies to the competitive weight lifter whose objective is to see how much weight he or she can lift. *Body building* involves lifting weights to build up muscles. *Weight training* is done to improve an individual's strength so that he or she can perform in other physical activities or sports. All three types of lifting might involve the same lifts but each lift would be tailored to the individual's objectives. A shot putter would do an *olympic lift* to improve putting, while a body builder would do a *power lift* to improve physique. Fitness programs to achieve adequate total fitness can be intelligently planned to meet the physiological needs and skill-performance goals for any individual—male or female.

As early as the preschool years, the growth and maturation of the neuromuscular system and the establishment of locomotor movement patterns laid the foundations for future learning and development of skills and attitudes of the individual toward physical fitness. Strong physical play forms the basis for a person's strength, agility, and coordination. To maintain these skills an individual must maintain a daily activity program throughout life. In school, activities for children can be planned with specific objectives to develop muscular strength, endurance, aerobic capacity, and skill; and to perform in sports and physical activities at a *social level* throughout life.

The development to the social level of physical fitness, or the redevelopment of fitness (for the individual who has been inactive for a number of years) requires regular periods of physical activity within individually designed programs. The individual must start with low-energy-use programs (such as walking) and gradually increase the stress placed upon the body in terms of speed, workload, and duration of activity (termed the *overload principle*) until the level of performance the individual is striving for is reached. High-energy-use programs such as tennis, running, swimming, bicycling, handball, and rope skipping are achieved through hard work and time.

Total fitness implies that a person is "in condition." Such a level of fitness is also called *overall fitness, endurance fitness,* or *working capacity* (the ability to do prolonged work without undue fatigue). If an individual is working toward a level of fitness needed for competitive sports he or she should do so only under the direction of a professional physical educator. In this section we are restricting our definition of "in condition" to that of the American Medical Association's Committee on Exercise and Physical Fitness. They stated in 1967 that fitness is "the general capacity to adapt and respond favorably to physical effort. The degree of physical fitness depends upon the individual's state of health, constitution, and present and previous activity." This is also our definition of a person's *total fitness*.

The Meaning of Total Fitness Many individuals may be classified as *nonexercisers*. These individuals possess only passive fitness, and make no effort to keep the body fit. They do only what is necessary during the daily routine. There is nothing physically wrong with this kind of person—not yet—nor is there anything really right with them. If lucky, they may remain like this for years. But without increasing physical activity, such an individual's body is, essentially, deteriorating.

Biological Aging The vitality and health of an individual is determined by many factors including optimum diet and total fitness. An estimation of normal aging becomes an estimate of the decline of the vitality of an individual. Under optimum conditions of energy supply, oxygen supply, waste removal, and periods of functioning and rest, the cells and the body tend to live longer. Body-age estimations based on such factors determine *biological age*. This bears no relationship to one's *chronological (year) age.*

The body shows biological age in terms of changes in structure and functioning of the major body systems. Various physiological functions change within these systems at different rates. Some changes take place rapidly. Others appear to be age-resistant. The biological aging process can be speeded up by a deficient food supply, inactivity (the nonexerciser), infection, traumatic injury, and physical irritation. Rapid biological aging leads to deterioration of the body, disease, and *premature death* (death prior to the estimations for the general population).

The struggle for a better life has brought about impressive improvement in the living conditions of humans. Our infant mortality rate has lowered and, over the last 100 years, the average length of life in the United States has increased. This has been due to the control of *communicable diseases,* such as pneumonia and influenza, which caused the majority of deaths in the past. With control of the communicable diseases (over the past 100 years), life expectancy in the United States has been extended from 40 to over 68 years for males and over 75 years for females.

However, these longer-living individuals often are not able to function normally or adequately in the later years and die of diseases that formerly were uncommon. Today's deaths are more commonly caused by various *degenerative conditions* (the outcome of biological aging). These diseases cause or are the result of biological changes in the structure and functioning of the body: atherosclerosis, coronary thrombosis (cardiac infarction), cerebral thrombosis (stroke), as well as cancer of various organs.

Total Fitness Exercise physiologists show that physical exercise, if sufficiently intensive and regular, can override the various phenomena of aging—such as the decrease in muscle mass, diminished oxygen intake, reduced heat production, and the fall in total blood quantity. Physical exercises are also intensive overall cerebral activities. They stimulate the neural controls of metabolism, respiration, blood circulation, digestion, and the activities of the glands of internal secretion. A correct combination of alert mental activity and physical exercise is at present the best method of preserving, for as long as possible, at a high level, the activity of the brain cells.

This control of the phenomena of aging—the desire for longevity—should begin as early as possible, before you have completed your physical development (between 14 and 22 years of age). It is considerably more difficult to control premature biological aging when it has already set in. A regular exercise program contributes to vitality and healthful good looks throughout the middle years. A person who has maintained a successful personal fitness program can enjoy middle and later years to the fullest. This is why the habits of physical exercise and total fitness should be formed from earliest childhood.

Total fitness is produced when someone engages in balanced activities, strengthening all body systems, particularly the cardiovascular system, the respiratory system, the nervous system, and the muscular system. But it is very important to realize that total fitness is produced by *optimum* intensity and duration of physical activity. The amount and duration of physical ac-

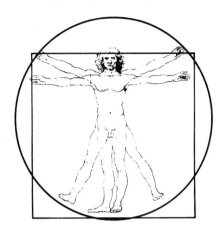

The proportions and symmetry of the totally fit human body attracted the scientific artistry of Leonardo da Vinci.

tivity required is different for every person. This is directed toward the female as well as the male. The value of total fitness is the same for both.

Contrary to some common thought, involvement in exercise programs and sports will not develop bulky muscles. A program that would *overdevelop* specific muscles would be unhealthy for males or females. Exercise improves the figure by "normalizing" it and causing it to become better proportioned. If the arms or legs are too heavy, exercise works toward slimming; if too thin, exercise develops them.

Activity Programs Your likelihood of maintaining a physical fitness program depends on how interesting it is to you. In order for people to maintain an activity program throughout the years it must maintain their interest. Most of the well-publicized physical fitness programs that stress exercises, machines, or rely on an athletic club need great motivation to be maintained throughout life. The best way for an exercise program to be fun is for you to take part in an individual activity or

dual sport. But you can not receive satisfaction out of a sport that you are not in condition to perform. Consequently, an individual must have a general conditioning program that is routine (usually 3 days a week) and that can be maintained easily to stay in condition for any sport.

An individual, while in school or college, should develop skills in several different activities to participate in throughout life. Five major factors should be considered as one plans physical fitness activities for later life. The individual should develop (1) muscular strength, (2) muscular endurance, (3) circulatory endurance, (4) flexibility, and (5) skill (coordination). Physical education courses should help the individual to gain knowledge in activities and sports that develop and maintain these factors.

The concepts of exercise, but not the principles, have changed drastically in recent years. Modern total fitness programs are the result of laboratory studies that have added greatly to our knowledge. Exercise is accepted today as being essential to counterbalance our overly sedentary life-style. Now, the question becomes, "how much and what kind of exercise?" Dr. Kenneth H. Cooper, in his book *The New Aerobics* (Bantam, 1970), points out that the body needs oxygen and the rhythmic physical activity that supplies the body with oxygen. During exercise, the blood is richer in oxygen and nutrients and more effectively eliminates wastes from the muscles and other organs. Activities that promote such efficient body functioning include walking, running, swimming, cycling, dancing, skiing, and tennis. Also, for exercise to be effective, it must be routine and done at one's capacity. But what is your capacity?

Before Starting an Activity Program If your current total fitness status is adequate and you are satisfied with your ability to function, then all you need is to maintain this level. But, if you are dissatisfied with your physical condition and capacity and want to improve it there are several steps to take prior to starting a total fitness program.

1. Have a complete medical examination, especially if you are over 30 years of age. (No one over 30 should ever start on any total fitness program without first consulting a physician.)
2. A major part of your medical examination should be an exercise *capacity test* (bicycle ergometer or treadmill test). It may be necessary to ask your physician for this test.
3. Recondition yourself before starting any regular exercise program. If you have not exercised regularly for a number of years, you must "recondition," as explained later in this chapter, on a warm-up basis to keep from injuring yourself.
4. Have an individual program worked out for you by a competent exercise physiologist or physical education specialist. It is important that you have a *balanced* activity program that improves the condition of your lungs, cardiovascular system, muscular system, and total fitness of your body.

Too often sedentary persons start an exercise program without considering these four points. Many individuals who die while exercising (jogging, running, or swimming) have rushed into a daily exercise program without consulting a physician or a physical educator. The least that can happen to such individuals is that they will become sore or injured because their muscles and joints are not ready for such activity or for carrying their body weight while exercising. To prevent sore and injured muscles, an individual should participate in a warm-up exercise program for a minimum of 6 weeks for each year they have been out of condition. A proper warm-up program helps to stretch and loosen ligaments, increase timing, improve muscular strength, and increase the cardiovascular activity in preparation for a more strenuous exercise program.

Principles of an Activity Program

Exercise tolerance is the level at which the body responds favorably to exercise. An individual's exercise tolerance is his or her ability to perform a series of exercises, participate in a sport, or enjoy a walk without undue fatigue. All exercises should be adapted to an individual's tolerance level. Activities that are too easy or are impossible should not be attempted.

The body has great ability to adapt to stress and increase one's exercise tolerance. Therefore, people who wish to improve their performance and physical condition should continually increase the duration and intensity of their exercises. Extending oneself beyond usual physical effort is called *overloading*, or, more recently, *interval training*. This involves increasing physical stress by:

1. Gradually and progressively increasing the speed of performing an exercise.
2. Gradually increasing the total *resistance*, amount of weight to be lifted.
3. Progressively increasing the total time that a given position, contraction, or resistance can be held or sustained.
4. Maintaining a constant resistance and progressively increasing the total number of *repetitions*, the total number of times a weight is lifted at one time or exercises are performed.

Fatigue may be delayed by reducing the work load (resistance), by slowing the rhythm, and by breathing regularly and deeply. In using interval training, a person may alternately run and walk to give himself or herself periods to recover from fatigue. The principles of overloading should help increase efficiency and performance. As you master an exercise program, progress to more strenuous exercises. All fitness programs should provide for progression. Generally, increasing the intensity or the tempo of a program is much more important than just increasing the time spent in your daily exercise program.

Pulse Rate   The intensity of an exercise program should be as great as possible, based upon the individual's current level of fitness and tolerance to fitness activities. The intensity of exercise should progress as the level of tolerance and fitness progresses. A good indication of one's current level of total fitness is *pulse rate* (a regular throbbing in the arteries caused by the contractions of the heart).

A good method of taking the pulse, especially while exercising, is at the carotid arteries on either side of the neck. Place your fingers (not your thumb; it contains its own pulse) on one side of the Adam's apple, and move around until you can feel a pulsebeat. Now, using the second hand of your wristwatch, count the number of beats in 10 minutes. Practice a few times before trying it while running. Now divide by 10 for the average pulse rate per minute.

Resting Pulse Rate   Your heart rate at rest is an indication of your basal level of total fitness. As your level of fitness increases, you strengthen your heart and your resting pulse rate *decreases*. To obtain an accurate measure of resting pulse rate, count your pulse for at least 10 minutes and then divide by 10 for an average pulse rate per minute. The *recovery pulse rate* is also important, because it indicates when an activity has been too strenuous for you. After exercising, if your pulse rate is 5 beats per minute or more above resting rate, after 30 minutes of rest, the physical activity has been too strenuous and you should reduce the intensity to an acceptable level at the next session.

Maximum Pulse Rate   The pulse rate taken during exercise indicates the intensity of the activity. The pulse rate increases during exercising and you should take it periodically during an activity. If an activity is to increase one's fitness, the pulse rate must reach *maximum pulse rate* (MPR) and be maintained for at least 15 minutes throughout the session. There are three methods for establishing maximum pulse rate:

1. More conservative exercise physiologists feel that a pulse rate of 151 beats per minute for a person under 30 years of age and 131 beats per minute for a person over 30 years of age may be taken as showing that the heart is working at 60 percent of capacity. After 30 years of age a person should not let his pulse rate go too much over 131 beats per minute, because of the greater chance of a heart attack or stroke with increasing age.

2. Many exercise physiologists use a rule-of-thumb method for obtaining maximum pulse rate. They never let the pulse rate increase above the age (after 30 years of age)—subtracted from 200. For example; 200 minus 50 equals 150 beats per minute is the MRP for a 50-year-old.

3. Dr. Kenneth Cooper, in his book *The New Aerobics*, uses the following table to determine what an individual's maximum pulse rate should be during an activity:

AGE	MPR
15–30	180
31–40	170
41–50	160
51–60	150
61–70	140
71–over	130

Remember, you should not try to reach a maximum pulse rate until you have gone through a warm-up period.

Muscular Fitness Exercises Before beginning any total fitness program, an individual must possess sufficient muscular strength to support the body weight easily and have the muscular endurance needed to complete the activities. Two types of muscular contractions, *isometric contractions* and *isotonic contractions*, have been used to develop muscular strength and endurance.

Isometric Exercises Isometric contractions are produced by pushing or pulling against an immovable object. The best results, if one is to use isometrics, appear to be obtained by using maximal contraction of the muscles, held for 5 to 8 seconds and repeated 5 to 10 times daily. Very few physical educators recommend the use of isometric exercises because of the increases in blood pressure they cause.

Isotonic Exercises Isotonic contractions are produced when an individual continues to raise, lower, or "move" a moderate load. Within isotonic exercise programs there are many combinations of *repetitions, resistance* and *sets* (the number of groups of repetitions of a specific exercise, to be done without resting). Muscular strength is best developed when the resistance is relatively high and the number of repetitions is low—such as in a weightlifting program. Muscular endurance, flexibility, and coordination, or the ability to control muscular movement, are best developed when the resistance is relatively low and the number of repetitions is high. Body weight is considered low resistance and calisthenic-type exercises best serve to produce these isotonic contractions.

Circulatory Endurance Exercises
Circulatory endurance exercises are activities that stimulate an increase in cardiorespiratory functioning, thus producing results known as *conditioning, training effect,* or *aerobic capacity.* Essentially, isotonic activities that are strenuous enough to increase the pulse rate to a maximum pulse rate and continued over a period of time (a minimum of 15 minutes) will improve circulatory endurance.

During such periods of sustained activity, heavy demands are made upon the heart, lungs, and circulatory system. Several months of such activity results in:
1. Increased oxygen-carrying ability of the blood due to an increase in the number of red cells and total blood volume.
2. Increase in the number or involvement of more capillaries.
3. Greater cardiac efficiency and output, which results in a lower pulse rate and a more rapid return to a normal pulse rate after physical activity.
4. Reduction of body fat by about 8 percent (overall weight loss of about 2 percent).

Women in a Fitness Program Women can participate in any fitness program in which men participate. A general conditioning program is as necessary for women as for men. And, as discussed earlier, a reasonable exercise program will not overdevelop muscles, but firms muscles, improves muscle tone, increases circulation, and promotes anyone's total health. The only precautions for women are that they should remember that they are generally smaller in bone and muscle structure than men and should start at lower levels of weight and intensity to keep from doing damage to muscles. A pregnant woman should consult her obstetrician about any exercise program. If she has been participating in a regular daily exercise program, which includes activities to strengthen abdominal and back muscles, she should be able to carry her child easily, deliver easily and swiftly, and recuperate rapidly after delivery. Normally, such a woman should be able to continue her regular exercise program, if it is not too strenuous, up to the sixth month of pregnancy. During the last three months, she may engage only in a simple walking program.

Fitness Programs For a total fitness program to be effective, the exercise should be regular (three times a week), and vigorous enough to raise the pulse to the maximum pulse rate. However, the value of exercise depends on how it is done. The three principles of physical fitness (muscular strength, muscular endurance, and circulatory endurance) should be incorporated into any total fitness program. Sufficient rest and sleep, an adequate diet, and regular exercise are all needed for total body fitness.

A professional physical educator can design a *balanced* total fitness program that does not overemphasize one aspect of physical development. Isometric exercises and weight training improve both muscular strength and endurance but they have minimal value for circulatory fitness. Brisk walking, jogging, and running are excellent circulatory exercises, but they do little for the abdominal, back, shoulder and arm muscles. Therefore, they should be accompanied by exercises which strengthen these regions. There are few activities in which all parts of the body are exercised equally well.

Yoga Yoga is more than a physical activity program. It is a program to unify spiritual and physical discipline. Yoga tries to establish within the individual the knowledge that:

1. Each person is solely responsible or his or her youthfulness and what is defined as the "vital force" necessary to continually regenerate the physical and emotional aspects and keep a person young and totally fit.
2. This vital force becomes dormant over the years.
3. Only the individual can stimulate and reestablish the vital force.
4. The stimulation of the vital forces comes through yoga—a means of manipulating the organs, glands, nerves, bones, and joints by methodically stretching and relaxing the body.

Like all exercise physiologists, a yogi (someone who practices yoga) feels that the major causes and symptoms of aging are caused by inadequate care of the body. The many poses, positions, and exercises are the specific types of movement necessary to strengthen every area of the body and activate the vital force of life. Certain types of movements relieve tension, strain, and stiffness, and relax the body. These specific movements, certain principles of nutrition, and meditation restore youthful characteristics. The final phase of yoga is to establish meditation, which is said to unify the spiritual and physical life, minimize conflicts and negative situations, and enable an individual to focus the whole mind on any given object instantly and completely. When yoga is mastered, efficiency increases, health improves, and complete relaxation becomes a normal part of life.

Twenty to 40 minutes a day is the average amount of time needed for a daily yoga program. Before meals or at least 90 minutes after meals are often suggested as ideal times. Some exercises are suggested for morning and others for evenings; consequently many programs are broken up throughout the day. Richard L. Hittleman in his book *Be Young With Yoga* (Warner Paperback Library, 1973) suggests a person should try at least 7 weeks of yoga to establish a program. Others feel 10 weeks are needed for a yoga course to become effective.

There are a wide variety of yoga programs (Hatha, Tantric, Zen, and so on), and books available. If you would like to try yoga as a total fitness program, find one of the many courses being offered through schools, YMCA's and YWCA's, and fitness studios. Or you may purchase one of the many books available and follow the course for the 7 to 10 weeks recommended by the author.

Warming Up—and Easing Off Each time one exercises or participates in a sport, the body should be warmed up by light conditioning and stretching exercises, such as those shown, before heavier, more strenuous activities are attempted. Proper warm-up increases body temperature, stretches ligaments, and slightly increases cardiovascular activity in preparation for exercise. The amount of warm-up necessary will vary between individuals and generally will increase with age. A warm-up program, of from 15 to 20 minutes at a very slow pace, starts with light, rhythmical calisthenics, accompanied by stretching and deep breathing. This helps to stretch and loosen the muscles and raise the heartbeat and body temperature enough to promote sweating. Following this with slow jogging and walking will help prevent soreness and muscle injury.

Just as the body needs warming up it also needs easing off after exercise. This helps return the blood to the heart and get the body temperature back to normal. One should keep moving for several minutes after vigorous activity until the breathing has returned to normal, the stress of the activity has subsided, and the body has cooled.

Calisthenics These exercises provide an opportunity to exercise specific groups of muscles or the whole body. The figures show a series of test exercises that can provide a foundation on which a calisthenic program may be developed. You should not, however, go on to more vigorous calisthenics (progression) until you can complete these tests. There are many basic calisthenic programs designed for the whole body. In the early 1960s the Royal Canadian Air Force originated two programs that have proved to be very successful. The 5BX (Five Basic Exercises) *Plan for Physical Fitness* for men and XBX (a series of ten exercises) *Plan* for women are simple calisthenic exercises that can be completed in 11 minutes each day. You should either follow an organized program such as this one or have a physical educator design a program especially for you.

Calisthenics _____

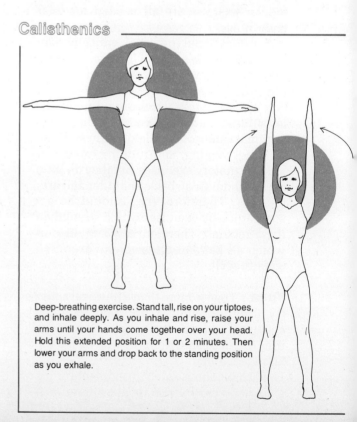

Deep-breathing exercise. Stand tall, rise on your tiptoes, and inhale deeply. As you inhale and rise, raise your arms until your hands come together over your head. Hold this extended position for 1 or 2 minutes. Then lower your arms and drop back to the standing position as you exhale.

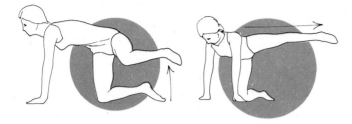

Leg extension. Start on your hands and knees on a soft surface. Keeping your left knee bent, raise it to the side until it is level with your hips. Extend the leg straight out to the side, keeping it at hip level. Then bend it back and return it to the floor in the starting position. Repeat with right leg.

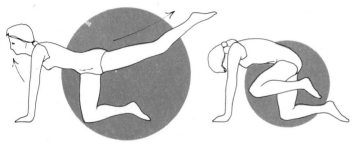

Knee-to-nose kick. Get down on your hands and knees on a soft surface. Bend your head down and bring your left knee as close to your nose as possible. Hold for 2 seconds. Next, extend the left leg back and up, at the same time bringing your head up. Hold for 2 seconds. Repeat action with right leg.

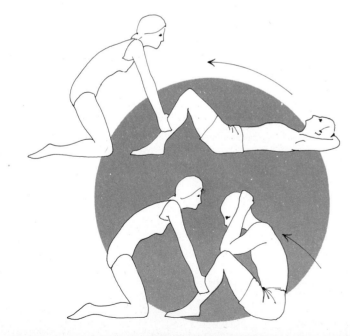

Bent-knee sit-ups. Lie on your back with your hands clasped behind your head, your knees bent, and your feet held down. Keeping your chin on your chest and your back rounded, roll up into a sitting position. When you are in a sitting position, straighten your back, lift your head, and press your elbows back. Hold for 2 seconds, then drop your head, round your back, and roll slowly down to the starting position.

Calisthenics (continued)

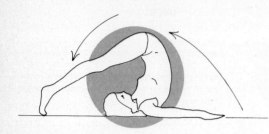

Yoga plow. Lie on your back with your arms beside your body. Lift both legs at once and slowly swing them up and over until your toes touch the floor behind your head. Your shoulders and arms should remain on the floor. Hold, then return to original position.

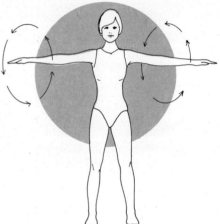

Arm rotation. Extend your arms straight out from the shoulders, and rotate them so that your hands are tracing circles about 1 foot in diameter. Rotate arms forward, then backward.

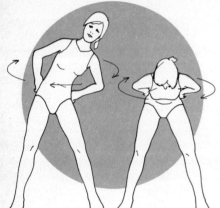

Body rotation. With your legs wide apart and hands on hips, lean forward and bend at the waist. Low rotate your body from the waist in great, slow circles. Lean far enough to the right, rear, left, and front so you feel the muscles stretch. Now rotate to the left, rear, right, and front.

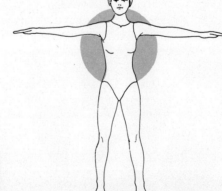
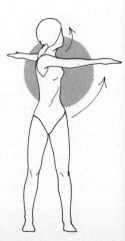

Standing body rotation. Stand with your feet well apart, and extend your arms at shoulder level. Twist your upper body all the way around to the right, following it with your eyes; hold for 1 second. Twist back to the left as far as possible; hold for 1 second.

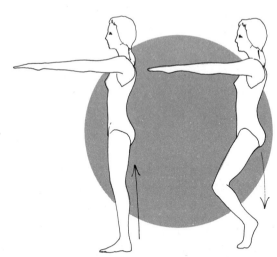

Windmill. Stand with your feet well apart and arms extended at shoulder level. Bending at the waist, touch right hand to left foot, keeping your left arm extended. Return to an upright position and repeat action, this time touching left hand to right foot.

Half knee bends. Stand with your legs together and feet parallel. Rise to the toes for a count of 1 and bring your arms forward for balance. Tighten the muscles of the seat, abdominal area, thighs, and knees. Keeping your back very straight, lower yourself until your knees are only half-way bent. Do not go into a deep knee bend. Rise again to your toes and then lower yourself to your heels.

Weight Training Lifting weights does not develop circulatory endurance. It does increase muscular strength and endurance through application of the principle of *progressive resistance exercises.* In other words, as strength increases, resistance is increased. Progressive resistance occurs when a person moves a given resistance (barbells or weights) a definite number of times (repetitions). Resistance exercise programs may be as extensive or as simple as the individual desires (competitive weight lifting, body building, weight training). However, no program should ever deviate from the principle of resistance progression. A person who simply wants to see how much weight he or she can lift may injure muscles and joints. Weights should be increased only as strength increases.

For an individual interested in increasing strength in order to participate socially in medium- and high-energy sports, weight training will help produce the strength needed for participation. Weight training combines weight lifting with calisthenics. Weight training takes time. A person may not reach the strength needed by some sports for months or years of continuous progression.

If you are interested in weight training, you may want to follow a trial program like the one presented in this section. You should remain in it for three months to determine whether there is an improvement in strength. Work out three times a week on alternate days. Start with a weight, such as those recommended in the suggested poundage table, that is light enough to do ten repetitions comfortably. Often, individuals starting their second workout find themselves stiff, sore, and tired, and the weights feel heavier than they did during the first workout. If this happens, reduce the weights by 5 pounds for one week or by 10 pounds for two weeks, or until the weights feel comfortable. Then return to the point at which you began, gradually increasing the weights once a week. Perform the exercises in numbered order, doing one set of ten repetitions at each workout. Rest 2 to 3 minutes between exercises. Increase the poundage whenever the weight in any one exercise feels light. Plan your program in writing; make out a "program card" such as the one shown listing exercises, poundages, and number of repetitions. Do not engage in any other regularly scheduled exercise program.

1. *Two-arm standing press.* Stand with weight at your shoulder. Now, using the strength of the arm, shoulder, and upper back only, push the weight above your head. Lower to your shoulder and repeat.
2. *Rowing motion.* Stand with your legs apart and your body in front bending position; keep your arms straight down. Without any body motion, pull the weights up until the bar touches your chest. Lower and repeat.
3. *Shrug.* Hold weight while standing with arms straight out. Keeping your elbows straight, pull your shoulders up toward your ears; do not move your whole body. Relax and repeat.
4. *Squat.* Stand erect with weight held across your shoulder. Keeping your heels on floor, bend your knees until your thighs are parallel to the floor. Keep your back as straight as possible. Rise to the standing position and repeat.
5. *Rise on toes.* After performing the squat, do not remove the weight from your shoulders. Rise up on your toes and lower your heels back to the ground. Repeat.
6. *Lateral bench raise.* Lie on your back on a bench. Start with a pair of dumbbells held straight up at arm's length.

Breathe in deeply, and slowly lower the weights to your side. Return to starting position and repeat.

7. *Barbell curl.* Hold weight at your thighs with both your hands. Without moving your body except to bend your elbows, raise the weight to the shoulders. Lower and repeat.
8. *Standing lateral raise.* Hold a pair of dumbbells down the sides at arm's length. Keeping your elbows stiff, raise the dumbbells straight out from your shoulders. Bring the pairs together above your head. Lower and repeat.
9. *Neck exercise.* Take a light dumbbell and wrap a towel around the handle. Place it on your forehead, and raise and lower your head up and down.
10. *Side Bend.* Hold a weight in one hand and place the other hand behind your head. As you hold the weight, bend as far as you can to the side. Return to a standing position and repeat. Do this exercise for both sides.
11. *Sit-up.* Lie on the ground and hook your feet under a barbell. Raise your body to a sitting position. Lower and repeat.

Remember that hard work is required to obtain results and results occur very slowly. The trial program outlined here should begin to increase your strength within three months. If you enjoy this program, ask a physical educator to design a weight training program for you. Weight programs are often part of a college or university curriculum, a men's club, the YMCA, or a gym. The YWCA and women's fitness and figure control studios are designing weight training programs for women. The same strength-building exercises performed by men to develop their muscles and reduce fat deposition may be performed by women. The only change is

Weight Progression Card

Exercises	May 1	May 2	May 3	May 4	May 5	May 8	May 9	May 10	May 11	May 12	Notes
Two-arm standing press	3 10 40	Skip	3 10 40	Skip	3 10 40	3 10 45	Skip	3 10 45	Skip	3 10 45	increase weight 10 lbs.
Rowing motion											
Shrug											
Squat											
Rise on toes											
Lateral bench raise											
Barbell curl											
Lateral raise											
Side bend											

NOTE: You may want to add the following to a weight progression card:
1. Dimensions of wrist, waist, thighs, and neck.
2. Holes so that the card can be put into a ring binder for future reference.
3. Space for notes on progress.
4. Charts should be for two-week periods.

Suggested Poundages at the Beginning of Weight Training

Exercise	Average Pounds To Start With	Range of Choice of Starting Weight
Two-arm standing press	40	30–50
Rowing motion	35	25–45
Shrug	45	35–60
Squat	45	35–55
Rise on toes	45	35–60
Lateral bench raise	7½ each	5–10 each
Barbell curl	35	25–45
Lateral raise (standing)	7½ each	5–10 each
Side bend	35	30–40

that women should start at a lighter weight (half of those found in the suggested poundage table) and progress at 5-pound increments.

Walking This is the most natural of all forms of exercise. A person may walk at any time with almost no medical risk. Brisk walking for a period of time or distance sufficient to accelerate the pulse strengthens heart, lungs, and leg muscles. Extremely inactive people may obtain endurance effects and begin a regular exercise program by walking; later, however, they must increase their rate of speed to obtain further benefits. Inactive, sedentary men (more than women) over 50 years of age should walk for exercise. They should not try jogging or running because of the increased chance of heart attack after 50.

Jogging The next step up from walking, jogging is steady, slow running. Jogging may be alternated with breath-catching

Schedule I and II

Week 1 (Total Distance: ½ Mile)

Monday	Warm up (always do warm-up exercises). Jog 55 yards in 25–30 seconds; then walk 55 yards.ᵃ Repeat four times.
Tuesday	Walk for 5–10 minutes after warming up.
Wednesday	Jog 110 yards in 55–60 seconds; then walk 110 yards.
Thursday	Walk for 5–10 minutes after warming up.
Friday	Jog 55 yards in 25–30 seconds; then walk 55 yards. Repeat two times.
Saturday and Sunday	Walk for 5–10 minutes after warming up.

ᵃYou need only estimate distances; they do not have to be accurate. A track is usually 440 yards in length with each straightaway and turn 110 yards. Using a car odometer or a pedometer, lay out a course beforehand. City blocks are about 220 feet by 500 feet. Telephone poles are about 100 yards apart. Any watch with a second hand is adequate for timing.

Schedule I

Week 2 (Total Distance: ¾ Mile)

Monday	Jog 55 yards in 25–30 seconds; then walk 55 yards. Repeat four times. Jog 110 yards in 55–60 seconds; then walk 110 yards. Repeat four times. Jog 55 yards in 25–30 seconds; then walk 55 yards. Repeat four times.
Wednesday	Jog 55 yards in 25–30 seconds; then walk 55 yards. Repeat three times. Jog 110 yards in 55–60 seconds; then walk 110 yards. Repeat three times. Jog 55 yards in 25–30 seconds; then walk 55 yards. Repeat three times.
Friday	Jog 55 yards in 25–30 seconds; then walk 55 yards. Repeat four times. Jog 110 yards in 55–60 seconds; then walk 110 yards. Repeat two times. Jog 55 yards in 25–30 seconds; then walk 55 yards. Repeat four times.

Week 3 (Total Distance: 1 Mile)

Monday	Jog 55 yards in 22–25 seconds, then walk 55 yards. Repeat four times. Jog 220 yards in 90–100 seconds, then walk 220 yards. Repeat one time. Jog 110 yards in 45–50 seconds, then walk 110 yards. Repeat two times. Jog 55 yards in 22–25 seconds, then walk 55 yards. Repeat four times.
Wednesday	Jog 55 yards in 22–25 seconds, then walk 55 yards. Repeat two times. Start a slow, steady jog for 2 or 3 minutes. The pace is 55 to 75 seconds for 110 yards. Walk whenever you need to; walk at the end of the 3 minutes. Jog again steadily for 2 or 3 minutes. Jog 55 yards in 22–25 seconds, then walk 55 yards. Repeat two times.
Friday	Jog 55 yards in 22–25 seconds, then walk 55 yards. Repeat two times. Jog 110 yards in 45–50 seconds, then walk 110 yards. Repeat one time. Jog your slow, steady pace for 2 or 3 minutes. Then walk until wind is back to normal. Jog 55 yards in 22–25 seconds, then walk 55 yards. Repeat two times.

Schedule II

Week 2 (Total Distance: 1 Mile)

Monday	Jog 55 yards in 25–30 seconds; then walk 55 yards. Repeat four times.
	Jog 110 yards in 55–60 seconds; then walk 110 yards. Repeat four times.
	Jog 55 yards in 25–30 seconds; then walk 55 yards. Repeat four times.
Wednesday	Jog 55 yards in 25–30 seconds; then walk 55 yards. Repeat three times.
	Jog 110 yards in 55–60 seconds; then walk 110 yards. Repeat five times.
	Jog 55 yards in 25–30 seconds; then walk 55 yards. Repeat three times.
Friday	Jog 55 yards in 25–30 seconds; then walk 55 yards. Repeat two times.
	Jog 110 yards in 55–60 seconds; then walk 110 yards. Repeat six times.
	Jog 55 yards in 25–30 seconds; then walk 55 yards. Repeat four times.

Week 3 (Total Distance: 1¼ Miles)

Monday	Jog 55 yards in 22–30 seconds, then walk 55 yards. Repeat four times.
	Jog 110 yards in 45–60 seconds, then walk 110 yards. Repeat two times.
	Jog 220 yards in 90–100 seconds, then walk 220 yards. Repeat two times.
	Jog 110 yards in 45–60 seconds, then walk 110 yards. Repeat two times.
Wednesday	Start to establish a steady, comfortable jogging pace for the required distance. Start at about 110 yards in 56 seconds. This is 4 miles per hour. See how long you can continuously jog with comfort. Walk when too winded to talk with companions. Jog and walk for 1¼ miles.
Friday	Jog 110 yards in 45–50 seconds, then walk 110 yards. Repeat four times.
	Jog steadily 330 yards in 2 minutes 48 seconds. Walk until wind is back to normal.
	Jog 110 yards in 45–50 seconds, then walk 110 yards. Repeat four times.

periods of walking. Jogging became popular in the late 1960s with the publication of *Jogging* by William J. Bowerman, track coach at the University of Oregon, and W. E. Harris, M.D., a heart specialist. This book presents a detailed, complete program for anyone interested in jogging as part of an exercise program. Jogging is pleasant, free, easy, relaxing, and fun. It can be done alone or in groups. Jogging will maintain a level of fitness and circulatory endurance. But to increase circulatory endurance, an individual must progress to running at some point in the schedule. To achieve this purpose, however, college students should alternate jogging with intervals of hard running after the first month or two of progression before entering a regular running program.

A jogging program begins with a short period of trotting and walking. As jogging progresses, the jogger covers greater and greater distances. You may want to attempt the following trial program for one month.

Schedules are planned for Monday, Wednesday, and Friday. You may rearrange them (Tuesday, Thursday, and Saturday) to fit your own schedule if you will remember the "hard–easy" principle of all exercise programs—exercise one day, rest the next when starting. If you jog for 55 yards and it leaves you gasping and too breathless to talk with your fellow joggers, you are running too fast or you have not worked yourself into the condition to perform in this program. If the 110-yard jogs were not too much for you, try Schedule II in the second week. If the first week's schedule seemed comfortable and you were pleased with your performance, continue on Schedule I for the second week.

By the fourth week you should know whether jogging is an exercise program that you enjoy. Also, you will know enough about it to use it for change of pace in other exercise programs. Exercise must be fun if an individual is to continue with it. Therefore, expose yourself to a number of different exercise programs. You may maintain your interest in fitness activities by alternating exercises if one set of exercises begins to bore you.

If you decide to continue jogging, refer to William J. Bowerman's book, *Jogging.* It provides schedules for reaching 4 or 5 miles a day. It also contains complete programs and many suggestions for varying your program to maintain interest.

Jogging may be satisfactory to an individual during the initial phase of conditioning. After the goal of a mile is achieved, however, running often replaces jogging. Running can provide a challenge as well as good circulatory endurance. The progression of jogging and walking outlined previously may be used to progress toward the goal of running a mile. Some people, however, may want to increase the time period in the schedule to two months. Before you try to run a mile, be sure that you can jog comfortably for this distance. Don't worry about your time at first. When you can jog for a mile, start pacing yourself and reducing your time. You should pace yourself so that you are running at a constant rate. Avoid any bursts of speed because they greatly reduce your efficiency and cause fatigue. Reduce your time by 10 seconds a week until you can run a mile in 6 minutes. This is considered excellent time for maintenance of circulatory endurance.

Running in Place

When space or weather restricts your ability to run, *running in place* can be a very effective means of maintaining circulatory endurance. The important factors in running in place are the cadence of the step and the duration of the activity. The most comfortable time length seems to be 5 minutes. To reach a

Running in Place

Number of Sessions	Running Time
1–5	1 minute
6–10	1½ minutes
11–15	2 minutes
16–20	2½ minutes
21–25	3 minutes
26–30	3½ minutes
31–35	4 minutes
36–40	4½ minutes
41–45	5 minutes

5-minute goal, begin by running in place for 1 minute. Then increase your time by 30-second intervals. Run for five sessions at each time level before progressing to the next interval.

When you can run in place for 5 minutes, you may begin to increase your step cadence.

Aerobics

Aerobics is a total fitness program for men first published in 1968. The originator of the program was Major Kenneth H. Cooper, M.D., of the U.S. Air Force Medical Corps. The key concept in this program is oxygen consumption. Because oxygen cannot be stored in the body, it must be continually replenished. Consequently, the fatigue level of an individual is controlled by the ability of his respiratory and circulatory systems to supply oxygen to the muscles.

Dr. Cooper's aerobics system consists of a point count assigned to different physical activities that increase circulatory endurance. An individual progresses to the point where he can perform activities worth 30 points each week. The number of points represents the amount of physical activity necessary for maintenance of the cardiorespiratory system.

Points are obtained by performing specific circulatory endurance activities in a specific amount of time. Such activities include running, swimming, bicycling, walking, running in place, and participating in strenuous games of squash, handball, and basketball. Dr. Cooper's book *The New Aerobics* (a revised version of the program published in 1968) provides standards against which a man may gauge his aerobic fitness. For beginners to the program the test of aerobic fitness is the distance that can be covered by running in 12 minutes.

Men should determine their fitness category and then refer to *The New Aerobics* and choose the schedule they should follow to obtain the 30 aerobic points per week.

Women's aerobic capacity is smaller than most men's. This is because of women's smaller physical size and lung capacity; they have less blood circulating

and fewer hemoglobin and red blood cells. In the book *Aerobics for Women* (Bantam, 1973), Dr. and Mrs. Mildred Cooper feel that a female needs 24 points a week for a satisfactory total fitness level. But, they do not discourage women from exceeding the 24 points, just as they do not discourage men from exceeding the 30 points-per-week, if they are physically able to do so. Point evaluations for women can be found in *Aerobics for Women*.

Circuit Training A *circuit* refers to a number of carefully selected exercises that are arranged and numbered consecutively; the exercises range over a given area. Each numbered exercise within the circuit is called a *station*. An individual moves at his or her own speed from one station to another until he or she completes the entire circuit. In most cases he or she repeats the total circuit more than once (usually three times) and records the total time of performance. This is a convenient and different approach to exercising—one that is physically, physiologically, and psychologically sound. Many cities are now establishing circuits in local parks. See if you can establish one in your area.

Circuit training involves two valuable activities; weight training and running. The best physical activity for development of muscular strength and muscular endurance is weight training. One of the most effective methods of developing and maintaining circulatory and respiratory endurance involves running (others are swimming, bicycling, and rope skipping). A well-planned circuit involves both weight training and running. Thus, circuit training increases muscular strength, muscular endurance, and cardiovascular endurance.

The value of circuit training lies in its extreme adaptability to a great variety of situations. A circuit can be designed to fit any individual, group, area, or condition

Distances Covered in 12 Minutes by Running

Age Groups	Fitness Categories	Age Groups
Under 30 years		30 to 39 years
Less than 1.0 mile	Very poor	Less than 0.95 mile
1.0 to 1.24 miles	Poor	0.95 to 1.14 miles
1.25 to 1.49 miles	Fair	1.15 to 1.39 miles
1.50 to 1.74 miles	Good	1.40 to 1.64 miles
1.75 miles and over	Excellent	1.65 miles and over
40 to 49 years		Over 50 years
Less than 0.85 mile	Very poor	Less than 0.80 mile
0.85 to 1.04 miles	Poor	0.80 to 0.99 miles
1.05 to 1.29 miles	Fair	1.00 to 1.24 miles
1.30 to 1.54 miles	Good	1.25 to 1.49 miles
1.55 miles and over	Excellent	1.50 miles and over

(it is even adaptable to medical rehabilitation). Circuit training enables an individual or a group of people to progress through a series of exercises and to check the progress against a clock.

Circuit training utilizes three variables: load, repetitions, and time. Weight training exercises provide the load, and sets provide the repetitions. Interval running, engaged in between stations, provides repetitions and time.

On a circuit, progression is produced by decreasing the time required to complete one circuit, increasing the work load (weight or sets), or a combination of both. Progression is assured because an individual works at his or her present capacity and can progress as capacity increases. Circuit training provides a series of progressive time goals that are achieved step by step. This time factor provides built-in motivation; it encourages a person to improve. The circuit layout in which a person moves from one station to another offers variety; this is appealing to most people.

The progressions used in weight training may be used in circuit training. Loads can be increased by progressively increasing the size of the weights to be lifted. In circuit training, it is not necessary to change weights as frequently as it is in weight training because weight training is only one of the variables involved in the program.

Calisthenic exercises may be used in a circuit. When this is done, the load is a person's own body weight. The load is increased by modifying the exercise. For example, the following changes will increase the work load in a push-up: standard push-up; push-up, pushing hands off the floor; push-up, pushing off the floor and clapping hands; pushing up, pushing off the floor and slapping the chest. Such modifications make calisthenic exercises very useful in circuit training. Load can

also be increased by increasing the number of repetitions, or sets, at each station or by increasing the number of times the circuit is run. Laps may be added; in that case, a person runs the length of the circuit without performing at the stations. Another way to increase the load is to decrease the time needed to perform a circuit. In maintaining good progression the most important factor is to increase the work load gradually and at a rate that can be handled with ease and safety.

An individual should set goals before beginning any exercise program. You should be able to say what purpose you want the program to serve. In planning a circuit, remember that your circuit must be based on your personal goals. Choose exercises that are strenuous. Each exercise should contribute toward progression by increasing both work load and work rate. This automatically eliminates the very light warm-up exercises that should be performed before the circuit is run. Also, do not include "duck waddle," deep knee bends, or any other exercise that can cause joint, ligament, or muscle damage if done too fast. Perform each exercise the same way every time so that you are able to observe and evaluate your improvement.

Select exercises that balance other exercises so that all groups of muscles receive proper exercise. Improper balance of strength between antagonistic muscle groups can produce permanent body damage. To avoid improper balance, classify the muscle groups into three categories: the arm, neck, and shoulder group; the abdomen, back and chest group; and the buttock, hip, and leg group. When arranging your stations, avoid consecutive placement of exercises that involve similar muscle groups. For example, both arm curls and chin-ups involve the arm, neck and shoulder muscle group. If you include both of these exercises in a circuit, separate

Recommended Circuit

Exercises (In the Order to be Done)	Repetitions 1	2	3	Weight in Pounds
Bench press	8	10	12	60
Side bends	7	9	11	
Chins	1	3	5	
Back extension	7	9	12	10
Two-arm curl	8	10	12	25
Squat	10	13	16	
Bent-leg sit-ups	15	20	25	
Three-quarter squat	9	12	15	25
Lateral raise	8	10	12	7½
Shuttle run	(5–10 yards)			

NOTE: This is a short 10-minute circuit that utilizes some of the exercises discussed in the *calisthenics* section. Follow the recommendations listed with each exercise for progression. Determine your own time limit by judging how well you perform the circuit when you first try it.

them. A circuit designed for general body conditioning should include exercises that involve all three of the muscle groups.

The amount of time you have available for performing a circuit is a factor in determining both the difficulty of exercises and the number of stations to be included in the circuit. The spacing and the arrangement of the stations are determined by the amount of space you have available and by the kinds of exercises you want to emphasize. If your basic purpose is general body conditioning (an emphasis on cardiovascular endurance), you should choose a large area for your circuit, allowing for distances between stations for running and movement. There should always be enough room for exercise that is strenuous, yet free-flowing and uninterrupted. Where there is available space and facilities, several circuits (or variations of one circuit) may be organized, utilizing the same area or equipment.

The *recommended circuit* is useful for general body conditioning. However, a person with a little experience, skill, and understanding may design circuits to meet the fitness needs of nearly any vigorous sport or activity.

Rope Jumping This is an excellent cardiovascular exercise. A person who jumps steadily for 5 minutes is getting a good workout. A 10-minute daily program of rope skipping improves and maintains cardiovascular endurance as well as a 30-minute program of jogging. Rope skipping may be either a program in itself or a bad-weather substitute for a jogging and/or running program.

Obtain a piece of rope that is anywhere from 6 to 9 feet long. An easy way to determine the correct length for you is to make the length of the rope two times the distance from your armpit to the ground, or a length that is comfortable. Tape the ends so they will not fray.

Variations within a rope-skipping program can add interest and incentive. They may also provide progression. (Progression may also be achieved by performing a specific number of jumps in a certain amount of time.) The normal skipping style may be modified by jumping on one foot, alternating feet, or jumping with both feet together. Running with skipping increases timing and coordination. Jumping backward is a simple maneuver in which various foot styles can be used. Make some forward-to-backward changes and then some backward-to-forward changes. This is difficult because you must jump an extra time as the turn is completed.

A double jump is challenging. This is done by spinning the rope faster and jumping a little higher. When you have increased your skill, shorten the rope slightly by winding it within the hand, and stay in the air longer by bending the knees

212

and keeping them high. You may achieve a triple jump. Double and triple jumps have an effect similar to that caused by sprints in running; they rapidly increase the heart rate.

A front cross may be achieved by crossing the arms when the rope starts downward. This makes a loop through which you may jump. On completion of the jump, the arms are uncrossed and the next jump is made in the normal manner. If you have difficulty performing a front cross, lengthen the rope slightly and either lower the hands as the arms cross or cross the arms far enough to bring the elbows together. These changes will give you a wider loop to jump through. A back cross may be done by performing a regular back jump with arms crossed in front of the body (cross your arms so your elbows touch each other).

Make your own modifications. Try jumps such as a double jump with a front cross, or try to run while you change jumping forms. Again, make some forward-to-backward changes and then some backward-to-forward changes.

Sports   Sports and other recreational activities may serve as conditioning programs. However, some individual and dual sports require such small amounts of physical activity that they are not adequate for a fitness program. Golf is such a sport. It has many psychological and social values but little physical value. The main energy expenditure in golf comes from walking. This walking is usually not vigorous enough to elevate the pulse significantly.

If a sport is to supply the requirements of a physical fitness program, it must be vigorous. Also, a person should participate in it for at least three sessions a week. Each session should last for a minimum of 30 minutes. Ideally, a person who is using a sport as the basis of a fitness program

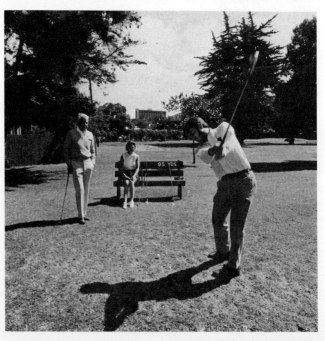

Photo by Mitchell Payne/Jeroboam.

should participate in the sport for 60 minutes every day.

When you participate in a sport, you should remember that your expenditure of energy depends on several factors:

1. *The number of participants.* In calisthenics, weight training, and running, you control the expenditure of energy. In dual sports, however, you must consider the number of participants. Handball may be least demanding in a game of doubles, more demanding in a game of singles, and most demanding in a game involving three people ("cutthroat").

2. *The skill of the participants.* Generally, a high level of skill is reflected in greater efficiency. Thus a skilled person can participate at a lower energy cost. As your skill develops, you should either increase the amount of time you devote to a sport or pit yourself against people who are more skillful than you are.

3. *The duration.* The longer the duration of an activity, the greater is the energy expenditure. Each participant should be vigorously active for 30 to 40 minutes. In a 60-minute game, then, you should be moving one-half to two-thirds of the time.

4. *The speed of the necessary physical movements.* Sports that require occasional bursts of speed are more demanding and require a greater expenditure of energy than are sports in which the participants can establish a steady pace. You should participate in such sports only after you feel your physical condition is adequate.

In choosing sports, remember the value of developing and maintaining circulatory endurance. Sports that improve circulatory endurance include individual activities such as swimming, scuba diving, snorkeling, hiking, running, and bicycling; dual activities such as wrestling and judo; and court games such as badminton, handball, squash, tennis, and volleyball.

Dual sports and court games require at least two participants. Court games further require a court. These requirements may limit your opportunities to engage in exercise. Individual activities usually offer more opportunities for participation.

Some sports are much more beneficial to fitness than are others. Golf is the least beneficial. It is followed, in increasing benefit, by court games, dual sports, individual sports, weight training, jogging, running, and swimming.

Use of Leisure Time The automobile, television, and beer are unfortunate tendencies we have of carrying our hectic work pace into our leisure activities. Abolition of these, however, would not cause us to become more involved in programs of physical conditioning. Whether one exercises regularly or changes one's life-style to be compatible with the environment depends on motivation. People must understand how to condition themselves and what certain activities do for total fitness to produce the motivation needed to exercise.

Psychological as well as physiological limits increase with exercise, making one feel better, be more decisive, and have a more positive and confident outlook on life. It enables one to actively participate in many activities that are part of a natural life-style.

Leisure time is well spent pursuing non-powered, nonspectator activities that reacquaint one with the environment. One should seek out activities that provide healthful exercise, are pleasurable, and cost much less than any form of motorized recreational vehicles, or seats at a spectator sport.

In Conclusion   How do we motivate you to exercise? We can't. You must motivate yourself. Also, are you likely to stay with an exercise program throughout life? Only you know. Anything that is enjoyable costs something. An active, enjoyable life costs energy. The energies of motivation and participation in a regular exercise program will pay off in a longer, more active, and more enjoyable life.

We can point out the importance of regular exercise in preventing or delaying chronic degenerative diseases (such as emphysema and heart disease). But only you will know what is a desirable level of exercise and fitness for you. Often, fitness programs are directed toward "big-time" athletics, not at an enjoyable level of "social athletics" for both males and females. It is very enjoyable to scuba dive, ski, hike, run on the beach, and grow *with* your friends and your children when you are in your 40's and 50's. This, however, requires exercise on a regular basis so that you can perform when you want to.

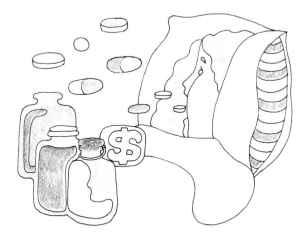

11

THE PATIENT AS CONSUMER

There is no doubt that Americans today place a high priority on living a long and disease-free life. It is generally conceded that freedom from pain and debilitation ought to be looked upon as a natural right of all human beings. Achieving this goal is facilitated by the proper selection of health products and services.

Of all consumer goods and services, none is more essential to one's welfare than health care. There are several excellent consumer magazines from product-testing agencies that may be helpful in choosing health care. Yet the array of products and medical facilities is huge, and the claims for the merits of each are confusing. Occasionally, we may visit a physician or dentist and receive specific care or advice, but few of us can afford professional counsel on *all* health matters.

Not only can we waste a great deal of money on ineffectual products and professionals, but our health, perhaps even our lives, may depend on getting *proper* treatment for disease and illness. There are times when self-treatment should not even be attempted. For example, some products—such as aspirin, laxatives, and antihistamines—are dangerous when used in excessive amounts, in the presence of certain physical disorders, or in combination with other medicines. In addition to the question of which products to select, there is always the question of whether any product should be selected without the consultation of a physician.

Obviously, people should not run to a physician for every little scrape, bruise, ache, or pain. If they did, our entire system of medical care would be swamped overnight and the doctors would be unable to take care of the more serious problems. How can we know, then, which of the hundreds of different symptoms that can develop require the services of a physician? There are several circumstances under which a physician should always be consulted:

1. *Severe symptoms.* Any type of attack in which the symptoms are severe or alarming—such as severe abdominal or chest pain, or bleeding—should obviously receive prompt medical attention.
2. *Prolonged symptoms.* Any symptoms —such as cough, headache, constipation, or fatigue—that persist day after day should be checked by a physician, even though the symptoms are minor. Serious chronic disorders are often revealed through persistent minor symptoms.
3. *Repeated symptoms.* Symptoms, even though minor, that recur time after time should be reported to a physician because, like prolonged symptoms, they may indicate a serious problem.
4. *Unusual symptoms.* Any symptoms that seem to be unusual, such as unusual bleeding, mental changes, weight gains or losses, digestive changes, or fatigue, call for a visit to a physician.
5. *If in doubt.* If in doubt, the safest action is to see a physician. If there is a serious problem, it can be corrected in its early stages; if there is no problem, then you have paid a very small price for your peace of mind.

Health Products—Good and Bad

There is a huge array of health products available on the market, from which the consumer must choose. The following discussion is in no way exhaustive. Several kinds of products are described to show the sort of information a person needs in order to make a safe and intelligent decision on the purchase and use of the product.

Aspirin Aspirin is probably the most effective medical substance that can be bought without a prescription. Aspirin, occasionally sold under its chemical name, *acetylsalicylic acid*, is the principal active ingredient of literally hundreds of nonprescription remedies. In many of these preparations, aspirin is the only effective ingredient, but the cost may be many times that of plain aspirin tablets. When advertisements refer to the "pain reliever that doctors recommend most," they mean aspirin. Although certain brands of aspirin have been highly advertised as being more effective than other brands, there is really no significant difference between brands of aspirin.

Aspirin has several beneficial properties. Its most common use is as a pain reliever, especially for headaches and muscular pains. It also has the ability to reduce fever and inflammation. For some people, aspirin may act as a mild sedative.

The "glorified aspirin" products often contain aspirin, phenacetin (another pain reliever), and caffeine (a mild stimulant), or just aspirin and caffeine, or aspirin with a buffering agent. These products have been shown to be no more effective for most persons than plain aspirin, though some people feel that buffers may reduce stomach irritation. Several products that originally contained phenacetin no longer contain this substance.

Although effective in relieving pain and reducing fever, larger doses over prolonged periods can produce kidney damage.

Patients receiving large amounts of aspirin over long periods may develop a condition known as *salicylism*, indicated by nausea, vomiting, ringing in the ears, trouble with hearing, and severe headache (which, of course, is not relieved by taking more aspirin). Although the moderate use of aspirin is generally safe, even here there are certain precautions to follow in its use. A few people suffer allergic reactions to aspirin (such as hives); other people find that aspirin causes stomach irritation. This latter problem can often be prevented by eating before taking aspirin. The dosage recommended on the label should not be exceeded. Dosages above this level are *not* more effective and may be harmful. Time-released aspirin has produced bleeding in the stomach lining in some cases.

Finally, aspirin should be used over long periods of time only on the recommendation of a physician, since it might otherwise be used to relieve the symptoms of a serious disorder that needed medical attention.

Aspirin is among the most common causes of poisoning of young children. It is important that aspirin, like any medication, be kept where children cannot get to it, preferably in a locked cabinet. Specially flavored children's aspirin is a particular problem, since children will want to eat it as candy. Manufacturers have attempted to devise lids that prevent children from opening the bottles, but this product should still be carefully kept out of the reach of children. Some authorities even recommend splitting adult aspirin tablets for use with children rather than keeping the flavored aspirin in the house.

A compound that is similar in its actions to aspirin is acetaminophen. It is contained in over 60 over-the-counter and prescription products, such as Excedrin and Tylenol. Acetaminophen is probably safer for people with aspirin allergy or bleeding disturbances. When acetaminophen is combined with aspirin, as in Excedrin, these advantages, of course, are lost.

Remedies for Coughs and Colds Every year new "miracle" cold remedies are offered to the public in massive advertising campaigns, only to drop quietly out of the market a few years later when their manufacturers release newer "miracles." The fact remains that, despite the many advances in other fields of medicine, there is still no way to prevent or cure the common cold.

A book by Nobel Prize winner Dr. Linus Pauling, *Vitamin C and the Common Cold*, (1970) has aroused much discussion and not a few warnings. Dr. Pauling recommends as prescription to prevent the common cold, the daily taking of 1 to 5 grams (1000 to 5000 milligrams) of vitamin C. This is well above the recommended 60 milligrams per day. Pauling actually did no research of his own. He just surveyed the literature, drawing heavily on uncontrolled experiments, talked to his friends (again, no controlled experiments), and reached his own conclusions.

According to the FDA and many scientists, Dr. Pauling's evidence fails to prove his point. In fact, the FDA warns that too much vitamin C (ascorbic acid) can cause severe diarrhea (especially dangerous for elderly people and small children). It may cause pregnant women to miscarry. Excessive vitamin C causes the body to form oxalic acid, an ingredient in some kidney stones, especially those related to gout. And the acidifying effect of vitamin C on urine could interfere with the treatment of diabetes.

The medical consensus is that the effects of massive doses of vitamin C on the human system are yet very poorly understood. But since the average person would like to believe in miracle drugs, it becomes almost impossible to ignore claims for a drug that sounds as harmless as vitamin C. A medical axiom bears repeating: "The taking of any drug not prescribed is unwise."

To put cough and cold remedies into their proper perspective, one needs to understand that a cold is caused by a virus and that, to date, only limited progress has been made toward producing drugs that will cure virus infections. In fact, no drug has been developed that will control cold-producing viruses.

A cough is a reflex action caused by the presence of foreign matter or other irritation within the respiratory system. The purpose of coughing is to remove the irritant. Cough and cold remedies may give symptomatic relief by deadening the cough reflex, opening a stuffed nose, or reducing fever, but they do not get at the basic cause of the trouble. By eliminating the symptoms, but not the source, the cough and cold remedies may in the long run prove harmful. For example, by relieving the symptoms, a person with a cold is tempted to go on with normal activities when he or she really should go to bed for

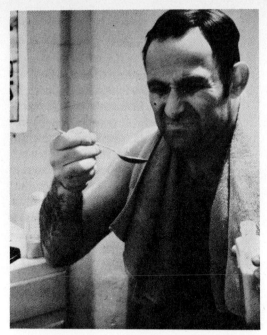

Potions, nostrums, elixirs, "wonder drugs," tonics. Man has swallowed all manner of things in the quest for good health.

Photo by F. Habicht.

24 hours. This rest period, early in the course of a cold, can often hasten recovery and prevent secondary infections and other complications. The result of "fighting" a cold is often secondary bacterial infection of the middle ear, sinus cavities, or lungs. Coughs can be the result of many serious conditions that need medical treatment rather than just a deadening of the cough reflex. For example, a cough could indicate tuberculosis, pneumonia, other infections of the lungs, or lung cancer.

The reputations of many products for "curing" colds come from the fact that most colds are gone in less than a week. If a cold lasts beyond a week, it is probably caused by a secondary bacterial infection, and should be treated by a physician. Antibiotics have no effect on the virus phase of a cold, but may be useful in clearing up the secondary infections. The cold sufferer should not pressure his or her doctor to prescribe antibiotics unless there is definite evidence of bacterial infection.

Most cold remedies contain an *analgesic* (aspirin, phenacetin, acetaminophen, or salicylamide) that can give relief from fever, aches, and pains. Many contain an *antihistamine* to dry up the mucous membranes in the nasal passages, and a *sympathomimetic* to stimulate nervous system functions. Nasal decongestants are most effective if applied directly to the mucous membranes by means of a spray or nose drops.

Antihistamines counteract the fluid release from cells that occurs during colds and allergy attacks. While this action may relieve the effects of a cold and certain allergies, antihistamines do not cure the cold. If they seem to cure it, there is a possibility that the actual problem was an allergy and not a cold at all. Antihistamines very commonly produce side effects such as dizziness and drowsiness, so they should not be taken when driving a car or operating machinery.

Sympathomimetics affect the blood supply to the swollen linings of the nose and throat. Major side effects may involve the cardiovascular system (causing increased heart action, tachycardia, and elevated blood pressure) and the central nervous system (causing anxiety and a fine tremor of the hands and fingers). Diabetics should avoid sympathomimetics since they may raise blood sugar. Patients with rapid or irregular heart action are advised against using them, because they may intensify high blood pressure and nervousness.

Products for the Eyes

Eye discomfort is one of the more bothersome problems a person can experience. The effects of air pollutants, wind, smoke, and sunlight are the target of a group of health products. The value of the eyes as essential sensory organs makes discretion in the selection of health products for eye care most important.

Eye Washes Many physicians warn against the self-treatment of the eyes with any kind of commercial eye wash or eye drops. The natural flow of tears through the eye is the best means of cleaning the eye of dust, dirt, and other irritating material. As is true with many kinds of self-treatment, eye washes may be used to try to relieve the symptoms of serious eye disorders that really need prompt treatment by a physician. If any of the symptoms for which eye washes are advertised (red eyes, sore eyes) last for more than a day or two, the eyes should be immediately examined by a physician.

Eyeglasses Eyeglasses should not be purchased from variety stores or by mail order. Anyone haviong difficulty with vision should have a thorough eye examination by an eye specialist. An *optometrist* (O.D.) is a nonmedical eye doctor, having attended a college of optometry. He or she can test the eye and prescribe lenses to correct focusing problems, but may not administer medications or perform surgery. Thus the optometrist cannot treat diseases of the eye. An *ophthalmologist* (M.D.) is a specialized medical doctor who can take care of any type of eye problem. The problem may need treatment other than glasses, and in any event glasses should be carefully fitted to the specific eyes of the individual and not purchased at random.

Contact Lenses Contact lenses are small plastic lenses that ride on a thin layer of tears directly over the cornea and under the eyelids. Recent improvements in their

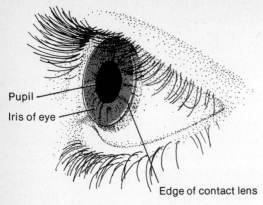

Pupil

Iris of eye

Edge of contact lens

Plastic contact lens, floating on a layer of tears over the cornea of the eye.

construction have increased their popularity. Practically invisible when worn, contact lenses are widely used by people in sports and entertainment, and by many others who dislike the appearance of regular glasses.

Contact lenses cannot be used by everyone. Certain types of visual defects can be corrected satisfactorily with "contacts"; others cannot. The lenses must be placed in the eye and taken out daily. They are easily lost, and some people find them too irritating to wear at all. In recent years, a soft, plasticlike contact lens has become available. Somewhat more comfortable, it is particularly useful for persons who are supersensitive to the hard contact lenses.

Contact lenses must be properly fitted to the eye by a qualified optometrist or ophthalmologist, and must often be adjusted before they can be worn comfortably. Poorly fitted lenses are very uncomfortable and may even damage the cornea.

Sunglasses Bright sunlight or glare can cause squinting, eyestrain, and headache, and may contain harmful amounts of ultraviolet rays that can gradually damage the lens and retina of the eyes. Sunglasses can reduce the discomfort of bright sun and screen out much of the ultraviolet.

Another reason for wearing sunglasses is that vision during the early evening hours is considerably reduced if the eyes have been exposed to bright sunlight during the day. This effect is hazardous if one is driving.

The prices of sunglasses range from very inexpensive to very expensive. It is wise to pay a little more and get a good pair of sunglasses. There are several requirements for a good pair of sunglasses. First, they should be fairly dark. Second, they should be properly ground, as optical flaws will create eyestrain and headaches just as severe as those produced by the bright sun. The figure illustrating a simple way of determining the optical quality of a pair of sunglasses before buying them shows how to test for distortion. A person who normally wears prescription lenses should

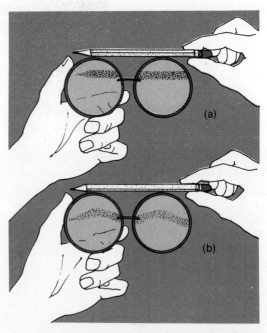

A simple test for optical quality of sunglasses. (a) Properly ground lenses reflect without distortion. (b) Poorly ground lenses reflect a distorted image and transmit it to the eye.

have sunglasses ground to his or her prescription or get the type that clip over regular glasses.

Sunglasses should never be worn for night driving, and should never be relied on to protect the eyes during a solar eclipse. There is no safe way of looking directly at the bright sun.

Pills for Sleeping, Waking, and Relaxing

Since most drugs that really affect the mind are under strict government control and are legally available by prescription only, you might wonder just what is in the nonprescription pills so openly advertised as being useful for going to sleep, staying awake, or relaxing, and relieving nervous tension.

Pills for Sleeping or Relaxing

Nonprescription pills for sleeping or relieving nervous tension are entirely different from the pills a doctor might prescribe for the same conditions. These advertised pills generally take advantage of one of the side effects of the antihistamine drugs. Antihistamines, which can be sold without a prescription, are useful in relieving the symptoms of certain types of allergies and are commonly contained in remedies for colds.

Certain of the antihistamines have the side effects of producing drowsiness, which may be rather severe in some people. For this reason, these antihistamines are sold as nonprescription sleeping pills. For many persons, these pills will really produce drowsiness. For some, they may be a psychological aid to sleep (since most sleeplessness is psychologically based). And for some others, there will be no effect at all. For a few people, antihistamines act as stimulants, producing nervousness and sleeplessness, thus contributing to the original problem. The nonprescription sleeping and relaxing pills often contain small amounts of other mild sedatives, such as scopolamine, but not enough to have any real effect.

If nonprescription sleeping pills are used, they should be taken *exactly as directed on the label*. Higher dosages (sometimes even the actual recommended dosage) can produce various side effects such as a dry mouth, dizziness, blurred vision, incoordination, loss of appetite, and nervousness. You should never drive a car or operate machinery after taking any antihistamine drug.

Pills for Staying Awake

The pills that are advertised as helping you stay awake usually contain caffeine. Caffeine, of course, is contained in coffee, tea, and cola drinks. Though not everyone reacts in the same way, many people do find that caffeine acts as a stimulant that can prevent sleep. Caffeine also makes some people feel nervous ("coffee nerves"). So the sleep-preventing pills will do for a person just what coffee does. The effect of one tablet is usually about equal to one cup of strong coffee.

The situations that justify taking these pills are rather limited. They do not serve as a substitute for sleep, but merely relieve the symptom of sleepiness. Their use has been compared to "whipping tired horses." They may help you study for an extra hour or two, but beyond that your ability to learn drops considerably. They should not be used to extend driving for more than an hour or two because driving becomes very dangerous beyond that point. A person who badly needs sleep may have hallucinations while driving or may just suddenly fall asleep at the wheel.

Cosmetics

In flipping through almost any magazine, the parade of cosmetic advertising demonstrates the importance people place in these products. But, what exactly, is a cosmetic? Are they in any way the same thing as, or similar to, drugs? According to the federal Food, Drug, and Cosmetic Act, cosmetics are defined as "(1) articles intended to be rubbed, poured, sprinkled or sprayed on, introduced into, or otherwise applied to the human body or any part thereof for cleansing, beautifying, promoting attractiveness, or altering the appearance, and (2) articles intended for use as a component of any such articles, except soaps." At present, there are more than 80 types of products considered cosmetics by the Food and Drug Administration.

Cosmetics may also be considered drugs when they make claims to alter a body function. For example, a deodorant is regulated as a cosmetic, because it is intended only to prevent odor. But an antiperspirant is regulated as a drug because it is intended to actually reduce perspiration, which is a normal body function. If a cosmetic is actually classified as a drug, its active ingredients must be listed ahead of all other ingredients. This is done, for instance, on the labels of dandruff shampoos, hormone creams, antiperspirants, sunscreen products, and all medicated cosmetics.

Skin Conditioners

Skin is nourished by the blood, and the way to make sure the necessary nutrients are available to the skin is to eat properly. Nutritional requirements for the skin are the same as the rest of the body—a balanced diet of fruits, vegetables, grains, meats, milk, and eggs. Dry skin will benefit from a simple oil, cream, or lotion. Since hormones can be absorbed through the skin in quantities large enough to have side effects, hormone skin creams should be used only on the recommendation of a physician. Exotic ingredients such as orchid pollen, royal bee jelly, and turtle oil are of no special medical or cosmetic value.

Persons bothered by skin irritations may reduce or eliminate the irritation by using some common sense. Underarm irritation may come from rubbing too hard when drying, as well as from a cosmetic or drug. Shaving too closely damages the skin. Clothing worn too tightly can chafe. Stiff, new clothing can also be a cause of skin irritation—especially some of the new permanent-press clothes. When a product containing alcohol, such as most deodorants, is applied to already irritated skin, a temporary burning sensation occurs.

Eye Cosmetics

Small amounts of carefully applied cosmetics can highlight a person's appearance and emphasize certain features, but the heavy application of cosmetics does not improve the appearance and may damage the complexion.

Cosmetics should be used around the eyes with extreme care. Some cosmetics cause rashes or other skin reactions for some people. (It is wise to test a new cosmetic on your arm before putting it on your face.)

More serious are possible eye infections brought on by the use and misuse of eye cosmetics. Preservatives in eye products retard the growth of hazardous bacteria. But during months of storage on the shelf of a pharmacy, the preservatives may lose their potency. Once the eye product is opened, microorganisms gain ready access to the cosmetic.

The human eye is bathed with secretions that keep in balance the normal skin microorganisms that migrate into the eye mucosa (underside of eyelid) and onto the eyeball surface. However, the introduction of large numbers of these same microorganisms that have grown in a contaminated eye product severely challenges these protective mechanisms. FDA studies have shown that if the cornea is scratched with a mascara brush, or irritated by wearing contact lenses or through the use of an eye-irritating shampoo, bacteria such as *Pseudomonas* (a type that can cause eye infections) infect the eye and pose a serious hazard to a person's vision. A scratch on the cornea (outer surface of the eyeball) allows the bacteria to invade and infect the cornea. Only products of good quality should be used near the eyes, and use should be as directed on the product.

Deodorants and Antiperspirants

The socially aware person not only wants to look good, but also wants to have a pleasant body fragrance. Conspiring against this are two problems—wetness and odor, each a product of a specific kind of sweat gland. Wetness comes from the eccrine sweat glands and odor from the apocrine sweat glands.

About three million tiny eccrine glands prevent the body from overheating. They secrete a clear, odorless liquid of 99 percent water and one percent sodium chloride salt. When the water evaporates from the skin, it removes heat from the body. The eccrine gland responds to two kinds of stimuli—thermal (heat) and emotional (fear, pain, tension, and sexual excitement). Eccrine glands on the palms, soles, and underarms respond to both stimuli. Those on the rest of the body respond only to thermal stimulation, except in extreme emotional stimulation, which brings on a "cold sweat" over the whole body. Wetness alone does *not* cause body odor.

The apocrine glands serve no known useful purpose. Far fewer, they function primarily in hairy underarm regions. Present at birth, they begin to function at puberty and respond only to emotional stimulation. Their activity reaches a peak with sexual maturity and diminishes with old age. When stimulated, they secrete a viscous, milky liquid composed of complex organic materials, which are decomposed by bacteria on the skin to form the end-products known as "body odor" or "underarm odor." Such bacteria are normal on the skin, and thrive in the warm, moist underarms.

Since sweating causes two problems—wetness and odor—two types of products are used. The *deodorant* works against body odor. The *antiperspirant* works against both wetness and body odor.

There are several ways to control body odor. You can wash organic material away before the bacteria can decompose it. You can try to mask the odor with another odor (perfumes are used for this). You can inhibit the growth of the bacteria by removing the moisture necessary for their growth (except that no products completely stop eccrine sweating). Or you can kill the bacteria or inhibit their growth with antibacterial agents. Such agents stick to the skin even after washing, so that deodorant effectiveness builds up over a period of days (or tapers off if use is discontinued). Antibacterial agents include zinc phenosulfonate and methylbenzethonium chloride.

The best way to control body odor is with a combination of methods. Regular use of a scented deodorant or antibacterial soap will keep you free of natural body odor for up to 24 hours. However, deodorants only kill or inhibit the bacteria, so a deodorant is not a substitute for washing. One warning—users of deodorant soaps may be more vulnerable to the effects of the sun and blister more easily.

An antiperspirant reduces the flow of perspiration from the eccrine gland through the use of metal salts such as aluminum. It also reduces body odor through the use of antibacterial ingredients. The most common antiperspirant ingredients are aluminum chlorhydroxide (or chlorhydrate or hydroxychloride) and aluminum chloride. To be effective, an antiperspirant ingredient must penetrate the sweat duct. For the greatest antiperspirant action, apply the product when you are not already sweating. Instead of applying it immediately after a bath, when the body is warm, apply it when you are at rest and cool. Then lie down for a few minutes—you sweat least then and consequently the antiperspirant penetrates better.

Deodorants and antiperspirant deodorants are available in many forms—liquid, pads, creams, roll-ons, sticks, powders, and aerosols. Read the label to be sure the product is actually an antiperspirant.

Suntans and Sunburns Many lightly pigmented people feel that they look better with a suntan. Almost everyone experiences a feeling of well-being when warmed by the sun. Yet the beneficial effects of this kind of sunbathing are almost nil, and there are in fact adverse effects.

If a person insists on getting a tan, there are several safety measures he or she can take. Human skins vary greatly in the amount of sun they can tolerate. Dark-skinned individuals have more immunity to sunburn than the fair-skinned. Yet even the person who tans well must be careful to avoid sunburn at the beginning of the summer. The key is to start with short periods of exposure and work up to longer periods. For a person with light skin, the first exposure early in the season should not exceed 15 to 20 minutes for each side, front and back. If you begin tanning later in the season, the length of first exposure should be even shorter. You can increase the exposure by about one-third each day. After a few days, exposures of several hours may be possible. Rays are reflected from sand and water, which means that you can burn even while sitting under an umbrella. You can burn on a hazy day, as well.

Suntan preparations are of varying val-ue. Many lotions contain chemicals called *sunscreens*, which absorb and block ultraviolet rays to some degree. The better lotions allow you to stay in the sun longer. They do not shut out all the radiation; otherwise you would never tan. Despite the claims of advertisements, there is no way to screen out the "burning rays" of the sun while admitting the "tanning rays" since they are one and the same. Read the label before purchasing any preparation. P-aminobenzoic acid, the salicylates, and benzophenone compounds are among the most effective sunscreens. Suntan lotions must be reapplied at least every two hours or after each swim. A word of caution—commercial sunburn preparations contain ingredients that may cause allergic skin reactions.

Those who like to tan very deeply every year should be aware of several possible effects of extreme long-term sun exposure. One is the development of premature wrinkles caused by the aging effects of ultraviolet rays on the skin. The skin may eventually look many years older than its true age. Another possible result is the development of skin cancer. Skin cancer is most common on the constantly-exposed parts of the skin, such as the face, neck, and ears. It is more common among people who suntan with difficulty than among those who tan easily.

Safe Use of Cosmetics According to the FDA, today's cosmetics are among the safest products available to consumers. Yet no rules, regulations or precautions by government or industry can protect the person who does not follow the label directions and warnings.

Some basic unwritten rules for good judgment that can prevent adverse reactions to cosmetics are:
1. Read and follow all directions and warnings on the product. If patch-testing (trying a portion of the product

first on a very small area of your skin) is suggested for any product, do not skip this wise step to determine your sensitivity to the product. And sensitivity can change: hair color, skin cream, or another type of product that should be patch-tested may irritate you the next time you use it, even though it has not in the past. Your body chemistry is always changing.

2. Basic cleanliness—in other words, washing your hands before applying a cosmetic—is important not only to your skin and appearance, but also to maintaining a clean product. Another point to remember is to close containers after each use; dust and germs can easily settle into any product left uncovered.

3. Never borrow another person's cosmetics. You may be swapping trouble.

4. When water must be added to a cosmetic before it can be used—such as cake eyeliner—it is a dangerous practice to substitute saliva for water. This practice can result in bacteria being transferred from the mouth to the eye, causing an eye infection.

5. If you do develop an adverse reaction, do not try to "wait it out." See your physician immediately. And to speed diagnosis, take the suspected cosmetic with you.

These actions are the consumer's own "voluntary program" for safety. They can be enforced only by the consumer at home.

Quackery

The colorful traveling medicine show may be a thing of the past, but medical quackery is still very much a part of the modern scene. Today's quacks are much more sophisticated than was the snake-oil salesman of the past, but their goal is still the same—to separate the suckers from their money. Many quacks seem to be sincerely interested in a person's health, but their real interest is in making money—lots of money. The cost of medical quackery in the United States today is estimated at between 1 and 2 billion dollars a year. Modern quackery takes several common forms. It may involve a direct "doctor–patient" relationship. It may involve the mail-order or house-to-house sale of worthless products. Or it may involve the sale in drug or "health food" stores of products that cannot do what is claimed of them.

Who Are the Quacks?   A quack may be defined as a boastful pretender to medical skill. A quack is anyone who promises medical benefits that cannot be delivered. Quacks may attempt to go beyond the limits of medical science or the limits of their own training.

Your own mental image of a quack may be that of an odd- or sinister-looking individual, but by actual appearance it would be impossible to tell a quack from an ethical physician. Any quack might be wearing expensive clothing or a white medical coat. A quack's personality is likely to be friendly, self-confident, and confidence-inspiring; his or her office walls are covered with "degrees."

Some quacks are well-intentioned persons who feel they have something to contribute to the health and well-being of other people, yet who are actually ignorant of the basic principles of health and nutrition. Such quacks are sometimes found in health food stores. While well-intentioned, their attempts to diagnose physical and nutritional problems can be as dangerous for the patient as the worst attempts by the most sinister of quacks.

Quacks have various kinds of training. Once in a great while, a licensed medical physician enters into an area that may be considered quackery. A few best-selling books have been written by such doctors. Much more common is the quack who has had more limited training, perhaps in methods of chiropractic or naturopathy (a mode of therapy using air, water, light, heat, massage, and so on). Many convicted quacks show no record of any formal higher education. College degrees and transcripts are obtainable from print shops and "diploma mill" colleges. The word *Doctor* in front of a name, or the letters of a degree after it, mean nothing in this situation. Sometimes the "quack" is not an individual at all, but a corporation that makes false claims for its products. And, of course, self-treatment is a form of quackery because most individuals are simply not qualified to diagnose and treat their own illnesses.

Who Turns to the Quacks? All kinds of people become the victims of quacks—the old and the young, the rich and the poor, and everyone in between. But quacks do seem to prey particularly on the extremes—the young, the elderly, the very rich, and the very poor.

The young person often becomes the victim of mail-order quackery. There are many deceptive advertisements in certain of the magazines that appeal to young people. The products offered promise good looks, popularity, and sex appeal. There are products that are claimed to help gain weight, lose weight, build muscles, enlarge the breasts, and cure acne. Seldom are these products of any real value.

Elderly people find appeal in products that promise to renew their lost youth and vigor. They often waste their limited money on useless treatments and products that claim to relieve arthritis, impotency, prostate conditions, gray hair, baldness, and "tired blood." The nutrition quack caters to elderly people who are led to believe that all their aches and pains can disappear through the use of certain food products or food supplements. In addition,

the elderly are attracted to so-called clinics and health ranches that claim cures for various chronic diseases through chiropractic, fad diets, and other limited methods.

Quacks are interested in the rich simply because they have money. The poor are receptive to quackery because good medical services are often scarce in low-income areas, and the cost of ethical care may seem prohibitive. For the urban minority resident who may not have a private physician and for whom a clinic visit may take upwards of three hours, reliance on self-perception and past experience in common illnesses is often necessary.

Much quackery preys on fear. People who have been told by a physician that they have an incurable disease live in fear—fear of death, fear of pain, fear of surgery, fear of the unknown. They may grasp at any straw of hope offered by the quack, no matter how unscientific or expensive the treatment may be. Sometimes fear keeps people from seeking an ethical physician in the first place. Afraid of surgery, they may turn instead to a quack who promises a cure without surgery. Sometimes quacks must create fear where none exists. They may, for example, tell perfectly healthy people that they have a serious disease and then recommend an expensive series of worthless treatments for the nonexistent disorder. The constant fear of imminent health disaster may lead to continuous self-treatment, an often bizarre regimen of self-administered "preventive medicine."

Ignorance and *gullibility* are strong allies to the quack. Millions of people are almost unbelievably gullible. These people unquestioningly accept almost anything they hear as reliable information and anything they read is accepted as absolute gospel. A quack can make a sales talk and literature seem entirely believable to such people. Even well-educated people who should know better often fall for quack schemes because no one can be completely knowledgeable in all areas. Most people lack sufficient medical background to know if what they have been told is reasonable or not, yet have just enough medical background to enable them to recognize a few names of diseases or medications. For this reason, quackery follows right on the coattails of science.

Major Types of Quackery Today

While quackery knows no seasons, the popular targets of quackery shift with the major causes of disability. Faithfully tagging behind public awareness of major health concerns are the "sure cures" and "money-saving self-treatments" of the quacks. There are several major forms of quackery about which a person should be well-informed.

Cancer Quackery Despite the intensive efforts of government agencies to control cancer quackery, millions of dollars are still being spent every year on worthless cancer treatments. Cancer quackery is one of the most tragic of all rackets because many persons with early, curable cancers waste vital time waiting for a worthless remedy to cure their cancer. By the time they seek ethical treatment using standard methods, their cancers have already progressed to an incurable stage. Early treatment by a competent ethical physician can often result in complete cure of a cancer.

There are many examples of cases where cancer patients have lost valuable time because of quacks. One actual case history is given here.

In this case, a chiropractor was ultimately convicted of second-degree murder in the death of a child he promised to cure of cancer, and is now serving a term of 5 years to life imprisonment. The patient (la-

ter victim) was an 8-year-old whose mother became concerned about a slight swelling over her daughter's left eye. When the child was taken to UCLA Medical Center, exploratory surgery revealed a tumorous mass in the left orbit, which was diagnosed as an extremely malignant and fast-growing form of cancer. An examination also revealed that there was no evidence of the spread of the cancer to any other part of her body. The parents were told that it was necessary to remove the eye and all of the surrounding tissue in the eye orbit. The parents consented to the surgery. But before it was performed, they met a couple who claimed their own son had been cured of a brain tumor without surgery by the chiropractor. Consulted by phone, he gave them absolute assurances he could help their daughter (without having seen the child or her medical records). His diagnosis for the cause of the cancer was a "chemical imbalance" that surgery would only make worse. Upon his insistence, the daughter was taken out of the UCLA hospital where, he claimed, the physicians would only use her as a guinea pig and "get their money." His own fee: $500 in advance plus $200 to $300 per month for medicine! The daughter was immediately examined by the chiropractor, and diagnosed as having hypochronic anemia, inflammation of the gall bladder, possible kidney disease, and hyperthyroidism—but no mention of cancer. Treatment included 124 pills (vitamins, food supplements, laxatives) daily, 150 drops of an iodine solution in a glass of water each hour for 11 hours a day, a 2-quart enema every other day, daily musculoskeletal adjustments in his office, and instructions for the parents to daily manipulate the ball of the daughter's foot with sufficient pressure to cause her to cry (which the parents refused to perform).

After over three weeks of "care," the

tumor had enlarged to the size of a tennis ball and had pushed the eye out of the socket and down along the nose. The parents discharged the chiropractor and brought the daughter back to UCLA, where her condition was now recognized as hopeless. Four months later, she died (John Minor, "A New Dimension in Murder," *American Cancer Society Volunteer* 16(2):4–5).

Cancer quacks often claim to use an effective treatment that is exclusively their own and unavailable to other physicians. Or they claim that regular doctors do not want to use effective cures for cancer because it would hurt their business. These claims are, of course, ridiculous. Effective medical treatments cannot be kept exclusive in the United States and the ethical doctors certainly do not need dying cancer patients in order to stay busy. There are very few ethical doctors in this country who are not already busier than they would like to be.

A strong ally of the cancer quack is the fear of surgery felt by many people. The quack always promises a cure without surgery, but in ethical medicine, surgery is one of the most important treatments for most kinds of cancer.

Arthritis Quackery Arthritis, sometimes called *rheumatism*, is an inflammation of the joints. (Rheumatism, broadly defined, includes some muscular conditions as well.) Millions of people suffer from some degree of arthritis, with great pain and crippling in extreme cases. Ethical medicine can offer a real cure for only a few of the many types of arthritis. About half of all arthritis sufferers are therefore led to try quack remedies, at a cost of about a quarter of a billion dollars a year. Many arthritis remedies are just aspirin with a fancy name and a high price.

Some types of arthritis tend to periodically come and go, even without treatment. Thus, quack remedies are often given credit for curing cases of arthritis that would have gone away even if nothing had been done. In arthritis, as well as any other disease, the ethical physician can still be relied on to offer the most effective, up-to-date treatment available.

Food Quackery Food quackery is a big business. Half the money spent on quackery is spent in the area of nutrition. Over 10 million Americans today are living in the shadow of confusion cast by the food faddists and health food quacks. These unfortunate people are encouraged to follow expensive, complicated, and often unpleasant diets. Rather than being better fed as a result, they are actually more likely to suffer from nutritional deficiency than those who eat ordinary diets, following the simple rules of basic nutrition.

Food quackery products are sold in several ways. They are often featured in health food stores, sold by door-to-door salespeople, advertised for mail-order sale, and promoted in "health" lectures. Regardless of the sales approach used, the food quack makes use of scare tactics, calculated to frighten people into buying certain products. Almost all operators in this field make use of certain modern myths. Each of these myths may contain some element of truth, but the conclusions drawn by the quack are not supported by scientific evidence. The following are some of these myths:

1. *All diseases are due to faulty diet.* Of course, such deficiency diseases as scurvy are entirely the result of poor diet, and a person's resistance to many infections is lower when the diet is poor. But no known diet can protect a person from all infectious diseases or from cancer, as is claimed by certain quack nutrition products.

2. *A particular product is indispensable.* Salespeople often represent their

products as being the only source of a vital food substance and imply that maximum good health is possible only if their products are used. The truth is that every substance known to be important in nutrition is available from a variety of common grocery-store foods. The salesperson will often answer this fact by saying that the product contains some substance not yet known to science. However, there is absolutely no basis for such a claim.

3. *Soil depletion causes malnutrition.* A common story is that repeated cropping of the land has removed some substance, which is therefore lacking from the foods produced. The only substance for which a deficiency in the soil is reflected in the crop produced is iodine. Since people today obtain adequate iodine through diet and the use of iodized salt, iodine deficiency is rare. If any other mineral is lacking from the soil, this deficiency is reflected in a lowered *quantity* of produce, but the nutritional *quality* is not affected.

4. *"Organic" or "natural" foods.* If there is a key word in the "health food" business, it must be either "organic" or "natural." According to the biological or chemical definitions of the word *organic* (see any dictionary), all foods are organic. The claim is often made that foods grown with commercial fertilizers are inferior to those grown with "natural" fertilizer (manure). The fallacy of this claim lies in the fact that a plant can absorb from the soil only certain simple inorganic nutrients. If manure is used as fertilizer, the organic compounds present must be broken down by bacteria into the same simple compounds present in commercial fertilizers before any absorption into the roots of the plant can take place.

A related claim is that the synthetically produced vitamins are inferior to naturally occurring vitamins. This statement is usually made by salespeople of high-priced food supplement products to indicate the superiority of their products over lower-priced products. Actually, the synthetic vitamins are chemically identical to the naturally occurring vitamins, are absorbed in the same manner, and function in the body in exactly the same way.

The very word *chemical* is often used in a derogatory manner by salespeople who apparently do not know or choose to ignore the fact that all food is nothing but a mixture of chemicals. They deplore the use of chemical food additives such as antioxidants, coloring agents, mold inhibitors, and numerous other additives important to modern food processing. Since the 1958 amendment to the federal Food and Drug Act, such chemicals have been screened by their manufacturers for any possible harmful effect before the federal Food and Drug Administration permits their use. In fairness, it must be pointed out that scientific debate continues over possible unknown effects of food additives. Caution must be exercised in allowing claims of proponents or opponents to replace substantial information.

5. *Myths about vitamins.* Recently there have been claims of unusual therapeutic effect for a host of conditions through the use of huge doses of vitamins E, B, and C. No claims have been more spectacular than those made for vitamin E. Because of the widespread confusion over contradictory reports on this vitamin, the National Academy of Sciences National Research Council (NRC) has issued a public statement regarding the misinformation.

The list of ailments claimed to be relieved by vitamin E is staggering. It includes most noninfectious diseases such as heart disease, sterility, muscular weakness, cancer, ulcers, skin diseases, burns, and shortness of breath. Beyond this, vitamin E has been claimed to promote physical endurance, enhance sexual potency, prevent heart attacks, protect against the health-related aspects of air pollution, and slow the aging process and alleviate its accompanying ailments.

Where do claims of such "miraculous cures" come from? Where do people get such ideas? To begin with, it is a fact that small amounts of vitamin E are necessary for normal life. But notions as to its miraculous powers come from unscientific interpretation of certain laboratory research. For instance, the sterility-prevention claims: While vitamin E has been shown in experiments (with vitamin E deficient rats) to prevent sterility and also abortion, studies with humans have failed to produce any evidence whatsoever that additional vitamin E does anything of the kind in people. Its reproductive effect was shown only in laboratory animals when they have been deliberately deprived of vitamin E for long periods of time. The same thing happened regarding muscular weakness in studies in animals. But according to the NRC, studies have produced no evidence that vitamin E has any effect on muscular dystrophy in humans.

The story was repeated in claims regarding heart disease and vitamin E. Large doses have been advocated for angina pectoris, coronary occlusion, congestive heart failure, thrombophlebitis, and thromboembolism. Although the dosage recommended by the NRC for adults is 30 units (1 milligram of synthetic vitamin E supplies one international unit, or IU) per day, hundreds of thousands of persons have been consuming up to one gram a day (about 35 times the daily requirement).

While insufficient amounts of vitamin E causes serious heart diseases in cows, sheep, and other grass eaters, no heart disease has ever been related to a vitamin E deficiency in man. To date, extensive tests have failed to demonstrate therapeutic benefit from supplemental vitamin E.

Ample supply of the vitamin is found in substantial amounts in the foods we eat every day. The chief sources of vitamin E in the diet are wheat-germ oil and other vegetable oils and vegetables, especially lettuce. About the only people lacking vitamin E are premature infants and people suffering from conditions that interfere with digestion or absorption of fats. Both of these groups should be, and usually are, under the care of a physician.

6. *Myths about food processing.* Some critics exaggerate the loss of food value through modern food-processing methods. Although some loss definitely does occur, it is minor in comparison with the benefit we receive from modern food technology. Today's processing methods are often less destructive to vitamins than were the methods used in the past. Highly nutritious "processed" fruits, vegetables, and meats are now available throughout the year, rather than just during limited seasons. The vitamin loss seldom exceeds 25 percent and is generally much less than that. At the same time, this is not meant to discourage the consumption of fresh foods. When fresh food is available and of good quality, people who can afford to buy it should be encouraged to do so.

7. *Advantages of "raw" sugar.* Most health food stores feature various types of raw or less processed sugar. There are two fallacies involved here. The first is that the nutritional value of less refined sugar is not significantly higher than that of pure sugar. The second is

that the sugar content is not much lower. The basic problem is that many people in the United States eat far too much sugar, a dietary factor that contributes to dental decay, obesity, malnutrition, blood sugar disorders, and possible heart disease. It makes no difference whether the sugar is "raw" or refined. In many of the cereal products that are highly promoted on children's TV programs, the most abundant ingredient is sugar. Even the more "natural" granola-type cereals often have an extremely high sugar content. It is believed that many of today's children are acquiring such a strong desire for sugar that their lifelong eating habits may be altered.

One of the most serious consequences of food quackery is that it frequently interferes with useful, scientific evaluation of nutrition, food processing, and preserving methods. There is presently a good deal of concern about food additives and their known and unknown effects—but this is a different concern from food quackery. In confusion over all the claims and counterclaims, congressional hearings testimony, industry press releases, and "muck-raking" reports, some people turn off their critical faculties and run straight in the other direction. Unfortunately, they usually do not improve their diet and general health in the process; they just substitute one set of myths for another.

Some Types of Quackery The following descriptions of types of quackery have been selected from recent issues of *FDA Consumer*, an official publication of the Food and Drug Administration. They should serve to illustrate the types of fraud and deception to which the public is being subjected. (See also the table listing products seized by FDA.)

Many people naively believe that they do not have to worry about quackery be-

cause the government does not allow it. In reality, there are and always will be some worthless treatments and products offered to the public. Although governmental agencies are active and successful in combating quackery, a quack may escape government detection for a period of time. The government must then gather evidence for a case. The burden of proof of the fraud is on the government's shoulders. The case may be tied up in the courts for many years until every possible appeal is exhausted. In the meantime, the fraud often persists.

It is therefore important for the individual to be able to recognize quackery and to know how to avoid it. Some of the signs of quackery are given below. Some of the signs discussed apply mainly to clinical quackery, where a "doctor" examines the patients and administers drugs. Other signs apply more to the sale of nonprescription remedies through mail order, drugstores, and health stores. Some of the signs apply to both forms of quackery.

Boastful Advertising The code of ethics of most medical, dental, and similar professional associations prohibits or greatly restricts the advertising of services by members. Generally, a simple announcement of name, address, and type of practice is all that is considered ethical.

Offer of Free or Low-Cost Diagnosis Less ethical practitioners often advertise complete physical examinations at very low costs ($10 or $15). Practitioners who give a free or low-cost diagnosis must make a living from the treatments they render, so they are naturally inclined to make a diagnosis that is going to lead to some of the treatments they provide. These practitioners often treat perfectly healthy persons or else fail to detect the serious disorders a person might have.

The low-cost diagnosis of the quack is in no way to be confused with free clinics set up in many urban locations. Low-cost treatment is not synonymous with quackery, nor high cost with quality. Nonetheless, some quacks *offer* low-cost diagnosis that in the long run may become much more expensive than ethical care.

Location Ethical practitioners usually prefer a professional environment for their offices. Medical offices, for example, are often near a hospital. The practitioner who rents space in a department store or discount store is not necessarily unethical, but one should be alert for other signs of quackery.

Claim to Cure Diseases that Others Cannot Cure The quack often claims the ability to cure some condition that the ethical physician cannot always cure, such as cancer, arthritis, or old age.

Guarantee of Cure or Satisfaction Ethical physicians never guarantee a cure; they do the best they can, but medical science has not progressed to the point where results are that certain. Even with a "guarantee," the quack is seldom known to refund any money.

Claims of Secret Treatments Claims of secret machines and formulas are meaningless because the ethical physician has knowledge of all the latest treatments and has access to their use. The secret remedies of quacks, upon investigation, always turn out to be worthless.

Testimonial Letters Quacks often make use of letters of testimonial; ethical practitioners seldom use this technique. No importance can be placed on these letters; many of them have been purchased or are written by ignorant people who really never had any disease. These people have no way of knowing why they may have felt better. Remember that 50 to 75 percent of all physicians' office visits are the result of

psychosomatic complaints that will often go away through psychological suggestion, even in the absence of any effective treatment. Some testimonials are written by people who later died of the disease of which they claimed to have been cured.

Attacks Against the Medical Profession Quacks often loudly attack the medical profession for its extensive use of surgery and drugs. These are, of course, the most valuable treatments for many disorders. But quacks cannot legally use drugs or surgery, so they claim the superiority of their own methods of treatment.

Quacks are often very defensive and claim that they are being persecuted by the medical associations and the government. Practitioners who make this claim should be regarded as possible quacks since it indicates that they have used unproven methods and have probably been in legal trouble as a result.

Public Protection At every level of government, efforts are being made to control fraudulent health practices. The Federal Trade Commission is active in cases involving fraudulent or deceptive advertising. The Post Office Department may move rapidly in cases of mail-order fraud. The Food and Drug Administration regulates the purity, safety, and proper labeling of drugs and food products moved across state lines. Certain state, county, and city governments are also active in suppressing quackery by enacting laws that make fraudulent practices a felony.

Several privately financed groups actively participate in the restraint of health frauds. Among these are the Bureau of Investigation of the American Medical Association, the Better Business Bureau, and the Chamber of Commerce. Although these organizations have no legal regulatory powers, they can bring cases of fraud to the attention of the public and the proper legal regulatory authorities.

When a person is in doubt about the merits of a particular product or treatment, it is often worthwhile to check with a local Chamber of Commerce, Better Business Bureau, local medical society, or licensed and registered physician.

Guidelines for Filing Consumer Complaints   When the top of a table is ruined by the furniture polish, when the canned tuna smells tainted, when a garage does not make promised repairs, or when a skin conditioner causes a rash, there is more to do than throw the product away and vow to buy a different brand the next time or shop elsewhere. You can, and should, report complaints to the proper government agency. The problem is in knowing how to register a complaint and to whom.

Here are some steps for consumers to follow *before* they report, *how* they report, and *where* they report.

Before You Report   Before consumers report violations or hazards, they should ask themselves these questions:
1. Have I used the product as directed?

Mail Fraud Cases Reported by the Post Office Department

"Firm advertises and sells by mail a bustline developer guaranteed to increase the size of the bustline 1-3 inches in 8 days. Promises total increases of 4-5 or possibly 6 inches." (November 7, 1974)

"Advertising and sale by mail of Vitamin E Cream for removing wrinkles." (October 24, 1974)

"Advertising and sale by mail of E-Z Slim Caps, represented to be effective for weight loss." (November 21, 1974)

"Advertising and sale by mail of the revolutionary new Youth Mask represented as equivalent to the effect produced by a miniature surgical face lift (mini lift)." (September 13, 1974)

"Advertising and sale by mail of "Hungrex with P.P.A." represented as the most powerful reducing aid ever released for public use." (September 18, 1974)

"Advertising and sale by mail of the Macobra bracelet represented to be effective in relieving or eliminating the pain and suffering associated with arthritis, rheumatism, or bursitis." (September 4, 1974)

"Advertising and sale by mail of the U.S. Women's Ski Team Diet represented to cause a weight loss of 20 pounds in 2 weeks." (September 4, 1974)

"Violation of Consent Agreement relating to the advertising and sale by mail of an RNA-DNA product represented to be effective for cellular rejuvenation." (December 18, 1974)

"Advertises and sells by direct mail advertising a formula and program which they guarantee will cause one to lose up to 7 pounds in the first 48 hours, 12 pounds first 2 weeks, 34 pounds first month, and 71 pounds in 3 months." (January 9, 1975)

"Advertising and sale via mails of a cure for depression." (January 16, 1975)

"Advertising and sale through the mail of a Vitamin E Shampoo represented to aid in scalp conditioning and in promoting vasolary circulation and vasodilation, and Vitamin E Capsules represented as being effective for healing stretchmarks and for helping to make the body beautiful from the inside out." (July 22, 1974)

"Advertising and sale by mail of Naturaid represented as an effective remedy for male impotency." (July 26, 1974)

"Advertising and sale through the mail of an electronic board designed to cure all ills." (July 24, 1974)

"Advertising and sale by mail of the Kicker Kit represented to be effective for breaking the smoking habit." (July 19, 1974)

"Advertising and sale by mail of X-11 Reducing Plan represented as an effective means for the user to lose 25 pounds or more without changing eating habits." (July 3, 1974)

"Advertising and sale by mail of Dr. Frank's Nutritional Skin Creme represented to be effective for skin maladies." (December 20, 1974)

Products Seized by the Food and Drug Administration

Product (date)	Charge
Potatoes (11/14/74)	Contain the added poisonous and deleterious substance chlordane.
Salmon, frozen king (1/13/75)	Decomposed.
Candy pacifier (2/7/75)	Unfit for food due to choking and aspiration hazards to those likely to use.
Pickles (1/13/75)	Labeling fails to state that the articles contain an artificial color.
Skin cleanser (8/5/74)	New drugs without an effective New Drug Application; inadequate directions for use.
Green beans, canned (8/5/74)	Held in rusty, leaky cans.
Cereal (1/22/74)	Held under insanitary conditions; rodent gnawed.
Candy (10/7/74)	Unfit for food, contains metal fragments.
Swordfish, frozen (11/4/74)	Contains the added poisonous and deleterious substance mercury.
Air purifiers (12/27/74)	Misbranded in that the labeling suggests device will purify air and is effective in treatment for respiratory problems; article is dangerous to health when used in accordance with directions.
Prophylactics (10/15/74)	Contain holes.
Peanut butter, organic (11/14/74)	Manufactured in insect-infested equipment.
Nail lengthener kits (9/26/74)	Article contains a poisonous and deleterious substance, which may render article injurious to users under such conditions of use as are customary or usual.
Dates (11/18/74)	Moldy.
Beans, pinto, split (9/10/74)	Contain dirty beans, animal excreta, insect-damaged beans, and rocks.
Pecans, canned, shelled (5/22/74)	Insect contaminated; not in conformity with the Fair Packaging and Labeling Act.

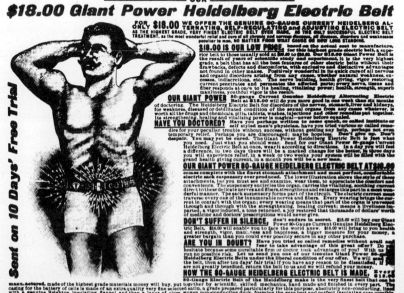

This rather overstated cure-all advertisement is taken from the 1902 Sears Catalogue.

2. Did I follow the instructions carefully?
3. Did an allergy contribute toward the bad effect?
4. Was the product old when I opened it?

Make sure all these factors have been taken into consideration first to confirm that the complaint lies with the product, not the consumer's misuse of it.

How to Report Report the complaint as soon as possible. Give your name, address, telephone number, and directions on how to get to your home or place of business. Clearly state the complaint. Describe in as much detail as possible the label of the product. Give any date or code marks that appear on the container (on canned goods these are usually stamped or embossed on the end of the can). Give the name and address of the store where the article was bought, and the date of purchase. Save whatever remains of the product or the empty container for your physician's guidance or possible examination by the FDA. Retain any unopened containers of the product you bought at the same time. If an injury is involved, see your physician at once. Report the suspect product to the manufacturer, packer, or distributor shown on the label, and to the store where you bought it.

Where to Report There are basically ten agencies with jurisdiction over products that one can turn to with a complaint. These agencies and their areas of responsibility include:

1. *Food and Drug Administration.* Drugs and medicines (human and veterinary); medical devices; cosmetics; and medical preparations made from living organisms and their products.
2. *Federal Trade Commission.* Promotion and advertising.
3. *Consumer Product Safety Commission.* Toys; laundry, cleaning, and polishing products; home repair and paint products; hobby items; and automotive fluids.
4. *U.S. Department of Agriculture.* Meat and poultry products.
5. *The Postal Service.* Mail-order frauds and unsolicited products by mail.
6. *U.S. Department of Justice and Bureau of Narcotics and Dangerous Drugs.* Illegal sale of narcotics or dangerous drugs (such as stimulants, depressants, and hallucinogens).
7. *Environmental Protection Agency.* Pesticides; air and water pollution.
8. *State Health Department.* Products made and sold exclusively within your state.
9. *State Board of Pharmacy.* Dispensing practices of pharmacies and drug prices.
10. *Poison Control Centers.* Accidental poisonings.

Consumers Union in Mt. Vernon, New York, which publishes a monthly periodical called *Consumer Reports*, also takes complaints and often relays complaints back to the manufacturer, packer, or distributor on items that have been tested.

Persistence of Quackery How does quackery persist in spite of intensive efforts by government and individuals to eliminate it? The answer is that, although quacks might not be very skilled in treating disease, they are very adept in other areas. They often operate at the very borderline of legality, perhaps obeying the letter but not the spirit of the law. When they are convicted, they usually serve a short jail sentence and pay a stiff fine (which they can well afford). Then, immediately they change location and perhaps their name and are back in business again.

Often, getting a conviction for a quack proves to be very difficult. Juries may be swayed by the emotional testimonies of former patients of the quack. Large corporations engaged in the sales of proprietary compounds retain excellent lawyers to fight their battles with the authorities, and the corporations often win. For example, it took the federal government 16 years to get the word *liver* removed from the name of Carter's Little (Liver) Pills on the basis that the pills had nothing to do with the liver.

The private citizen can aid the campaign against quackery through reporting incidents of suspected quackery to the local district attorney's office or the local medical society. It is often only through such complaints that authorities are alerted to a fraudulent operation. It is apparent, then, that today, as always, it is the responsibility of the individual to be alert to both health fraud and quackery and to avoid them.

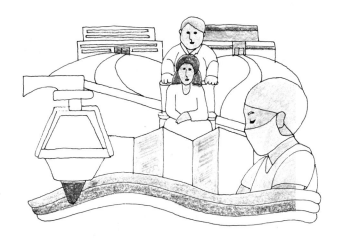

12

SELECTING HEALTH SERVICES

In this chapter there will be an attempt to analyze the health services and their problems in making good on the delivery of these services. Just as quackery was exposed in the last chapter, the health services professionals are viewed critically in this one. This statement is necessary lest the approach in these two chapters appear contradictory. Such a stance is taken in the hope that the student will be encouraged to view the health services more objectively.

A reflection of the high priority Americans attach to freedom from disease is the fact that more is spent per person for health care in this country than anywhere else in the world. Unfortunately, enjoying a completely healthy life remains a clouded and uncertain hope for millions in our population. In the enlightened mid-1970s, many people are bewildered as to who they should seek out for health counsel; or, once informed, are unable to locate the professional help they need; or find they are too poor to pay the professional fees asked. People are shocked and dismayed to learn of skyrocketing malpractice insurance rates, physicians' boycotts and strikes, closing hospitals, and escalating fees.

The present system of financing health care is both inadequate and chaotic. Different levels of care exist for the poor and the nonpoor. Economic incentives have resulted in a relative oversupply of physicians in suburban areas and a relative undersupply in the inner cities and in rural areas. The private insurance structure tends to pay for (and thus encourage) expensive care of illness in hospitals, but usually fails to pay for (and thus may discourage) preventive care in physicians' offices.

The federal government's first attempts to provide national health care for selected high-need groups have been inadequately funded. Some are advocating a national health program for *all* Americans. Yet the rhetoric continues, and with it, the hopes of those in need remain unanswered. A rational means of financing adequate health services is vital to an improved general level of health in this country.

The Health of Americans

A greater proportion of personal income is spent for health care in the United States than is spent in any other country in the world. Yet this country has been falling behind other nations in the key criteria used in measuring national health. In infant mortality, we presently rank 20th. In the number of years adults live, we rank 25th. While we spend over 10 percent of our gross national product for health services, Sweden spends only 5 percent.

Loss of Work Days Americans lose millions of days from work every year due to illnesses and injuries that last less than three months and that involve either medical attention or restricted activity. In 1972, according to the United States National Health Survey, wage earners lost 297 million work days as a result of some acute condition. This amounted to an average of 3.7 days off the job per worker.

Injuries resulted in an average of 1.0

Infant Mortality per Country

Rank	Country	Infant Mortality Per 1,000 Births
1	Finland	10
2	Sweden	10
3	Iceland	12
4	Japan	12
5	Netherlands	12
6	Norway	13
7	Switzerland	13
8	Denmark	14
9	Spain	15
10	New Zealand	16
11	France	16
12	Luxembourg	16
13	Australia	17
14	Belgium	17
15	Canada	17
16	Hong Kong	17
17	East Germany	18
18	Ireland	18
19	United Kingdom	18
20	United States	18
21	Singapore	20
22	West Germany	20
23	Czechoslovakia	21
24	Israel	21
25	Austria	24

Taken from *1975 World Population Data Sheet*, Population Reference Bureau (Washington, D.C.: 1975).

work days lost per person per year. The survey showed that home accidents were the most frequent single cause of injuries, followed in order by injuries from motor vehicles and on the job.

This survey reflected a distinct difference in days of disability between the low- and middle-income brackets. The average American had 16.5 days of restricted activity as a result of an acute and/or chronic condition. The average number of bed-disability days was 6. Persons from families with an annual income of less than $3,000 averaged 33 restricted activity days, while those from families with an income of $10,000 to $14,999 had an average of 13 days. Those with incomes under $3,000 had an annual average of 7 days away from the job, while in the $10,000 to $14,999 bracket, workers averaged 5 lost days. Average bed-disability days for the less than $3,000 income group was 12 days, while the average for the $10,000 to $14,999 class was 5 days.

Causes of Death in the United States

Causes of death differ with different ages in life. Accidents top the list from childhood through age 45. The five leading causes of death, arranged by age group and ranked from one (most frequent) through five, are:

1. *Infancy (under 1 year of age):* (a) congenital malformations; (b) postnatal asphyxia; (c) premature birth; (d) influenza and pneumonia; and (e) birth injuries.
2. *Preschool children (ages 1 through 4):* (a) accidents; (b) influenza and pneumonia; (c) congenital malformations; (d) cancers; and (e) meningitis.
3. *Elementary and junior high school students (ages 5 through 14):* (a) accidents; (b) cancers; (c) congenital malformations; (d) influenza and pneumonia; and (e) heart diseases.
4. *Senior high school and college-age persons (ages 15 through 24):* (a) accidents; (b) homicide; (c) suicide; (d) cancers; and (e) heart diseases.
5. *Young adults and parents (ages 25 through 44):* (a) accidents; (b) heart diseases; (c) cancers; (d) homicide; and (e) suicide.
6. *Middle-aged persons (ages 45 through 64):* (a) heart diseases; (b) cancers; (c) stroke; (d) accidents; and (e) cirrhosis of the liver.
7. *The elderly (ages 65 and over):* (a) heart diseases; (b) cancers; (c) stroke; (d) influenza and pneumonia; and (e) hardening of the arteries.

Life Expectancy per Country

Rank	Country	Life Expectancy At Birth (Years)
1	Denmark	74
2	Iceland	74
3	Netherlands	74
4	Norway	74
5	Belgium	73
6	East Germany	73
7	France	73
8	Japan	73
9	Sweden	73
10	Australia	72
11	Bulgaria	72
12	Canada	72
13	Ireland	72
14	Italy	72
15	New Zealand	72
16	Puerto Rico	72
17	Spain	72
18	Switzerland	72
19	United Kingdom	72
20	Austria	71
21	Cyprus	71
22	Israel	71
23	Luxembourg	71
24	Malta	71
25	United States	71

Taken from *1975 World Population Data Sheet,* Population Reference Bureau (Washington, D.C.: 1975).

The High Cost of Medical Care

Medical care is an increasingly costly item for the American public. The total national health bill now stands at over $100 billion a year, or more than $475 per person per year. In terms of the Consumer Price Index, medical costs have increased faster over the years than any other major category of personal expenses. From 1963 to 1973, medical costs rose 61 percent. In 1973, personal expenditures for health care were $61 billion, up from $22 billion ten years earlier. For the same period, the amount spent for all personal needs rose from $375 billion to $805 billion. In order words, the percentage of total personal expenditures of the average person for health care rose from 6.1 percent in 1963 to 7.6 percent in 1973.

Individual medical care items have increased at differing rates during the past decade. As of 1973 semiprivate hospital room rates are up 165 percent; physicians' fees, up 66 percent; dentists' fees, up 57 percent; optometric examinations and eyeglasses, up 44 percent; and the cost of prescriptions and drugs, *up only 5 percent*. For the same period of time, the amount spent for all personal care items, such as toothpaste, cosmetics, and so on, increased *only 34 percent*.

There is no question but that much of this higher cost represents proportionately better care. A study from Massachusetts General Hospital is a case in point. It is a comparison of patients coming into the hospital with heart attacks in terms of cost per patient and fatalities for years 1920, 1940, and 1970:

Year	Patients	Fatalities	Cost Per Patient
1920	100	40	$200
1940	100	30	$400–600
1970	100	16	$3500

In spite of past increases in medical costs, all indications are that if medical services are to be improved to any extent, the costs will go higher. Some are even suggesting that by 1980 hospital costs may rise to at least $300 per day per bed. Already costs of $100 per day per bed are common, with intensive care beds now averaging about $300 to $500 per day.

Why the great increase in medical costs? Answers are multiple. Costs per square foot on new construction have soared. Hospital employee salaries and benefits are up (63 percent of the hospital budget goes into salaries and benefits). New equipment becomes obsolete before it is worn out. It is estimated that every year about half of the major equipment in a hospital becomes obsolete. Hospitals are expected to be open and available 24 hours a day, 365 days a year, emergencies or not. A high-quality acute-care hospital hires an average of six employees for every patient.

There is public apathy about hospital costs. People are confident that, unreasonable cost or not, their health insurance will bail them out (often unaware their insurance will pay only one-fourth to one-third of most hospital bills). Welfare payments are rarely enough to pay the true cost of public care. To make ends meet, hospitals overcharge private patients (and their insurance companies). Some private insurance policies provide coverage only if the patient is admitted to the hospital overnight (although overnight admission may not be required for the emergency). People abuse their health insurance—figuring the care is coming to them, forgetting that each such unnecessary use helps boost the cost of health insurance. People go to the hospital when the same care might be provided just as well and with much less cost in a physician's office or clinic.

Although disturbing, there is evidence that the medical profession (at least the

AMA) has been opposed to both better and cheaper medical care. Many physicians are guilty of greater concern over maintaining their high income than providing medical service their patients can afford. Medical care costs everyone. It should be used discreetly and only at those times it is required.

Paying Medical Bills   The traditional method of financing health costs has been for each family to pay off their medical bills as they arise, always hoping that there is sufficient money available in the bank to cover major episodes. For some families this amounted to a "pay-as-you-go" method, hoping the money for the week held out. For others it was a matter of budgeting, reserving money each month for medical costs. If all medical expenses were "average," it would not be too difficult for a family to budget money each month for such a purpose, just like a budget for other household expenses. But medical expenses are often erratic, with times of great expense separated by times of lesser expense, so budgeting becomes almost impossible. All of us know of some families that seem to be hit repeatedly by heavy medical expenses that go way beyond the average. As a result of the erratic, unpredictable nature of medical costs for a family, there has been a greatly increasing trend toward collective financing of medical expenses.

It is the boast of the health insurance field that over 89 percent of our population holds some form of health insurance. Studies show that in the long run medical care tends to be a little cheaper in the form of a prepaid plan. In this manner people are protected somewhat against sudden large medical expenses by being forced to lay away funds systematically.

The current methods of collective financing of medical costs fall into one of two basic categories—public (tax-supported) and private (voluntary) health insurance.

Public Medical Care   Tax-supported health care programs have been available for certain groups for years. Starting in 1798, when health care was provided for the U.S. Merchant Marine, services have expanded into the array of services now available to select age, economic, and residence groups. Further expansion of public health services is being proposed.

Care of the Poor   Most of the first organized medical programs were those for the poor. In the mid-1930s, Congress passed the federal Social Security Act. Among other things, this act provided medical services for several categories of poor people: the elderly, the blind, and dependent children. In January 1966, *Medicaid* (Title 19 of the Social Security Act) gave funds to states to expand their public assistance programs to persons, regardless of age, whose incomes are insufficient to pay for health care. Medicaid greatly increased medical care for the poor.

According to the Bureau of the Census, over 15.3 percent of all Americans live *below* the poverty line. By federal definition, the "poor are those who are not now maintaining a decent standard of living—those whose basic needs exceed their means to satisfy them."

While 69 percent of the poor are white, 31 percent are nonwhite. But the number of poor whites and nonwhites to their total populations is another picture. Nine percent of *all* whites are poor, but about 32 percent of *all* nonwhites are poor.

A part of the basic needs of people is adequate medical care. Those poor living in urban areas generally have greater access to such services than rural poor. However, only about 40 percent of all poor families live in metropolitan areas, and about 60 percent in nonmetropolitan areas.

Although pressures on health facilities exist everywhere, they tend to be greater for the rural poor. They include the presence of a hospital or clinic, the lack of physicians in the rural places, transportation—general accessibility. Also important is the difference in level of welfare provisions in the various states. Southern states tend to provide less state health care than other regions of the United States.

Medicare Medicare, a government program of health insurance under Social Security that helps the elderly (those 65 years of age and older) pay for medical care, became effective July 1, 1966. It has two parts: compulsory hospitalization financed by contributions from employees and employers, and voluntary medical insurance.

1. *Hospital Insurance.* The hospital insurance portion of Medicare helps pay for medical care received as a hospital inpatient and for certain follow-up services. It does not pay physicians' bills. Its basic coverage includes: (a) up to 90 days of inpatient care in any participating hospital in each benefit period (a new benefit period begins after a person has not been an inpatient for 60 days); (b) a "lifetime reserve" of 60 additional hospital days; (c) up to 100 days of care in each benefit period in a participating extended-care facility, such as a nursing home, after the patient leaves the hospital; and (d) up to 100 medically necessary home-health "visits" by nurses, physical therapists, home-health aides, or other health workers.

2. *Medical Insurance.* The medical insurance part of Medicare helps pay physicians' bills, as well as a number of other medical items and services not covered under hospital insurance. The plan is voluntary. Those who are drawing benefits before age 65 are enrolled in the medical insurance automatically. The monthly premiums, or payments, are shared equally by those who enroll and by the federal government. A person can sign up for it at age 65 whether or not he or she is eligible for other services of Medicare under Social Security.

Medical insurance benefits include payment for: (a) physicians' services; (b) up to 100 home-health visits each year furnished by a home-health agency taking part in Medicare, if a physician arranges the treatment; (c) other health services prescribed by a physician, such as x rays, radiation, artificial limbs, surgical dressings; and (d) office medical supplies, outpatient physical therapy services and ambulance services.

A subscriber pays the first $60 of medical expenses each year, and then 20 percent of the balance. A person can drop out of the medical insurance program any time simply by filing written notice.

Military Coverage A military veteran may receive care for any condition inflicted or activated during service. The veteran will be taken care of at government expense through the Veterans' Administration hospitals. Spouses and children of military personnel who are on active duty or who are retired from the service are eligible for the Aid to Military Dependents Program. Children are covered until they are 18 years of age.

Special Diseases There are tax-supported medical programs for certain noncommunicable diseases that are of particular social concern. State hospitals for the mentally ill and neurologically disabled have been provided for almost 100 years. Clinics and hospitals for drug problems are being built both by the federal government and by individual states.

Communicable Diseases Communicable diseases are of high public concern. Sexually transmitted diseases (syphilis and gonorrhea) are of epidemic proportions in this country. Public medical care centers, often city or county, provide both public education, diagnosis, and treatment. For example, there is a public hospital for lepers at Carville, Louisiana. In some of the larger cities there are special hospitals for other infectious diseases.

General Hospital Care Most counties and larger cities in the country provide a county or general hospital for their citizens. Although these hospitals usually provide general medical care, they tend to be strongly oriented to the care of poor persons or those with chronic illnesses.

Local or County Health Departments Virtually every county government in the United States supports some kind of county health department. Services provided vary from county to county, but usually include some or all of the following: (1) communicable disease control, (2) tuberculosis control, (3) sexually transmitted disease control, (4) local community health offices, (5) public health nursing services, (6) public health social services, (7) public health nutrition services, (8) child and maternal health consultations, (9) public health dentistry, (10) sanitation inspection and supervision, (11) maintenance of vital records, (12) public health education, (13) air pollution control, (14) school and industrial health services.

Eligibility for services from county health departments and general hospitals varies from place to place and depends on the restrictions thought necessary by the local agency.

Private Health Insurance

Over 89 percent of the total population within the United States is covered, to some extent, by some form of private health insurance. The whole reason for the existence of private health insurance programs is that individuals cannot successfully budget against the potential costs of all illnesses. This is especially true with certain illnesses, such as cancer, that may require long hospitalization and much medical care and that could easily bankrupt the average family. The best hope for protection against these larger medical expenses, then, lies in large numbers of persons pooling the risks through health plans so insurance companies can spread both the chances and the costs.

Unlike the public insurance plans, the costs of private health coverage are maintained solely by the beneficiaries. The major advantage of private health insurance at the present time is that it does permit the insured to select specific provisions and types of coverage that might be unavailable through public plans. Another advantage of private health insurance coverage is that it encourages the insured to take better care of themselves—to see a physician or have necessary diagnostic work done, knowing that they are already allotted a specific amount of money for this purpose. With Medicare in effect, most health care policies now terminate at age 65, or when the insured individuals become eligible for Medicare.

Many insurance companies now sell medical insurance (also known as *hospital* or *surgical insurance*) through employee groups, professional organizations, and directly to individuals.

Kinds of Subscriptions The most favorable premium rates (the cost of insurance) have been gained through the formation of groups of subscribers. A group is composed of a number of individuals or families who subscribe to a similar insurance plan. Group plans are generally available only through an employer, educational institution, or fraternal organization. Typically, only one type of plan is available to the group, with a similar premium charge to each subscriber within the group who holds a similar contract. (There may be some small differences in premium rate depending on the size of the family.) It generally costs more for an unaffiliated individual to buy insurance of the same type and coverage, or else his or her policy might provide fewer benefits. The graph on health insurance premiums demonstrates the greater amount of dollar volume being placed by subscribers into group policies. Group policies paid out in 1973 over five times as many dollars in benefits as did the individual or family policies.

Types of Benefits In terms of benefits (the services on which the insurance plan makes payment), there are two general plans: *service* and *cash indemnity* plans. Service plans are generally in the form of contracts between the policyholder and the hospital or physician. The hospital agrees to provide certain services to anyone who is a policyholder under such a plan and who can present a policy identification card. The hospital or physician then agrees to accept the fees allowed under the plan as full or near-full payment for the care that is given. After the hospital (or physician) has completed its service, its office fills out a claim form and sends it to the insurance company. Reimbursement is then made directly to the hospital or physician according to the provisions of the policy.

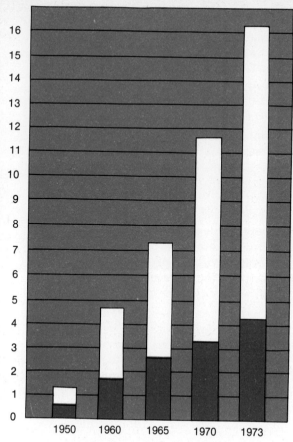

Health insurance premiums of insurance companies by type of policy. Group policies, white; individual policies, shaded.

Adapted from 1974–1975 Source Book of Health Insurance Data, Health Insurance Institute (New York: 1974).

Cash indemnity plans pay benefits in the form of cash to the policyholder, whereby the insured person is paid a specified sum of money toward the covered expenses. (These payments can also be made directly to the provider of care through an arrangement called an *assignment of benefits*.) The patient is generally required to present either a physician's or hospital's statement showing the exact amount due or a receipt confirming payment already made.

Types of Insurers No two health insurance plans are exactly alike. There are several hundred different health insurance companies in the country today. Their plans, however, tend to fall into several main categories.

Blue Cross Blue Cross is a nonprofit operation with over 68 million members. This represents about 38 percent of the population, and 84 percent of all Blue Cross members belong to a group plan. Through seventy-eight plans in the United States, Blue Cross insures members against costs of hospital care, physicians' services, drugs, and laboratory tests. Even though all these plans bear the name Blue Cross, each is sold exclusively within a given geographical area, and is governed independently by a local board made up of community, hospital, and medical leaders.

Types of coverage range from several weeks to a full year of hospital service. The most widely sold policies cover the partial or complete cost of 30 days of hospital care. Other plans also cover services of physicians, anesthesiologists, x-ray diagnosis and therapy, drugs, and laboratory tests. Most plans also now include extended coverage (benefits payable in the event of a long siege of illness). Hospital claims are paid directly to the contracting hospital. Physician claims may be mailed to the subscriber (who endorses the check and mails it to the physician) or directly to the physician.

Blue Shield Set up along the same general lines as Blue Cross, Blue Shield plans claim over 83 million subscribers through seventy-one different plans. Organized in 1946 and endorsed by the American Hospital Association, Blue Shield plans are designed to provide prepaid coverage for physicians' services and at the same time help to assure the collection of physicians' fees.

Blue Shield is available in most states. Payments of claims are made to physicians based either on their usual, customary, and reasonable (UCR) fee for the treatments or by allowing a fixed dollar amount for a given type of care. In some areas, such as Southern California, Blue Shield prepays both physicians' and hospital costs. Blue Shield is available in most states.

Commercial Most of the health insurance plans available are being written by commercial insurance companies. Although their coverage is similar to Blue Cross and Blue Shield, the approach of the commercial companies is often quite different. Their plans tend to be of the cash indemnity type or are a combination of service-cash indemnity. The commercial health insurance companies in no way engage in setting up contracts with hospitals or physicians and thus do not seek to control the quality of medical services rendered to their policyholders. A wide variety of plans is available, even from one given company; thus a family can select a policy that is tailor-made to its needs.

Commercial companies have helped in the development of certain other forms of health insurance such as the following:

1. *Major medical.* Just as the name implies, these plans are set up to give large amounts of coverage for major expenses. They are not designed or intended to pay for smaller medical expenses that the insured individual can easily pay out of his or her own pocket or that can be covered by the regular type of health insurance plan. Accordingly, major medical plans usually contain a deductible clause, excluding payments on medical expenses under $100 for a given period; this figure can range as high as $500. The policyholder is expected to pay this amount. Beyond this, some policies provide coverage for 75 to 80 percent of the costs above the

deductible amount; the policyholder agrees to pay the remainder.

2. *Comprehensive plans*. Contracts of this type are designed to provide regular (basic) medical care *plus* major medical coverage. They are designed to combine the best features of the other types of policies. They can be purchased either on a group or individual basis. Some Blue Cross plans now offer comprehensive coverage.

3. *Income (disability) insurance*. People may not realize their need for income protection until income ceases. Many look upon accident and serious illness as things that happen to "other people." This coverage may be in the form of short-term or long-term protection. (Short-term policies are those with a maximum benefit period up to 2 years; long-term plans have benefit periods greater than 2 years.)

Most income contracts are written on a scheduled basis. The insured people elect to take such coverages as they believe will benefit them. They can tailor their contract to their particular needs and their ability to pay. Their total premium will be determined by the kinds and amounts of coverages they take, and by their occupation, age, and sex. Accident coverage may include total disability, loss of life, limb, or sight, and blanket medical expense. Sickness coverage may include total disability, hospital room and board, surgical operation, inhospital physician, and nurse expense.

The most important part of the contract is the provision for total or partial disability. Most companies use a 30-, 60-, or 90-day clause requiring that disability commence within this time period following the accident.

It is important that a person look carefully at the insuring clause in accident policies, since policies are not uniform. Some refer to injury, while others refer to "accidental means" or "accidental bodily injury." Sickness policies may make no distinction between "the patient's occupation" and "any occupation" as found in most accident contracts, and most are limited to a maximum payment period of 52 or 104 weeks.

Partial disability payments are usually available in accident policies either automatically or for an additional premium. Benefits may be 40 to 50 percent of total disability benefits, payable only if the insured is able to go to work.

Income benefits for sicknesses are not sold separately from accident income protection. It is likely that both will be issued in the same contract; a separate contract covering accidents usually is drawn up only for those who specifically request such a policy.

Independents There are, in addition, several hundred smaller local plans. They have been organized by labor unions, corporate managements, physicians, and laypeople. They tend to be unique in that most of them provide their own salaried physicians, their own clinics, and sometimes their own hospitals. They go under such names as the Health Insurance Plan of Greater New York, the Kaiser Foundation Health Plan, and the Community Health Association of Detroit. Patients are expected to use the staff physician who is provided and not to bring a nonstaff physician into the clinic or hospital. Plans lacking their own hospitals have agreements with specific hospitals to provide services. Although the independents are generally local, it does not mean they are small. Many are large organizations. New York, California, and other states have a number of such plans.

Dental Plans   Health plans are now available that provide coverage for specific items such as dentistry, drugs, and contact lenses. Dental care, as an example, has usually been excluded from health care plans except as necessary in cases of accident. Increasingly popular dental insurance usually provides coverage for oral examinations (including x–rays and cleaning), fillings, extractions, inlays, bridgework, and dentures, as well as oral surgery, root-canal therapy, and orthodontia.

Dental plans are commonly set up as group plans. One leader in this field has been Group Health Dental Insurance, Inc., in New York. Rates depend on the type of coverage provided and the makeup of the particular group. Most coverage provides a limited amount of care, with the patient paying the balance of the cost. Usually excluded are dental services not considered necessary for normal chewing, such as cosmetic care. Further information describing available dental care plans can be obtained by checking the Digest of Prepaid Dental Care Plans, U.S. Public Health Service, Washington, D.C.

Purchasing Health Insurance   The novice can easily be totally confused by the first attempt at purchasing health, hospital, surgical, or accident insurance. It is literally a concern of life and death and should not become a battle of wits between the buyer and seller. In purchasing health insurance the buyer must be careful not to end up with a policy that does not give the coverage needed, or requires payment for additional provisions that are not needed.

Generally, a person should begin the purchase of health insurance by first determining (1) the type of health care expenses he or she desires to be protected against, and (2) the extent (proportion) to which he or she desires these expenses insured. One should have a clear picture of the regular, periodic payments one is obligated to pay—such as auto loans, rent or loan payments on a house, educational fees, furniture payments, and so on. A family must be sure that the expected health insurance premiums can be added to the budget and be paid. It is also wise to remember that the family with more financial obligations has as much, if not more, need for health insurance than the family with fewer financial obligations. If a financially obligated person were to encounter huge unexpected medical bills and not be able to keep up payments on a car, refrigerator, or house, these could be taken away through repossession or foreclosure. Therefore, the financially obligated person particularly needs adequate health insurance. It must not be something a person plans to buy when all the rest of the bills have been paid.

Observing these points should enable a person to make a wise selection of health insurance. In certain types of employment the health insurance is automatically provided as a fringe benefit, and an employee does not have the problem of selection.

Here are some questions that should be asked of the insuring company:

1. Is the company or prepayment plan licensed to do business in your state?
2. What is the organization's reputation for fulfilling its obligations to its policyholders?
3. Is there a claims payment office located either in the state or otherwise reasonably near?
4. Does the company's agent have a good reputation in the community?

There are three classes of medical expenses—hospital costs, physicians' fees, and paramedical costs (laboratory, x–rays, nursing, physical therapy, and pharmaceuticals). The first two lend themselves more readily to the provisions of health insurance. A prospective buyer of health insurance should be aware of the prevailing costs for these services in the community and measure these costs against the benefits offered by specific policies.

There is a wide range of contract provisions that limit the insuring companies' liability and that frequently are discovered only too late by the subscriber. Among these are:

1. *Insuring clause.* Be sure the coverage includes the types of benefits you desire.
2. *Exclusions or conditions not covered.* Most policies exclude certain types of costs including (1) cosmetic or plastic surgery; (2) elective surgery (operations performed at the patient's convenience); (3) occupational illnesses and accidents covered by public insurance programs, such as Workmen's Compensation; (4) conditions resulting from acts of war and riot; (5) preexisting illnesses; and (6) dental work.
3. *Waiting periods.* There is usually a time interval between the issuing of a contract and the date certain benefits are payable. Examples of such benefits might be maternity, elective surgery, or preexisting illness.
4. *Benefit reductions.* Benefits might be reduced if services are performed in a nonparticipating hospital or by a nonparticipating physician.
5. *Persons covered.* Usually policies include coverage for spouses and unmarried dependent children. These names must be specified in the policy.
6. *Age limits.* Some policies specify maximum and minimum age limits; most policies will cover a dependent child only up to a stated age.
7. *Cancellation and renewal provisions.* Many policies are cancellable by the insuring company; some policies state that the company can elect not to renew the policy at any premium-due date.
8. *Limited choice of a physician or hospital.* All limits should be explicitly understood, such as the restrictions on selection of a physician and the coverage of a nonparticipating physician's costs.

Your own physician's advice in the selection of a health insurance plan can be very useful. He or she can advise you of the record of the specific company in honoring its commitments.

It is wise periodically to review your health insurance policy. Changes in income, marital status, obligation to dependent children, and employment might substantially affect your policy and your needs for certain types of coverage. It is particularly important to be aware of employee plans that are carried by the employer. A change of job might terminate your coverage.

Regardless of how a family provides for its medical care, it is obvious that some form of payment planning is essential. Most people are directly dependent on a continual income, and financial protection against physical disability is a most important asset. Not only must a family protect its ability to earn money, it must also protect its savings and investments against large unanticipated medical and hospital costs. A well-planned, well-balanced health insurance program can do just this.

The People in Medicine

A major problem facing the public today is the shortage of physicians. Because of population increases, it is estimated that the current number of physicians in the United States is about 50,000 fewer than considered necessary to maintain a high level of general health care. The situation is, however, improving. In 1950, there was one physician for every 671 persons. By 1972 it had improved to one physician for every 575 persons. Such ratios are encouraging compared to those of some Third World countries that have one physician for every 25,000 to 30,000 persons.

In addition to the need for more physicians, the ones available are not always evenly distributed throughout the population. The physician–patient ratio is more favorable in urban areas and less favorable in rural areas. Some physicians prefer to practice in urban locations close to modern medical facilities where their incomes may be higher, and where there may be

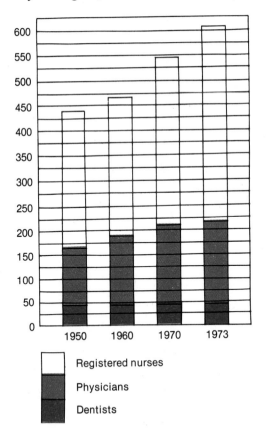

Health professionals per 100,000 people. Note: Nurses refer to employed nurses. Physicians refer to all physicians, active and inactive. Dentists refer to dentists in private practice.

Taken from 1974–1975 Source Book of Health Insurance Data, Health Insurance Institute (New York: 1974).

more cultural advantages both for themselves and their families. The upshot of such concentration, of course, is that scattered rural populations are often deprived of adequate medical personnel. A further problem is that not all physicians are available for general health care.

Although the number of physicians per 100,000 people has increased in recent years, more and more physicians have restricted their practice to specialized fields of study because of the flood of new medical information. Specialists outnumber general practitioners by almost six to one. This results in reduced numbers of general practitioners per 100,000 people, depriving many of adequate medical care. Consequently, a change is taking place from reliance on a family physician (who was usually a general practitioner) to reliance on group practice or clinic medicine, composed of a group of specialists. This has caused some confusion as to what kind of physician to consult. Compounding the problem is the increasing demand the American public is making on the physician's services. Today the average American sees a physician five times a year, twice as often as in 1930.

The Specialties The more physicians concentrate their attention on a given system of the body, the less time they have for the whole person and the less proficient they are in general practice. To thoroughly know one area of medicine, physicians must confine themselves to it to the exclusion of other areas. Such concentration has been necessary for medicine to make its great strides in heart surgery, cancer treatment and prevention, psychiatry, orthopedics, surgery, and other areas. A recognized specialist must have completed a full program of medical training and passed the written examination required of a particular specialty. Brief descriptions of several fields of specialization follow.

Family Practice The need for better-trained physicians who can give patients long-term comprehensive care led to the creation of this specialty in 1969. The training varies somewhat from one hospital to another. Some programs emphasize internal medicine, psychiatry, and surgery, whereas others stress obstetrics and pediatrics. The main concern in family practice is getting to know the family, rather than being most concerned with a particular disease or organ, as in internal medicine. Thus the main goal of family practice is to provide physicians who can take care of most of the patient—family illnesses and injuries.

Internal Medicine The internist specializes in diagnosis and is particularly suited for both preventive medicine and coordinating the work of specialists needed to treat the specific problems the patient faces. Generally, internists do not deliver babies, practice surgery, deal with eye diseases or refractory corrections, or treat children.

Obstetrics and Gynecology Obstetrics is the care of the woman in pregnancy and child birth. It is frequently combined with gynecology, the care of women's diseases. Stressing preventive medicine, the obstetrician sees the mother early in pregnancy, supervises her health, and handles the delivery. Such attention has reduced infant mortality in this country and assures the best possible health for both the child and the mother.

Pediatrics Pediatricians specialize in the care of infants and children. They advise parents, give checkups, diagnose congenital deformities, administer immunizations, and treat childhood diseases. Some pediatricians confine themselves to certain types of children's diseases, such as cardiovascular disorders or pediatric allergies.

Surgery The work of the surgeon involves surgically operating on a patient to correct some physical condition. It may involve removing a cancer, repairing a defective heart, setting a broken bone, or attempting to correct a damaged brain. Since the body is so intricate, this specialty is subdivided into specific areas, such as neurosurgery, thoracic surgery, orthopedic surgery, and abdominal surgery.

Psychiatry The psychiatrist deals with emotional illnesses and disturbances and mental retardation through the use of verbal contact as well as by the use of drugs, surgery, convulsive therapy, and hydrotherapy. The psychiatrist is a medical specialist who holds an M.D. degree. Some are also specialists in neurology. By distinction, a *psychologist* generally holds a graduate Ph.D. or M.A. degree (nonmedical degrees) and may engage in experimental, teaching, or clinical work. The *clinical psychologist* has had further training in a medical setting and diagnoses and treats emotional and neurological disorders by the use of verbal/nonverbal methods rather than by medical measures. (By contrast, a *counselor* could be anyone giving advice to people with normal problems.)

Some other fields of medical specialty are:

1. *Anesthesiology*, the science of administering general and local anesthetics.
2. *Dermatology*, the science of treating diseases of the skin.
3. *Neurology*, the science dealing with physical diseases of the brain and nervous system.
4. *Ophthalmology*, the medical branch treating the eye and its diseases.
5. *Otorhinolaryngology*, the medical branch treating diseases of the ear, nose, and throat.

6. *Pathology*, the study of the disease process, including the examination of functional changes in tissues and organs of the body, and identification of the disease causing the change, such as cancer. The pathologist may serve as a coroner and perform autopsies.
7. *Proctology*, the medical branch treating diseases of the rectum and anus.
8. *Radiology*, the science of using x–rays, radium, and other radioactive materials for the diagnosis and treatment of disease.
9. *Urology*, the science of treating diseases and abnormalities of the urinary tract in the female and the urogenital tract in the male.
10. *Emergency Medicine*, the newest specialty; the administering of emergency medical procedures of all kinds; practice usually confined to the emergency room of a hospital.

Overall, there are over thirty recognized fields of medical specialization today. Each is governed by its respective board for purposes of examination and certification.

The General Practitioner (GP)

In the past, many Americans looked almost solely to a single physician to diagnose and treat all the family's illnesses. The physician practiced general medicine and attempted to handle the full range of health conditions. In 1931, 74 percent of the physicians in the country were GP's. But today, specialists outnumber general practitioners by almost five to one.

Physicians are entitled to practice general medicine after they have completed medical school training, have served one year of internship in general hospital practice, and have passed the state or national board examinations required for licensure in that particular state. Although not required, most recent graduates take additional, or postgraduate, training of some kind. Today, many practicing GP's have completed at least two years of residency training.

Some unique problems face general practitioners today. The principal one has been that in order to maintain a high-quality practice, they must keep abreast of the mass of new medical information and changes in medical techniques.

Requirements for the M.D.

Before a person is licensed to practice medicine, he or she must meet certain professional and ethical requirements. Although training standards vary somewhat from state to state, he or she must take 3 to 4 years of premedical college work, and then complete a 4-year training program in a medical school approved by the Association of the American Medical Colleges and the Council on Medical Education of the American Medical Association. In addition, most states require that he or she serve a 1-year internship to gain hospital experience. Before being allowed to practice in a given state, a physician must be licensed by a board of medical examiners. This license is granted only after either a state or a national board examination has been passed. In addition to these basic requirements, if a physician desires to take a residency in a hospital to receive advanced training, or to meet the requirements of a given specialty in medicine, he or she must spend additional years (2 to 5) in training.

Some standards for the training of physicians as well as the ethics of medical practice are set by the medical profession itself. The medical profession also assumes the responsibility for regulating the professional conduct and ethics of its members. Much of this regulation is handled through local and county medical societies. Most of these societies have adopted standards for their members, such as prohibiting advertising, refraining from guaranteeing cures, adhering to all legalities regarding the taking of human life and the administration of drugs, cooperating with legal authorities, and giving evidence, through all public and private contacts, of their trustworthiness. Not all physicians meet such standards. In this respect, physicians as a whole are no different from other professional groups. In choosing our physicians, we should have the privilege and the right of being satisfied both with their reputation, private and public, and professional qualifications. To them we entrust our lives.

Osteopathy Osteopathy is considered another field of medicine, and those trained in it are referred to as physicians. This practice of medicine was started around 1870 by a physician named Dr. Andrew Still. He held that disease could be based on disturbed nerve functions that resulted from a pinching of the nerves as they leave the spinal column. According to this theory, a disease or condition in any particular organ of the body could be traced to a lesion in the nerve supplying that organ.

The medical profession considers this theory unfounded and contradictory to its knowledge of human anatomy and pathology. Over the course of years, however, osteopathic physicians have been quietly abandoning many of the peculiar tenets originally held in osteopathy and have increasingly emphasized the place of drugs in the practice of sound medicine. This change has progressed to the point where, today, their training and practice is similar to that of traditional medicine but with more emphasis on musculoskeletal manipulation. Nonetheless, osteopaths are usually barred from practicing in medical hospitals.

Depending on the state in which a person resides, he or she will have greater or lesser interest in osteopathy. Moves have been initiated in various state medical societies to unite the medical and osteopathic professions, but only one has been accomplished so far. California, in 1962, recognizing that the quality of osteopathic training was closely similar to that of medicine, passed legislation enabling osteopaths in the state to be considered M.D.'s. All former osteopathic colleges in California now bestow the M.D. degree upon their graduates. Significantly, this move came about as the result of a joint effort between osteopathic and medical societies within that state.

Some families prefer the services of an osteopathic physician. A qualified osteopath can satisfactorily serve as a family physician.

Selecting the Right Physician In selecting medical care, a person must determine his or her personal family needs and then must find out what is available.

Those individuals belonging to independent health groups may take one of a number of physicians rather than making a choice of physicians.

Some people prefer a general practitioner, while others select several specialists in selected branches of medicine. Since some general practitioners restrict themselves to a narrow branch of practice, it is necessary to know the nature of a physician's practice. If the family includes young children the physician chosen should enjoy working with children. The same point should be applied to elderly people. A person who cannot find one ideal physician for the entire family may prefer settling for several specialists, such as a pediatrician for the children and an internist for the adults.

In selecting a private physician, either for general practice or to deal with a specific problem, there are certain procedures worth following that may help guarantee you will find a physician well suited to your needs and temperament.

1. Consider the reputation of various physicians in your community. Contact a local *accredited* hospital for the names and addresses of the physicians who practice through that hospital. There is usually a relationship between the quality of a hospital and the quality of the physicians who practice there.

   If considering physicians who have been recommended by friends and relatives, you should be prepared to do some independent investigating. Other people's attitudes toward their doctors and their illnesses might not be useful to you. It is wise, however, to stay away from doctors who consistently cause dissatisfaction among people whose judgment you respect.

2. Visit the office of the physician you are considering. The office should be within easy commuting distance. Find out if the physician is accepting new patients; see if the office is neat, clean, and orderly. Discuss with the physician such general questions as whether he or she can furnish you or your family general medical care; whether he or she makes house calls; if he or she is usually available for emergencies; what other physician provides these services in the event the physician is out of town; the fee schedule and how it compares to that of other physicians in town.

   The physician should be a person you can confide in and who appears interested in your family's health and well-being. If you are satisfied regarding these points, you have found your physician.

The Patient-Physician Relationship

Patients are entitled to receive careful, professional service from their physician including laboratory test results and consultations with any medical specialists necessary for adequate medical treatment. It may not always be possible for the physician to cure, but the patient should feel confident that the physician is using the best skills.

A physician should be as concerned with preventing disease as curing it. Patients should be well informed as to when inoculations and periodic examinations are due. In the practice of preventive medicine, it may be difficult for patients to understand the full benefit of medical care and justify the cost of it. Prevention of illness is not only easier, but less painful, cheaper, and less time consuming. A careful physician would much rather keep patients from getting ill than attempt to bring them back to health once they are ailing.

Patients should understand the physician's fee schedule. If the cost of medical care is imposing a genuine hardship on a patient or the family, the physician will want to know about it. The physician may be willing to adjust his fees in the case of hardship. The patient should feel no embarrassment about raising such a discussion.

In return, the physician may expect certain courtesies and cooperation from patients. In nonemergencies, patients should make appointments and then keep them punctually. They should be prepared to pay medical bills promptly or make arrangement to pay them as soon as possible. Patients should follow the physician's instructions exactly. If medication is prescribed it should be obtained immediately and taken as directed. The physician has a right to expect the confidence of patients.

Physicians are not necessarily under obligation to answer emergency calls from unknown individuals late at night. The physicians will have no medical history of the patient, may be subjecting themselves to physical hazard, or may be greatly fatigued. Some individuals moving into a new community may fail to contact a new physician until they need one in emergencies or late at night. Then, if difficulty in obtaining care is encountered, they make complaints against the medical profession. In such emergencies, the nearest general hospital should have physicians on duty who can provide care.

A physician can give the best service when confident that patients appreciate the service. As much as he or she would enjoy being able to cure every physical ailment, medical research has not provided all the necessary answers to accomplish that aim. But a good physician will go just as far in diagnosis and treatment as ability, training, available facilities, and patients allow.

Chiropractic It is necessary to make some mention and clarification of *chiropractic*. It is a system of treatment based on the belief that the nervous system largely determines a person's state of health and that any interference with this system impairs normal functions and lowers the body's resistance to disease. Patients are treated primarily by specific adjustment of parts of the body, especially the spinal column. X—rays are used extensively to aid in locating the source of the difficulty. Supplementary treatment measures such as diet, exercise, rest, water, light, and heat are used. Chiropractic treatment by law may not include the use of drugs or surgery. The training of chiropractors, although ranging from 2 to 4 years, consists in most states of 4 years of training in a chiropractic school following graduation from high school. Graduation does not qualify a chiropractor to practice in all states, since not all states license the practice of chiropractic.

Since many of the body's ailments are caused by infections or degenerative diseases, any field of the healing arts that does not qualify a practitioner in the diagnosis

and treatment of these kinds of maladies restricts their usefulness. Most chiropractors are better trained in body manipulation and adjustment than they are in adequate understanding and diagnosis of the underlying disease. As interpreters of x—rays, their qualifications are not to be confused with those of the radiologist, a medical specialist. The academic and professional training beyond high school for the chiropractor may be only 6 years, whereas it is 12 years for a radiologist (who also holds the M.D. degree). Accordingly, a chiropractor should not be chosen as a family physician. It is the official position of the American Medical Association that "chiropractic is an unscientific cult whose practitioners lack the necessary training and background to diagnose and treat human disease."

Dentistry Dental training consists of 4 years of professional training following 2 to 4 years of required college work. A dental specialty usually requires two or 3 years of additional professional training. The majority of dentists are general practitioners who provide many types of dental care. If an individual is in need of a dental specialist a general dentist will be more than glad to recommend one who will provide the required treatment.

Although there has been an actual increase in the number of dentists in the United States, the number has not kept pace with the increasing population. Since 1950 there has been a 27 percent increase in dentists, but a 4 percent *decrease* compared to the population as a whole.

Nursing The nursing team is led by the professional or *registered nurse* (R.N.) but also includes the vocational nurses, nursing aides, medical technologists, orderlies, and attendants. Registered nursing training requires 2 to 4 years of professional training beyond high school. Additional training can be taken to qualify a nurse in a nursing specialty (such as obstetrics, pediatrics, psychiatry, or surgical nursing).

Since 1950 the number of nurses has increased 117 percent. About 29 percent of all professional nurses work on a part-time basis. The number of male nurses is slowly increasing, and today accounts for over 1 percent of all professional nurses.

Ancillary Professional People Various other professional people serve in an auxiliary, or *ancillary*, manner on the health team. *Midwives* are professional people who help care for women during pregnancy, labor, delivery, and the post-partum period. The *nurse-midwife* is a registered nurse who has completed advanced training in midwifery. Successful completion of the American College of Nurse-Midwives certification examination entitles the nurse-midwife to use the title certified nurse-midwife (C.N.M.). Nurse-midwives function as a part of the obstetrical team of medical centers. In contrast, the *lay* or *granny midwife* provides assistance to women during childbirth in the absence of a medical practitioner. Trained largely through apprenticeship, the lay midwife generally serves in low-income or rural areas, where the delivery of the baby usually occurs in the home.

The *physician's assistant* is qualified by academic and practical training to provide patient services under the supervision and direction of a licensed physician who is responsible for the performance of that assistant. Following a period of training, the physician's assistant works in physician's offices, hospitals or clinics. Graduates are also known as *physician's associates, clinical associates, MEDEX's, child health associates*, and *community health medics*.

Facilities for Patient Care

As medical techniques have improved, so have facilities for patient care. Today's physician makes few home visits, particularly in urban areas. The home no longer needs to serve as a hospital for delivery of babies or for treatment of tuberculosis and pneumonia, or as a nursing home for elderly people suffering from chronic diseases. Today, only minor illnesses are cared for at home. Improved standards of diagnosis and treatment require facilities that are only available in physicians' offices, clinics, nursing homes, and hospitals.

Nursing Homes Providing health services for patients who are convalescing, who have chronic illnesses, or who are elderly is the niche occupied by nursing homes. Care here is less intensive as well as less expensive than that of a hospital. Developed as a result of the 1935 Social Security Act, private nursing homes have become both numerous and profitable. Later the act was extended to provide for care in public nursing homes.

Although many of the more than 13,000 nursing homes in the country provide excellent care, it is important that one be aware of wide differences in care when making a selection. Many are really quite poor. In some parts of the country, nursing homes have been guilty of drugging patients to keep them docile. Elsewhere they have been largely understaffed so that critical medical problems have gone unrecognized. Since many of these homes survive through Medicaid payments, they are proprietary enterprises, more dedicated to making a profit than providing adequate health care.

One assurance of quality is accreditation of the home by the Joint Commission on the Accreditation of Hospitals. Granted on a one- or two-year basis, such accreditation assures that certain standards such as fire and safety laws are being met and assures cleanliness of patient care, accurate and up-to-date records, a staff dietician, menu planning and food storage, and a planned activities program. Beyond such assurances, an individual should check fee schedules, proximity, and available openings.

Hospitals Population increases, along with greater physician use of hospitals, have substantially increased the demand for available hospital facilities. Hospitals are usually constructed with funds from community sources, private philanthropists, local or state taxes and federal funds. Because of the increased demand for hospital services and the greatly increased costs of new hospital construction, many hospitals are being built with the aid of public funds. Providing up-to-date hospital equipment and paying new increases in salaries have greatly raised the operating costs of existing hospitals. For these reasons, some parts of the country either lack or have substandard hospital facilities. Before an older hospital is enlarged or a new one built, it is important that the community consider its needs and the ability of the area to support modern hospital facilities, both financially and professionally.

Today there are more than 7,000 hospitals of all kinds in the United States. The three basic types are the government, voluntary, and proprietary hospitals.

The federal government has established hospitals for military personnel and their dependents, American Indians, merchant seamen, veterans, lepers, and drug addicts. Individual states have built specialized hospitals for emotionally and neurologically ill patients and for those with tuberculosis, as well as general hospitals, which are usually associated with a state-supported medical school. Most local city or county hospitals offer general medical care. Funds for these hospitals are provided by state and local taxes and/or federal taxes.

Voluntary hospitals are private hospitals set up on a nonprofit basis. They provide inpatient beds for more than two-thirds of all hospital admissions in this country. Established by local communities, charitable organizations, churches, or philanthropic individuals, they are run by governing boards, usually selected from the community. They receive their funding from patients, insurance carriers such as Blue Cross, or government programs such as Medicare or Medicaid.

Proprietary hospitals are owned and administered by individuals or corporations, and are set up to make a profit. Some are even established by real-estate promoters and then leased to physicians at no construction cost to the community. Proprietary hospitals may have a questionable reputation. They tend to prefer the most profitable types of hospital cases, while taking few, if any, charity cases. The majority of these hospitals are small and only about one-third of them are accredited.

The Accreditation of Hospitals In 1952 a Joint Commission on Accreditation of Hospitals (JCAH) came into being to judge the operations of hospitals. It is sponsored by the American Hospital Association, the American Medical Association, the American College of Surgeons, and the American College of Physicians. It has set up national standards for hospital care, it accredits hospitals meeting these standards, and it periodically reviews accredited hospitals. To qualify, the hospital must have a tissue review committee that reviews the pathology of tissue removals and transfusions, and physician committees that review the surgical procedures and medical care of other physicians and that take disciplinary action if required. Upon application, a hospital is thoroughly examined for cleanliness, laboratory operations, food handling, and records, as well as the practice of its staff physicians. The hospital may be accredited for one or two years depending on how well it qualifies.

It is increasingly important for a hospital to have JCAH accreditation. A nonaccredited hospital may not train interns, residents, or nurses. There may be no doctor's review committee overseeing the treatment that takes place as a check against unnecessary or inappropriate surgery or other treatments. In some nonaccredited hospitals much needless surgery takes place merely to increase the income of the surgeons. Some medical insurance companies have refused to make payments to nonaccredited hospitals. Today, hospitals representing over 89 percent of the country's total hospital bed space are accredited. Most of these hospitals are voluntary ones.

When choosing between these forms of patient care, it is important to examine the patient's need carefully. Some conditions require hospital care, and in most cases the patient is admitted to a hospital upon application by the physician. In fact, some hospitals will not admit a nonaccident patient unless recommended by a physician.

Those conditions, especially those of the elderly, that require medical attention but not necessarily hospitalization can frequently be accommodated in a nursing home. Some elderly people have a strong aversion to entering hospitals. Cost is a consideration, and because the level of treatment is usually less intense in a nursing home, and less expensive, most medical insurance plans provide payment for more days in a nursing home than in a hospital.

FURTHER READINGS

AMA Committee on Exercise and Physical Fitness and the Medical Aspects of Sports, ed. *Sports and Physical Fitness*. Chicago, Ill.: American Medical Association, 1970. The best authorities on physical fitness put together their definitions and recommendations on what is physical fitness.

Better Homes & Gardens magazine. *The Better Homes & Gardens Calorie Counter's Cookbook*. New York: Bantam Books, 1972. An excellent book for the person who wishes to change eating habits and reduce or maintain weight.

Bogert, J.L.; Briggs, George M.; and Calloway, Doris Howes. *Nutrition and Physical Fitness*. Philadelphia, Pa,; W.B. Saunders, 1973. An excellent textbook on nutrition.

Carper, Jean. *All-in-One Calorie Counter*. New York: Bantam Books, 1974. An up-to-date, very complete calorie counter.

———. *The Brand Name Nutrition Counter*. New York: Bantam Books, 1975. An excellent book listing the calories in brand name products. A short introduction presents excellent information of foods, additives, and processing.

Cooper, Kenneth H. *The New Aerobics*. New York: Bantam Books, 1970. A classic study in physical fitness. A must for individuals wanting to improve their physical condition.

Cooper, Mildred, and Cooper, Kenneth H. *Aerobics for Women*. New York: Bantam Books, 1972. Applying the principle of aerobics to women's physical fitness.

Cureton, T.K. *Physical Fitness Workbook for Adults*. Champaign, Ill.: Stipes Publishing, 1970. A workbook for fitness programs from an established expert in exercise.

Gawer, Herman, and Michelman, Herbert. *Body Control and Physical Fitness*, 1972. Illustrates a number of exercise programs for both males and females.

Harris, W.E.; Bowerman, William J.; and Shea, James. *Jogging: A Complete Physical Fitness Program for All Ages*. New York: Grossett & Dunlap, 1967. The best reference available on jogging and its use in physical fitness programs.

Healey, Colin. *Methods of Fitness: A Complete Guide to All Methods of Attaining Physical Fitness*. New York: A.S. Barnes, 1973. A very complete book on physical fitness.

Jones, Kenneth; Shainberg, Louis; and Byer, Curtis. *Foods, Diet and Nutrition*, 2nd. ed. San Francisco: Canfield Press, 1975. A guide to nutrition for young people who would like to improve their diets and need a reasonable education to attain a better nutritional level.

——— . *Total Fitness*. San Francisco: Canfield Press, 1972. A reference explaining the balanced activities needed for overall fitness.

Lowenberg, Miriam E., et al. *Food and Man*. New York: John Wiley & Sons, 1974. Textbook on food and nutrition.

Magnuson, Warren G. *The Dark Side of the Market Place*. Englewood Cliffs, N.J.: Prentice–Hall, 1968. An exposé of modern-day quackery.

Pyke, Magnus. *Synthetic Food*. New York: St. Martin's Press, 1971. A book describing the "nonfood" being sold.

Royal Canadian Air Force Exercise Plans for Physical Fitness. New York: Pocket Books, 1972. All exercise programs in one book.

U.S. Department of Agriculture. *Food For All, Yearbook of Agriculture 1969*. Washington D.C.: U.S. Government Printing Office, 1969. A very complete book on all aspects of food.

——— . *Shopper's Guide, Yearbook of Agriculture 1974*. Washington, D.C.: U.S. Government Printing Office, 1974. A must for all shoppers who wish to understand the federal labeling laws and how to buy food.

Winter, Ruth. *A Consumer's Dictionary of Food Additives*. New York: Crown Publications, 1972. An important guide for everyone on the additives in food.

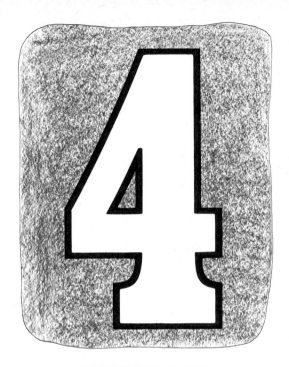

HUMAN
SEXUALITY
AND
REPRODUCTION

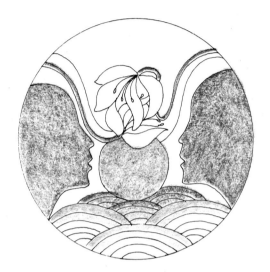

13

HUMAN SEXUAL BEHAVIOR

Only in recent years has human sexuality begun to emerge as a "respectable" field for physiological and behavioral research. Prior to this time, little objective research was accomplished, because of a variety of obstacles. For example, some people felt that sex was "dirty" or "sacred" or that its "mystery" was best preserved as such. Some scientists whose background and training could have led them into sex research were often inhibited in their own sexual insecurity or prudishness.

The sexual attitudes held by individuals cover a wide and contradictory range; what seems right and appropriate to one may seem wrong or inappropriate to another. The issues of male and female sex roles, sexual freedom, sexual ethics, nonmarital sexual adjustment, marriage and its alternatives, and the presentation of sex in the arts and media are exceptionally complex.

Objective sex research is of value to society for several reasons. It places sexuality in its proper perspective as a normal healthy part of human physiology and behavior. It removes the cloak of secrecy from sexuality, helping to reassure people that their own sexual feelings, responses, practices, and problems are typical of millions of other people, or if not, how they differ. It helps to dispel anxiety-producing misconceptions and inhibitions. And it provides a sound basis for overcoming sexual problems.

Much of the information in this and the following two chapters has been established relatively recently. The Kinsey group did most of their research in the late 1940s and 1950s; Masters and Johnson in the 1960s and 1970s; and current research by many others. We have tried to avoid imposing our own behavioral standards on this information. Rather, we have attempted to provide the reader with the factual basis on which he or she may make sound personal decisions about nonmarital, marital, and extramarital sexual relations, contraception, abortion, and so forth.

Let us begin by making some distinctions between various types of sexual relations. *Nonmarital* indicates sexual relations of a person who is not married. *Premarital* refers to relationships preparatory to or affecting eventual later marriage. *Marital* are those relations between spouses during marriage. *Extramarital* are those sexual relations carried on by either spouse with someone outside of the marriage during the time the couple is married.

Nonmarital Sexual Adjustment

The sexual behavior of the unmarried person has been a source of interest throughout history. A traditional approach to sexual development and adjustment was to pretend that sexual tensions, if ignored, would somehow just go away. This attitude, of course, was unrealistic because the biological sexual drive of the unmarried person is no different from that of the married person of the same age. But the traditional attitude has been to condemn any form of sexual satisfaction outside of marriage.

This restriction of sex to marriage has forced millions of people to marry who really should have remained single. Additional millions have been forced to marry years before they were really ready, but at an age when their sexual drive was at a level they could not ignore.

Today, American society is hardly in agreement in what it considers right or wrong on matters of sexual conduct. During the past 50 or 60 years, there has been a definite liberalization in attitudes toward sex. But individual codes of behavior still range from total sexual freedom to strict prohibition of nonmarital sexual contact. Today, as always, unmarried individuals and couples must still decide on their own course of sexual conduct.

Petting There are various degrees of sexual relationship. One is *petting*, which might be defined as all relations more intimate than kissing but short of actual sexual intercourse. Petting typically includes fondling the breasts and sexual organs. It may or may not lead to orgasm in either the male or female. The stimulation may be manual (with the hands), or oral (by means of the mouth).

Any value judgment regarding petting should be based on such considerations as the age and emotional maturity of each individual and the individual's attitudes and backgrounds. Petting is a normal step in the development of sexual and emotional maturity and enables one to learn his or her own sexual responses and those of the opposite sex.

Petting generally stimulates sexual desire more than it relieves sexual tensions. Petting is sexually arousing; the natural tendency in petting is to gradually become more and more intimate until it culminates in actual sexual intercourse. Consequently, the sexually aroused couple finds it very difficult to stop short of intercourse. It is such unplanned intercourse that most often results in nonmarital pregnancy, since adequate birth control has not been considered or may not be readily available. Many couples develop techniques of petting to mutual orgasm as an alternative to intercourse. If this is done, it is important that no semen be allowed near the vaginal opening, since pregnancy can occur even without actual entry by the penis.

Masturbation Bringing on sexual orgasm by manipulating one's own or someone else's genitals is called *masturbation*. Despite the elaborate mythology about the supposedly harmful effects of masturbation, it is now recognized as perfectly harmless and a part of normal sexuality in both the male and the female. Over 90 percent of all males masturbate at some time in their lives, as do over 60 percent of all females. There may be various reasons for this. The female genitals, being less externally apparent than the male genitals, may receive less self-stimulation. Males are often more intensely sexual in their teens than females and find the need for the release of sexual tensions more compelling. Females may be subject to more parental counsel and may come to view masturbation as either unnecessary or undesirable.

Most individuals resort to masturbation only as a substitute for sexual intercourse when the latter is unavailable. As a result, masturbation is more common among unmarried individuals, although married and otherwise sexually active men and women may masturbate when their partners are pregnant, menstruating, or unavailable for intercourse. When sexual partners have died, as with widows and widowers, or when partners are unable to respond sexually, as may happen with advancing age, masturbation may provide a necessary release of sexual tension without the need to seek out new sexual partners.

The old wives' tale that masturbation leads to insanity probably originated from the fact that emotionally disturbed individuals sometimes masturbate compulsively. The fear that masturbation would lead to impotence was based on the erroneous notion that the lifetime supply of semen was limited and could be exhausted through masturbation.

Masturbation may begin at any age. The frequency of masturbation among normal unmarried males varies considerably, from about once a month to several times daily. Females typically masturbate less frequently than males.

Prostitution Prostitution is the exchange of sexual favors for a fee—usually promiscuously and without affection. While the most common form of prostitution is female and heterosexual, there also exists male heterosexual prostitution as well as male and female homosexual prostitution. The distinction between prostitution and amateur sex is sometimes vague, as when a person exchanges sexual favors for personal gain, such as job advancement, or accepts expensive gifts or living expenses from a wealthy friend.

Prostitution is illegal throughout most of the United States. It is often singled out as a prime example of victimless crime since it involves a mutually agreed-on exchange of fee for service rendered between two consenting persons. Both enter into the relationship voluntarily and, theoretically, both benefit. Those who favor the prohibition of prostitution usually cite as their grounds religious beliefs, fear of organized crime, suppression of sexually transmitted diseases, degradation of the sex act, and the possibility of robbery and blackmail under the guise of prostitution.

Nonmarital Sexual Intercourse

Nonmarital sexual intercourse is a subject of considerable interest today. It is apparent that in the last few years there has been some increase in its prevalence and a great increase in discussion about it. Nonmarital sexual relationships are now entered into more openly than in any time in the recent past. Despite improved contraceptive methods, the illegitimacy rate is at an all-time high, a possible indication of increased sexual activity.

As with petting, there is no universal answer to the question of whether or not to engage in intercourse outside of marriage. Many individual factors must be considered. For some, religious beliefs forbid premarital sex. For others below the age of consent, state laws proscribe such behavior. But, for the young adult of legal age and holding no strong religious beliefs, it becomes a highly individual question to be decided on the basis of personal values and philosophy, giving due consideration to all possible (positive and negative) results of such action. The following are some of the considerations that should be kept in mind for those making this decision.

Pregnancy The basic motivation behind most of the legal, religious, and social regulations pertaining to marriage and most sexual behavior is to provide a stable family environment for the child and to determine who is responsible for its support. Although attitudes towards sex have changed considerably, pregnancy out of marriage is regarded as a serious problem by many people.

Modern contraceptive methods can reduce the chance of pregnancy to a very low level if they are used properly and consistently. Anyone engaging in nonmarital sexual relations should choose a highly effective contraceptive method and be certain that it is used properly. Even when a normally foolproof method (such as the "pill") is chosen, there should be a definite plan and agreement on the action to be taken in case accidental pregnancy occurs. If a couple is not mature enough to discuss this problem realistically, then it is questionable whether they are mature enough to engage in sexual relations at all. Some of the paths available to the unmarried parents are:

Abortion According to the U.S. Supreme Court, every woman in the United States has the same right to an abortion during the first 6 months of pregnancy as she as to any other minor surgery. In other words, during this period of time *any* pregnant woman is entitled to abortion on demand. During the first 3 months, a state may require that it be performed by a qualified physician. During the second 3 months the state may further require that facilities in which it is performed be properly equipped, but the legal option to seek an induced abortion is a right of the woman.

The Supreme Court decision was rooted in the right to privacy, a part of everyone's liberty and protected under the "due-process" clause of the 14th Amendment.

The Court opinion was that a state may not use abortion statutes to regulate sexual conduct, directly or indirectly. In addition, they concluded that a fetus is *not* a person under the Constitution and thus has no legal right to life, a conclusion that antiabortionists strongly condemn.

An induced abortion is one that occurs as the result of medical intervention of the pregnancy. It may be *therapeutic* (for medical reasons), *on demand* (at the option of the woman and without medical reasons), or *illegal* (if in violation of existing laws). An abortion tht occurs naturally and without medical intervention is known as a *spontaneous abortion* or *miscarriage*.

Some precautions are in order if an abortion is being considered. An induced abortion may temporarily interfere with the body's hormonal system, and some women may need postabortion medical care. Repeated induced abortions may later lead to the inability to carry a child to full term.

A woman should be certain that an abortion is philosophically and ethically acceptable to her. Because of religious or personal philosophical viewpoints, some find abortion an unacceptable option. Abortion should be avoided if it is going to cause feelings of guilt or emotional recrimination. Regardless of her decision, a woman may still have questions. This is natural. She must make the best personal decision and then let the matter rest.

"Right to Life" Various "right-to-life" organizations have opposed the U.S. Supreme Court decision on abortion. Although not unified, groups in various parts of the country share common positions. In opposition to the legal right of a woman to acquire an abortion, members hold that from the moment a sperm cell fertilizes an egg, new life has been created. They believe that the developing embryo or fetus is a separate growing organism, and as such can never be considered an integral part of the mother's body. They hold that this developing embryo is not only human, but that it also has legal rights including the "right to life" at any stage of its development. On this premise, they oppose abortion *on demand,* reject it as a method of curtailing population increase, are convinced it poses both emotional and physical hazards to the woman, and feel that it constitutes a denial of basic moral and religious principles.

Single Parenthood The prospect of keeping and raising a child out of wedlock is not necessarily desirable or pleasant for most women, although in recent years, increasing numbers of unmarried women are taking this option. It is probably preferable, for both mother and child, to the option of marrying just "to give the child a name" and then divorcing after a few years of bitter marriage.

Marriage Though pregnancy is one of the most common reasons for getting married, it may be one of the poorest. A high percentage of forced marriages turn into disasters, leading to divorce or, perhaps even worse, to meaningless, bitter relationships. Unless both parties truly want to marry, it is far better to take one of the other options.

Adoption In many cases, adoption is the best course of action. Often it assures the child a loving home where it is welcome rather than resented. In many areas, there is currently a strong demand for newborn infants for adoption. This may not be so with all children from minority backgrounds. An unwed minority mother whose child may end up in a foster home or orphanage may feel compelled to keep her child. With the easier access to public financial aid for dependent children, more unwed mothers have chosen to retain custody of their children.

Sexually Transmitted Diseases The risk of sexually transmitted diseases depends on the pattern of previous sexual relationships. If the only relationship involves a mutually faithful couple, of course, there is no risk of infection (assuming neither is infected to start with). If a person has casual sexual contacts or has intercourse with anyone who does have such contacts, then the risk of sexually transmitted diseases is greatly increased, as syphilis and gonorrhea are presently at epidemic proportions in this country.

Psychological Motivation A multitude of subtle factors motivate the expression of sexuality, in addition to the more obvious need for release from sexual tensions. These nonsexual motives are not always undesirable, since they are generally present to some extent in any sexual relationship, within or outside of marriage. Among the more universal motives in sexuality are the needs to feel wanted as a sexual partner (sexually attractive) and to feel successful as a lover. The ego reinforcement obtained through successful sexual relationships is very important for the total emotional adjustment of most adults. The expression of love is another nonphysical aspect of sexuality.

One of the less desirable sexual motives is the use of sex for bargaining power, where sexual privileges are traded for various emotional and/or material rewards and withheld as punishment for failure of the partner to provide such rewards. Another misuse of sex is as a trap to force an expression of commitment from a partner who does not really feel any great degree of love.

It is important for each sexual partner to understand the motives of the other. If it is going to be "pure" sex—sex for physical satisfaction alone—then both partners should share this feeling, and no pretense of love or other commitment should be made. Deception amounts to exploitation and can only lead to someone feeling used and hurt.

Effect on Future Marriage One of the traditional concerns about nonmarital sex has been whether it might affect the success of any future marriage. This is really a very difficult question to answer, for several reasons. First, so many factors relate to marital happiness that it is really impossible to determine cause and effect. In addition, it is fruitless to make statistical comparisons of the divorce rate, orgasm rate, or any other "indicator" of marital happiness between groups who have and have not had nonmarital sexual experience.

The problem is that people who have nonmarital sex also differ statistically in many other ways from those who do not. For example, they tend to have more permissive attitudes on all phases of sexuality, are more likely to use alcohol, tobacco, and marijuana, are less likely to hold strong religious beliefs, and feel less bound by the traditional sanctity of marriage. If one wants to "prove" that premarital sex has either a positive or a negative effect on future marital success, it is easy to find statistical studies to support either point of view. In reality, few of these studies can be considered valid, since it is impossible to separate nonmarital sex habits from all the other associated habits or attitudes. About the only safe conclusion is that premarital sexual experience seems neither essential nor detrimental to marital happiness.

Social Considerations As noted earlier, different societies and different elements within a particular society hold varying attitudes toward nonmarital sexual intercourse, ranging from total permissiveness to total prohibition. In the United States, we find an ambiguous situation, with many people disapproving the sexual activities of others but excusing their own. The "official" attitude here is prohibitive of sexual activity before marriage. The "unofficial" attitude is still the highly discredited double standard, which is much more tolerant of the sexual activities of men than of women. This is an unfortunate carry-over from the era when women were not expected to enjoy sexual intercourse and were expected to be subservient to men.

The "sexual revolution," or however we choose to designate the recent rapid changes in social attitudes towards sex, has included a dramatic shift away from the double standard. As women expand their roles beyond those of wife, mother, and homemaker, the restrictive implications of the double standard are falling way to a more realistic view of the female sex drive and sexual behavior.

Legal Considerations In a few states, any sexual intercourse between unmarried persons is illegal, but such laws are seldom, if ever, enforced. Of more importance are laws that prohibit intercourse with a woman below the age of consent, which varies among the states from 14 to 21, but is most often 18 years of age. A male having intercourse with a young woman below this age can be prosecuted for statutory rape, a felony offense. Even if she appears to be older and lies about her age, the male can still be convicted.

Still another problem can arise when an unmarried woman becomes pregnant and sues for child support. Any male who has had intercourse with her during a given period of time may be named in the suit.

Sexual Orientation

In Alfred Kinsey's studies of the human male and female (Kinsey, Pomeroy, and Martin, *Sexual Behavior in the Human Male,* 1948; Kinsey, Pomeroy, Martin, Gebhard, *Sexual Behavior in The Human Female,* 1953) it became apparent that the extent to which people participated in homosexual activities varied greatly. This led Kinsey to employ the concept of a heterosexual–homosexual behavior rating scale. It was apparent that males and females do not each represent two separate populations, heterosexual and homosexual, but that there is a kind of line (continuum or scale) running from the entirely heterosexual person at one extreme to the entirely homosexual at the other. Moving toward the center from the entirely heterosexual extreme would next be those who, although primarily heterosexual, had had some homosexual experience. At the very center of the scale would be those who have as much heterosexual as homosexual experience, or the *bisexual* person. These people claim that they are not basically oriented one way or the other and do not simply alternate sexual objects occasionally. Rather, they claim a permanent need for relations with both sexes, "to enjoy the best of two worlds," as it were.

Homosexual Orientation

Homosexuality is the sexual attraction to members of one's own sex. Significant numbers of both males and females experience it to at least some degree during their lifetime.

While different authorities give somewhat varying figures on the incidence of homosexuality, a fair estimate based on a consensus of opinions seems to be that about 2 percent of American men and a similar percentage of American women are exclusively homosexual during adult life. A considerably larger group of both males and females (variously estimated at 25 to over 50 percent) passes through a transient period of homosexual feeling and/or activity during the preadolescent or adolescent years before settling into exclusive heterosexuality.

Many homosexuals give no obvious indication of their sexual orientation. Since the opinion of the general public is still negative about homosexuality and the risk of social and professional difficulties when a homosexual orientation becomes known is still great, there are valid reasons to be guarded in its display. However, both male and female homosexuals run the gamut from masculine to feminine in appearance and the vast majority are not identifiable as such. Generally, homosexuals meet each other at bars, parties, and through friends where they can be fairly certain of each other's sexual orientation. This is similar to the way heterosexuals meet, except that homosexuals often cannot meet each other in work situations or in other places where it might be hazardous to be open about their sexual orientation.

Homosexual Behavior Patterns The typical pattern of homosexual relationships differs considerably between male and female homosexuals. The female tendency is to establish long-term homosexual relationships lasting for months, years, or even a lifetime. This is in accord with the socialization of women in our society towards love and long-term relationships. One recent psychological research study (Mark Freedman, *Homosexuality and Psychological Functioning*, 1971) that compared homosexual and heterosexual

women found that both groups put more emphasis on the romantic and "love" aspects of their relationships than did men of either orientation.

The typical pattern of male homosexuality is quite different. Among males, the emphasis is generally on variety in sexual partners, as is also generally true of heterosexual men in our society. Because men in our society are trained to be assertive and powerful, it is much more difficult generally for two men to live together than it is for a dominant man and a submissive woman in a traditional heterosexual relationship. However, many male homosexuals form close, long-term relationships with another man. When two men or two women live together in a love relationship, they often see the inadequacy and futility of traditional sex roles where one partner is dominant and the other submissive. In many of these relationships, there may be as much or more give-and-take and sharing as in many modern heterosexual marriages.

Among the practices used by male homosexuals to achieve orgasm are mutual hand manipulation of the penis, oral-genital contacts, and anal-genital contacts. Techniques used in female homosexual contacts include kissing, manual and oral stimulation of the breasts, and manual or oral stimulation of the genitals.

Some homosexuals enter into heterosexual marriages, for a variety of reasons. Sometimes the individual is truly bisexual and enjoys relationships with both sexes. More often, the marriage is the homosexual's attempt to live a "straight" life, thinking that marriage may counteract homosexuality (it seldom does). Or marriage can be a "front" for homosexual activity, a disguise to appear socially acceptable while privately engaging in homosexual activities. The mates chosen for these marriages are often individuals with low sex drives who make few heterosexual demands on the homosexual.

Viewpoints on Homosexuality Many homosexuals view their orientation merely as an alternative life-style, presenting no more difficulties than the typical heterosexual person encounters. Homosexuality meets with varying responses from academics and professionals. Psychiatrists and other physicians, for example, disagree greatly on how to regard homosexuality. Is it an illness, a maladjustment, a neurosis, or an alternative life-style? Should treatment be suggested for homosexuality in itself? Or should treatment be considered only if a patient's homosexuality is creating problems? In the latter case, should the goal of treatment be to reorient the patient sexually or merely to help the patient adjust to homosexuality and its associated problems? There are no clear answers to these questions, and controversy continues to rage in many medical and psychiatric journals. In a significant recent move that indicates present trends, the prestigious American Psychiatric Association dropped homosexuality from its list of mental disturbances.

An extremely important factor in the current professional view of homosexuality is the fact that almost all research conducted in the past 20 years has occurred in the clinical setting. That is, the people being studied as representative of the homosexual orientation were those who, for reasons of problems of adjustment, sought psychiatric care. Obviously, this kind of sampling could not give a balanced and adequate view of the entire homosexual population. In the past three years, numerous studies, including a major one funded by the Kinsey Institute for Sex Research, have been published that have concentrated on the homosexual orientation of people living in various American communities.

On the other hand, as many as 80 percent of people in the general population consider homosexuality wrong. Typically, better-educated city-dwellers of the East and West Coasts are more likely to accept it than are less educated rural people.

The law's response to homosexuality is now being critically examined. The simplistic assumption that homosexuality is strictly a legal question, calling for arrest and imprisonment, is clearly being put aside. The professional composition of the National Institute of Mental Health's Task Force on Homosexuality, which published its final report in 1972, indicates the recognized complexity of the problem: the commission included social historians, sociologists, psychologists, judges, and lawyers.

Across the United States, larger communities are currently considering legislation to outlaw discrimination against homosexuals in housing and employment, as well as other denials of civil rights based on sexual preference. Within the next several years, it is likely that tensions between the heterosexual and homosexual communities will continue to ease. This trend has been heralded by the Institute for Sex Research. Preliminary results of the Intitute's massive study of homosexuality indicate that homosexuals are more and more interested in coming "out of the closet" and into the open to assume the equal place in society so long denied them.

Transsexuality *Transsexuality* is a psychological condition in which the person feels a difference between gender and physiological sex. The transsexual feels he or she belongs to the sex opposite the one that is anatomically apparent. A transsexual thinks, feels, and acts like a person of the opposite sex. He or she may feel trapped in a body and social role of the wrong sex.

Transsexuality is often confused with transvestism (wearing clothing of the opposite sex) and with homosexuality. Although many transvestites and many transsexuals dress like the opposite sex, transvestites are not transsexuals. Similarly, passive homosexuality in the male transsexual is common. However, most male homosexuals have a normal gender role. They feel themselves to be true males, not females caught in a male body. The male homosexual enjoys his penis as well as the interest other homosexuals have in it; he derives genital pleasure from his sexual contacts. The transsexual male, on the contrary, hates his penis and derives no pleasure from it at all. Usually he does not experience erection or ejaculation.

The transsexual is usually a biologically normal male or female. With rare exceptions, there are no anatomical, chromosomal, or hormonal abnormalities. Transsexual attitudes can sometimes be traced back to a childhood background of parents whose own sexual roles were unclear or who were disappointed that the child was not of the opposite sex. Some also indicate there may be prenatal factors that influence the development of the transsexual.

Psychotherapy has not been highly successful in the treatment of adult transsexuals, though it is obviously preferable to more radical treatment. Many transsexuals have achieved happiness only after surgical and hormonal sex change procedures. While this is undeniably an extreme measure, the alternatives for many transsexuals are continued suffering or even suicide. Several ethical sex change clinics have been established within the United States, and the majority of their patients have expressed satisfaction with their sex changes. Those changing from male to female (the more common procedure) may be provided with breasts and a vagina, and they may experience sexual pleasure and even orgasm. In the reverse change, it has been possible surgically to construct an artifical penis that can remain in a semi-erect state, but that of course would transmit no semen. Some may attach an artificial penis just for intercourse. Of course, natural parenthood is impossible after either sex-change procedure.

Variant Sexual Behavior

There are many patterns of sexual behavior that are contrary to the standards of at least some members of our society. Some forms of sexual behavior are condemned by almost everyone. Other sexual practices are condemned by some and accepted by others. For example, if a truck driver eating lunch in a truckstop café pinches the waitress, she may typically wink at him and promptly forget the incident. If a diner in a hotel dining room pinches the waitress, she will tell him to "watch it" or maybe even call the manager to talk to him. If a man pinches a woman on the street, she is apt to call a policeman and have him arrested. As another example, if a man peeks through a bedroom window at a partially dressed woman, he may be arrested and convicted of a sex offense. But looking at even more scantily clothed women in a nightclub act is perfectly acceptable behavior to many members of our society. In these two examples, the major factor seems to be the context, rather than the details of the act itself.

Our definition of variance also includes the psychological component. Specific patterns of variant sexual behavior can be readily associated with particular mental illnesses and poor social adjustment. The most common forms of variant sexuality can be discussed in terms of four types of psychopathology: (1) feelings of sexual inferiority, (2) mental incompetence, (3) developmental abnormalities, and (4) an orientation toward violent behavior.

Sexual Insecurity The fear of sexual inadequacy can be associated with certain types of variance. For any one of a number of reasons, the sexually insecure person has been made to feel ashamed or disgraced because of a real or imagined inability to function satisfactorily in heterosexual relationships. From this single foundation, a range of variant behavioral patterns can arise.

Exhibitionism Legally, exhibitionism is when an adult man obtains sexual gratification by the purposeful exposure of the penis to an unsuspecting female or child, who is an involuntary observer, usually a complete stranger. The exposure must be intentional and not incidental as in the case of a drunk urinating. The object of the act must be female, either child or adult. Exposure to other males is commonly an overture to homosexual activity and is not related to exhibitionism as defined by the law. The penis may be flaccid or erect and the exposure may or may not include masturbation.

Although most exhibitionists cannot give a valid account of their feelings at the time of the exposure, the apparent intention of the act is to arouse an emotional expression in the victim. The most common intention of the exhibitionist seems to be to evoke fear and shock rather than pleasure from his victim. An amused reaction often sends the exhibitionist into a state of depression. It is important to note that the exhibitionist is not soliciting further contact with his victim. On the contrary, he is afraid of any closer contact. If a woman approaches him for sexual contact, he is likely to run away. The exhibitionist is one of the most harmless of sex offenders.

The most significant psychological finding in exhibitionists is a deep feeling of inferiority and sexual inadequacy. Thus, through exposing themselves, they seek a feeling of power, dominance, and sexual adequacy—the reaction they are striving for is shock at the large size of their sex organs. This probably explains why they often expose to children, who are more likely to be shocked than adults. In addition, this is probably the reason why an amused reaction can be so crushing. In most cases, the safest and best response for a person encountering an exhibitionist is merely to ignore him.

Obscene Phone Calls Obscene phone calls are anonymous communications with a woman without intention of further sexual contact. Like the exhibitionist, the caller finds sexual release in the act itself or in masturbation during the call. The hoped-for reaction is shock and consternation on the part of the victim. The fact that the victim is both inaccessible and unknown protects the caller from a possible sexual confrontation. The best way to deal with an obscene phone call is for the woman simply to hang up. The longer she stays on the phone, the more she is likely to encourage the caller. If she demonstrates fear or shock, she is playing his game and inviting further calls.

Voyeurism A *voyeur* is a person who attains sexual gratification by looking at sexual objects or situations. One of the complications in studying voyeurism is the fact that almost all people have some degree of voyeuristic tendency. Society accepts such forms of voyeurism as viewing "topless" shows at bars, reading sex magazines, and watching attractive people in brief bathing suits. The true sexual variant is the peeper or "peeping Tom" who looks into a private room or area with the hope of seeing nude or partially nude females without their knowledge or consent. The peeper wants to see the female behaving in presumed privacy. A few peepers call attention to themselves by such actions as tapping on a window, but the vast majority of peepers try to avoid detection. They often masturbate while peeping.

Peepers are generally shy with women and have strong feelings of inferiority. Their interests are heterosexual but their overwhelming fear of being rejected keeps them from seeking normal heterosexual activity. Some are men who quite by accident came upon the opportunity to observe a nude woman and happened to get caught. Some were drunk at the time of their arrest. A few are mentally deficient. It is unusual for a peeper to be at all dangerous.

Mental Incompetence Some sexual variations result from mental inadequacy. The two examples discussed below are generally associated with rural communities and undereducated individuals.

Bestiality Bestiality is engaging in sexual contact with animals. This is apparently a common occurrence among rural boys, yet this is one of the most taboo forms of sexual outlet. Even in rural areas, bestiality is the object of both condemnation and ridicule. There are apparently no important deviant psychological motivations behind typical bestiality. It is usually engaged in only as a substitute for more normal sexual relationships. The animal is generally used as an aid to masturbation, rather than as a true sexual stimulus.

Incest Incest is sexual intercourse between individuals too closely related to marry legally. The relationship can be father-daughter, father-stepdaughter, mother-son, mother-stepson, or brother-

sister. Incest is one of the most ancient and widespread of the sexual taboos.

Most incidents of incest develop either within a subculture, which takes less strict attitude toward such behavior, or as a result of the mental incompetence of one of the partners. Even in the contemporary United States, there remain certain subcultures in which incest is thought of as unfortunate, but not a grave or unexpected situation. Paul Gebhard, et al. (*Sex Offenders*, 1965) found that incest is most common among impoverished, unintelligent, uneducated individuals living in rural surroundings. They come from a cultural background wherein sexual morality is publicly emphasized, but privately breached with impunity.

Developmental Abnormalities Some forms of sexual variation are associated with the failure of the individual to develop normally. Either because of an inability to attain normal sexual maturity or because of regression (return) to earlier, immature sexual habits, this type of variant is likely to show one of the following behavior patterns.

Pedophilia Pedophilia is sexual involvement of an adult with a child. It may be either homosexual or heterosexual. Pedophilia is probably the least acceptable form of sexual behavior in our society. Since the variation lies in the sexual immaturity of the child, the natural break-off point for classifying an act as pedophilia would be the onset of puberty.

Pedophiles are usually characterized psychologically as suffering from an arrested development (fixation) in which the offender has never grown psychosexually beyond the immature prepubertal stage or from a regression back to this stage of development. As a result, the great majority of sexual acts in pedophilia consist of the sex-play type found in children, such as looking, showing, fondling, and being fondled. The nature of the sexual act usually corresponds to the maturity expected at the age of the victim rather than at the age of the offender.

In the vast majority of heterosexual pedophilia cases (J.W. Mohr, et al., *Pedophilia and Exhibitionism*, 1964) the offender is part of the close environment of the child. The offender is usually known to the child and the family of the child. The offenders are most commonly neighbors, family friends, or relatives. Less than one-fifth of the offenders are strangers or only casual acquaintances. In homosexual pedophilic offenses, the offender is more often a stranger.

Parents, police, and the courts can minimize the harmful effects on victims of pedophilic offenses by skillful handling of these cases. It has been found (Mohr et al., 1964) that the child is often damaged more by the events following the offense than by the offense itself. The effect on the child depends greatly on the reaction of parents and other adults on discovery of the offense. If the parents react with obvious fear, anger, disgust, or hysteria, the child is more likely to suffer lasting effects. An additional problem is the appearance of the child as a witness in court. Interrogation and cross-examination can be far more damaging than the offense itself.

Fetishism Fetishism is sexual arousal from perception of inanimate objects. Fetishism is a displacement reaction, a sexual response not to a living being, but to a symbol of that being. A certain amount of fetishism is entirely normal—certain items of clothing, such as black lace panties, have so universally been equated with sex appeal that some sexual arousal from the sight of them is neither surprising nor abnormal. At what point, then, does a fetish become abnormal? Some possible criteria for fetishism are (1) the fetish item is used in masturbation; (2) the fetish item is necessary for erection for intercourse; (3) sexual partners are chosen on the basis of possession of the fetish item; (4) the fetish item is collected (through purchase or theft).

As one might expect, the most common fetish items are lingerie, such as panties, brassieres, and stockings. More surprising is the rather common fetish with shoes. There is a thriving mail-order industry offering fetish items through advertisement in certain sex-oriented magazines. A fetishist encounters legal problems only if he or she is caught stealing the fetish item.

Transvestism Transvestism is wearing the clothing of the opposite sex. The practice exists among both men and women. Transvestism usually indicates a distorted and confused sociosexual life that often, but not always, includes homosexuality. There are several possible motivations behind transvestism.

First, there is the true homosexual. He or she dresses in garments of the opposite sex as an outward sign of homosexuality (to attract persons of the same sex) and as a symbol of the wearer's preferred role in homosexual acts. In this case, the clothing has no emotional or sexual value to the wearer. It is a means to an end, not an end in itself.

Second is the true transvestite who wears the clothing of the opposite sex for the emotional or sexual gratification it provides. This type of transvestism is an end in itself and often involves fetishism.

Violent Behavior A disposition towards unnecessary violence and an orientation to use force to deal with emotional needs and desires is the basis of certain types of variant sexual patterns. For this reason, these variations pose the very real danger of physical and psychological harm.

Forcible Rape   A detailed study of men convicted of forcible rape (Gebhard et al., 1965) indicated that they fall into several distinct groups. The most common type of rapist was found to be a man whose entire way of life includes the use of unnecessary violence. This type of rapist does not commit rape because of a lack of willing sex partners. Instead, he prefers rape to conventional sex. For this type of individual, sexual intercourse is most gratifying if it is accompanied by physical violence or the serious threat of violence. This indicates a strong sadistic element in the personality of this most common type of rapist. He dislikes women and gains satisfaction from punishing them. Often more violence is used than would be necessary to complete the rape. In some cases, the violence seems to substitute for sexual release or at least diminish the need for it. In fact, these rapists sometimes become impotent and are unable to complete the sex attack.

A second type of rapist is the amoral delinquent. Such men pay little attention to normal social controls and operate purely for their own gratification. They are not sadistic—they simply want to have intercourse, and the contrary wishes of the female are of no importance. They are not hostile toward females, but look upon them solely as sexual objects whose role in life is to provide sexual pleasure to men.

A third type of rapist is the drunken variety. The drunk's aggression ranges from uncoordinated efforts at seduction to hostile and truly vicious behavior released by his intoxication.

A fourth type of rapist is the explosive variety. These are previously normal individuals who have suddenly snapped into a psychotic state as a result of emotional stresses. An example might be a mild-natured college student who suddenly rapes and kills.

A final category of rapist is the "innocent" male who in attempting to gain a voluntary relationship has misinterpreted the true feelings of the woman. He may be accustomed to the socially approved pattern of behavior in which a girl says "no, no" but means "yes, yes" and not realize that this particular woman really means no.

A woman can best reduce her chances of being a victim by avoiding those situations that most often lead to forcible rape. Of these, touring bars alone is the most frequently mentioned by women who report forcible rape. Hitching rides is another dangerous practice.

There can be no clear answer to the question of what to do when faced with a rapist. This question can be answered only on the spot, since circumstances can vary so much. Among approaches that sometimes work are calmly talking the rapist into changing his mind, making lots of noise, or tricking him in one way or another. But even the best planned defense may fall apart in the suddenness and fear of the actual attack. A rapist can be extremely dangerous. Distasteful as it sounds, if rape seems unavoidable, it is highly advisable for the woman to yield to and cooperate with her assailant. It is far better to be raped and alive than raped and dead.

Historically, rape has been one of the most difficult charges to prosecute successfully. Most rapes are unreported by their victims. This failure to report is caused by the embarrassment and humiliation inflicted by unsympathetic authorities and by the fact that women were long considered to be wholly responsible for their own rape.

Fortunately, public health officials and many police departments are realizing that rape is one of the most traumatic of crimes.

A victim of rape requires understanding and professional care to avoid permanent emotional damage. Women's groups have been establishing rape treatment centers that serve to aid the victim through the experience and to encourage her to assert her legal rights.

Gradually through recent court decisions and enactment of restructured state laws, the atmosphere for the prosecution of rape is slowly changing in favor of the victim. Defendants are facing increased chances of successful prosecution through new legal provisions limiting the probing that can be done into the previous sex life of the victim. Defense lawyers, by dredging up the past sex life of the victim, have often attempted to make her appear as the community whore, and the defendant as someone she enticed into this unfortunate liaison. Such antics have been used to discredit the complaint of the victim. Even with the new changes, much still remains to be done to fully protect women from the rapist, and to ensure successful conviction.

Sadism Sadism is the attainment of sexual gratification from the infliction of cruelty upon another person. The sexual sadist is often unable to achieve orgasm without the use of some form of violence. There are both male and female sadists and heterosexual and homosexual sadism. As was mentioned in the discussion of forcible rape, sadism is often a motivating factor in rape. The rapist frequently uses more force than is necessary to complete the rape, and elements of torture are sometimes involved. Many men use sadistic cruelty in their relationships with prostitutes or even their wives, being unable to gain satisfaction without this cruelty. Sadism can take forms that have no apparent relationship to its sexual basis.

Masochism Masochism is the attainment of sexual gratification from suffering physical pain. There are men and women who must be physically punished in order to achieve sexual arousal or orgasm. The punishment often involves beating, whipping, biting, pinching, scratching, burning, and similar painful treatments. Various psychological explanations have been offered for masochism. It has been interpreted in terms of the destructive impulses carried in the unconscious mind. It has also been related to subconscious guilt feelings from which the masochistic punishment gives temporary release.

Sexual Anatomy and Physiology Reproduction of the whole individual in humans is achieved by the sexual process—the fusion of the female sex cell, the egg (ovum), and the male sex cell, the sperm. This fertilized cell (zygote) then develops into an adult individual.

The singular significance of sexual reproduction to humans can be seen when we compare ourselves with our parents. Each fertilization of an egg by a sperm brings together new genetic combinations. No one of us is exactly identical to either of our parents. Throughout human history, this type of reproduction has made possible the mutations that, over thousands of years, have permitted adaptation to changing environments.

This form of reproduction contrasts with the asexual process found among more primitive plant and animal forms, where reproduction is by a mere division of a single cell or organism into two smaller, but similar, cells. Such a process involves no genetic recombining.

The Female Organs of Reproduction The female genital organs are both internal and external. The internal parts of the system include the ovaries, fallopian tubes, uterus, and vagina. The external organs consist of the hymen, labia majora and minora, and clitoris.

Ovaries The production of female sex cells, eggs (ova), is accomplished by the ovaries (the female gonads). They are situated deep in the pelvic cavity, one on either side of the uterus. The ovaries serve a dual function, producing both eggs and hormones. Within the ovary are many vesicles called *ovarian follicles*. At the time of birth, it is estimated that the ovaries contain about 400,000 immature follicles. Beginning with puberty these immature fol-

licles mature at the rate of 1 about every 28 days and develop into *graafian follicles*. Each month, usually midway between menstrual discharges, a graafian follicle ruptures and releases a mature egg. Since the reproductive life of the female extends about 35 years (ages 12 to 47) and about 1 egg per 28 days is produced (or 13 a year), only about 450 eggs out of a possible 400,000 ever mature.

The graafian follicle begins develop-

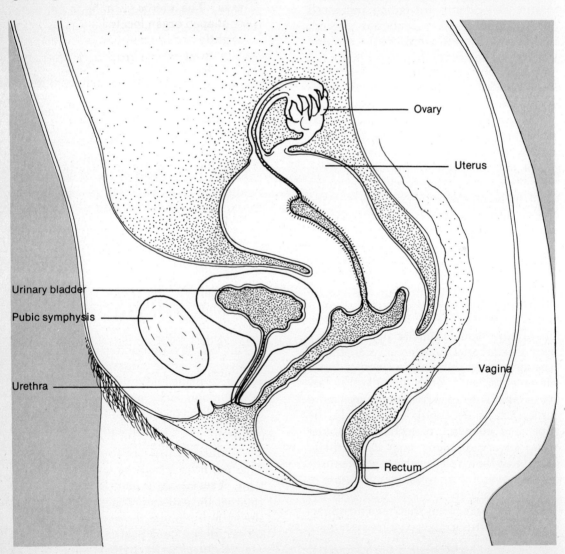

The female reproductive system

ment near the center of the ovary. As it enlarges, it moves toward the surface until it finally appears like a little blister on the surface. Near the midpoint between menstrual discharges, it ruptures and releases the egg enclosed within it, a process called *ovulation*. Actually ovulation may occur as early as the eighth day and as late as the twentieth day. After ovulation, the blood clot is soon replaced by yellow-colored cells and is called the *corpus luteum*. This body remains about 14 to 15 days after which it degenerates into a fibrous body (*corpus fibrosum*).

Fallopian Tubes The fallopian tubes, or oviducts, are about 4 inches long and extend from the uterus out to the ovaries. The outer end of each tube is fringed (fimbriated), and these fingerlike fringes are adjacent to each ovary. When the egg ruptures through the wall of the graafian follicle, the fimbria catch the egg and pass it into the tube. The inner lining of the fallopian tube is covered with minute, hairlike structures called *cilia*. Once inside the fallopian tube, the egg is propelled toward the uterus by the movement of the cilia and contractions in the walls of the tube. The egg has no powers of movement of its own.

Once the egg is released from the ovary, it can be fertilized by any sperm that may be present. Three to four days is normally required for the transport of the egg from the ovary through the fallopian tube to the uterus. An egg is believed to remain viable for about 24 hours, after which it begins to degenerate. Since both the egg and the sperm have a limited life, fertilization must take place within about 24 hours after ovulation if conception is to occur that month.

Usually fertilization occurs within the fallopian tube. Although the ovum is normally picked up by the fallopian tube on the same side as that on which the ovulation occurred, it has been clearly shown that eggs have, on occasion, migrated across the pelvis to be picked up by the opposite tube. Sperm present around the ovary at the time of ovulation (from a recent insemination) have been known to fertilize an egg outside of a fallopian tube in the pelvis. In the event such a fertilized egg is not picked up by a fallopian tube, it might develop in the pelvis completely outside the uterus.

Uterus The uterus (womb) is a hollow, pear-shaped organ located in the pelvis. It is slightly above and behind the bladder, but in front of the rectum. It is loosely suspended in position by several ligaments. Its normal position is a forward tilt. Loosening of these ligaments due to childbearing may cause the uterus to tilt backward. Other causes of misplacement can be pelvic diseases (such as cancer) and congenital deformity. In the adult it may be about 3 inches long and 2 inches wide. Its walls are thick and very muscular. In pregnancy it stretches to over 12 inches in length as it expands to accommodate the growing baby. The upper half of the uterus is the corpus (body), the lower half is the *cervix*, and the lower opening is the *os*.

The inner layer of the uterus, the *endometrium*, is richly supplied with blood vessels and glands. Following ovulation, the egg descends through the tube into the uterus. If the egg has been fertilized, it becomes embedded in the endometrium within 3 to 4 days.

Vagina The vagina is a tube extending from the external genitalia to the uterus. This muscular tube is 4 to 6 inches long, and lies between the bladder and the rectum. It serves as the excretory duct for the uterus, the female organ for intercourse, and the birth canal. The tissue lining it gives off a mucus-like secretion during sexual arousal. The rhythmic contractions of its muscular walls during the climax of

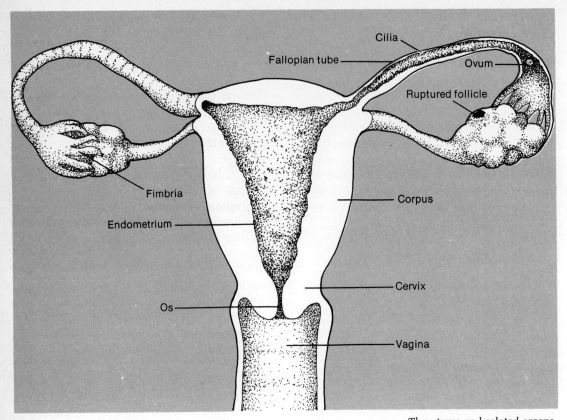

The uterus and related organs.

intercourse produce an intensely pleasurable sensation called *orgasm*. Only the outer portion of the vagina is sensitive, and orgasm is induced by the sensations of the clitoris, although felt in the vagina as contractions.

Hymen In young girls the external opening of the vagina may be partially closed by a membrane called the *hymen*. This membrane varies in size and thickness, and may remain intact until the first sexual intercourse. It may, however, be greatly reduced in size before mating as the result of the use of tampons (vaginal insertions used during menstrual discharge), by a physician as a part of a medical examination, or through participation in active

sports. In rare cases it may need to be surgically cut or stretched by a physician before intercourse can be accomplished. Contrary to common belief, its rupture may not involve bleeding. Its absence should not be taken as a sign of lack of virginity.

Labia Two pairs of liplike structures surround the external opening of the vagina. The outer and larger pair are the *labia majora*; the inner and smaller pair are the *labia minora*. The space between the labia minora into which the vaginal passageway and the urethra open is the *vestibule*.

Clitoris At the front terminus of the vestibule is a small erectile organ called the

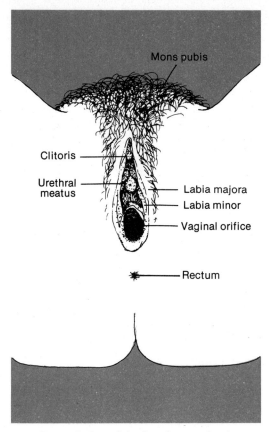

External view of the female reproductive organs.

clitoris. Somewhat similar to the penis in the male, it is rarely longer than 1 inch. As with the penis, the clitoris has many nerve receptors. During sexual play it becomes erect and is the chief site of sexual excitement in the female. Unlike the penis, the clitoris does not contain the urethra.

The fatty cushion on the surface of the body directly anterior to the labia majora is the mons veneris. During puberty it becomes covered with curly hair.

Menstruation Menstruation is the periodic discharge of blood, mucus, and cellular fragments from the uterine endometrium, occurring at more or less regular intervals (except during pregnancy and lactation) from the time of puberty to the menopause.

The onset is commonly between the twelfth and thirteenth year, but may occur as early as the tenth year or as late as the sixteenth. The onset of the first menstruation is referred to as the *menarche.* Since puberty is the broad range of physical changes that occur between childhood and maturity, menarche represents just one sign of puberty.

The cessation of menstruation, *menopause,* commonly occurs between 45 and 50 years of age. As the menarche represents just one sign of puberty, so menopause is just one sign of the climacteric, sometimes referred to as the "change of life."

Although menstrual discharge most commonly occurs every 28 days, women vary considerably in the length of their menstrual cycles—the interval of days between discharges. Some women are known to have cycles as short as 21 days, and others as long as 38 days. In fact, with many women the length of the menstrual cycles varies from cycle to cycle.

The duration of the menstrual flow is usually 4 to 6 days, but periods ranging from 2 to 8 days in length may be considered normal for some women. For a given woman, the duration of the flow is commonly similar month after month.

Usually the blood is liquid, although clots may appear if the flow is excessive. The average amount of blood and tissues lost ranges from 60 to 180 milliliters (about 2 to 6 tablespoonfuls) each menstruation. Some women report a weight gain of 1 to 3 pounds just before the beginning of menstrual discharge. This is retained water rather than fat. The average weight gain, however, is only about ¼ pound.

The Menstrual Cycle The cycle of events in the uterus from the beginning of one menstrual discharge until the next is called the *menstrual cycle.* Four distinct phases occur during the typical 28-day cycle:

1. *Proliferative or follicular phase.* After menstruation has stopped (days 3 to 5 of the cycle), the endometrial lining is thin. The glands contained within the endometrium are straight, short, and narrow. In the ovary the graafian follicle is maturing. During this phase, which lasts about 10 days, the follicle produces a hormone, estrogen, which causes active growth in the endometrium. The endometrium becomes quite thick and dense.

2. *Ovulatory phase.* Ovulation usually occurs between days 12 and 16, but most commonly on day 14. During the day of ovulation, there is little change in the endometrium. As soon as the ovum ruptures through the graafian follicle, the remains of the follicle become a corpus luteum.

3. *Secretory or luteal phase.* Under the influence of hormones given off by the corpus luteum, the endometrium continues to increase in size. The glands in the endometrium become quite enlarged and tortuous (twisted) and become very active. This phase of the cycle lasts 13 to 14 days. In the event the egg is not fertilized, the corpus luteum disintegrates. With the disintegration of the corpus luteum the hormones it has been producing decrease, and the cells and glands of the endometrium begin to die, causing the destructive phase, or menstrual flow. In the event the egg is fertilized, it becomes embedded in the thick endometrium, where it continues its development.

4. *Destructive or menstrual phase.* This phase occurs because of the death of endometrial cells. This layer has a very rich blood supply. With the tissue disintegration, both blood and cell fragments are discarded together. This phase usually lasts 4 to 6 days.

Gonadotropic Hormones

Hormone	Effect
Follicle-stimulating hormone (FSH)	FSH directs the development and activity of the graafian follicles. It causes the follicle to secrete causing it to secrete estrogen.
Luteinizing hormone (LH)	LH helps to prolong estrogen production. It triggers ovulation, thereby initiating formation of the corpus luteum and causing it to secrete both estrogen and progesterone.
Luteotropic hormone (LTH)	LTH, also called *prolactin*, helps to prolong estrogen and progesterone production by the corpus luteum. It causes milk secretion by the mammary glands after the birth of a baby.

Hormones and the Ovarian Cycle

The ovarian cycle is under the control of two sets of hormones, those from the anterior pituitary gland, called *gonadotropic hormones,* and those from the ovary. The table on gonadotropic hormones names and describes the effect of the three hormones.

Ovarian Hormones Under the stimulation of the gonadotropic hormones, the ovaries secrete two hormones, estrogen and progesterone.

Estrogen is produced by the graafian follicle before ovulation and by the corpus luteum after ovulation. It brings about the maturation of the secondary sex characteristics. These are changes that occur during puberty and include the development of the breasts, the deposition of fat around the hips, a change in hair distribution, the maturing of the reproductive tract, and the female sexual drive. Complete removal of the ovaries (oophorectomy) before puberty prevents the development of secondary sex characteristics and the sexual organs remain immature. Removal after puberty causes the cessation of menstruation and causes the body to become masculine.

Estrogen also stimulates the growth of the endometrium during the proliferative phase of the cycle. Increased amounts of estrogen through the combined action of the follicle-stimulating hormone (FSH) and the luteinizing hormone (LH) feed back to the pituitary gland causing it to slow down FSH production and speed up

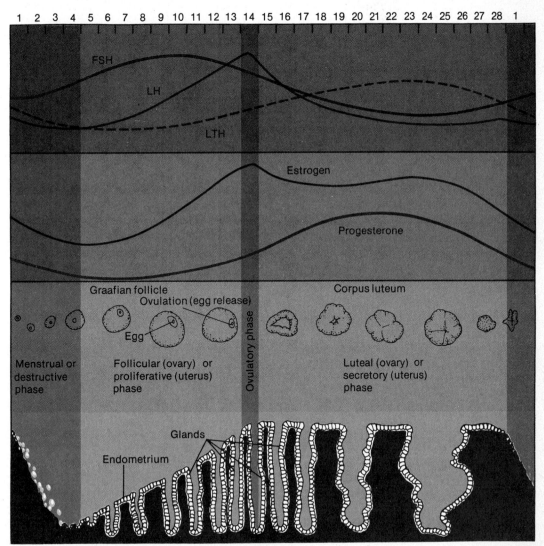

The menstrual cycle. The upper portion of the graph shows the hormone levels through the average 28-day cycle. The lower portion shows the changes in the endometrium that are oc-curring simultaneously in response to differing amounts and combinations of these five chemicals.

LH production. As seen in the figure of events in a typical menstrual cycle, this occurs during the proliferative phase.

Progesterone is produced by the corpus luteum. These are its effects: it prepares the endometrium for the implantation of a fertilized egg. In pregnancy, it maintains the endometrium in good condition. During pregnancy, it is produced by the corpus luteum during the first 2 to 3 months and by the placenta thereafter for the course of the pregnancy. If there is no pregnancy, increased amounts of progesterone in the blood feed back to the pituitary gland causing it to slow down LH and LTH (luteotropic hormone) production.

It should be apparent by now that the ovarian hormone estrogen is antagonistic to the pituitary hormone FSH. FSH initiates and stimulates the ovary to produce estrogen, but then estrogen inhibits further FSH production. FSH cannot be abundant again until the amount of estrogen in the body drops off. Likewise, the ovarian hormone progesterone is antagonistic to the pituitary hormone LH. LH stimulates the corpus luteum in the ovary to produce progesterone, but then progesterone feeds back to the pituitary and inhibits further LH production.

This raises a question. If progesterone is essential to maintaining the endometrium, but if progesterone can be cut off (and the endometrium discharged) by the action described above, how does a pregnant woman maintain her pregnancy? The answer is that in the event an egg is fertilized, the outer cells of the developing embryo (which by this time is implanted in the endometrium) give off a new hormone that serves the same function as did LH and LTH. This new hormone, chorionic gonadotropin, serves to keep stimulating progesterone production by the corpus luteum, thus maintaining the endometrium and retaining the pregnancy. The

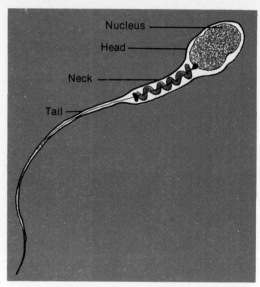

A human sperm cell.

corpus luteum continues to produce progesterone until about the thirteenth week of pregnancy. At this point the corpus luteum "gives out." The massive amounts of progesterone needed to maintain the endometrial lining for the remaining weeks of pregnancy must be supplied by the placenta.

The Male Organs of Reproduction

The male genital organs are less complex than those of the female. The male does not need to provide for the fate of the fertilized egg. The sole task of the male genital organs is to see that sperm cells are produced and introduced into the female tract. Thus the male genital organs are more external and more obvious.

Sperm Production Sperm cells are produced in the testes (testicles, male gonads). Each testis is an oval gland about 1½ inches long. The testes are suspended from the under side of the body in a bag, the scrotum. Sperm production cannot occur at normal body temperatures. The scrotum allows the testes to be suspended from the body. Thus, their temperature is 3 to 4 degrees lower than normal body temperature, which appears to be ideal for sperm production. In cold temperatures, the thin scrotal muscles contract and pull the testes closer to the body wall. In hot temperatures the muscles relax allowing the testes to be suspended farther away from the body.

Not only do high temperatures prevent sperm production, they also may destroy sperm cells, causing infertility (temporary inability to reproduce) or even sterility (permanent inability to reproduce). Low temperatures inhibit sperm production, but do not destroy sperm cells.

During pregnancy, the testes of a male fetus are formed in the abdominal cavity. About the eighth month of pregnancy, the testes of the fetus migrate from the abdominal cavity into the scrotum. Failure of this descent to occur leads to sterility. Such a condition is called *cryptorchidism* (*crypt* meaning "hidden" and *orchid* meaning "testis"). This condition can be corrected surgically.

The testes serve as endocrine glands as well. The male sex hormones they produce begin to flow in large amounts at about 13 years of age. This occurs with the onset of puberty and marks the beginning of the physical changes leading to sexual maturity. Such changes (secondary sex characteristics) include the development of broad shoulders, lowered voice, the growth of hair on the face, chest and pubis, and the development of the male sex drive.

Within each testis are a great number of very small tubes called *seminiferous tubules*. Sperm cells are formed inside these tubules. Beginning during puberty, these sperm cells are produced without let-up for the lifetime of the male. Initial production starts slowly, then increases, until, in the sexually mature male, the in-

credible number of 10 to 30 billion sperm cells are produced each month. The number of sperm produced during a man's lifetime defies imagination.

Each sperm cell is microscopic in size. The length of each cell is about 50 microns (it would take 480 of them end to end to cover an inch). Each cell consists of a head, neck, body, and tail. One set of chromosomes (23) is carried in the head.

Sperm Release The passage of the sperm from the testes to ejaculation from the penis is through particular ducts, with secretions from specific glands added at certain points to activate the sperm.

Epididymis As the sperm mature they move out of the seminiferous tubules and collect in a coiled tube called the *epididymis*. It lies on the upper side of each testis and would be about 20 feet long if uncoiled. Here sperm are stored until released from the body by ejaculation or until they disintegrate and are reabsorbed by the tubules.

Vas Deferens The *vas deferens* is a duct about 18 inches long that carries sperm from the epididymis to the ejaculatory duct. Near the ejaculatory duct is an enlarged section called the *ampulla*, which, like the epididymis and vas deferens, stores sperm. During ejaculation, the walls of the deferens contract, propelling sperm cells through the duct.

Seminal Vesicles The seminal vesicles are a pair of glandular structures located at the base of the bladder in front of the rectum. They empty into the vas deferens to form the ejaculatory duct. During ejaculation, the vesicles contract and add their glandular secretions to the semen.

Prostrate Gland This large organ is located directly below the bladder. It sur-

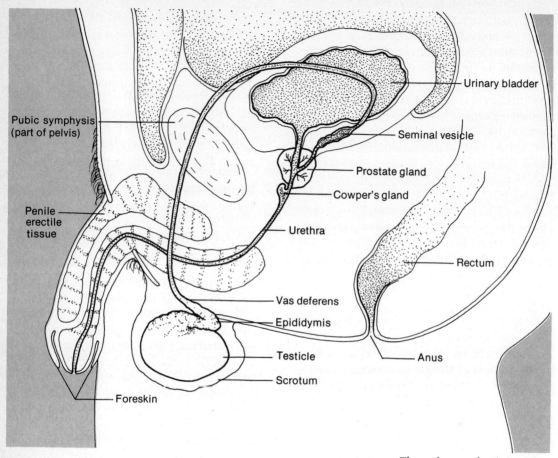

Pubic symphysis (part of pelvis)

Penile erectile tissue

Foreskin

Urinary bladder

Seminal vesicle

Prostate gland

Cowper's gland

Urethra

Rectum

Vas deferens

Epididymis

Testicle

Scrotum

Anus

The male reproductive system.

rounds the urethra (the duct carrying urine from the bladder to the end of the penis). The ejaculatory ducts pass through each side of the prostate gland to join the urethra. During ejaculation the gland contracts to add its secretions to the semen.

In older men the prostate gland commonly enlarges so that it obstructs the urethra, thus hindering urination. This condition occurs to some degree in over half of all elderly men and can usually be corrected surgically.

Cowper's Glands Two small glands about the size of peas lie on either side of the urethra slightly below the prostate gland. These glands produce an alkaline secretion that precedes ejaculation and is evident at the tip of the penis as a drop of clear, sticky material. This secretion serves to remove any urine that may still be in the urethra and to lubricate the vaginal canal in intercourse.

Penis The male organ for copulation is the penis. Containing the urethra, the organ is used for urine excretion and, in the erect state, for semen ejaculation. As with other physical dimensions, its size varies. In an erect state it will average about 6 inches in length and 1 inch in diameter. Passing through the length of the penis are three columns of erectile tissue: two corpora cavernosa, side by side, and a smaller corpus spongiosum, beneath and housing the urethra. At the tip of the penis the corpus spongiosum enlarges to form the glans penis. The glans penis is richly supplied with nerve receptors, making it especially sensitive to external stimulation. A free fold of skin, called the *foreskin* or *prepuce*, overhangs the glans penis when it is relaxed. Surgical removal of the foreskin to prevent infection is known as *circumcision*.

The corpora of the penis are richly supplied with blood vessels, which are empty of blood when the penis is limp but engorged with blood during an erection. An erection may be brought about by physical manipulation of the penis, by sexual thoughts, by pressure from a full bladder or rectum, by wearing clothing that fits too tightly, or by any event that causes congestion of blood in the region of the penis. The inability to attain an erection is called *impotence*. It is not to be confused with sterility, which is either an insufficient number or total lack of sperm cells. A man may be sterile, yet fully potent.

Semen Semen, or seminal fluid, is the fluid ejaculated during the male sex act. It consists of fluids from the testes, seminal vesicles, prostate gland, and Cowper's glands. The sperm is a grayish-white sticky fluid, which contains 60 million to 120 million sperm per milliliter.

Ejaculation Physical stimulation of the penis not only causes it to become erect, but finally results in forcible expulsion of semen, called *ejaculation*. Ejaculation usually results in the discharge of about 2.5 milliliters of semen. In sexual intercourse ejaculation occurs at the climax and sperm cells are placed in the vaginal canal. It is usually accompanied by a feeling of intense sexual excitement and emotional release called *orgasm*. Shortly after ejaculation the orgasm subsides, the penis becomes limp, and the male feels sexually satisfied.

Male Reproductive Hormones The male hormones are collectively called *androgens*. A principal androgen, called *testosterone*, is produced by the testes. It is formed by cells between the seminiferous tubules, called *interstitial cells*. It is responsible for the development of the male secondary sexual characteristics as well as the development of the reproductive organs.

Testosterone production is, in turn, under the direct control of two gonadotropic hormones from the pituitary gland, namely follicle-stimulating hormone (FSH) and interstitial-cell-stimulating hormone (ICSH). ICSH is considered analogous to luteinizing hormone (LH) produced in the female. FSH causes the seminiferous tubules to produce sperm cells. ICSH causes the testes to produce testosterone. When the amount of testosterone becomes too great, it reacts against the ICSH, which is then reduced. Testosterone can also serve to control FSH.

The absence or removal of the testes may cause hormonal deficiencies in the male. Since the production of testosterone becomes increasingly important to male sexual characteristics after the time of puberty, the effects of insufficient testosterone would depend on when the deficiency occurs. If it occurs before puberty, the male fails to develop male secondary sex characteristics. A boy who loses his testes prior to puberty is known as a *eunuch*. If a male loses the testes after the onset of puberty, he will retain some male secondary sex characteristics and lose others. The removal of the testes is called *castration*.

Sexual Stimuli Sexual responses are a basic element of human physiology and psychology. Not surprisingly, they can be induced by a wide range of stimuli.

The sounds, smells, touch, sight, and indeed even the thought of sexual situations can sexually arouse most people. The sexual response of both male and female can be divided into identifiable phases, each with its physical and emotional characteristics.

The *excitement phase* is the first, accompanied by the initial signs of physical arousal. The *plateau phase* follows, in which the sex organs further change in size and shape. Breathing and cardiac rates increase. The *orgasm phase* brings the intensely satisfying sensations of sexual climax. In the *resolution phase*, the organs return to their normal sizes and shapes, and the intense feelings of climax subside.

Female Sexual Response The response of a woman's body to sexual stimulation is widespread, involving organs besides the genitals. In the excitement phase, the clitoris tip swells and the shaft elongates two or three times in size; the labia majora and labia minora expand and spread. The vagina may begin to lubricate within 10 to 30 seconds, the outer two-thirds lengthening and distending. The uterus moves away from the vagina. Lubrication varies among females, yet for a given woman it usually depends on how aroused she is. During excitement, the breasts enlarge, and the nipples erect, stiffen, become highly sensitive to touch, and flush. The areola (the dark ring around the nipple) is engorged with blood. Skeletal muscles contract throughout the body. Pulse and breathing rates increase.

At the plateau phase, the clitoris moves under its hood and becomes so tender that efforts to touch it directly may be painful. The labia minora increase in size and turn bright red. The outer one-third of the vagina contracts, while the inner two-thirds expands.

In the orgasm phase, strong contractions occur in the outer half of the vagina (three to five in a mild orgasm, eight to twelve in

an intense one). The uterus contracts as it does in labor, and the anus contracts tightly. The intensity and duration of orgasm in the female varies more than in the male.

In the resolution phase, the clitoris and labia slowly return to normal size and position. The outer one-third of the vagina quickly returns to normal, while the inner two-thirds returns to normal more slowly (5 to 8 minutes). Following orgasm, the sex flush of the breasts rapidly disappears, and the breast size slowly (5 to 10 minutes) returns to normal.

The period of sexual stimulation preceding orgasm varies from woman to woman and from time to time for the same woman. The experience of many couples is that the woman needs a longer period of stimulation in intercourse to achieve orgasm than does the man. But Alfred Kinsey *et al.* (*Sexual Behavior in the Human Female*, 1953) reported that the average woman can masturbate to orgasm almost as fast as the average man. They attributed the difference to the fact that the masturbating woman can manipulate her sensitive areas more specifically than is possible in intercourse. This conclusion seems to be confirmed by Masters and Johnson (1966), who found the measurable physiologic intensity of female orgasm greatest in masturbation, moderate in partner manipulation, and lowest in intercourse.

The subjective experiences of a woman during orgasm, as reported by Masters and Johnson, begin with a feeling that orgasm is imminent, followed by an intense sensual awareness of the pelvic region. The woman becomes almost completely oblivious to the surrounding environment, focusing on her own sensations. The next feeling, reported by almost every woman, is that of warmth, starting in the pelvic region and spreading throughout the body. A final feeling, reported consistently, is that of a pelvic throbbing.

During and directly following orgasm

there is a marked coolness of the lips of the mouth and surrounding areas. This is due to sudden release of blood vessels. Muscular and psychological relaxation accompanies orgasm.

Caressing of the clitoris plays an important role in achieving orgasm for many women, yet clitoral stimulation is not essential in achieving orgasm. A sexually responsive woman whose clitoris is removed surgically will remain capable of orgasm in intercourse. Some women can achieve orgasm when a part of the body distant from the clitoris, such as the ear canal, the small of the back, or the anus, is stimulated. Even where the clitoris is not stimulated directly, it enlarges and participates fully in the total response. A woman's body responds to stimulation consistently regardless of the source of that stimulation. There is neither a purely clitoral orgasm nor a purely vaginal one, but from the body's point of view only one kind, a sexual orgasm.

Many women are multiorgasmic (experiencing three or more orgasms within a few minutes) if stimulation is repeatedly resumed before sexual arousal drops below plateau-phase levels. Masturbation often best contributes to multiorgasmic ability, because it frees the woman from dependence on her partner's abilities. In lovemaking, the woman's ability to be multiorgasmic depends to a greater extent on foreplay and other forms of stimulation than on prolonged intercourse. In intercourse, the possiblities for multiple orgasm depend somewhat on the partner's ejaculatory control—his ability to engage in prolonged, vigorous intercourse without ejaculation and subsequent loss of erection. Many women also enjoy reaching multiple orgasms through oral or manual stimulation by their partners.

Male Sexual Response The excitement phase in the male is signaled by erection of the penis. The erectile tissue is a spongy mass of blood-filled spaces. During sexual arousal, the small arteries supplying blood to the penis dilate, letting more blood in, while the small veins draining the erectile tissue contract, letting less blood out. Thus blood accumulates in the penis, producing erection—an increase in the length, width, and firmness of the organ. The scrotum tightens, and the testes draw up close to the body.

Erection may be brought on by physical contact, sexual thoughts, sights, or sounds, or by involuntary activity of the nervous system during sleep. When sexual arousal is prolonged, the penis may erect and relax and then erect again, several times.

In the plateau phase, the fully erect penis may increase in diameter as orgasm approaches, particularly around the glans, and may turn a reddish-purple color. A few drops of preejaculatory fluid from the Cowper's glands are gradually emitted from the penis. The testes become further elevated (the more complete the testicular elevation, the greater the ejaculatory pressure), and they increase in size. A sex flush (reddening of the skin) may appear, the rate of breathing and heartbeat increase, and muscular tension increases throughout the body.

The increase in sexual arousal to the point of orgasm (ejaculation) requires, in all but a very few males, tactile stimulation of the penis. Masters and Johnson divide the male orgasm into two stages. The first stage is a period of 2 or 3 seconds before ejaculation during which the man can feel the ejaculation coming and can in no way restrain or control it. The second stage is the actual ejaculation of semen from the penis by contractions of the urethra and related muscles. The first three or four contractions expel the semen under great pressure. During orgasm, the breathing rate may increase as much as 40 times per minute, and the heart rate to from 110 to 180 or more beats per minute.

Sexual Response Cycle of the Human Female—Extragenital Reactions

	I. Excitement Phase	II. Plateau Phase	III. Orgasmic Phase	IV. Resolution Phase
Breasts	Nipples erect Breast size increases Veins become visible Areolae swell	Nipples turgid Further increase in breast size Areolae engorge	No observed changes	Rapid return to normal of nipples and areolae; slow decrease of breast volume and normal vein pattern
Sex Flush (Not all women have this)	Raised reddish rash appears first on upper abdomen, spreads rapidly over breasts	Rash spreads to rest of body	Degree of flush parallels orgasmic experience (estimated at 75% incidence)	Rapid disappearance of flush in reverse order of its appearance
Muscle Tensions	Voluntary muscles tense. Involuntary: vaginal wall, abdominal and rib muscles tense	Further increase in both voluntary and involuntary tension. May show spastic contractions of facial, abdominal and rib muscles	Loss of voluntary control; involuntary contractions and spasms of muscle groups	These spasms and involuntary contractions may last up to 5 minutes into this phase, slower return to normal
Rectum	No observed reaction	Voluntary contractions of anus (sometimes)	Involuntary contractions of anus simultaneously with contractions of orgasmic platform	No observed changes
Respiratory Rate	No observed reaction	Appearance of reaction occurs late in phase	Respiratory rates as high as 40 per minute. Intensity and duration indicative of sexual tension	Resolves early in phase
Heart Rate	Rises parallel to tension regardless of technique of stimulation	Rises to average 100–175/min.	Range from 110–180 plus high rates indicate variation in orgasmic intensity	Return to normal

Sexual Response Cycle of the Human Female – Genital Reaction

	I. Excitement Phase	II. Plateau Phase	III. Orgasmic Phase	IV. Resolution Phase
Blood Pressure	Elevation parallels rising tension	Elevation rise above normal by: Systolic: 20–60 mm Hg. Diastolic: 10–20 mm Hg.	Elevations rise above normal by: Systolic: 30–80 mm Hg. of mercury Diastolic 20–40 mm	Returns to normal
Labia Majora	Lifts up and out—away from vagina—in woman who never had a child. Moves slightly away from midline in woman who has children	May become engorged with blood during prolonged phase	No observed reaction	Returns to normal slowly.
Labia Minora	Slight thickening and expansion that extends vagina outward by 1 cm.	Vivid color changes ranging from bright red to deep wine. Signals impending orgasm.	No observed reaction	Color subsides to normal light pink in 10–15 sec. Returns to normal size slowly
Clitoris	Tip of clitoris (glans) swells. Shaft elongates and its diameter increases Clitoral color deepens due to extra blood	Clitoris withdraws and retracts against pubic bone and under hood.	No observed changes	Returns to normal position 5–10 sec. after orgasm; slower return to normal size and color
Vagina	Vaginal lubrication appears 10–30 sec. after initiation of any form of sexual stimulation. Vaginal barrel expands and distends. Vaginal wall color deepens markedly	Orgasmic platform develops in outer third of vagina. Gross distension by blood reduces the size of opening by 1/3. Inner 2/3 of vaginal barrel widens and deepens	Orgasmic platform contracts at .8-second intervals for 5–12 times. After first 3–6 times, contractions slow down and are less intense	Swelling and engorgement of orgasmic platform rapidly subsides, vaginal wall relaxes and slowly (15–20 min) returns to normal color
Uterus	Uterus begins to elevate to upright position from anterior one. Uterine muscles show response to stimulation	Full uterine elevation producing tenting effect over vagina. Increased reaction of uterus to stimulation	Contraction of uterus starts at top and spreads down to cervix; parallels the intensity of orgasm. Usually begins 2–4 seconds after she is aware of orgasm	Widening of cervical opening continues for 20–30 min. Cervix dips into seminal pool. Uterus returns to normal position

Sexual Response Cycle of the Human Male—Extragenital Reaction

	I. Excitement Phase	II. Plateau Phase	III. Orgasmic Phase	IV. Resolution Phase
Breasts	Nipples erect (inconsistent—may be delayed till second phase)	Nipples erect and turgid (inconsistent)	No observed change	Slow return to normal
Sex Flush (Not always present)	No observed reaction	Raised, red rash late in phase (inconsistent; starts on upper abdomen, spreads to chest, neck, face, and maybe arms)	Well-developed rash, parallels intensity of orgasm (estimated at 25% incidence)	Rapidly disappears in reverse order of appearance
Muscle Tension	Voluntary muscles tense; involuntary show some signs, testes begin to elevate, abdomen and rib spaces tense	Increase of both voluntary and involuntary tension; semispastic contractions of face, abdomen, and rib musculature	Loss of voluntary control. Involuntary contractions and spasm of muscle groups	May take up to 5 minutes to subside
Rectum	No observed reaction	Voluntary contraction of rectal sphincter (inconsistent)	Involuntary contraction of rectal sphincter at 8-second intervals.	No observed changes
Respiratory Rate	No observed reaction	Reaction appears late in phase	Rate rises to as much as 40 per minute. Intensity and duration indicates sexual tension	Resolves during refractory period
Heart Rate	Increases parallel to rising tension regardless of technique	Rates range from 100–115 beats per minute	Rates range from 110–180 beats per minute	Returns to normal
Blood Pressure	Elevates directly parallel to rising tension regardless of technique of stimulation	Elevates from normal by Systolic: 20–80 mm Hg. Diastolic: 10–40 mm Hg.	Elevates from normal by Systolic: 40–100 mm Hg. Diastolic: 20–50 mm Hg.	Returns to normal

Sexual Response Cycle of the Human Male – Genital Reaction

	I. Excitement Phase	II. Plateau Phase	III. Orgasmic Phase	IV. Resolution Phase
Penis	Rapidly becomes erect; may be partially lost and regained during prolonged phase·or impaired by introduction of non-sexual stimulation	Increase of circumference at coronal ridge. Color deepens at coronal ridge (in estimated 20% of men)	Expulsive contraction entire length of penis at 0.8 sec. intervals. After first 3–4, frequency and force lessen. Minor contractions continue for several seconds	Two-stage return to normal 1. rapid loss of congestion to 1–1½ times enlargement 2. Slowly subsides to prearousal size
Scrotum	Loses its folds and free movements; sac constricts, becomes congested and appears tense	No specific reactions	No specific reactions	Rapid loss of tense appearance; return of folds and free movement sometimes delayed
Testes	Spermatic cord shortens, causing testes to partially lift toward body	Testes enlarge to 50% increase. The longer this phase lasts the greater the increase in size due to congestion. May be 100% full elevation of testes, particularly the left or lower testicle signals impending ejaculation	No recorded reaction	Return to normal size and position in relaxed scrotum may occur rapidly or slowly, depending on length of plateau phase
Secondary organs (Vas Deferens, Prostate, Seminal Vesicle, and Ejaculatory Duct	No observed changes	No observed changes	Secondary organs contract creating sense of pending ejaculation, initiates ejaculatory process.	No observed changes
Cowper's Glands)	No observed changes	Emits 2–3 drops of mucoid fluid containing active sperm	No observed changes	No observed changes

(All charts adapted from Masters and Johnson, *Human Sexual Response*, Little, Brown & Co., Boston, 1966)

In the resolution phase, following ejaculation, the penis usually reduces quickly to about half its erect dimensions, then more slowly to its unstimulated size. During the few minutes immediately after ejaculation, the glans of the penis may be painfully sensitive to touch. The scrotal sac gradually returns to its relaxed state, and the testes descend.

The majority of men are incapable of another erection for a period of time after ejaculation. However, the minimum time interval required before repeated male erection and orgasm varies greatly, both among different men and for the same man at different times. It may range from minutes to days. This time interval increases with the age of the man and with general physical or emotional fatigue. It decreases with the degree of original sexual arousal, the degree of sexual restimulation after ejaculation, and the period of sexual restraint prior to the first ejaculation. If the man is young, has been without sexual release for some time, or is restimulated after ejaculation, he may be ready for further sexual intercourse within just a few minutes.

Nocturnal Emissions   Nocturnal emissions, commonly called "wet dreams," are involuntary discharges of semen, often accompanied by sexual dreams. Almost all males experience these emissions at some time. They are perfectly harmless and serve to relieve the pressure of fluid in the seminal vesicles if no other sexual outlet is available. Women may also come to orgasm in dream states.

Techniques of Intercourse   It is not the intention of this book to give detailed instructions for achieving sexual satisfaction, because attempts to follow such instructions can hinder rather than help a couple in attaining their goal. We will, instead, give a few general comments that may or may not be useful to a particular couple. We feel that a good sexual relationship can be achieved if each partner has an adequate knowledge of sexual psychology and physiology, a positive attitude toward sex, and a concern for the sexual satisfaction of the partner. Open and uninhibited discussion of sexual desires and responses is more important than any effort to follow "rules" in a book. Each partner should feel free to tell the other which practices increase sexual enjoyment and which decrease it. An interest in sexual experimentation is good, especially after several years of marriage. If a couple is satisfied with their conventional sexual patterns, they may not feel the need to experiment with the varied positions and practices that they might find in diverse books. As long as open, honest communication exists, and the couple is aware that their own desires and interests may change with the passing years, then they should practice whatever is comfortable for both of them.

Preparing for Intercourse   There is no set routine that is universally necessary or useful in preparing for intercourse. The sexual responses of individual men and women are highly variable and individual, so a technique that is ideal for one couple might have no value for another.

It is common, however, for the woman to need a longer period of stimulation before intercourse than the man in order to prevent pain upon first penetration and increase her chance of achieving orgasm. While a man may attain erection in a few seconds, a woman may need several minutes to become fully aroused and produce adequate vaginal lubrication.

Most women enjoy a few minutes of sex play before actual penetration of the vagina as it prepares them physically and psychologically for successful intercourse. Premature penetration is a complaint expressed by many women. Every woman will discover particular types of caresses and stimuli that provide her with the most intensive sensations, and she should freely communicate this information to her partner. Among the types of sexplay that stimulate many women are kissing various parts of the body, gently fondling or tightly squeezing the breasts, lightly rubbing, pinching, pulling, sucking, or lip-biting the nipples, squeezing or lightly rubbing the buttocks, lightly stroking the insides of the thighs, and manipulation of the genital organs. Genital manipulation is mentioned last because many women prefer to become somewhat aroused before this begins. Many books recommend direct manipulation of the clitoris, but William Masters and Virginia Johnson (*Human Sexual Response*, 1966) suggest that indirect clitoral manipulaton by stimulating the mons area is preferred by most women as direct clitoral stimulation can be painful. Women who are fatigued or under emotional stress may need more than usual stimulation prior to intercourse, or may not need to have intercourse.

One important test of whether a woman is ready for penetration of the vagina is the extent of lubrication of the vaginal walls. The man can readily determine this with his fingers. If a woman is ready for penetration before the vagina is adequately lubricated, the penis can be lubricated with one of the water-soluble vaginal jellies that are readily available in drug or grocery stores.

Men similarly respond to a great variety of stimuli, such as kissing; licking and kissing the ears; body kisses, and oral and manual stimulation of the nipples, penis, scrotum and testes, and anus. In sex play, any practice accepted and enjoyed by both partners has its place.

In all types and phases of sexual relationships, open and honest communication is important. Many people are very reluctant to talk about sex, even to the ex-

tent that they fail to tell their partners just what pleases or displeases them sexually. Therapists report many cases where the primary cause of sexual problems is lack of communication between partners. It is of utmost importance that couples develop the ability to openly and honestly communicate their sexual feelings.

Sexual Intercourse   There are almost innumerable different positions that have been successfully used in sexual intercourse. There has been a tendency in many of the "sex manuals" to stress positions that place the penis in direct contact with the clitoris, based on the assumption that if the clitoris is the most sexually responsive part of the female body then it should receive direct stimulation. But the research of Masters and Johnson and the personal experience of many couples have indicated that such contact actually decreases the sexual pleasure of both the man and the woman. Sexual positions in which the clitoris receives indirect stimulation are more satisfactory for the majority of women and probably all men. Any position that allows a full penetration of the vagina by the erect penis will often provide an adequate amount of indirect clitoral stimulation. There are some women who cannot reach orgasm by any indirect method. With such women sexual positions or methods of stimulation should be chosen that provide satisfaction.

A couple who try many different positions for intercourse will probably find several that seem particularly good for them and will probably use all of these positions from time to time. Some of the more common basic positions are discussed briefly below. Each of these positions has many variations.
1. *The man-above position.*   This is probably the most common position in use in the United States. It seems to be the most natural and comfortable posi-

tion for many couples. The woman lies on her back with her legs spread apart, either drawn up or straight out. The man lies facing her, between her thighs. If guidance of the penis into the vagina is necessary, either the man or woman can give this assistance. This position allows most couples to kiss freely, but is more restrictive of breast manipulation than some of the other positions.

2. *The woman-above position.* In this common position, the man lies on his back while the woman lies above and facing him. Some couples roll from the man-above position to the woman-above positon, or vice versa. Some women can achieve orgasm more easily in the woman-above position by controlling the pelvic thrusts while the man lies more or less passively.

3. *Face-to-face positions.* There are many of these positions. They offer several advantages. Neither partner must support the weight of the other, so they are good for prolonged sexual connections. Kissing is easy, as is breast manipulation or any other type of caress desired.

4. *Rear-entry positions.* There are several different rear-entry positions. The woman may lie on her side or face down or may kneel on her hands and knees. In any case, the man approaches from behind, passing his erect penis between her legs and into her vagina. These positions facilitate breast manipulation, but, of course, kissing is more difficult.

5. *Other positions.* The variety of sexual positions is limited only by the imagination and agility of the couple. Many couples occasionally enjoy a more unusual position, for variety in their love-making. The sitting positions are enjoyed by some couples. In one of these, the man lies on his back while the woman sits astride him, feet forward.

This position allows very deep vaginal penetration. In other sitting positions, the man may sit on a chair or the edge of a bed while the woman sits astride him. Some couples even enjoy intercourse while standing up, using front or rear entry. There is no reason why any position that affords mutual pleasure should not be used.

After the penis has been fully inserted into the vagina, a man is often at the very peak of his sexual arousal and near orgasm. In order to prevent premature ejaculation, many couples find it desirable to lie together quietly for a short time before beginning the pelvic thrusts of intercourse. By lying quietly at this time and any subsequent time that orgasm seems near, many men can delay ejaculation.

One criterion in the choice of positions is whether they allow for greater or lesser penetration. Depending on differences in length of penis and vagina, the level of sex drive, and the absence or presence of pain during a given lovemaking, the woman may or may not desire greater penetration. Subtle changes in position can allow for this. For instance when the woman is on her back she may, after initial penetration, bring her legs together to prevent too deep a penetration. A creative couple can usually find the preferable position for a given lovemaking technique.

Certain marriage manuals place a great emphasis on the importance of simultaneous orgasm. We feel that simultaneous orgasm is not an important goal in sexual intercourse and that concentration of efforts toward this goal may decrease the pleasure received by each partner, rather than increase it. Since the orgasm of the male is usually assured (except in impotence, as discussed later), all efforts should be concentrated toward helping the woman achieve orgasm. However, a man may maintain even prolonged erection in lovemaking without reaching an orgasm. As with the female, intercourse without orgasm can on occasion be satisfying for the man.

Women vary in the ease with which they can achieve orgasm. The difference may be either physical or psychological, but it is very real. Every study made has shown that significant numbers of women can achieve orgasm only with difficulty, if at all. Kinsey's classic study indicated that after 5 years of marriage, only 40 percent of wives reached orgasm over 90 percent of the time, and that 17 percent of wives never reached orgasm. After 20 years of marriage, 11 percent of wives still had failed to reach orgasm in intercourse. More recent studies indicate that the young women of today are much more successful in achieving orgasm than those of 1953, but that many women still reach orgasm only with difficulty.

The majority of women do not expect to achieve orgasm with every intercourse. But the woman who reaches orgasm too infrequently is likely to lose her enthusiasm for sex. The man who wants to keep his sexual relationship happy and vigorous should try to satisfy his partner as often as possible.

There is no single pattern of orgasm that is best for every couple, though many couples find, through experimentation, a pattern that seems best for them. Many couples develop a pattern whereby the woman reaches one or more orgasms first, followed by the ejaculation of the man. In other couples, the woman finds that the stimulus of the penis throbbing in ejaculation is just what she needs to push her to orgasm.

Oral and Anal Sex Many couples greatly enjoy oral and anal sex practices, whereas other couples never even experiment with them, perhaps feeling they might be unhealthy, abnormal, or immoral. Actually, there is no medical or moral reason to avoid oral or anal sex, and many couples or individuals who try these practices enjoy them and at least occasionally include them in their lovemaking.

Oral and anal sex are useful in adding variety and new heights of excitement to lovemaking and in stimulating a less responsive sex partner. Oral practices include fellatio (oral stimulation of the penis), cunnilingus (oral stimulation of the female organs), and "69" (combination of fellatio and cunnilingus). Oral sex may be a preliminary to genital coitus or may proceed to orgasm by either or both partners.

Anal practices include insertion of a finger into the anus of either partner, prior to or during coitus, and anal intercourse in which the penis is inserted into the female's anus (pederasty). In the latter practice certain precautions are necessary. It is usually advisable to lubricate the penis with a vaginal jelly to prevent tearing the delicate anal tissues. A further precaution is necessary—if the anus is tense (when the person fears pain), it must be slowly relaxed, or penetration may in fact be painful. Many physicians also recommend washing the penis if vaginal intercourse is to follow anal penetration to avoid possible vaginal infection with rectal bacteria. As in oral sex, anal sex may progress to orgasm or lead to vaginal coitus.

Oral and anal stimulation are especially useful whenever there is a low level of arousal. Such may be true with some older males. A man reaches his peak of sexual desire and capacity at about age 18 and gradually declines thereafter, while a woman may not reach her peak of sexual desire until about the ages of 35 to 45. Thus, in middle age the desire of the woman may exceed the capacity of the man to fulfill it, especially if he is several years older than her. In such cases, the

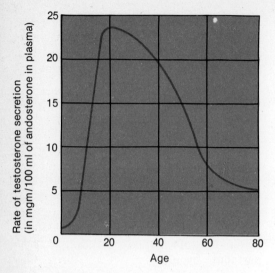

The rate of testosterone secretion in the male, by age. Note peak at age 17–18.

woman's skillful oral and hand stimulation of the man's penis, scrotum, and anus will often assist him in attaining and maintaining an erection at times when he might not otherwise. However, in the adult male sexual arousal is not tied completely to the levels of testosterone. Men who have been castrated as adults are able to respond to sexual arousal, though at a diminished level.

Frequency of Intercourse The frequency of sexual intercourse is a source of conflict in many relationships. In almost any marriage, there will be times when one partner would like sexual intercourse and the other partner is either not interested or incapable of responding. Such situations may place a great burden on the marital relationship unless both partners are understanding and tolerant. Some of the sex manuals have portrayed the ideal relationship as being a continuous sexual spree with each orgasm coming bigger and better than the previous one. In reality, sex is only a part of any total relationship, and

the success of a couple's sexual relationship is often a reflection of their total ability to communicate and relate to each other.

It is very difficult to make direct comparisons of the basic sex drive of men and women, due to the fundamental differences of these drives. The woman who is sexually arousable must be sensitive to tactile stimuli and be able to enjoy the psychological awareness of penile penetration. She experiences compelling sexual drives that demand release, particularly if she becomes sexually aroused, with blood engorging her genital organs.

The man experiences an inherent physical sexual stimulus. The accumulation of fluids within the seminal vesicles and prostate gland acts as an internal sexual stimulus. The longer these fluids build up, the greater becomes the need for their release. The man who has not ejaculated for an extended period of time may experience an extraordinary level of sexual tension.

Various research projects have indicated that the average man would like to engage in intercourse a little more often than would his female sex partner. Of course, in a particular couple there may be a great similarity in sexual desire or a very great difference, with either the man or the woman having the greater desire. Further, the effects of cultural and social factors on both the male and female sex drives cannot be objectively measured.

There is no particular "normal" frequency of intercourse that is most desirable. Among happy and physically healthy couples, the frequency of intercourse ranges from once a month or less to several times a day. Statistically, the average frequency, though this should not be interpreted as a goal for an individual couple, is between two and three times a week. A young couple is likely to exceed this frequency, whereas an older couple may not engage in intercourse that often.

If disagreement over frequency of intercourse is creating conflict within a relationship, each partner should try to evaluate the situation, rather than just fighting about it. Let us first consider the more likely situation—a couple wherein the man desires intercourse more often than does the woman. First, there are several things the man should ask himself: Am I keeping myself physically attractive? Am I pleasant and loving with my partner at all times, or just in bed? Do I spend enough time in precoital sex-play? Do I seriously try to help her reach orgasm as often as possible? (The woman who is too often disappointed soon learns to avoid frustration by avoiding sex.) Are the conditions right for privacy and freedom from interruption during intercourse? Is she inhibited by fear of pregnancy? (Many women fail to respond because either consciously or subconsciously they fear pregnancy. A change in contraceptive method may be helpful.) Am I expecting too much of her? Few men appreciate the amount of energy the modern woman must spend on a career, housework, child care, and community activities. There is often just too little energy left for sexual activity. In the past, the tired woman often took a passive role in sexual intercourse, but today many men expect their wives to take an active part. The woman, herself, may expect to reach orgasm if she engages in intercourse and may be reluctant to begin intercourse if she feels she lacks the energy to achieve orgasm.

The woman in this situation might ask a few questions of herself: Why do I refuse him? Am I trying to punish him for something that is beyond his control? Do I honestly find him a satisfactory sex partner? Would I be more confident with another contraceptive method? Have I honestly explained to him why I sometimes refuse him?

The situation in which the woman wants intercourse more often than the man is more difficult, since the man must attain an erection and generally take a fairly active role in order to satisfy her. Again, the woman might consider possible reasons for his reluctance. Does she try to be sexually appealing? Are her demands excessive? As a man grows older, his biological capacity for sex diminishes. The man in this situation is in a particularly bad emotional position. He is faced with the demand and perhaps derision of his partner in addition to his own feelings of inadequacy. One of the most important needs of the ego is a sense of sexual adequacy. This man may easily develop anxieties that will increase his sexual problems. The man who feels sexually inadequate is often reluctant to make any attempt at intercouse, for fear of impotence. He avoids the risk of ego-damaging impotence by avoiding sex. This situation becomes worse with the passage of time, so prompt efforts should be made to remedy it. A physician should be first consulted to rule out the possibility of any physical cause. If no physical cause is found (most impotence is psychological), then a qualified marriage counselor should be consulted.

Compulsive Sexuality   Common among both sexes are people whose sex lives consist of an endless series of brief encounters with ever-changing partners. Seldom is any level of emotional intimacy established, and there is often a hollow or "something-is-missing" feeling. Although these people may engage in seemingly normal intercourse quite frequently, they often gain no emotional satisfaction from it.

In males, this problem is sometimes called the *Don Juan complex*—if the emphasis is on the number of different sexual partners—or *satyriasis*—if the emphasis is on the frequency of sexual contact. The term *nymphomaniac* is sometimes applied to women who seem to have unusually high numbers of heterosexual encounters.

Several personality traits are commonly associated with compulsive sexuality. The foremost is probably a feeling (which can be unconscious) of sexual or personal inadequacy. The person needs to constantly "prove" his or her ability to attract lovers and function sexually. But regardless of the number of lovers attracted or orgasms reached, the fear of inadequacy remains.

Fear of intimacy is also common. Many people, perhaps as a result of past emotional hurts or their feelings of inadequacy, lack the confidence required to establish a close relationship with another person. Lacking intimacy, their sexual relationships always seem incomplete, so the search for satisfaction must continue.

Many people have been raised in sexually repressive atmospheres. Sexual guilt or inhibition, perhaps as a result of childhood conditioning, may act to deny sexual satisfaction, even though full physiological orgasm may occur.

Finally, compulsive sexuality may be a part of a broader antisocial or sociopathic personality. Someone with an antisocial personality is unable to postpone immediate pleasure or gratification of an impulse, lacks the capacity for maintaining a close relationship with another person, and feels no guilt or anxiety over antisocial acts. Such a person would probably have a history of job problems and regular run-ins with the law in addition to compulsive sexuality.

Like other forms of sexual dysfunction, compulsive sexuality can often be treated successfully by a qualified therapist. Treatment may involve building a sense of personal or sexual adequacy, developing the ability to establish intimacy with another person, or extinguishing feelings of guilt or inhibition. People with antiso-cial personalities generally require more basic therapy since their compulsive sexuality is just one symptom of a larger personality disorder.

Anxieties Many people, more sexually inexperienced ones in particular, suffer needless anxieties over the appearance of certain parts of their body. They are concerned lest the shape and or size of their breasts, vagina, or penis, or fears of pain during intercourse, interfere with their sexual attractiveness or in some way limit their sexual expectations.

Male Anxieties Many young men suffer needless anxiety regarding the size of their penis. Some worry that it may be too small to satisfy a woman. Some fear that it may be too large to be accommodated by the vagina. All of these fears are really groundless because of the nature of the vagina and of female sexual sensitivity. The size of the penis and whether or not it is circumcised has little to do with the sexual satisfaction of the man or of the woman. Sexual technique, experience, and care about the partner's needs are the important things.

The vagina can accommodate a penis of virtually any size. Masters and Johnson found that even in very small women the vagina, when sexually aroused, lengthened sufficiently to accept the largest fully erect penis. Thus there need be no apprehensions over sexual intercourse between a man with a large penis and a woman with a small vagina.

In the case of a man with a short penis, it should be remembered that there are very few sensory receptors in the deeper part of the vagina. These receptors are concentrated in the clitoris and labia and outer vagina. As a result, the sensory satisfaction a woman receives will be as great with a short as with a long penis.

Some young men even worry about the fact that their penis seems to curve (most of them do curve) or have some other irregularity. Every man should realize that the size or shape of the penis is of negligible importance in sexual intercourse.

Female Anxieties Because of the erotic significance our culture has attached to a woman's breasts, some women carry undue concern over the development of their breasts. Breast size has no bearing on a woman's responsiveness. Flat-chested women report as much response to sexual stimulation as big-bosomed ones. The size of the breast has no relation to its sensitivity. Nor is there any relationship between breast size and the consistency of attaining orgasm, or to the frequency of intercourse. The onset of breast development relates in no way to the woman's ability to achieve orgasm.

Certain myths regarding menstruation and pregnancy may frighten women. There is no physiological reason for refraining from sexual intercourse during the menstrual discharge, nor will it cause distress. In fact, sexual activity during that time may provide relief from pain and discomfort. Masters and Johnson showed that few women object to sexual activity during menstruation.

Sexual activity during pregnancy does not need to be avoided. Many women experience the same or an increase in erotic feelings during the first and second trimesters of pregnancy. Such feelings may decline during the third trimester, but intercourse does not need to be discontinued until some time during the third trimester.

Some women with no coital experience hold unconscious, irrational fears of mutilation from penetration of the penis. With sufficient partner tenderness and sex play, the entry of the penis brings great pleasure to the woman in the absence of some pathological condition or psychological problem. In fact, during sexual arousal a woman is less sensitive to pain than she is when not sexually aroused.

Sex in Menstruation, Pregnancy, and Old Age There is no important medical reason for refraining from sexual intercourse during menstruation. Most couples do, however, avoid intercourse during the 2 days of heaviest flow for personal reasons. But during the 2 or 3 days of limited flow that follow, intercourse may be enjoyed by both the man and the woman. Some women seem to enjoy especially intercourse at this time due perhaps to their hormone levels or the freedom from fear of pregnancy.

Sexual intercourse can usually be continued in pregnancy until about two or three weeks before delivery, unless some condition arises that causes the physician to recommend against it. Some women find their sexual drive increased during pregnancy, while others experience a decrease. Intercourse should definitely be discontinued as soon as it causes the woman any pain or discomfort. Following childbirth, the couple should refrain from intercourse for two to three weeks, or until any torn or cut tissue has healed. This prevents infection or the tearing of stitches. During the period before and after delivery when intercourse is prohibited, the woman may wish to provide her partner with periodic sexual release by caressing him to orgasm.

Old age need be no barrier to an active sexual life and, according to Kinsey et al. (1948, 1953) and Masters and Johnson (1966), many older persons continue to be sexually active, though the frequency of activity drops considerably. Those individuals who were most sexually active in their youth are generally more active in their old age. In both sexes, a continuity of sexual activity is important. It is easier to remain sexually active than it is to resume sexual activity after a long period without it.

Common Sexual Problems

The sexual relationships and even the marriages of many couples are damaged or destroyed by problems of sexual function. Most of these problems are actually of psychological origin and can be overcome through mutual understanding, open communication, factual knowledge, and, if necessary, professional help. In this section, we will consider a few of the more common sexual dysfunctions.

Female Orgasmic Dysfunction The variety of problems related and unrelated to female sexual function has long been known, incorrectly, as *frigidity*. The term has been used as a catch-all. At one extreme it describes the woman who, though responsive, never displays or feels any sexual interest or arousal. At the other extreme it could describe the woman who does not attain orgasm on every occasion of intercourse, or the woman who does not respond instantly to a man's sexual advances. The term *frigidity* has been used both for the woman who is rarely sexually aroused as well as for the woman who is easily aroused but seldom or never to the point of orgasm.

Masters and Johnson have thus discarded the rather meaningless word *frigidity* for the more descriptive phrase *female orgasmic dysfunction*. According to them, the phrase should be used for the woman who is not able to achieve orgasm in her sexual response. (William Masters and Virginia Johnson, *Human Sexual Inadequacy*, 1970.)

The nonorgasmic woman can be placed in one of several categories. One, the woman who has never achieved an orgasm in her life through any method of sexual stimulation, suffers from *primary orgasmic dysfunction*. Two, the woman who has experienced at least one orgasm in her life (by coitus, masturbation, or some other form of sexual stimulation), but who no longer experiences orgasm, suffers from *situational orgasmic dysfunction*.

A third example would be the woman who can regularly achieve orgasm through masturbation, but is unable to in intercourse. Although this might be looked upon by some as a dysfunction, how it is viewed depends on a woman's expectations. If she is satisfied in her relationship with her sex partner, does not feel frustration, and feels free in alleviating her sex tensions through masturbation, such behavior can be considered completely normal.

When orgasmic dysfunction seems to be a problem, the first step taken should be a physical examination to rule out any physical cause of interference with sexual pleasure. While such cases are not common, a physical problem such as a tough, intact hymen can make intercourse painful or impossible. Such physical problems can usually be easily corrected. Another problem with which a physician can help is fear of pregnancy. Many women are inhibited in their sexual responses by conscious or unconscious fear of pregnancy. The change to a birth control method in which a woman has greater confidence can often improve her sexual responsiveness.

Many women (and men as well) suffer from long-term residual sexual inhibitions as carryovers from childhood indoctrination by parents, religious groups, and even other children that sexual pleasure is in some way wrong or immoral. If such inhibitions are deeply ingrained into the personality, professional counseling may be necessary.

But many women who do not suffer from obvious conflicts still do not respond adequately. For example, a woman may find that she is "turned off" by her husband, yet is highly "turned on" by other men. In such a case, the cause must lie either in some trait or traits of the man to which she does not respond, or in the quality of the total relationship between them. Certainly, when the relationship between a man and a woman starts to deteriorate, the sexual responsiveness of the woman toward that man is often quickly extinguished.

A common complaint of women is that "the romance is gone." The various media of communications have led many women to believe that marriage should be all youth, beauty, glamour, and excitement. This picture does not match well with the man who comes home from work wanting his dinner, the newspaper, and his favorite television program. He wants to go to bed, have intercourse, roll over, and go to sleep. As a result, many women complain of a lack of intimacy, feeling used and useless, and resent being merely a sexual object. The outcome is that they are no longer sexually responsive (at least to that man). Their anger and resentment is expressed in withdrawal.

Impotence and Premature Ejaculation Impotence is the inability to attain or maintain erection of the penis. Premature ejaculation is male orgasm and loss of erection before the reasonable sexual desires of the sex partner are satisfied. Impotence and premature ejaculation are the most common forms of male sexual dysfunction. These problems are often related to one another and, according to some definitions, premature ejaculation is a form of impotence.

Impotence, like frigidity, is generally the result of emotional, rather than physical causes. In cases of severe or persistent impotence, however, a physical examination should be obtained to rule out possible physical causes.

Impotence exists in all degrees. In its most severe form, called *primary impotence*, the penis never, under any circumstances, becomes erect nor has it ever, during the life of the man. This is the form of impotence that is most likely to have an organic (physical) cause. This is especially true if the penis is never erect during the rapid eye movement (REM) or dream phase of sleep or on awakening from REM sleep.

Much more common is a transient or secondary form of impotence in which erection sometimes occurs, though not necessarily when intercourse is desired, or ceases to occur in a formerly potent male. This form of impotence is almost always the result of emotional factors. There are probably few men who escape having at least a few episodes of transient impotence at some time during their lives. Guilt, anger, conflict, anxiety, jealousy, depression, fear, and hostility are among the emotions that commonly result in impotence.

The incidence of transient impotence increases with age, though younger men are certainly not immune from this problem. The first incident of impotence usually occurs during a period of emotional stress, and is especially likely to occur following heavy drinking. Any kind of emotional problem may be involved, but job problems and love conflicts are very common causes of transient impotence. Also, fatigue must not be overlooked as a cause of temporary impotence. Other frequent causes of impotence are anxiety growing out of fear of sex as something bad and immoral that may be punished (a common problem in extramarital affairs); feelings of inadequacy as a man; and excessive fear of or hostility toward women.

The reaction of a woman to a man's impotence will greatly influence his success in that and future attempts at intercourse. Her immediate feelings may be those of hurt and rejection and her natural impulse may be to hurt in return, perhaps making fun of the man, ridiculing him, or accusing him of having an affair. Such a reaction will produce enough feeling of anxiety and inadequacy to practically insure that the next attempt at intercourse will also fail. On the other hand, a reassuring partner response, perhaps including gentle hand or oral stimulation of the male organs, may result in immediate potency or in any case will not interfere with future efforts at lovemaking.

Premature ejaculation, while seeming to be just the opposite of impotence, may have similar emotional causes. Even fewer men are likely to get through life without ever experiencing an incident of premature ejaculation. In fact, under certain conditions, premature ejaculation must be considered an entirely normal and predictable event. For example, it is unrealistic to expect a young man who has been without sexual release for many days to withhold ejaculation while the partner thrusts vigorously in efforts to achieve orgasm. Similarly, the first attempt at intercourse with a new and highly exciting partner may be normally expected to result in premature ejaculation.

How do we define *premature*? Certainly, ejaculation before penetration of the vagina is premature, as is ejaculation immediately thereafter. But what about ejaculation after the woman has had one orgasm when she would really like to have three? What about the woman who takes an hour to reach orgasm? Obviously, there can be no clear-cut definition.

How do you distinguish "normal" premature ejaculation from the "problem" variety? The distinction here is that if a man has regular and frequent intercourse with the same partner, and it often ends in premature ejaculation, it is a problem. In such a case there may be underlying psychological causes, which may be quite

similar to those of impotence. Examples: hostility toward the woman, in which premature ejaculation is used to deny her sexual satisfaction; guilt about sex, in which premature ejaculation is used to "get it over with"; feelings of sexual inadequacy, in which there is a rush to prove that the penis is still working; fear; and love conflicts.

A variety of solutions for the problem of premature ejaculation are available. Of prime importance, as in impotence, is for both the man and woman to minimize the problem, rather than making a big issue of it. If the premature ejaculation is of one of the "normal" types described, then the male is likely to be young enough and highly enough aroused that a second erection will soon follow the first and, with seminal pressure reduced, prolonged intercourse should be possible. Regular sex partners can learn to delay male orgasm by both holding very still when premature ejaculation threatens. This is especially useful just after penetration when premature ejaculation is most likely to occur. Some doctors recommend that a topical anesthetic ointment be applied over the glans (head) of the penis to delay ejaculation. The stimulus to the penis can similarly be reduced by wearing a condom (rubber). Masters and Johnson, in *Human Sexual Inadequacy*, recommend an "exercise" for premature ejaculation in which the woman's hand stimulates the male penis almost to the point of orgasm, then, with the thumb and forefinger, tightly squeezes the shaft of the penis about an inch below the glans. Done repeatedly, this often solves long-term problems of premature ejaculation. A more basic approach is psychotherapy. Since the more persistent cases of premature ejaculation are of psychological origin, this is sometimes the only method of treatment that can produce lasting results.

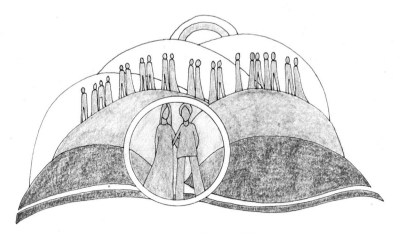

14

A PERSONAL AND SOCIAL INSTITUTION

People are still getting married. In fact, they are doing so in near-record numbers, despite the predictions during the past few years that conventional marriage was on its last legs. While many correctly choose not to marry, the majority of young people still have faith in the institution of marriage and are willing to try it, though perhaps in a form different from their parents' marriages.

At the same time that more people are marrying, a record number of existing marriages are ending in divorce. Many divorces result from marriages that should never have taken place—the seeds of failure were present at the time of the marriage. Marriage should be entered into rationally as well as emotionally. Both individuals should objectively evaluate their own readiness for marriage and the nature of their relationship.

Are You Ready for Marriage?

In many ways, readiness for marriage is a subjective quality. There is no single criterion of age or physical development or emotional makeup that qualifies one for matrimony. However, certain objective standards taken together may serve as an index of marital readiness.

Age at Marriage The age at which a couple marries allows one to predict the chances that the marriage will succeed. Many studies have shown that the level of satisfaction and success in marriage increases with the age of the couple at the time of marriage. Emotional conflict, sexual problems, money problems, in-law trouble, and divorce are all much more common among those couples who marry in their teens. Marriages where the husband was in his teens are particularly unhappy.

Some people feel pushed to marry at a fairly early age to avoid getting "left out." Such fear is not warranted because at any age, numerous individuals eligible for marriage will be found. In fact, some excellent marriage prospects delay marriage for several years in order to reach educational or career goals. The national average age at first marriage is 23 years for men and 21 years for women, and is rising. This statistic may reflect the fact that an increasing number of couples live together before marriage.

One of the sources of problems with young marriages is that many people greatly change their value systems and life-styles between the ages of 16 and 22. During this period, one's interests, tastes, ideals, standards, and goals often change completely. If people marry before this change, there is a strong possibility that they will no longer meet each other's emotional needs six years later.

A related problem is that early marriage often interferes with the development of a mature philosophy. There is a tendency for the intellectual growth of an individual to stop at the time of marriage. This can be prevented, of course, but many young people fall into a deep philosophical and intellectual rut from which they never escape. Or one partner grows while the other stagnates, a sure formula for unhappiness.

Emotional Maturity The emotional demands of marriage are much greater than those a couple experiences during dating. Thus, an important requirement for marriage is emotional maturity. This generally increases with age, but some individuals remain emotionally adolescent even though they have legally become adults.

Before marriage, a person should be as free as possible of emotional maladjustments, such as moodiness, jealousy, anxiety, depression, and insecurity. The presence of such traits in a marriage can be destructive. A person who is subject to such maladjustment should seek qualified professional counsel.

The truly mature person has skill in establishing and maintaining good interpersonal relationships. He or she recognizes the needs of others and is willing to assume some responsibility for meeting these needs. Each partner in a marriage must have such a concern for the other if happiness is to result.

Social Maturity Social maturity develops through social interaction. Before marriage, social maturity should be built through dating many different individuals. This gives a better basis for the selection of a marriage partner and helps satisfy social curiosity. The person whose dating is more restricted may later, after marriage, feel he or she has missed something and may try to compensate through extramarital affairs.

It is important to experience a period of single, independent life before marriage, a time of freedom between the dependence of living with one's parents and the responsibilities of marriage. It is only through living away from parents that one can really come to know oneself, develop full social competency, and learn to manage one's own affairs. A strong argument can be made that anyone who is too immature, insecure, or otherwise incompetent to live independently is, for the same reason, not ready for marriage. Many people, after enjoying their independence, feel a desire to "settle down" into marriage. Others find the single life permanently satisfying and prefer not to marry. There is absolutely no reason why anyone should feel an obligation to marry.

Financial Resources Although less important than the preceding personal characteristics, financial factors must be considered before marriage. The minimum amount of money a couple needs to live on is highly variable. Most young couples enter marriage without great amounts of money. But if either or both of the young married people is to be a student, there must be a careful evaluation of the marriage situation to avoid the unfortunate situation of an educational program terminated for financial reasons.

Often the parents of student couples offer some financial help. But the couple should evaluate this possiblity in terms of their sense of independence. If such help is going to be a source of conflict, then some other financial arrangement must be developed. If the couple is to rely on the earnings of the wife, then obviously it is important that a highly reliable method of contraception be used. A pregnancy in this situation would be a serious financial and emotional burden. Pregnancy may also interrupt the wife's studies, seriously delaying her career.

Because few couples ever have what they consider to be enough money, a couple's attitude toward money and how to use it is likely to be more important than the size of the paycheck. A given amount of spendable income for one couple may be sufficient to meet common interests, while the next couple may be suing for divorce because the same amount of money is not enough. The relation of income to happiness must be relative to expectations. When a couple feels committed to an occupational field where income is lower, they can be happy if they are content to live at that level. If, however, their expectations run higher than income, their marriage may be troubled.

Selecting for Happiness Chances of a happy marriage are determined by your own personal traits, those of your partner, and how these traits act upon each other. Consider, then, some of the traits to look for in a potential mate. Right away, let us dispel the notion of "the one and only" or the "marriage made in heaven." For every person there are thousands of potentially good mates. If the person you might be considering for marriage seems to have a serious deficiency in some respect, just keep looking. On the other hand, if no one seems to fit your ideal for marriage, you might well be overcritical or just not inclined towards marriage.

Positive Personality Traits By far the most important characteristic in a potential marriage partner is his or her personality. Some people have positive personality traits that enable them to enjoy life to its fullest and to bring joy to anyone in contact with them. Others are so burdened with negative reactions that their own happiness is impossible, as is that of anyone who must live with them. Traits that help produce happiness in marriage include the ability to adjust easily to changes in conditions, optimism, a sense of humor, an honest concern for the needs of others, a sense of ethics, and freedom from such negative traits as anxiety, depression, insecurity, and jealousy.

Mutual Need Satisfaction The happy and lasting marriage is one in which the needs of each individual are adequately satisfied. While the idea may not appeal to romantics, the basic reason why people marry is to satisfy their needs. A good marriage satisfies many needs—sex, love, companionship, security, and subtle psychological needs. Since everyone is unique in his or her psychological needs, the characterization of the imaginary ideal partner for each person is a highly individual matter. Only through knowing each other very well, over a long period of time and in a variety of situations (both pleasant and unpleasant), can two people learn whether they are able to fulfill each other's needs.

Genuine Mutual Love The distinction between genuine love and infatuation is not always clear. Infatuation is frequently a kind of substitute for love until a person has the capacity to love someone fully and deeply. It tends to involve sexual attraction more than personality attraction. Infatuation is unrealistic, a fantasy. The object of the infatuation is seen as a "dream mate," lacking any undesirable traits. Infatuation is often immediate, whereas love develops with time. Usually, infatuation wears off quickly. Yet it may, with time, develop into mature love.

A person truly in love is concerned with the loved one's happiness and well-being. He or she is tender, protecting, loyal, and is willing to sacrifice some pleasures in order to bring pleasure to the loved one. There is a desire to share ideas, emotions, goals, and experiences. Love continues to grow with the passage of time.

There should definitely be a strong sexual attraction between any persons considering marriage. It would be an unusual couple who would want to marry in the absence of a sexual attraction. However, many people mistake sexual attraction for love, when it is actually just a part of love. A couple can have a very good sexual relationship without loving each other, but such a relationship would make a poor basis for a happy marriage.

Now let's get back to the point about love as a factor in deciding to marry. Obviously, it is difficult to tell you what love is, though we have tried to demonstrate what love is not. Above all else, true mature love is the one factor that will inspire a couple to look at all the factors conducive to a happy marriage with care, and with respect for themselves and each other.

Hereditary Traits Some individuals carry obvious hereditary defects. Others seem perfectly normal, but come from families in which such defects are known to occur. The latter individuals may or may not be carrying undesirable hidden genes. If there is any question regarding the possibility of transmitting defective genes, it is wise to seek genetic counseling, either from a physician or a specially trained genetic counselor recommended by a physician. Any decision to marry and have children, marry and not have children, or not to marry should be based upon such guidance and not on the advice of well-meaning, but uninformed friends and relatives.

Agreement on Parenthood Any couple considering marriage should reveal their feelings about having children. Ideally, they should agree on whether they want children and, if so, how many. It is always unfortunate when a person who wants children marries one who would rather remain childless. Automatically, one or the other of them is destined to be unhappy. If there is serious disagreement on this matter, it would be a good idea for each individual to look for another mate.

If neither person wants children, there is no reason to feel guilty about a decision to remain childless. Studies have shown that children are not essential to happiness. In fact, they have been shown to place additional strain on already unhappy marriages. A couple need feel no obligation to themselves or to society to produce children. Many people now feel an obligation to limit the number of children produced.

Similarity in Background

It is important for any couple considering marriage to take a critical, objective look at their differences in personality and family background. These differences may be minor and insignificant or major and may have a great bearing on the marriage. Many studies have shown that the more similarities between two individuals, the greater their chances of marital success. Significant differences may involve age, nationality or ethnic background, economic status, education, intelligence, religion, or previous marital status. Most marriages can be successful despite these differences, if the couple is willing to work out the special problems involved.

Age

When there is a wide difference in age, the individuals must examine why they want to marry a person considerably older or younger. Is it the inability to find a partner close to one's own age? Is it the desire for immediate economic security? Is it a feeling of flattery at commanding the attention of a more mature or more youthful person? Is the older person seen as a "father" or "mother" figure? Does the older person need to dominate or the younger to be dominated? On the average, marriages are happiest when the man and woman are within a few years of each other

in age. However, if the marriage with a wide age gap fulfills a great need for each person, then such a marriage may also be happy.

Ethnic Differences

Marriages between members of different ethnic groups face the most difficult problems of any type of mixed marriage. Not only may there be problems within the marriage, but the couple may experience resentment and prejudice from family members and unenlightened members of society.

The internal problems in these marriages may revolve around customs, standards, and points of view. For example, the attitudes toward women and their rights, duties, and status may be quite different. Family patterns of authority and the role expected of each member may conflict. Attitudes on raising children and care of elderly relatives may be another area of disagreement. These problems do not appear in all mixed marriages, but such topics should be discussed objectively before marriage.

The problems caused by prejudices of family members and society are particularly frustrating, because they should not exist in an enlightened society. The source of many of these problems is the ethnocentric attitude of groups that guard their ethnic heritage to excess and often sincerely believe in the supremacy of their group over all others. The elders of some of these groups encourage their youth to maintain a distance from outsiders, to continue to respect the traditions and customs of the group, and to marry within the group. The young man or woman who marries outside the group may experience total rejection by even immediate family members.

Other problems may arise in finding housing and employment, especially in black-white marriages. There may even be problems in finding friends who will honestly accept both partners. The amount of social prejudice felt by the interracial couple will vary from city to city and with the part of the country. Interethnic couples may find their best acceptance today in college towns and large cities, where the general attitude is usually more enlightened and liberal than in many other places.

It is likely that the number of interracial marriages will continue to increase, if the trends of the past few years can be projected into the future. The breakdown of social prejudices is painfully slow, but it can be hoped that the need for a discussion such as this will eventually be a thing of the past.

Economic Status   Even though our society has always claimed that one of its goals is social equality regardless of economic status, patterns of behavior do vary greatly with the economic level. Behavior that is "correct" at one economic level may meet with disapproval at another level. Attitudes toward authority, freedom, ethics, education, and other values may differ. Marriage of individuals of different economic backgrounds may require some adjustment of these attitudes.

A problem area in a marriage involving widely different economic backgrounds may be in-law relationships. The wealthier set of in-laws may not entirely accept the son-in-law or daughter-in-law who comes from a less affluent background.

Other problems can arise when a person who has been raised in affluence marries another person of limited income. This couple has two choices. One is to accept financial aid from the wealthy in-laws (if it is offered), which may be psychologically damaging to the poor person. Or they can live within their income, which may require a difficult adjustment. While this may be no problem, it should be discussed and agreed upon before marriage.

Education   Even with the increasing educational opportunities available today, it is not unusual for a couple to have a wide difference in level of education. Changes in values, personal goals, and social sophistication often accompany more education. Compatibility in marriage is largely a matter of common interests and differently educated persons are likely to have few common interests. There is a tendency for boredom to develop and for each to go his or her own way. Yet there are individuals who, though short on formal education, have horizons that are wider than many college graduates who confine their interests to a specialized major field of study.

Intelligence   Perhaps a similarity in level of intelligence is even more important than similarity in level of education. In marriages in which there is a wide contrast in basic intelligence, the partners tend to drift apart. Not only may the more intelligent partner long for stimulating exchange of ideas with someone else, but also the less intelligent person may develop feelings of inferiority. Each may grow lonely. These marriages can be successful if each partner recognizes the other's strong points and allows each to excel in his or her own way. Common interests can be found and cultivated.

Religion   Religious differences can be one of the most disruptive influences in a marriage. The important factor is not simply the fact of difference in religious affiliation, but the significance the individuals attach to their beliefs. To some, religion means nothing. To others, it is the unifying force in their lives. A religion shared in marriage can form a powerful bond between husband and wife. Religious conflict can act as a powerful wedge, forcing them apart.

Most of the differences we have discussed thus far can be worked out satisfactorily. However, in certain combinations of religious beliefs, if each person remains faithful to a different religion, there may be constant conflict throughout the marriage. Such marriages should be entered into only after the couple has reached mutually acceptable answers to all possible questions and problems of mixed marriage life. Nothing should be left to chance or to be settled after marriage. The couple should go together and discuss their decisions with their parents and the clergy of each faith. Their decisions should be clearly in mind and well stated (in writing, if necessary), so there can be no possibility of misunderstanding. This last point is particularly important in regard to the religious education of any children they might have. If, after such discussions with parents and clergy, there still seem to be conflicts, it would probably be better for each to look for someone else whose religious beliefs are more similar. This may seem to be a pessimistic view of the problem, but it does seem that the best way to avoid the problems of a religiously incompatible marriage is to avoid such a marriage.

Previous Marriages   One out of every five to six marriages today involves a person who has been married before. The chances of falling in love with a divorced or widowed person are not remote. Marrying a person who has been divorced or widowed is not the same as marrying one who has never been married before. A past marital experience affects the attitudes a person brings to a second marriage. These attitudes may be the product of memories of a happy marriage, the bitter aftertaste of marital disappointment, or more maturity than the person who has never been married.

Second marriages can turn out to be very desirable and happy. Or the problems that were causes of trouble in the first marriage may reappear. Before marrying a previously married individual, there must be definite answers to several questions, such as, "Has the divorced or widowed person recovered sufficiently from the feeling of loss to make a wise choice or is he or she desperate? If the former mate is still living, what are his or her attitudes toward that person? What are the chances of the former mate coming between the new partners? Can the new mate be content to live in a home previously occupied by the former partner? Are the real causes of the divorce, rather than simply the legal grounds, known to the new mate? (Remember that you have just heard one side of the story.) Is there any assurance that the same problems will not recur? Has the person been divorced more than once? (Third and subsequent marriages are usually poor risks.)

If the divorced or widowed person has custody of children from a prior marriage, a prospective mate should want to feel confident of the relationship to them. Also, one's own attitude toward these potential stepchildren should be honestly appraised. In the event there are children born into the second marriage, in addition to children present from the first one, the parents must make every effort to avoid any showing of partiality toward one set of children.

Danger Signals in a Relationship

Many people are married only a short time before they realize that their marriages are mistakes. As a result, the divorce rate is very high during the first few years of marriage. It is obvious that many divorces result from bad choices of marriage partners. Much misery could be prevented if these incompatible couples could be identified before they made the commitment of marriage. The following characteristics of the premarital relationship signal danger.

Quarreling   Quarreling is a very serious danger signal in any relationship moving toward marriage. Such quarreling is almost certain to continue after marriage, probably at an increased frequency and intensity. Quarreling almost always means that the needs of one or both partners are not being fulfilled in the relationship. As long as needs are mutually met, there is no need to quarrel, and a relationship runs smoothly. Couples must not rely on the folk belief, so often reinforced by movies, television, novels, and other media, that true love seldom runs smoothly and that they should not be concerned over their "lovers' quarrels." The theme of lovers fighting, breaking up, making up, marrying, and living happily might be entertaining in the popular media, but it has little to do with real life. Constant quarreling calls for serious evaluation, in which the real reasons for the quarrels are determined through open and honest communication of feelings. If an area of conflict cannot be clearly resolved, it would seem foolish for a couple to marry.

Lack of Communication   If either partner cannot openly and freely express his or her feelings on any subject to the other, this casts considerable doubt on the chances of a happy marriage. Not only is lack of communication a problem in itself, but it can also be an outward symptom of a personality problem in one of the individuals or a basic incompatibility of the two. It is important that any couple considering marriage thoroughly discuss their feelings about sex (roles, frequency, techniques, and so on), parenthood, contraception, family finances, the role of each partner in a marriage, in-law relationships, and general life-style. Any inability to communicate or open disagreement in one of these areas can only be interpreted as a danger sign and portent of an unhappy marriage.

Lack of Confidence in the Marriage   Another prime indicator of unhappy marriage is doubts by either partner that the marriage is likely to succeed. Retrospective surveys of married couples have shown that the happiest married couples are those who had the fewest doubts before marriage that they would be happy. In contrast, a large percentage of unhappily married couples recall serious premarital doubts about the ultimate success of their marriages.

Off-Again, On-Again Relationships   A history of temporary breakups in a relationship is strongly predictive of failure in marriage. Such breakups indicate that one or both partners may lack a strong commitment to the relationship, that needs are not being well fulfilled, or that other serious problems exist. The same problems that cause temporary breakups are likely to remain after marriage, leading to continued trouble. Couples with a history of breakups should carefully consider the underlying causes before entering into marriage.

Society and Your Marriage

In the rigid cultures of the past, marriage was important for familial and economic reasons. Today such concerns are viewed as of secondary importance. The couple's goal now is personal happiness, arising from personal intimacy. This represents a shift from a social and legal control of marriage to an increasingly individual-centered view of sexual and emotional responsibility and accountability.

Cultures have built basic codes and customs to protect marriage. Those who may or may not marry are restricted by social custom, religious tenet, and legal statute. Once married, one is expected to honor the marital commitments unless released by the state and, for some, by one's religion.

Marriage Laws   Every state has laws regulating marriage. Although these laws vary somewhat from state to state, there are certain similarities among them.

Minimal Age for Marriage Every state has a minimum age requirement for marriage. The age ranges from 14 to 17 for women and from 15 to 18 for men. The most common age requirements are 16 for women and 18 for men. All states require parental consent for marriage if either partner is below a given age. Most commonly, such consent is required if the age of the man is below 21 or the woman below 18.

In the past, the major reason for the difference in age of consent between the sexes was based on the assumption that the young man's career and educational goals should be given precedence over the responsibilities of marriage. By implication, the young woman's orientation towards marriage and homemaking did not require this kind of restriction. In numerous states, the differences in ages of consent are coming under review, as more young women pursue educational and career goals.

Physical Examination and Blood Tests In all but a few states, a medical examination that generally includes a blood test is required. In most states, this is only for the detection of sexually transmitted diseases. About two-thirds of the states require that the examination must be given not longer than 30 days before the issuance of the marriage license. In some cases, the blood test must be within 10 days of the issuance of the license.

Prohibited Marriages Every state prohibits marriage between close relatives such as brother–sister, father–daughter, mother–son, and marriages between step-parents and step-children, and in some states, between first cousins. The marriage of a person who is already married to one living spouse (bigamy), and the marriage of a person who is legally judged to be mentally ill is prohibited in all states. A marriage that involves force or willful misrepresentation is invalid and usually grounds for annulment of the marriage.

Engagement Engagement today means the private agreement between a man and a woman to marry each other. The engagement may or may not be made "formal" by public announcement. If such a formal announcement is made, it is usually after a period of informally testing the arrangement. If there is no formal announcement, it is easier to break off the engagement if the couple later desires to do so.

Purposes of Engagement One of the main purposes of engagement, whether informal or formal, is to let each partner learn how he or she reacts to a prolonged relationship with the other. During this time the couple can test their reactions to the new relationship in a more intense and exclusive manner. Since many people feel that a marriage should involve exclusive sexual fidelity between the couple, they may also reason that a similar fidelity should exist during the engagement. The person who does not recognize the exclusivity during engagement may not recognize it in marriage. Yet during engagement, the two people need not seal themselves off from society. If, for example, one of them is away, or otherwise unavailable, the other should feel free to carry on social dating. Such dating may be limited to enjoyment and convenience without serious interest or sexual activity, and may not involve only one person. Such dating can relieve some of the loneliness of separation and can be a good test of a couple's devotion. If their love relationship can withstand a minor test like this, the chances are better that it can withstand the test of marriage. If the relationship cannot stand such a trial, and either jealousy or a new interest develops, then it is good to discover it before marriage, as the same thing may likely happen after marriage. It is always far easier to break an engagement than a marriage.

Other purposes of engagement are to allow time to answer the many questions essential to a successful marriage. Often the attempts to answer these questions will indicate that no marriage should take place. Some of these questions include: When and where will the wedding be held? Who will be invited to attend? Where should the honeymoon be and how much money should be spent on it? Do the partners adequately understand sexual intercourse and contraception? Are they going to want children, and if so, how many? What are their attitudes on the use of contraceptives? Where is the couple going to derive its income and how much will it be? How will the money be spent? Where does the couple plan to live? Will either be continuing with college? These questions and many more require definite answers before marriage.

Sexual Relations During Engagement

The extent of intimacy during engagement is a matter for each couple to decide. Some couples feel that sexual intercourse during engagement is desirable and engage in it without any apparent problems. Other couples question the advisability of intercourse at this time, agree on definite limits to their lovemaking, and then respect these limits. The training of other couples places them in a dilemma— they want to have intercourse, but do not think they should. If intercourse is going to result in guilt feelings, then it is probably better to wait for marriage. That is, after all, one of the reasons for marriage.

Some people approaching marriage worry about the effect that any past sexual relationships may have on their marriage. They may wonder if their own marital adjustment will be difficult or if they will experience rejection by their partners. The best way to avoid any such problem is not to dwell on the past and to build on the future. What is done is done. The past need not interfere with the present and the future.

There may be a question of how much detail should be exchanged about past sexual experiences. There certainly is no need to discuss everything. Uncalled-for "confessions" may only arouse suspicions and create doubts. Minute details regarding the past are better left untold. However, anything that could affect the marriage should be told before, not after, the wedding.

While there is no definite length for an engagement, it should, of course, last long enough so that all of the functions discussed can be carried out. The divorce rate is higher among couples who know each other for only a short time before marriage.

Breaking Engagements

Although broken engagements can be unpleasant, they are certainly preferable to broken marriages. If the partners are incompatible, it is far better to admit it before marriage than after. If, at any time, either partner wants to break an engagement, it should be broken. Once a person decides to break an engagement, it should be done promptly and kindly. The opinions of the family or friends, the fact that the wedding plans are underway, or embarrassment or pride should not be allowed to alter one's decision. Any pleas, promises, or threats the other person might make should be disregarded. The wishes of the other party should not be "given in to" out of pity or fear. In time, both parties will get over the experience and an unhappy marriage may have been avoided. No person should ever assume a "this-one-or-nobody" attitude. There are thousands of good marriage partners available to anyone who will seek them out. To the jilted party, this advice:

do not act "on the rebound" to hastily start another serious relationship, either for spite or to salvage your own hurt feelings. Such swift actions can lead to an even worse marriage than was avoided.

Premarital Counseling Increasing emphasis is being placed on premarital counseling to assist couples in making an adequate marital adjustment. It has been found that the probability of happiness in marriage can be predicted by examining the couple's background, personality traits, engagement relations, engagement adjustment, and other factors.

The counselor may be a professional marriage counselor, a member of the clergy, or a physician. Some marriage counselors use personality tests to indicate a person's suitability for marriage or the couple's likely compatibility. The couple should discuss with the counselor any fears or inhibitions they may have regarding sex. They should be counselled regarding financial plans, housing, budgets, and any other phase of marriage that may require adjustment.

Some states, such as California, require premarital counseling for couples seeking a marriage license whenever one or both of the individuals are under 18 years of age. Even though a state law may require only a blood test for syphilis, each prospective partner should have a thorough physical examination to detect any condition that might interfere with sexual relations, childbearing, or earning a living. There should be a consultation with a gynecologist regarding the preferred method of contraception for the couple.

Adjusting to Marriage

Starting a marriage should be one of the more pleasurable and memorable stages in life. There is the excitement of setting the date, deciding on where to live, making wedding plans, the actual ceremony, and the honeymoon.

The Wedding Ceremony The particulars of the wedding ceremony are usually determined by the couple. The role of the parents of the couple can be small or large. Although many couples want their weddings to be something they and their friends will remember, no wedding should place a heavy financial burden on either the couple or their families. A wedding is merely the beginning of a relationship and is not an end in itself. It does not need to be a big "production." Plans should be made carefully so that, in the effort to carry out an impressive ceremony, the couple does not become so nervous, confused, and fatigued that the setting for a good honeymoon adjustment is lost. The wedding should fit the desires of the couples, not the social aims of the parents.

The wedding rite may be a brief statement before a judge or justice of the peace or may be a modest-to-elaborate religious ceremony. Regardless of the form chosen, the ceremony should fit the social and emotional needs of the couple, affirming their goals and their commitment in terms that are meaningful to them.

Elopement and Secret Marriage In an elopement the fact of the marriage is made known only after the wedding. In a secret marriage both the fact of the wedding and the marriage are kept secret for an extended period. There may be valid reasons for elopement. Parents may have an unjustified opposition to the marriage, in spite of the reasonable age and maturity of the couple. The couple may elope to save the cost of the typical wedding ceremony and reception. Many couples elope as an expression of the new sense of freedom felt by many young people.

There are arguments against elopement and secret marriage, especially the latter.

The couple may be acting too hastily because of fear or pregnancy. They may be by-passing some of the important functions of engagement (the divorce rate is higher after elopements and secret marriages). Parents, friends, and relatives, whose support is needed during married life, are sometimes hurt and alienated. If the marriage is to be kept secret for a period of time, the couple may face frustration in keeping it quiet, and yet fulfilling their marriage.

The Honeymoon A honeymoon is a special period during which, in privacy and isolation, a couple takes the first steps of adjustment to shared living. Although not every couple can or does have a honeymoon, such a period can help smooth the transition from single to married life. A honeymoon should be well planned to make the adjustment as easy as possible. Ideally, it should allow the partners to concentrate on each other, sexually and socially, rather than on business, extended travel, or crowded activity schedules. The place chosen for the honeymoon should be one that both can enjoy, but the cost should not create an undue burden. The honeymoon should last long enough to allow for adjustment, yet not so long that it leads to boredom.

Marital Sexual Adjustment The sexually inexperienced bride and groom will very likely have some anxieties about their wedding night. Each partner hopes for a mutually satisfactory sexual experience, but has many doubts. Much of this anxiety can be reduced with proper preparation. The bride's premarital consultation with a gynecologist can help considerably. At that time, a contraceptive method should be prescribed that minimizes the fear of pregnancy and that will not interfere with total freedom in sexual expression. Oral contraceptives and IUD's are widely prescribed for this purpose. The gynecologist

may also check the virginal bride-to-be for any genital problems that may make intercourse painful or unpleasant.

Even with these precautions, the couple should not expect their first efforts at sexual intercourse to be entirely successful. The inexperienced groom may seldom have adequate sexual control and, on the first attempt at intercourse, may ejaculate and lose erection almost immediately after vaginal penetration, or even before. After a while, he should be able to attain erection once again and, with seminal pressure reduced, delay ejaculation for some time.

An inexperienced bride may be disappointed in her failure to achieve orgasm on her wedding night. But many studies have shown that a virgin bride often does not reach orgasm through intercourse for a matter of several days, weeks, or even months. In fact, a significant number of women achieve orgasm only after a year or more. Marital adjustments take time. Time is required to break down fears and inhibitions and to learn sexual techniques. The sexual success of a marriage depends greatly on the quality of communication and sharing between the husband and wife. Doubts, fears, and uncertainties can be dispelled or reduced by open expressions of love and tenderness. Patience and sensitivity to the partner's needs are an essential aspect of this adjustment.

Sexual satisfaction is not the only aim of marriage. The success of a marriage cannot be measured by the number of orgasms per month, as some of the handbooks to marital sex seem to indicate. Sex must be viewed as only a part of marriage. On the other hand, a couple should not neglect working toward a satisfying sexual adjustment.

Extramarital Sexual Relations A majority of Americans still consider sexual exclusiveness in marriage an important value. At the time of marriage, most people plan to remain faithful and expect their new mates to do the same. Yet recent surveys show that infidelity occurs at some time in over half of all marriages. Thus there seems to be a definite gap between what we believe (or say we believe) and what we actually practice.

Often it is difficult to pinpoint the real causes of infidelity, because most people try to justify their behavior with elaborate rationalizations. Though infidelity is often attributed to an unsatisfactory sexual relationship within a marriage, it also occurs when the marital sexual adjustment is entirely satisfactory. In fact, the real motivations for infidelity are probably more often nonsexual than sexual. Among the more common reasons given for infidelity are boredom with the marital partner or the home situation in general, lack of sexual interest by or in the marital partner, and lack of warmth, love, or affection in or for the partner. Some people even rationalize their extramarital affairs as evidence of their true love for the partner, since their affairs enable them to remain married and to tolerate both the marriage and the spouse. Others explain their infidelity as a healthy heterosexual interest in a variety of partners.

The amount of guilt associated with infidelity varies greatly. Those most bothered by guilt would be people whose behavior contradicts their own values and standards. But guilt presents little or no problem for other people, sometimes because there are no conflicting values to induce it. Some so thoroughly rationalize their infidelity that they escape all guilt. For many people, the worst psychological problem associated with infidelity is some degree of anxiety related to a fear of getting caught by either their own or a lover's spouse—an unpleasant situation at best.

When the rationalizations are stripped away, three principal causes of infidelity emerge. All are interrelated, and all reveal an underlying inability to be fully committed to a relationship of love and mutual regard and respect. It is a mistake to always assign the blame to the partner who is unfaithful, as the problem may involve characteristics in the supposedly "innocent" partner that almost force the infidelity of the other as a matter of ego preservation. Thus the problem may lie in either partner or in both. Any lasting relationship requires commitments and compromises that one or both partners may be unable or unwilling to make. The three basic problems (adapted from Leon Salzman, "Female Infidelity," *Medical Aspects of Human Sexuality* 6 [February 1972], pp. 118–136) include:

1. *Lack of commitment.* Some people marry even though their degree of love and commitment is uncertain. Such marriages may be motivated by financial, social, religious, or psychological factors. An often-expressed attitude is, "Well, if it doesn't work out, I can always get a divorce." Any expectation of fidelity in such a case is totally unjustified. Obviously, anyone so weakly committed should avoid marriage.

2. *Failure in adjustment.* Marriages in this category begin in love, loyalty, and commitment, but the partners gradually drift apart, until one or both must go outside the marriage in order to fulfill emotional needs. A cause of such problems may be the unrealistic expectations that so many people hold for marriage. Almost from birth, we are conditioned by various media and the national folklore to expect to marry and live happily ever after. The ideal marriage is portrayed as a state of perpetual euphoria in which problems just do not exist. Sex is supposed to be supremely enjoyable, with both partners always in the mood for sex at the same times and each sexual act ending in earthshaking

orgasms, each bigger and better than ever before. Nonsense. In every marriage there are going to be problems: money problems, in-law problems, sexual problems, illnesses, child-raising problems, role and identity problems, conflicting interests, conflicting careers, and, if the marriage lasts that long, problems of aging and retirement. When the realities of married life are compared with the unrealistic expectations that most of us hold, then even a very good marriage can look like a dismal failure. In our disappointment, we feel entirely justified in going outside of marriage to satisfy our various needs. Into this category fall the millions of people who excuse their infidelity on the basis that it sustains their marriage.

3. *Personality disorders.* A variety of personality structures can make fidelity impossible. Included are the sociopathic, the paranoid, the jealous, the immature, and the egocentric types. A very common trait associated with infidelity is insecurity about one's sexual attractiveness or adequacy. The person who has numerous short-term affairs is often motivated by a need for reassurance that he or she can attract lovers and perform well sexually.

In conclusion, it seems that while infidelity is occasionally part of a neurotic or psychotic personality development, it more often represents a rational and understandable form of behavior in a normal person. It may occur in people who are basically loyal and faithful, in response to compelling emotional needs. It may occur as a single brief affair, as a series of occasional brief affairs, or as a chronic situation.

While the incidence of infidelity has traditionally been higher among men than among women, this is believed to have been the result of social pressures rather than any basic biological or psychological differences. Such factors as fear of pregnancy, and the double standard by which society has winked at male infidelity while frowning at the same behavior in women, have tended to create the different patterns. Improved contraception, readily available abortion, and the general liberation of women are acting to remove these restraints on the expression of female sexuality. As a result, infidelity is becoming equally common among both sexes.

The infidelity of either partner need be no reason to terminate an otherwise satisfactory marriage. It may, however, be taken as evidence that the needs of the unfaithful partner are not being adequately met within the marriage. If the marriage partners can calmly and rationally discuss their needs and feelings, then the resulting mutual understanding can often result in each partner's being better able to satisfy the needs of the other, so the need for infidelity ceases to exist. A realignment of unrealistic expectations for marriage is often necessary. If a couple cannot work out their own problems, they should not hesitate to seek the help of a qualified marriage counselor.

There are many, however, who have strong religious convictions. For these, infidelity on the part of the spouse may be a very serious blow to the marriage. Clerical counsel may be sought by those spouses who are faced with this situation. If both partners are willing to "forgive and forget" and work to correct their shortcomings, then even a very shaky marriage may be returned to a state of relative happiness.

Divorce

In some marriages, it becomes apparent that unresolved conflicts have destroyed any basis for continuing the relationship. Marriage can be broken either formally or informally. It may be broken informally by desertion, in which one partner simply disappears, or by separation, in which the couple agrees to live separately. Neither desertion nor separation constitutes a legal divorce nor terminates the marriage. A marriage can be legally terminated by annulment if it can be established that some legal requirement for marriage was never met (because of fraud, deception, illegal age, bigamy, or some other violation). Or divorce can be obtained if it can be established that one partner violated the marriage rights of the other partner. Technically, in most states, divorce must be based on such grounds rather than on simply mutual agreement. Other states, such as California, have introduced reformed no-fault divorce laws, under which the couple need have no grounds other than irreconcilable differences.

Grounds for divorce in the various states include irreconcilable differences, adultery, cruelty (physical or mental), desertion, nonsupport, alcoholism, drug addiction, impotence, insanity, pregnancy at time of marriage, bigamy, fraud, force or duress, felony conviction, and imprisonment. A particular state might recognize many or few of these grounds. Persons seeking divorce often go to extremes to establish complaints within these categories, even though the actual cause of failure was something entirely different. This practice is so common that the number of decrees awarded in certain categories tells very little of the true nature of the marital conflicts among the couples involved.

The majority of divorce decrees are awarded to women for several reasons. Generally, women have access to more grounds for divorce than men. The courts tend to be more sympathetic to the divorce suits of women and tend to award alimony more readily to them. It is also more common for the woman to be awarded custody of the children, if any, than the man. The man typically makes child support payments to his ex-wife until the children reach a given age.

The first major divorce reform in the nation, California's Family Law Act, became effective in 1970. It is expected that other states may follow California's lead. This act eliminated the term *divorce* and substituted *dissolution of marriage*. Its most important reform changed the legal termination of marriage from an adversary action in which one party must be found "guilty" and one "innocent" to a neutral petitioning requiring no finding of misconduct. Cruelty, adultery, and other previous grounds for divorce were eliminated. A marriage may be dissolved now only on a finding of irreconcilable differences or incurable insanity, the latter being the only grounds remaining from the old law. The act also details more enlightened child custody rules, emphasizing the quality of the parent-child relationship instead of the personal character of the parent, as in the past. Finally, the interlocutory period was shortened from one year to six months.

Incidence of Divorce The divorce rate is at an all-time high. The trend in recent years has been a gradual rise in the divorce rate. Between 1957 and 1974, the rate climbed from 2.2 per 1,000 people to about 4.3. The current divorce rate represents one divorce for every 2.5 marriages, and it will probably continue to increase in response to more liberal attitudes toward divorce and the reform of laws in many states.

The incidence of divorce can be correlated with several characteristics of the marriage. Divorce occurs more frequently in cities than in rural areas. Divorce has traditionally been a "luxury," available generally only to those in the middle and upper classes who could afford the legal expenses. Desertion was more common in the lower socioeconomic classes. How-

318

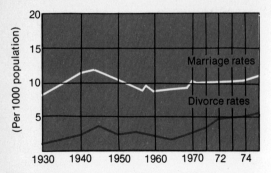

Marriage and divorce rates in the United States, 1930–1972.

Taken from Public Health Service, U.S. Department of Health, Education, and Welfare.

ever, this is changing. Legal assistance and "do-it-yourself" divorce procedures in many states have made divorce a relatively simple and moderately priced option. It is more common during the first five years of marriage than later. Marriages in which one or both parties were less than age 20 at the time of marriage are more likely to end in divorce.

It must be remembered that divorce rates are only a partial indication of marriage failure. There are many couples whose marriage has failed but who have not obtained a divorce for economic or religious reasons, fear of loss of social or professional standing, the presence of children in the home, or fear of admitting failure. The increase in divorce rates is due to many factors, which may or may not include increasing unhappiness in marriage. The evolving criteria for success in marriage place a greater importance on love and companionship, without which a marriage today is more often considered to be a failure. Public opinion toward divorce is increasingly liberal. More and more people are deciding that the temporary pain of divorce is better than living in the continuing turmoil of an unhappy marriage. The increasing independence and freedom of women to be self-supporting

has probably been influential also. On the other hand, a woman who is not prepared to enter the labor market, who has not developed marketable skills, may find the loss of financial security a greater threat than is the undesirable relationship. This is perhaps more relevant for the female reared with marriage as the only adult goal. The older female or male may also have health problems that further threaten the prospect of being alone or able to remarry.

Effects of Divorce on Partners The emotional effects of divorce are greater than the average person who has never been through it realizes. Both parties involved usually find it a painful experience emotionally, socially, and financially. It usually does not solve the basic human problems that were its true cause. New problems are created for both the divorced couple and any children they might have had. There is often a mixture of feelings of guilt and resentment. For some, the readjustment demanded is severe enough to call for the outside help of friends, clergymen, or a psychiatrist.

Effects of Divorce on Children Particularly bewildering is the effect of divorce on children. They are pulled in two directions. The best affection the divided parents can bestow is not compatible to the security children should feel in a warm home relationship. Children are helpless in resolving their position with each of their parents, since children feel loyalty to both. Any court battle over custody only aggravates the damage. Some children become so emotionally disturbed that their attitudes toward their school work and friends are noticeably affected. Their world has collapsed. Children often develop a feeling that somehow they were responsible for the divorce. As children mature, it becomes necessary for them to achieve an outlook on the matter that does not warp their own chances for successful marriage. They must be convinced that their parents' problems do not reflect upon them. Most of all, they must learn from their parents' experience so that they do not make similar mistakes.

Divorce Prevention   The most effective divorce prevention takes place before marriage. This includes the development of desirable attitudes toward marriage and the selection of the right marriage mate. There is a need for a reemphasis on the place of stable marriage as the basis of the social order in this country. One's success in marriage influences the success with which he or she can creatively accomplish goals of all kinds. For many people, a successful marriage is essential to personal fulfillment.

Remarriage   Divorce need not be the end of marital pleasure. The remarriage rate among divorced people is high, indicating that few of them are completely soured on the idea of marriage. According to the U.S. Bureau of the Census, a divorced man or woman of any age is more likely to remarry than the never-married person of the same age is to get married initially. The bureau reports, for example, that at age 30 a single woman has a 50 percent chance of marrying, while a divorcee of that age has a 94 percent chance of remarriage. An interesting statistical fact that has been noted in very recent years is that, particularly among younger divorced people, men are somewhat more likely to remarry—and to do so sooner—than young divorced women of the same age.

The divorce rate among second marriages is somewhat higher than in first marriages, but the divorce rate soars in third and subsequent marriages. On the other hand, a remarriage may result in much greater happiness than the original marriage. Remarriages can turn out well if the new partners earnestly try to avoid the problems that destroyed the first.

The Decision to Have a Child

Whether or not a couple wants children is a crucial decision. To have children represents a long-term commitment that will be most demanding on the couple in all ways.

There are some excellent reasons for deciding not to have a family. Children are not needed to perpetuate the species. The world is already suffering from the effects of enormous overpopulation. Many well-adjusted couples feel sufficiently rewarded with their understanding of themselves, each other, and their professions to more than compensate for the emotional rewards of children. Children, particularly when infants, place heavy demands on a couple. A person may not be prepared emotionally or physically to provide these. Some couples see that it may be impossible to raise children the way they feel they should be raised because costs are too high, congestion too great, and resources too few.

Yet, many couples desire children despite these conditions. As they assess themselves and their resources they are willing to provide, or sacrifice, for a child. They look forward to the emotional rewards that come from creating a new person and from helping this child reach its emotional and intellectual potential.

The decision to have or not have children is as important as is the decision to marry. Questions the couple should answer in reaching this decision should include: Is our marriage stable enough to bear the stresses of a family? Do we love children enough to sacrifice for their welfare? Do we both agree on wanting a child or will it create hostility in one of us? Are we known carriers of undesirable genes that may cause abnormality in a child (see next chapter)? (An unwanted child may not only lead to a disturbed parent, but to an emotionally disturbed child.) Rather than making a decision to *not have* a child, couples should assume they are not going to have a child until they decide *to have* one.

Alternate Life-Styles

Increasing numbers of people are choosing to live in other than the traditional marriage arrangement. They are generally motivated by a search for individual freedom and fulfillment. Actually, most of the life-styles being adopted are not really new at all, but have long existed in various forms and at various periods of history. In many cases, though, the motivations behind these alternate life-styles are new, and in almost every case the openness of these arrangements and their acceptance by society is growing.

Certainly the simplest alternate life-style is just to remain single and live alone. If a person is satisfied with this arrangement, then there is no psychological or sociological reason why he or she should not pursue it.

Long-term homosexual "marriage" is another possibility and for many individuals proves to be a satisfactory life-style. As is true for several other life-styles, persons choosing homosexual marriage should be strong enough to withstand the stigma, however unwarranted it may be, that some elements of our society still direct toward certain life-styles.

The alternate life-style that has attracted the greatest following in recent years is the common practice of "living together," which in many respects resembles the old-fashioned common-law marriage. In this arrangement, a heterosexual couple sets up housekeeping in a fashion that greatly resembles marriage, the principal difference being the absence of license or ceremony. The motivations for living together are what distinguishes this as a separate life-style. While old-fashioned common-law marriage is often associated with lower income levels and is usually motivated by economic expediencies, living together is a middle- and upper-class phenomenon with various motivations. It may be based on a philosophic rejection of marriage as being too confining and restrictive for individual growth. It may be motivated by the romantic view that the love relationship remains stronger when it is maintained voluntarily, rather than enforced by the legal contract that marriage represents. In still other cases, living together is viewed as a trial period that, if successful for a period of time, will lead to legal marriage.

Most couples living together expect of each other the same degree of fidelity as is typically expected by marriage partners, with neither person free to engage in outside sexual relations or even to date. Thus, the degree of freedom in the relationship of living together is really little greater than in marriage, with the exception of the legal ease with which the relationship can be terminated. Of course, the emotional trauma in breaking up can be as great as in terminating a marriage.

Even among the strongest advocates of living together, there are many who feel that legal marriage should accompany the birth of children. The commitment involved in legal marriage, while not guaranteeing a lasting relationship, at least indicates an intention on the part of each person to make a stable partnership. In addition, the great majority of people in our society still stigmatize the child born of unmarried parents. While this stigma is terribly unfair to the child, it is a reality and will probably continue to be so for some time.

The most revolutionary of the alternate life styles is *group marriage*—a catch-all term applied to a wide variety of polygamous living arrangements in which small groups of adult males and females, and their children, live together under one roof or in a close-knit settlement, calling themselves a *family, tribe, commune,* or *community.* All property is generally collectively owned and all the members work for the common good. Many group marriages represent utopian minisocieties largely opposed to the mores and values of contemporary American society.

The collectivism of group marriages usually extends to their sexual relationships. While some communes consist of conventionally faithful married couples, more commonly there is some degree of sexual sharing.

Most group marriages, as well as most other utopian schemes, fail. Many of the problems of traditional marriage are merely multiplied in group marriage. Considering the difficulty in finding just two people who can live together compatibly, it becomes a near impossibility to find larger groups of people who can live harmoniously and lovingly together. A marriage of one man and one woman involves one interrelationship, which we all know is difficult to keep in working order. But the smallest possible group marriage, three people, involves three interrelationships; four people make six relationships; and fifteen people results in 105 relationships. Jealousies and love conflicts are

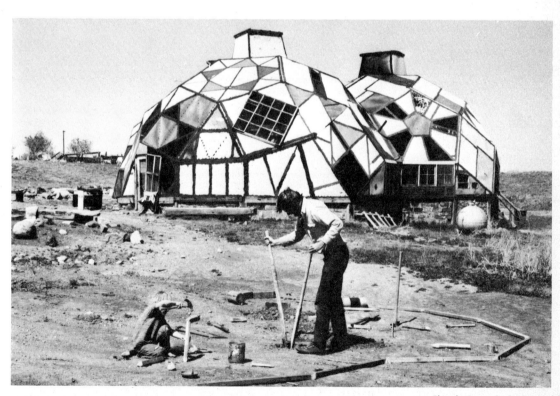

Photo by Dennis Stock, Magnum.

similarly multiplied in group marriages, and considerable individual freedom must be sacrificed in the process of coordinating and scheduling many lives. Thus, most group marriages are unstable and typically last for only a few months.

In Conclusion   While essentially defending marriage, the book *Human Sexuality, A Psychosocial Perspective* (Richard Hettlinger, 1975) welcomes serious reflection in suggesting another alternative:

Marriage of the future, while preserving the central concept of a union between two people, will be different from its past. Open marriage will allow much more opportunity for personal development and separate interests, putting an end to the assumption that one partner has to subordinate his or (more commonly) her individuality to the other. . . . While the ideal of a lifelong commitment will probably persist, a couple will be free to terminate a marriage that has ceased to be satisfying or beneficial to themselves and their children.

The concept of open marriage may be realized in many different forms in the future. People should feel free to create new marriage forms, providing only that the essence of the relationship is not lost—the firm and loving commitment of two people to each other.

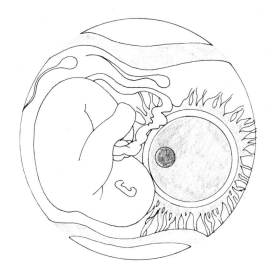

15

HUMAN REPRODUCTION

Most people have at least a practical interest in heredity as shown by their frequent attempts to associate traits of a child with similar traits of his or her parents, grandparents, aunts, uncles, and so forth. But recent advances in the scientific study of heredity have made it important for the enlightened person to have some basis for understanding the actual mechanisms whereby hereditary information is stored in cells, is passed on to offspring, and works to create desirable or undesirable hereditary traits. Many authorities believe that the science of genetics is reaching the point where it may be eventually possible to modify human heredity—perhaps eliminating "undesirable" traits and increasing the frequency of "desirable" ones. Parents may someday (perhaps soon) have considerable control over the genetic makeup of their children. It is possible that even the genetic material of the adult may be alterable. The entire course of human evolution may be changed. Thus, genetics will become not a matter of curiosity, but a topic of vital concern and, most likely, of controversy. Let us therefore consider some of the basic mechanisms of heredity.

Heredity The story of the transmission of traits from parent to child is revealed within the cell contents and functions. What happens inside the cell is the basis for the normal and, sometimes, abnormal functioning of the person.

The Cell All plants and animals are made up of the microscopic units of living material called *cells*. A human being, for example, contains about 2 trillion (2 × 10^{12}) cells.

Cells from the diverse tissues of the body may appear to be quite different from one another. Although all cells are similar in the first day of embryonic life, as they develop into different kinds of tissues, they become differentiated in order to carry out their specialized tasks, such as carrying oxygen in the blood, transmitting nerve impulses, contracting on signal, or supporting the mass of the body.

However, most cells of the body maintain a similar structure (see figure of "typical" cell). The cell consists of a nucleus

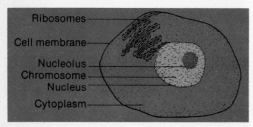

The major parts of a typical human body cell are: the nucleus, enclosing filamentous chromosomes (chromatin material) and one or several spherical nucleoli; the semifluid cytoplasm surrounding the nucleus and suspending organelles such as the ribosomes and endoplasmic reticulum; and the enveloping cell membrane.

surrounded by cytoplasm, all of which is enclosed within a cell membrane. Within the nucleus are twisted, rodlike structures called *chromosomes*.

Chromosomes The number of chromosomes within the nucleus varies with different species of organisms. The 46 chromosomes normally found within the nucleus of each human cell actually represent two similar sets of 23 chromosomes each. Each set of 23 chromosomes is referred to as the *haploid number*; two sets are referred to as the *diploid number*. The diploid number is found in almost all cells of our body. Only the sex cells (sperm and eggs) possess the haploid number. Thus, when a sperm unites with an egg, the new, united cell (the zygote) will contain the same number of chromosomes as all other cells. (If the sex cells possessed the diploid number, the zygote would possess 92 chromosomes and would thus double with each generation.)

Each chromosome in a haploid set (23) is different from the others in shape and size, but all haploid sets of human chromosomes are similar. In other words, each chromosome in one haploid set matches a similar chromosome in any other haploid set (except for chomosome number 23).

At fertilization, each sex cell (sperm or egg) contributes a haploid set. We can think of one set as being the paternal set (from the sperm) and one set as being the maternal set (from the egg). The two comparable chromosomes from each haploid set can be thought of as a pair. We could think of each diploid set of chromosomes as consisting of 23 comparable pairs.

Fertilized eggs receiving an abnormal number of chromosomes (more or less than 46), tend to develop abnormally and die early. In the event that the embryo fully develops and the child is born, it may be abnormal, as in the case of mongoloids (who may possess 47 chromosomes).

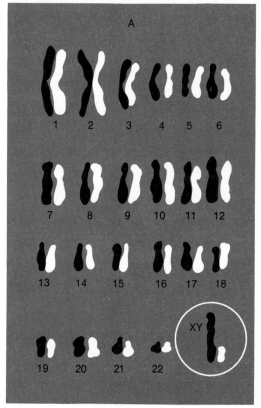

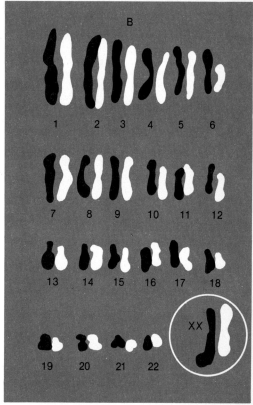

A schematic view of human chromosomes: (A) normal male; (B) normal female. Note the XY pair in the male; these are each diploid sets. In each pair of chromosomes the dark chromo-some represents that contributed by the father (paternal set), and the light represents that contributed by the mother (maternal set).

Genes Chromosomes are highly important to human reproduction. They are made up of theoretical units called *genes*, which in turn are composed of DNA (deoxyribonucleic acid). Through DNA, genes express themselves as traits. Since each body cell contains two sets of chromosomes, each cell possesses two genes for each characteristic. These genes occupy the same position on each chromosome. The two genes for a given characteristic may express themselves in the same way or differently. If the action of the gene pair is alike, the genes are said to be *homozygous* for that trait. If the action is different, they are said to be *heterozygous*.

In the event the genes are heterozygous, one gene of the pair will commonly be dominant over the other, and the trait it determines will be apparent in the individual. In such a case, the gene not creating a visible effect is recessive, or concealed. A homozygous gene pair may be dominant or recessive.

An example of a dominant-recessive relationship can be seen in the trait for tasting. Most individuals have the ability to taste the organic compound phenyl-thiocarbamide (PTC), while a few have no taste for it. Those who have taste for PTC know it, for when they get some in their mouths they sense a very bitter taste. The

Some Human Traits Known to Be Inherited According to Dominance and Recessiveness

Dominant	Recessive	Dominant	Recessive
Hair and Skin		**Skeleton and Muscles**	
early baldness (dominant in male)	normal	short stature	tall stature
pigmented skin, hair, eyes	albinism	dwarfism	normal
ichthyosis (scaly skin)	normal	midget	normal
dark hair	blond hair	polydactyly (more than 5 digits on hands and feet)	normal
non-red hair	red hair		
curly hair	straight hair	syndactyly (webbing of 2 or more fingers or toes)	normal
normal	absence of sweat glands		
		brachydactyly (short digits)	normal
		progressive muscular atrophy	normal
		Circulatory System	
Eyes		blood groups A, B, and AB	blood group O
brown	blue or gray	hypertension (high blood pressure)	normal
congenital cataract	normal		
nearsightedness	normal	normal	hemophilia (X-linked)
farsightedness	normal	normal	sickle-cell anemia
astigmatism	normal		
glaucoma	normal	**Excretory System**	
		polycystic kidney	normal
		normal	diabetes mellitus
Features		**Nervous System**	
broad lips	thin lips	tasters (PTC)	nontasters (PTC)
large eyes	small eyes	normal	congenital deafness
long eyelashes	short eyelashes	normal	phenylketonuria (PKU)
broad nostrils	narrow nostrils	Huntington's chorea	normal
"Roman" nose	straight nose	migraine headache	normal

ability to taste PTC is the effect of a dominant gene. A person can taste PTC either by possessing two dominant genes for the trait (homozygous dominant) or by possessing one dominant gene and one recessive gene for the trait (heterozygous). Any person who cannot taste PTC possesses two recessive genes for the trait (homozygous recessive).

In the example selected, the usual trait is expressed by a dominant gene and the exception by a recessive gene. It is considered normal for a person to be able to taste

PTC. However, dominant genes do not determine only normal traits. The table on inherited traits shows that some dominant traits can also be abnormal.

Undesirable Genes Traits determined by genes may be desirable or undesirable. Undesirable genes cause physical development that obviously deviates from the norm. If the deviation is slight, the person may be able to survive in spite of the abnormality. If the deviation is severe, the person may be unable to survive. In other words, the effects of the gene are lethal, but they are lethal only if their effects are manifest. Dominant genes that are lethal are easily spotted and can perhaps be counteracted. There is a greater concern with lethal genes that are recessive. Such recessives will not be noticed unless they are present in the homozygous state. It is possible for undesirable recessives to be concealed for a number of generations. They need be of little concern as long as they are masked by a dominant gene.

Concealed recessive genes may become visible when close relatives produce children. If one possesses a given recessive gene that is concealed, since they have similar hereditary backgrounds, it is likely that the other also carries the same concealed recessive. Therefore, there is a great chance that their offspring will be homozygous for these recessive genes. The only biological problem in the marriage of close relatives is that their children might inherit and manifest undesirable homozygous recessive genes that were concealed. An example of a condition in which a person possesses two particular homozygous recessive genes is phenylketonuria (PKU), which usually causes permanent neurological damage.

The Determination of Sex and X-Linked Traits

As previously mentioned, one haploid set of chromosomes is similar to any other set. This is true for chromosomes pairs 1 through 22. In the male, pair 23 is not well matched; in the female pair 23 appears to be matched. In the female these two chromosomes are both called the *X-chromosomes*. In the male there is only one *X-chromosome*; the odd mate is called the *Y-chromosome*. Although different in shape and size, in meiosis this pair acts as though it were similar.

Only one chromosome of each pair goes to one egg or sperm. When the female

produces an egg, it gets only one X-chromosome. When the male produces sperm, the X-chromosome goes to one sperm, the Y to another. Thus, while all eggs possess an X-chromosome, this is not true for all sperm. There will be both X- and Y-sperm cells. When an X-egg unites

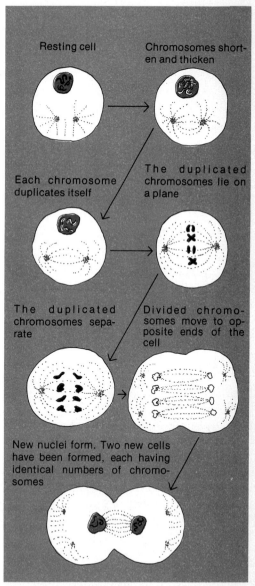

Resting cell

Chromosomes shorten and thicken

Each chromosome duplicates itself

The duplicated chromosomes lie on a plane

The duplicated chromosomes separate

Divided chromosomes move to opposite ends of the cell

New nuclei form. Two new cells have been formed, each having identical numbers of chromosomes

Mitosis, the formation of two genetically identical cells, is the method of reproduction of all human body cells except sperm and egg.

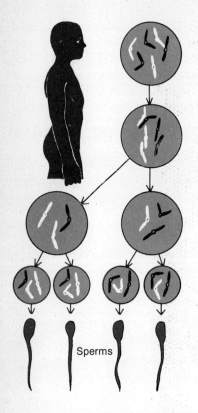
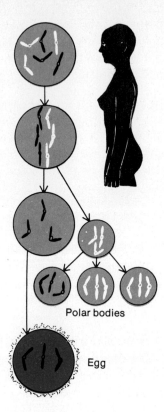

Cells in testes and ovaries possess 23 chromosomes from mother (white) and 23 from father (black). Only three of each shown

Each chromosome duplicates. Similar duplicated chromosomes from mother and father pair off and line up on center plane of cell

In first division each new cell receives one duplicated chromosome of each pair, or 23

In second division each duplicated chromosome divides, forming two new cells, each with 23 chromosomes

Above cell matures to become sperm or egg. Each male meiosis forms four sperms; each female meiosis forms one egg and three useless polar bodies.

Sperms

Polar bodies

Egg

Meiosis, the production of sperm and egg cells. Note: the number of pairs of chromosomes shown here has been reduced to 3 (6 chromosomes) for simplicity. Remember that each body cell in a human has 23 pairs (46 chromosomes) and that a germ cell has only one member of each pair (23 chromosomes).

with an X-sperm, an XX-zygote is formed; this develops into a female. When an X-egg unites with a Y-sperm, an XY-zygote is formed; this develops into a male. Sex is thus determined by chromosomes.

By this system, we could expect males and females to appear in about equal numbers. Actually, records show that more male than female babies are born. In the United States, the proportion is about 106 to 100 among whites; about 103 to 100 among blacks. Among Koreans, it is 112 to 100; among Cubans, 101 to 100.

Being determined by chromosomes, the sex of a child is fixed at the moment of conception. This determination is the work of the father, not the mother. Although the chance of producing males to females is about one to one when thousands of cases are considered, the sex of the children in a given family may not be so well divided. There are some families in which there are four or five girls and no boys, or vice versa. It is simply a matter of chance.

Inherited Versus Acquired Traits

There are some women who, during pregnancy, make efforts to not look upon one-eyed individuals or other sorts of physical deformities, believing that what they experience or think about during pregnancy affects the fetus. Nothing of the sort is true. Sons of lumberjacks are not born with well-developed muscles. Even though Jewish boys have been circumcised for centuries, they are still born with a prepuce. The old practice of binding the feet of Chinese girls was repeated anew with each generation. Traits that are developed through diligent effort and in response to a person's environment are described as *acquired characteristics*, and are not inheritable.

Such physical traits as sex, intelligence, height, color of skin, and blood type are inherited characteristics. The full expression of certain physical traits will depend on one's education, medical care, and diet. Thus, both inheritance and environment are important in development. But the physical traits as such are determined by chromosomes.

Genetic Counseling Providing and interpreting information on the effects of human genetics is an increasingly essential medical service. Of great importance to future parents, its primary purpose is to prevent the occurrence of inherited birth defects that cause abnormalities of body structure or function, or of mental development that often preclude the healthy start of a life. This not always being possible, the further hope is to reverse or at least reduce their damaging effects.

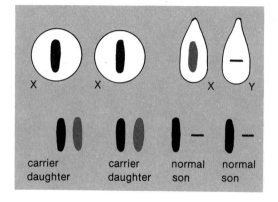

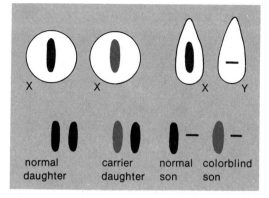

The pattern of inheritance involving X-linked traits. The black chromosomes represent dominant genes for normal color vision; the color ones represent recessive genes for color blindness; the dashes represent Y-chromosomes which bear no genes for color vision.

Today well over 1,200 genetic diseases have been described and the list is growing. Yet the incidence of affected persons may appear quite small. Cystic fibrosis, the most common genetic disease among whites in the United States, occurs once in every 2,000 births. Phenylketonuria (PKU) occurs once in every 10,000 births. Some occur more commonly among certain population groups. Tay–Sachs disease appears among Jews of Eastern European origin, and sickle-cell anemia occurs among blacks. Because the typical physician seldom sees a case of a genetic disease, and because the methods of handling these conditions are so complex and expensive, genetic counseling is a fragmented field of medicine. Because no medical staff can afford to be expert in more than a handful of genetic diseases, or because of the inordinate cost of trying to set up centers for each condition, there is a good measure of cooperation between medical geneticists. The National Genetics Foundation provides a central telephone number in New York that any physician may call for information and referrals to centers that can help. The National Foundation March of Dimes lists genetic counseling centers throughout the United States.

Various groups of people are targets for genetic counseling. A number of major inherited disorders occur with some frequency because there is a relatively large proportion of carriers of harmful genetic traits in the general population. While having the gene usually poses no health problem for a carrier, there is always the chance of serious genetic disease in any child of two carriers of the same harmful trait. When both partners are carriers, genetic counseling provides information as to the advisability of their deciding to have children. At present, carrier tests are available for a large number of genetic diseases.

Other times, the counselor may need to make a prediction about certain defects after conception, but well before birth. A relatively simple procedure, *amniocentesis,* can be performed after the 16th week of pregnancy. This process involves withdrawing, with a needle through the abdominal wall, a small amount of amniotic fluid, which surrounds the developing fetus in the uterus. Since this fluid contains fetal cells, it can provide important information for genetic analysis. If a defect is identified, the physician has firm information to provide the parents on the advisability of continuing the pregnancy.

Not all genetic defects appear during pregnancy or at the time of birth. Some appear in the affected person months or years later. Cystic fibrosis may appear any time from birth to 6 months of age; Tay–Sachs disease from birth to 6 months; sickle-cell anemia after 6 months; Duchenne muscular dystrophy from 2 to 4 years; and glaucoma and Huntington's disease from the late 30's on. When a genetic disease has appeared in an adult, genetic counseling provides information on the advisability of that person parenting a child.

To obtain genetic counselling, interested persons are usually referred by their physicians to a counselor or to a center. Such specialized counseling services are often to be found in medical centers, teaching hospitals, or in satellite clinics set up to provide counsel in more distant locations.

Tay–Sachs Disease Occurring almost exclusively among young Jewish children of Eastern European ancestry, Tay–Sachs is an enzyme deficiency disease caused by a recessive gene. The infant appears normal and healthy for the first 6 to 9 months; then its development slows down. By 1 year, its natural and acquired skills begin to deteriorate and the child loses mobility and speech is impaired. During the next year the deadly Tay–Sachs symptoms occur, including infrequent seizures, loss of sight and destruction of the central nervous system. Death usually occurs before the fifth birthday.

One in every 30 Jews of Eastern European extracton is a Tay–Sachs carrier. Because the gene is recessive, both parents must carry it for their children to be in danger. Even if both parents are carriers, the chances of an affected child are 1 in 4. Carrier adults can now be identified by a simple, inexpensive blood test and can be counseled on whether to have children or, if pregnant, to continue the pregnancy. In pregnancy, amniotic fluid may be drawn from around the fetus and tested, revealing if the fetus has Tay–Sachs. The expectant parents can then make the decision of whether to seek an abortion.

Phenylketonuria (PKU) PKU is caused by a recessive trait, which is marked by the absence of a liver enzyme needed for the conversion of phenylalanine (an amino acid) by the body. Where both parents are carriers, there is a 1 in 4 chance of the child having the disease. Between the ages of 4 and 24 months, the affected child may show a progressive mental decline. It is generally fair, lighter in both skin and hair coloring than either its parents or siblings, tends to have a smaller head size, is often clumsy, with hyperactive reflexes, and may suffer an occasional seizure.

The disease is identifiable in newborns, by a testing that is now required by law in most states. When the disease is detected, the newborn is placed on an immediate, long-term therapeutic diet to largely reduce the effects. If untreated, the victim often becomes severely mentally retarded.

Another concern with PKU is the PKU victim who herself becomes pregnant. The fetus ends up being bathed in high levels of phenylalanine, is more severely affected than the mother, and often carries congenital malformations. Genetic counselors advise a PKU victim against conceiving, and if pregnant, may advise her to seek an abortion. However, if she delivers a child, such a mother is advised not to breast-feed the infant in order to reduce the chances of more severe damage to the child.

Sickle-Cell Anemia Another inherited disorder, one that is particularly common among blacks, is sickle-cell anemia. A description of it may be found in Chapter 18, in the section explaining anemias.

Congenital Defects Abnormal conditions present at the time of birth are called *congenital defects*. The incidence of these conditions is relatively high. Approximately 6 percent of all newborns, or 1 in every 16, carries a congenital defect. Not all of these conditions are inherited. Some defects cause physical or mental handicap, disfigurement, shortened life, or death. Of the 190,000 babies born each year with congenital defects, about 13,000 die before

they reach their first birthday. Some malformed embryos do not reach full development but are aborted before birth. Some authorities estimate that about one-third of all miscarriages are caused by malformed embryos.

Kinds of Congenital Defects Many kinds of defects have been observed. Some of the more common include clubfoot, extra fingers and toes, cleft lip (harelip), cleft palate (opening in the roof of the mouth), albinism (absence of pigment in the skin, hair, and eyes), missing limbs, cretinism (dwarfism with mental retardation), mongolism, hydrocephaly (head enlargement caused by accumulation of cerebrospinal fluid), cystic fibrosis (a mucous gland deficiency disease), open spine, congenital urinary tract defects, diabetes, erythroblastosis fetalis (destruction of red blood cells), and congenital heart disease. Some defects may be medically corrected or modified at birth by surgery (extra fingers and toes, clubfoot, cleft lip and palate, erythroblastosis fetalis, and hydrocephaly); others may not (mongolism, albinism, and diabetes).

Erythroblastosis Fetalis The Rh factor is a chemical substance found in the red blood cells of about 85 percent of the American population. People who carry this substance are Rh positive (+); those who lack it are Rh negative (−). If, in any way, Rh+ blood enters the bloodstream of an Rh− person, the Rh factor stimulates the production of an antibody called *anti-Rh*. This antibody can destroy any red blood cells containing the Rh factor.

The Rh factor is of potential importance when an Rh− woman is pregnant with an Rh+ fetus (the father has to be Rh+). In such cases, the anti-Rh antibody may diffuse across the placenta from the mother's blood to the fetal blood, where red blood cells may be destroyed. This is seldom a

problem in the first such pregnancy (Rh−
mother, Rh+ fetus), but may become quite
serious by the second or third. The result is
a severe form of anemia (*erythroblastosis
fetalis*). The infant may be born dead or
may die shortly after birth. If it survives, it
may be mentally retarded.

In cases where tests during pregnancy
indicate a dangerous anti-Rh level in the
mother's blood, damage can often be prevented by giving the baby blood transfusions immediately after birth or even in the
uterus before birth.

The sensitization of the Rh− mother
(stimulation of her antibody production)
does not usually take place during pregnancy, but at the time of delivery, miscarriage, or induced abortion of an Rh+ baby.
Thus the problem can be prevented with a
reverse vaccine sold as RhoGAM and
under other trade names. This vaccine (actually an injection of anti-Rh antibodies)
will neutralize any Rh factor that might
enter the mother's blood at the time of delivery of an Rh+ baby. The vaccine should
be injected into an Rh− woman within 72
hours after such a delivery or after any
miscarriage or induced abortion. This procedure protects the next pregnancy from
Rh antibodies with over 90 percent effectiveness.

Causes of Congenital Defects Faulty
genes cause about 20 percent of all birth
defects; a faulty environment in the uterus
another 20 percent; and combinations of
the two, 60 percent. Hereditary defects
may cause chemical disturbances in the
fetus that may result in conditions such as
phenylketonuria, galactosemia, and cystic
fibrosis.

The uterine environment includes those
things that happen to the mother during
pregnancy and the things that take place in
the uterus around the fetus. Virus infections in the mother, particularly during the
first three months of pregnancy, may cause

defects. One such infection is rubella
(German measles). Most dangerous during
the first 4 weeks of pregnancy, it may cause
deafness, heart and eye defects, and even
mental retardation.

Drugs the mother takes during pregnancy may cause abnormalities. Such
was true of thalidomide, a tranquilizer-
sedative, which was available in Europe
during the early 1960s. It may cause severe
deformity of the long bones, so that children are born with both arms and legs missing. The deformity occurred when
mothers took the medication during the
second month of pregnancy.

Most defects start during the first 90
days of pregnancy. Drugs (sedatives, tranquilizers, and other drugs) that might be
safe to take under most circumstances may
be dangerous in light of the rigorous demands of early pregnancy. This is especially true of the unplanned pregnancy in
which damage may be done before the
woman even knows she is pregnant.
Knowing that there may be other causes for
a missed menstruation, a woman may take
insufficient precaution in her exposure to
x-rays, virus infections, or drugs. She may
not see a physician for several months, by
which time she has already passed the
time of greatest fetal damage.

Prevention of Congenital Defects
Here are some simple suggestions on how
prospective parents may reduce the
chances of birth defects in their children.

1. Do not have sexual intercourse with a
   close relative; this increases the risk of
   producing a defective child. Such increased risk is the basis for state laws
   prohibiting close relatives from marrying each other.
2. All couples should have a family
   physician who should be made aware
   of any known history of family defects
   or sources of complication such as an
   Rh-incompatibility so he or she can

correctly counsel the couple or refer them for genetic counseling. They should both seek the physician's counsel before planning a pregnancy, and then the woman should see the physician at regular intervals during pregnancy. Since premature babies are more likely to be defective than full-term babies, medical care during pregnancy is essential to avert premature delivery.

3. The physician treating other conditions should be told of any suspected pregnancy, even though the woman may only think she is pregnant. A woman who either is pregnant or apt to become pregnant should take only those medications prescribed by her physician.

4. The pregnant woman should avoid contact with diseases. If there has been known contact, she should inform her physician.

5. Except in emergency, x-rays should be avoided during the first 90 days of pregnancy.

6. Smoking should be avoided during pregnancy. The more a mother smokes during pregnancy, the less her baby will weigh. The weight of a baby at birth can relate to its chances of survival, especially if it is exceptionally small.

7. The age of the mother must be considered. A high correlation exists between birth defects and the age of the mother, and in some cases, the father. Mothers under 18 and over 40 produce a greater percentage of defective children than those between the ages of 18 and 40.

8. Since diet affects growth, pregnant women should learn to eat properly. Diet must be thought of both in terms of the woman's own health and the future growth and development of her children. The fetus depends entirely on the diet of its mother.

Fertility Control

One of the most basic needs a baby carries with it into the world is a need for love and acceptance, the need to be wanted. An unwanted child often suffers lifelong emotional problems resulting from an unhappy childhood as the unloved and rejected product of an unplanned pregnancy. These emotional problems may be reflected in problems at school, delinquency and crime, and personal and social maladjustments. In addition, national and world population problems demand some birth control measures.

At the same time that children need to be wanted, adults need to be able to freely express their sexuality without fear of an unwanted pregnancy. It has been estimated (Elizabeth B. Connell, "The IUD: Sex Without Pregnancy," *Medical Aspects of Human Sexuality* 6 [January 1972], pp. 42–167) that in only about one in a thousand acts of sexual intercourse is pregnancy a desired goal. Thus the effective use of safe and adequate contraceptive methods is of obvious importance both to adults and to their children.

Unwanted Pregnancies Numerous studies have clearly shown that unwanted pregnancies among unmarried college students seldom result from a lack of knowledge, but from a lack of motivation to use birth control methods. This lack of motivation is closely related to internal conflicts about accepting oneself as a sexual person or about the propriety of nonmarital intercourse. Most effective birth control methods require some advance planning—a prescription must be obtained and filled, or a product purchased. Such advance planning entails conscious and rational acceptance of the likelihood of sexual intercourse. For someone who cannot accept himself or herself as a sexual, adult person or who has strong conflicting emotions about sexual intercourse, such conscious acceptance may be impossible. If sex just "happens" rather than being planned, the person can avoid the emotional discomfort or guilt involved in a conscious decision.

Selecting a Method Methods of controlling birth fall into four general categories: sexual abstinence, contraception, sterilization, and abortion. Sexual abstinence is the avoidance of sexual intercourse either temporarily or permanently. Contraception is the interference, either by chemical or physical means, with ovulation, fertilization, or implantation of the fertilized egg. Sterilization is the surgical alteration of the reproductive system to eliminate the possibility of impregnation. Abortion is the surgical or chemical termination of a pregnancy before term. Each of these methods has its advantages and disadvantages.

In selecting the best method for a given situation, an important factor is *safety*. The ideal method would neither harm health nor reduce the capacity for future parenthood. It should be free from harmful or unwanted side effects, both for the person using the method and for the partner. A second factor is the *rate of effectiveness*. It must be effective in preventing pregnancy for the particular person. It should also have "use-effectiveness," or a high probability of continued use. The third factor is *ease of administration*. It is expected that any permanent device, like an intrauterine device (IUD), will be inserted by a professional. If a temporary device is used, the person must find it easy to apply. Ideally, the device will be one that is applied at some time other than during actual preparation for intercourse. A fourth element is *acceptability*. Acceptance must include medical factors (one's medical history, absence of side effects, physical comfort); social factors (prevailing religions, cultural

hesitations); and psychological factors (personal aesthetics, one's own habits and attitudes). *Reversibility* is a fifth element. Sixth is *expense*. Some devices (such as the IUD) require only an initial expense, while others involve a recurring cost (pills, condoms, foams). Even in the United States, economy is a factor for many couples; in some countries several cents a day may be a prohibitive cost. Last is the effect the device has on sex drive and the pleasures of intercourse. It is natural to want the assurance that such feelings will not be reduced. A couple must be satisfied they have chosen the method of birth control that best suits their needs.

Sexual Abstinence Abstinence requires that a couple avoid sexual intercourse either temporarily when pregnancy is most likely to occur, or permanently.

Withdrawal (Coitus Interruptus) This method consists of withdrawing the penis from the vagina just before ejaculation. It is an ancient technique and is mentioned in the Old Testament. Withdrawal was a common method prior to the development of mechanical and chemical contraceptives.

For this method to be effective, the man must be alert to the first signs of orgasm and be prepared to terminate intercourse at any moment. For some couples this does not seem to produce any ill effects. For others this interruption of intercourse just before the moment of greatest pleasure may disturb the entire sexual relationship.

In terms of its effectiveness, withdrawal presents a serious problem. As seen from the table on the effectiveness of various fertility control techniques, for every 100 couples practicing withdrawal for a full year, 23 women are likely to become pregnant. One reason for this is that some of the first fluids emitted from the penis, even before orgasm, may contain sperm. Another reason is that any mistake in timing withdrawal may permit some semen to be deposited in the woman. One drop of semen may be sufficient to cause pregnancy. The first drops of semen discharged by the male contain a higher concentration of sperm than later semen. Not only is timing essential, but distance as well. Due to the mobility of the sperm, it is necessary to prevent sperm from contacting any part of the woman's external genitals. Another necessary element is trust, a trust on her part that she can rely on him to withdraw in time. On the positive side, this method takes no preparation, no equipment is necessary, no medical supervision is required, and it costs nothing. For couples desiring to be successful in limiting their family size, this method would be used only in an emergency or as a last resort.

Effectiveness of Fertility Control Techniques

Method	Pregnancy rate[a]
rhythm	38
jelly alone	25
withdrawal	23
condom alone	14
diaphragm	12
intrauterine devices	6
foam alone (two applications)	5
condom with foam	3
sequential steroids	2
combined steroids	0.2
sterilization	0.003

[a]based on the number of pregnancies per hundred years of exposure for a given method. In other words, for every hundred couples practicing a given method for a full year, this is the number of women who would be expected to become pregnant. (Adapted from information from the World Planned Parenthood Council.)

The Rhythm Method This method is based on the fact that a woman usually produces a mature egg once a month with some predictability. If the egg fails to meet a sperm within 24 hours, it begins to degenerate. Sperm inseminated into the woman's body and kept at normal body temperatures can remain alive for 24 to 72 hours after intercourse and still fertilize an egg. Conception can occur only if intercourse takes place slightly before or during the time in which the egg is alive. Thus, there should be a single 3-day period in each menstrual cycle during which pregnancy might result. This is all simple enough. The big question each month is, when does this period occur?

Ordinarily a woman produces a ripe egg about 14 days before the start of the next menstruation. Ovulation is tied more closely to the next onset of menstruation than to the last one. But even assuming that a woman has menstrual periods that are invariably 28 days apart (the mature egg may be released anywhere from the 17th to the 13th day before the next menstruation begins) there is little way of predicting in any given cycle when ovulation will occur. To be safe, a woman must refrain from intercourse on these 5 days. Yet intercourse 2 days prior to earliest ovulation could still leave sperm to fertilize the eggs, and intercourse a day after the latest possible ovulation could mean an egg was still present to be fertilized. Thus, for a regular 28-day woman to be safe, it is recommended she refrain from intercourse from the 19th to the 12th day before her next menstrual discharge, or from the 10th to the 17th day after the beginning of her last discharge. For a period of 8 days each month she must not have intercourse.

Unfortunately, most women do not menstruate with such clocklike regularity. Some women have menstrual cycles as short as 21 days and others as long as 38

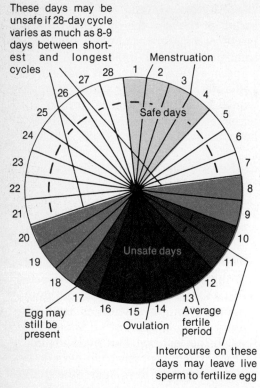

These days may be unsafe if 28-day cycle varies as much as 8-9 days between shortest and longest cycles

Menstruation

Safe days

Unsafe days

Egg may still be present

Ovulation

Average fertile period

Intercourse on these days may leave live sperm to fertilize egg

The theory of the rhythm method. The shaded sections indicate days of greatest chance of pregnancy (the darker shading, the greater the chance). This chart is based on an average 28-day menstrual cycle.

days. The average woman may vary as much as 8 to 9 days between her shortest and longest cycles. Few women realize how irregular their menstrual cycles are. Following childbirth the cycles may be upset for several months and ovulation time may be unpredictable.

The major drawback to the rhythm method is detecting the day of ovulation. Around the day of ovulation about 25 percent of women sometimes experience a low abdominal pain called *mittelschmerz*, occuring as a result of irritation from the ruptured follicle. Few women experience this with every cycle.

Another clue to the approximate day of ovulation is the shift in basal body temperature (BBT). This is measured with a special thermometer that shows tenth-of-a-degree graduations relatively far apart. The readings are based on the fact that ovulation causes changes in the normal body temperature of a woman each month. The BBT figure shows the typical pattern as a function of the day of cycle.

This method of calculating sex life each month is a major disadvantage to many couples. Regulating sex according to the calendar rather than to the way a person

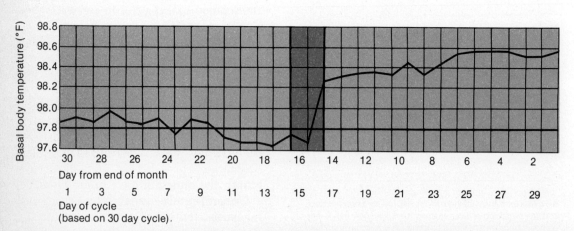

Basal body temperature (BBT) during typical menstrual cycle. Ovulation will commonly occur 14 days before the end of the cycle. Since the length of menstrual cycles varies, the days on the chart are listed in reverse order.

feels does not appeal to most young couples. Even faithful adherence is not highly effective in preventing pregnancy. Thirty-eight out of 100 women practicing this method for a year could be expected to become pregnant.

Contraception Contraception today amounts to one of two things. It may either prevent fertilization or prevent ovulation. The types of contraceptive methods available fall into three categories: mechanical, chemical, or hormonal.

The Condom The condom is usually a synthetic rubber sheath worn rather tightly over the erect penis and fitted with a rubber ring at the open end to help hold it in place. The function of the condom is to prevent the sperm from reaching the vagina. It is almost as effective as the diaphragm in preventing pregnancy. Its effectiveness can be increased if it is used in conjunction with a contraceptive jelly applied to the outside of the condom or foam inserted into the vagina before intercourse.

The condom is used widely around the world both for the prevention of sexually transmitted diseases and the control of pregnancy. Its use also combats *Trichomonas* infection and reduces the chances of transmission of *Herpes* virus. It is sometimes useful to men bothered by premature ejaculation since it reduces penile sensations. It is one of the handiest methods to use and can be purchased almost anywhere for $.10 to $1.50 per condom. It has no side effects and is fully reversible once discontinued. Until the availability of the pill and the IUD, it was one of the more effective methods of birth control. Even today the use of a quality condom with a contraceptive foam (by the woman) offers good protection.

However, there are drawbacks. The condom interferes with the full enjoyment of

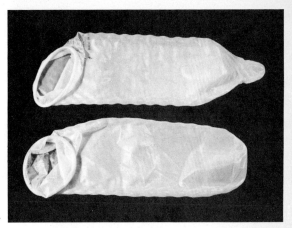

Condoms. Top, receptacle end; bottom, plain end.

intercourse by dulling the man's sensations, and it requires interruption of the act to put it in place. Condoms are subject to breakage and they can come off during intercourse.

The failure rate of the condom can be reduced by taking several precautions. First, only high-quality condoms should be purchased. The U.S. Food and Drug Administration has found that as many as 5 percent of cheaper condoms have holes in them. Since condoms are made of very thin rubber, they should be handled with care. To avoid damage, the condom should be placed on the penis just prior to vaginal penetration.

The condom, like other contraceptives, should be used throughout the menstrual cycle, rather than just when the woman's fertility is most likely greatest. Otherwise a couple is, in effect, taking the same risk of pregnancy as if the rhythm system were used.

The penis should be withdrawn from the vagina promptly after ejaculation to prevent semen from working out over the top of the condom. Some condoms have a small saclike receptacle end that helps prevent this type of leakage, but with-

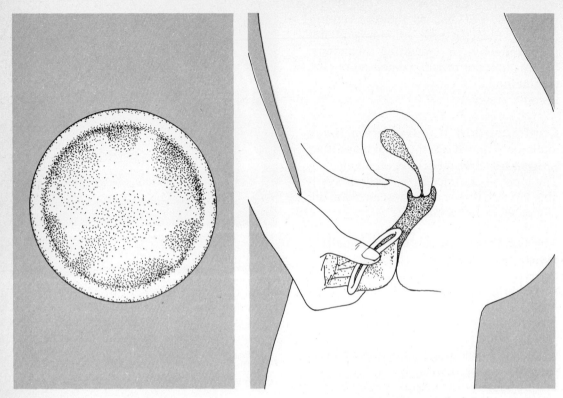

Typical diaphragm (left) and its proper insertion prior to intercourse.

drawal should still be prompt. Use a new condom for each act of intercourse.

The effectiveness rate of the condom when used by itself is about 14 pregnancies per 100 women years, but the effectiveness improves at about 1 pregnancy per 100 years when a foam spermicide and the condom are used together. (Contraceptive effectiveness is measured in the number of pregnancies that would result when 100 women use a given kind of contraceptive device as recommended for one year, or the number of pregnancies per 100 woman-years.)

The Diaphragm The vaginal diaphragm, used widely in the United States, is a shallow rubber or synthetic cap designed to be covered with spermicidal jelly and to cover the neck of the uterus, thus preventing sperm from entering. It has a flexible metal spring or coil to hold it in place. A diaphragm ranges in size from 2 to 4 inches in diameter to allow for variations in the distance between the pubic symphysis and the posterior portion of the cervix. Since a diaphragm of the wrong size may slip out of place or be displaced during intercourse, a woman must be fitted for a diaphragm by a physician. The woman can then purchase the diaphragm by prescription at a drugstore. Since a woman's vaginal dimensions change as a result of childbirth, the diaphragm should be checked for fit after delivery. A woman should never borrow a friend's diaphragm.

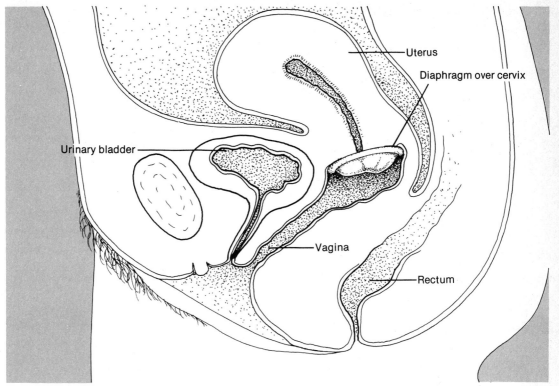

Correct positioning of the diaphragm.

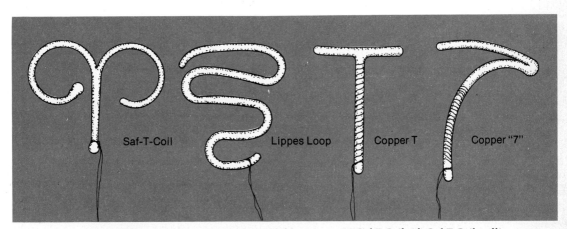

Saf-T-Coil   Lippes Loop   Copper T   Copper "7"

Intrauterine devices commonly available: (a)   (c) Saf-T-Coil; (d) Saf-T-Coil nullip.
Margulies spiral (with stem); (b) Lippes loop;

Two women of the same height and weight may have quite different vaginal dimensions.

A contraceptive jelly containing a *spermicide* (material that kills sperm on contact) should always be used with the diaphragm. Jelly should be applied around the edge and the cup side of the diaphragm prior to insertion. Masters and Johnson have shown that the vagina widens and elongates during sexual excitement and that even the best-fitting diaphragm moves quite freely in the vagina. The diaphragm can be inserted 2 to 4 hours in advance and must be left in place for 8 hours after intercourse.

A diaphragm properly fitted and inserted will not be felt by the woman and will not impair sexual sensation for either partner. It may be left in position for 24 hours without any harm or discomfort to the woman. After removal, the diaphram should be washed and dried. With such care it should last for several years.

The use of the diaphragm requires continuous, high motivation. While the diaphragm was once quite popular, today less than 10 percent of couples use this technique. Nor is its effectiveness very high. Out of 100 women using it for one full year, 15 to 25 are likely to become pregnant.

Intrauterine Devices The intrauterine device (IUD) has been used for a long time. Although it has been known for centuries that a foreign object in the uterus prevents pregnancy, only recently have researchers developed materials that the body can accept.

The devices vary in shape, size, and kind of material. They range in size from 7/8 to 1 3/8 inches. They may be made of stainless steel, preformed plastic, or copper. The plastic devices, shown in the figure on intrauterine devices, are inserted by being pushed through a small tube into the uterus. The IUD is inserted by a physician or specially trained nurse. It is usually inserted during menstruation when the opening of the cervix is dilated. Physicians will also commonly do a Pap smear to check for uterine cancer, and a pelvic examination to determine the position and size of the uterus so the IUD can be safely inserted. Insertion may cause cramping for a few days and may cause longer, heavier periods. The physician will want to check in a month or so to be sure insertion was performed correctly. Some women may spot-bleed during the first few weeks after insertion. If pains are severe and persist, the IUD may have to be removed.

Once inserted, the device can remain in place indefinitely. Some obstetricians recommend that the CU–7 and Tatum T (both of which use copper) be changed every two years because the copper dissipates. No other contraceptive protection is necessary, and usually neither partner is aware of its presence. The devices have a nylon thread attached that protrudes from the opening of the cervix. Prior to intercourse a woman should feel with her finger to be certain the device has not been expelled in severe cramping or slipped into the vagina.

The IUD is completely reversible. If the woman decides to become pregnant, she goes to her physician and has the IUD removed. A woman should never do this by herself. Before long the uterus is again functioning in a normal way, and within one month to a year most women become pregnant. An occasional pregnancy may occur with the device in place. If pregnancy is confirmed, the FDA advises the removal of the IUD.

Older women and those with a greater number of children tend to tolerate an IUD better and have fewer expulsions than younger women and those with fewer children. Newer designs, however, are proving successful for childless women. When bleeding and cramps are reported, this may be corrected by changing to a smaller IUD. There are fewer expulsions from the uterus with larger IUDs, though there are more pregnancies with smaller ones. Because of the possibility of intestinal obstruction, the FDA advises against the use of any closed-ring type of IUD. With the FDA-approved IUDs, perforations of the uterine wall are rare and deaths from the IUD are quite low. The incidence of uterine cancer is no higher than with women not using the IUD. Of course, the IUD offers no protection against sexually transmitted diseases. In spite of these affirmative endorsements regarding the IUD, it is necessary for the user to be aware that all of the data, pro and con, are not yet in on the IUD.

As to effectiveness, of 100 women using the device for one year, about six can expect to become pregnant. The use of the IUD is unrelated to sexual intercourse, requires no daily motivation, involves no cost beyond that of initial insertion, and has no effect whatsoever on a woman's hormone levels. There is great hope for worldwide use of the IUD today in terms of its low cost, ease of insertion, and long-term effectiveness once in place.

The Douche Some people believe that pregnancy can be prevented by washing away the semen after intercourse by douching, or washing out, the vagina. Various douches have been used—hot water, cold water, vinegar, lemon juice, soap chips dissolved in water, or washes available in drugstores. A large rubber bulb, or syringe, is filled with the fluid and emptied into the vagina.

Unfortunately, sperm are safely within the uterus within 30 seconds after ejaculation. A douche can wash out the vagina but not the uterus. Following unprotected ejaculation, regardless of how soon the douching is done and what substance is used, it is too late. In addition, the necessity for postorgasmic douching deprives both the man and woman of a warm and tender time together. Douching does not prevent pregnancy and should not be considered acceptable for that purpose.

Vaginal Spermicides Various chemical preparations kill or impede the movement of sperm. These vaginal spermicides are available in the form of creams, jellies, aerosol foams, and suppositories.

Creams and jellies are usually used with a diaphragm, while the other spermicides, which tend to be somewhat stronger, are usually used without any other contraceptive device. The woman inserts a measured amount of the spermicide into the vagina with a special applicator one hour or less prior to each intercourse. The applicator deposits the preparation high in the vaginal tract at the opening into the uterus. One application is good for only one intercourse. The action of the preparations is twofold: the spermicide acts to kill the sperm on contact and the chemical base of the preparation forms a coating that keeps surviving sperm from reaching the egg. The effectiveness of jellies alone in preventing pregnancy is not very good. Of 100 women using this method for one year, 25 are apt to become pregnant.

Vaginal foams are a variation on the creams. They are packaged in a can under pressure and the contents are released into a plastic applicator, by which the foam is applied high in the vagina. When used as directed, with an application prior to *each* intercourse (with a reapplication if intercourse is repeated in the morning following intercourse the prior night), 5 of every 100 users can expect to become pregnant. When used along with the condom, its effectiveness improves to about 3 pregnancies out of every 100 users.

Suppositories are small pencil-shaped glycerin-gelatin preparations containing a spermicide that melts at body temperature. They are inserted deep into the vagina a few minutes to an hour before intercourse.

Foaming tablets dissolve on contact with the moisture in the vagina when inserted. They release a carbon dioxide gas to produce a foam that spreads the spermicide over the upper vaginal area. A tablet should be inserted several minutes to an hour before intercourse.

The action of the vaginal spermicides is completely reversible when discontinued. They do require use at some time relatively close to intercourse and require memory and motivation on the part of the woman to insure effectiveness.

Hormonal Contraception

The female oral contraceptive pills are designed to prevent ovulation. These pills, which are highly effective in preventing pregnancy, are composed of female hormones. You will recall from an earlier discussion that the pituitary gland produces the hormones FSH and LH, which are necessary for the production and release of a mature egg in the ovary. The follicles in the ovary produce both estrogen and progesterone. Among other functions, the estrogen inhibits the production of FSH, and progesterone inhibits the production of LH. When the pill is taken daily starting with day 5 (the fifth day after the beginning of menstruation), the presence of progestin and estrogen inhibit the body's production of FSH and LH before they are able to produce a mature egg. Ovulation does not occur and no egg is present to unite with the sperm that are released during intercourse. The woman then fails to become pregnant. This suppression of egg production is very much like the suppression of egg production that takes place while a woman is pregnant. Under the influence of natural estrogen and progesterone, no other mature eggs are produced until after the pregnancy has terminated.

The Combined Pill The first pills produced combined estrogen and progestin. Most combined pills are designed to be taken for 20 or 21 days of the menstrual cycle, starting on day 5 and ending on day 24 or 25. Then for 7 or 8 days, the pill is omitted, or placebos or iron supplement pills are substituted for a week. Menstruation is allowed to occur. The menstrual periods tend to become regular 28-day events. Only one type of pill is taken. Some women experience side effects such as nausea, headache, swelling of the breasts, and bleeding. Commonly these symptoms diminish or disappear after the first several months. In addition to preventing ovulation, the combined pill also makes the uterine lining less receptive to a fertilized egg, thus making the pill even more effective than it might otherwise be. Out of 100 women usng the combined pill for one year, only about 2 are apt to become pregnant.

The Sequential Pill Because of some complaints regarding the side effects of the combined pill, the sequential pills were developed. They amount to two different pills, one taken from day 5 through day 19 and the other from day 20 through day 24. (The days differ slightly for different brands.) The pills taken the first 15 days contain estrogen only; the pills taken the last 5 days contain both estrogen and progestin (like the combined pill). The sequential pills are packaged so that the pills are easily taken in the right order. The action of both pills is similar. The effectiveness of the sequential pill is less than that of the combined pill. Of 100 women taking the sequential pill for one year, 1 or 2 are apt to become pregnant.

As with the combined pills, depending on the brand used, there are minor variations in the dosage and number of pills taken. There are 20-, 21-, or 28-pill packages. For 7 out of 28 days the latter utilize placebo tablets, which have no chemical effect but keep the woman in the habit of taking the pill every day.

The pill is a prescription drug and requires a visit to a physician, which includes a physical examination to determine what birth control pills are relatively safe to take. The exam should include a Pap smear, a breast exam, a blood pressure check, and taking of a medical history. *Do not get pills from a physician who does not examine you.* A regular checkup twice a year is recommended.

Take only the pills for which you have a prescription—one kind of pill may affect you differently from another. In the event you may want to change pills after a couple of months, do not buy too large a supply. Never give them to a friend unless she is taking exactly the same pill to begin with. Keep an extra package on hand to replace pills that get lost.

Take the pill about the same time each day. This makes it easier to remember and helps to maintain a more constant level of hormones in the blood. If you forget to take a pill, take it as soon as you remember and take the next pill at its scheduled time. If you miss two pills, take two each day for the next two days and use an additional contraceptive (foam, condom, diaphragm) for the next week.

There is no evidence that the pill produces cancer. Since most physicians require a routine Pap smear (to detect uterine cancer) and breast examination every six months, there may be fewer deaths from cancer for women on the pill. In some cases, women with blood type A may run a somewhat higher risk of blood clots. The pill should never be prescribed for women with persistent headaches, swelling of the legs, vein tenderness, and chest pains. Even so, the mortality risk from full-term pregnancy is ten to fifteen times greater than from pill-formed clots. *But it is most important that the pills be taken only under a physician's supervision.*

The major advantage of all pill methods is their effectiveness and simplicity. The pill is taken at a time other than during sexual intercourse. Obviously, for the method to work, the woman must be motivated to take the pill and remember to do so. When a woman wants to become pregnant, she merely stops taking the pill, and she should become pregnant with at least the same likelihood as before taking the pill.

Minipills These are low-dose progestin pills with no estrogen. They do not impair a woman's glucose tolerance (causing a diabeteslike condition) as occasionally happens in women taking regular birth control pills. Their effectiveness in preventing pregnancy is similar to that of an IUD.

Morning-After Pills A woman may find herself in a situation where she engages in sexual intercourse and a condom tears, or she has unprotected intercourse during her fertile period. Faced with the very real possibility of pregnancy, the "morning-after" pill may be used to insure against pregnancy *after* she has had intercourse. In a woman, once an egg is fertilized, several days are required to move it to the uterus and several more for it to become implanted in the uterine lining. A woman in this predicament should not panic, but should contact a physician, hospital, or school infirmary. Implantation and pregnancy may be prevented if two 25-mg tablets are taken twice a day for 5 days, starting within 24 hours and no later than 72 hours after unprotected intercourse. Consisting of diethylstilbestrol (DES), a synthetic estrogen, the pill causes contraction of the uterus and the expulsion of its contents. The woman may experience severe nausea.

There has been much concern over the cancer-producing potential of DES. It has been banned as an animal feed additive used to speed growth in beef cattle because illegal residue levels remained in the livers of slaughtered animals. The drug has been linked to scores of cases of vaginal and cervical cancer in young women whose mothers took it during pregnancy to prevent miscarriages. Its effectiveness for that purpose later was disproved. The FDA has, however, approved the use of DES as a "morning-after" birth control pill. According to the FDA, there is no significant risk to women under prescribed dosages and if not taken for prolonged periods. They stress, however, that it must be taken exactly as prescribed, and should be used *for emergency only* and not for routine birth control. Although the drug has been very popular for postcoital contraception

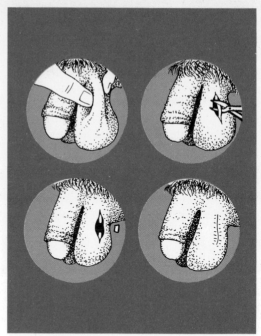

Vasectomy, or sterilization by severing the vas deferens.

for several years, its use for this purpose had not been officially approved by the FDA until recently.

Three-Month Contraceptive Injection
There is limited use in the United States of a contraceptive drug that can be given by injection. Called Depo Provera, and containing synthetic progesterone, it is taken by an injectable contraceptive, and can prevent pregnancy for up to 3 months at a time with one injection. Women using it report menstrual irregularity, sometimes having no period for months. When stopped, many women may become pregnant within 3 to 9 months. However, there is a chance it may cause temporary or permanent sterility. Some women regain their fertility after having quit the injections for a number of months. In addition, it has most of the other adverse side effects associated with the oral contraceptives. It is

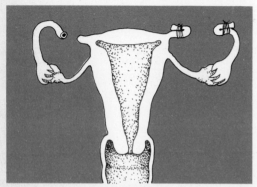

Tubal ligation, or sterilization by severing the fallopian tubes.

recommended for women who cannot use the pill or IUD, who do not remember to take the pill, or who do not like either the pill or the IUD. The Food and Drug Administration has approved its limited use in this country at present.

Experimental Contraceptives Other hormonal contraceptives are now under investigation. A long-term capsule is injected into the arm or buttock and offers contraception for as long as two years. A male birth control method is being investigated that makes conception impossible by preventing the development of sperm. It can be administered either by injection or by oral doses. Vaccination appears to be another possibility. The idea of making the woman immune to sperm by injecting her with antibodies that would attack and reject sperm is being studied. A unisex birth control pill, which can be taken by either partner, is being researched. Its study has been prompted by the need for a "rest period" for some women on the pill.

Sterilization Sterilization is a permanent method of fertility control that is virtually 100 percent effective. A man or woman who has been properly sterilized can have children only if a second operation is successfully performed to undo the work of the first. Sterilization does not remove any of the sex organs or glands and has no effect upon sexual desire or performance.

For a woman, the operation, called a *tubal ligation*, consists of cutting the two fallopian tubes and closing off the cut ends. It can be done as part of a cesarean delivery, by abdominal incision, by a laparoscope, or by way of the vagina. Once the tubes have been tied, the sperm can no longer reach the egg, and the egg can no longer reach the uterus.

For a man, the operation, called a *vasec-tomy*, consists of cutting and tying the vas deferens, the passages through which sperm travel from the testes to the genital passages. It requires only small cuts on both sides of the scrotum and can be safely performed in a physician's office. Following vasectomy, mature sperm may remain in the passages for up to six weeks. Contraceptives should be used for sexual intercourse until a sperm count confirms the absence of sperm in the semen. The man continues to produce seminal fluid as before; it is still ejaculated upon orgasm, but it contains no sperm. The sperm disintegrate and are absorbed by blood vessels in the testes.

Once sterilization is performed, no daily motivation or remembering is required to prevent pregnancy. The main problem is its low rate of reversibility. Only 35 to 50 percent of sterilized people can be restored to fertility.

Sterilization is legally permissible in every state of the union, as well as in many countries throughout the world. A few states require a medical reason for the operation.

Abortion The removal of a growing embryo or fetus from the wall of the uterus to which it is attached is defined as an *abortion*. A natural abortion, commonly called a *miscarriage*, is the spontaneous termination of pregnancy by the body. It is believed that about one of every ten pregnancies ends in this manner. About 75 percent of these occur during the second and third months of pregnancy. Common causes are an abnormally developing fetus, abnormalities of the placenta, and maternal disease. An induced abortion is the expulsion of the embryo or fetus by artificial means. An induced abortion is legal or criminal, depending on state laws.

regardless of existing state laws, has the same right to an abortion during the first 6 months of pregnancy as she has to any other minor surgery. During the first 3 months of pregnancy, the abortion decision must be left to the medical judgment of the pregnant woman's attending physician. After the first trimester, a state may regulate the abortion procedure in ways that are reasonably related to maternal health, for instance, by requiring hospitalization. But it is illegal to demand that a panel of physicians approve the abortion. Only after the fetus has developed enough to have a chance of survival on its own, usually during the seventh month, may a state regulate and even proscribe abortion except where it is necessary for the preservation or health of the mother.

The court has held that a woman's right to privacy overcomes any state interest in using abortion statutes (as some states have) to regulate sexual conduct, even though indirectly. It also holds that a fetus is not a person under the Constitution and thus has no legal right to life. Legal abortion during the first trimester is decidedly safer than childbirth. After the first trimester, the danger to the mother increases, hence the states' authority to protect the health of the mother. The United States has joined Japan, India, the Soviet Union, and the majority of Eastern European countries in making abortion freely available.

There are several common ways of aborting pregnancies. The most common is the classic D and C (dilatation and curettage) in which the cervix is dilated and the inside of the uterus is merely scraped clean. Up through the twelfth week, when performed by a physician under aseptic conditions, the D and C is a safe procedure. Another method that can be safely used before the twelfth week is the suction curettage. A machine that builds up a negative pressure sucks out the products of conception. As with the D and C, care must be taken not to perforate the uterus. From the fourteenth to the sixteenth week, there is no method that will be used. The woman will be told to wait until the sixteenth week until enough amniotic fluid has developed. Another method that may be used from the sixteenth to twenty-fourth week of gestation is to introduce a hypertonic solution of saline or glucose into the uterine cavity. Not without risk to the mother, this should be performed only by a skilled physician. Improper administration can result in the rapid death of, or serious infection to, the woman. A physician may perform a curettage afterward to clean out the uterus. Occasionally, for a pregnancy of more than 12 weeks' gestation, an abdominal procedure may be performed. The physician may remove the fetus by cesarean section, or may remove the entire uterus (a hysterectomy). Before the removal of the uterus, evidence of medical pathology must be present.

Properly performed by a qualified physician in an aseptic setting, these methods may present little hazard to the woman, often less than allowing the pregnancy to continue to full term. While some women do suffer from emotional problems following the abortion, many women do not. Most important is for the physician to make an individual determination and recommendation for each patient based on the factors in each case.

Regardless of the type of abortion, few people would argue that it should take the place of contraception. Many people feel, however, that abortion must be readily available as a backup method of fertility control for those who find themselves with an unwanted pregnancy.

A Personal Decision Fertility control is a highly individual matter that must rest upon a private decision between a man and a woman. It is plainly a matter of which method to choose, not whether or not to choose one. During a normal adult life, a woman may have four hundred chances to conceive. Such a woman could give birth to thirty or forty children.

The choice of a method must be satisfactory to both partners. A choice ought to be made in terms of a couple's taste and preferences, their emotional dispositions, their physical requirements and any medical limitations, and their moral standards and religious attitudes. Methods ought to be discussed with a physician as part of any premarital counseling. Information may also be obtained from family planning clinics or from qualified agencies. (One such agency is Planned Parenthood Federation of America, 515 Madison Avenue, New York, New York 10022.) Ask for the address of your state or area organization. The address may also be obtained through a local telephone directory.

Infertility

For most couples, family planning means limiting the number of children they have, or at least spacing their arrival. The majority of young couples who desire children have little difficulty in producing them. Physicians estimate that at least 50 percent of all fertile couples can achieve pregnancy within 1 month of regular intercourse, and 75 percent are successful by the end of 6 months.

Yet for a significant minority, the problem is just the opposite. Some couples who practice no form of birth control would like to have children but have none at all. Other couples wish for more children than they have but are unable to have them. Out of every one hundred married couples, ten are unable to have any children at all and fifteen have fewer than they would like. This means about 25 percent of the population is troubled with insufficient fertility.

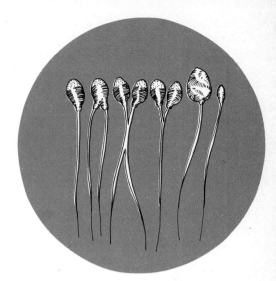

Various forms of human sperms: left, normal; others, abnormal. Sterility will result if the percentage of abnormal sperm reaches 25 to 30 percent of the total sperm.

There are two degrees of insufficient fertility. The total inability to produce children is termed *sterility*. A temporary inability to produce children is called *infertility*. A couple should consider themselves infertile until they are shown to be sterile.

Causes of Infertility Infertility may be due to physical defects, emotional stress, a mistiming of ovulation, or a sperm allergy. It may be traceable to one partner or to both. For every hundred cases of infertility, the wife is unable to conceive in fifty cases, the husband is unable to induce conception in thirty, and the problem is shared by both partners in twenty.

The Man In the male the problem is a failure to discharge enough active sperm to reach and fertilize the egg. This difficulty has no relation to the man's masculinity, since the male hormones and the sperm are produced by different cells. A man may be sterile and still have normal sexual performance in all other respects.

Normal semen amounts to a minimum volume of 3 milliliters of ejaculate. (1 milliliter is approximately ¼ teaspoon.) There should be at least 60 million sperm per milliliter of semen, of which 60 percent must be normal sperm. (See figure showing normal and abnormal sperm.) Sixty percent of the sperm should be motile 2 hours *after* ejaculation. If the sperm count falls below 10 million per milliliter or the percentage of normal sperm falls below 70 percent, the male is considered sterile. Thus too frequent coitus, once or several times daily, may prevent the buildup of sufficient volume of semen. Such couples may be advised to wait 36 hours or more between each act of intercourse.

Failure in sperm production may be caused by illnesses (mumps or other diseases), occupational hazards (exposure to x-rays, radioactive substances, certain metals or chemicals, gasoline fumes and carbon monoxide, or excessive heat), sedentary living, obesity, tight underclothing, infrequent coitus, unhealthy habits (excessive smoking or drinking), poor health, inadequate nutrition, or emotional stress. Other causes for male infertility can be blockage of the ducts (from birth defect or infection) or varicocele (a swelling of the veins on the vas deferens). These conditions may often be corrected surgically.

Techniques have been devised to increase the concentration of sperm. The first drops of semen contain a far greater number of sperm than the later discharge. In some cases a man is advised to withdraw the penis after the first portions of ejaculated sperm have entered the vagina to prevent dilution of the first drops. Some physicians have collected first semen drops from several ejaculations, combined them, and introduced them artificially into the uterus of the woman.

The Woman The female reproductive system is not only more complicated anatomically than that of the male, but it must also respond to the interaction of some critical hormones. Thus, the causes of infertility in the woman can be more extensive.

The first fact that must be known is whether a mature egg, which can be fertilized, is available each month. Basal body temperature readings and tissue examinations from the uterus can be used to help detect the course of ovulation. Depending on the cause, failure to ovulate may be treated surgically, hormonally, or by other medication. Some women begin ovulating after taking an oral contraceptive for several months and then stopping.

Infertility can also be caused by abnormal functioning of the genital system, abnormal genetic development of ova, undersecretion of gonadotropic hormones, salpingitis (inflammation and fibrous formation within the fallopian tubes), or vaginal fluids that kill the sperm. The egg may be fertilized properly, but be unable to attach to the uterine wall. This may be caused by a hormonal imbalance that alters the nature of the uterine lining.

There is also some evidence that secretions from the vagina and/or cervix in some women may inactivate sperm. In these women, the chances for conception appear to improve if the woman is removed from contact with sperm for a period of time through either abstinence or by use of a condom. It is believed that there may be an antisperm activity in some women, perhaps the production of an antibody or antibody-like substance. If so, the man's use of a condom can eliminate the sperm contact with the woman, yet allow for frequent intercourse.

Emotional Factors In some underprivileged countries, diseased, half-starved humans existing in filthy conditions seem to have little trouble reproducing. Other women who are near physical collapse or who have undergone the psychological trauma of rape (and who would prefer not to be pregnant) bear children. Yet, strangely enough, the fertility of some couples desiring children seems to be upset by subtle emotional matters.

Some women have become pregnant after they have moved out of an annoying neighborhood or after they have taken leisurely vacations. Women who apparently could not conceive have become pregnant shortly after adopting a child.

With some, emotional tension may be the basis of the problem. Tension may prevent the release of the ripe egg or prevent its movement. It may interfere with the production of sperm. Low sperm counts have been revealed among male college students during examination periods, among airplane pilots during wartime combat, or in men who are in a state of nervous exhaustion caused by overwork. Such sperm counts have changed when the emotional stress has been relieved. Some couples become fertile when they begin visiting a fertility clinic, but before they have actually received treatment.

Timing of Intercourse To achieve pregnancy, it is important to have intercourse near the time of ovulation. Physicians frequently suggest methods of improving the chances of fertilization during this period. For example, the couple might refrain from intercourse in the few days preceding ovulation in order to conserve sperm, and then repeat intercourse in 48-hour intervals during the fertile period.

A couple ought to consult their family physician if they are unable to conceive after several months. In the event the physician feels his or her training is insufficient for the problem or is unable to find the cause, he or she may refer the patient or couple to a specialist or clinic. Medical

schools often have fertility clinics. Help may also be obtained from a local Planned Parenthood Clinic. If the couple does not know where to find such a clinic, they may write to Planned Parenthood, 515 Madison Ave., New York, N.Y. 10022.

Artificial Insemination Many couples, where one of the partners is sterile (either naturally or surgically) and who desire children, turn to artificial insemination. In this process sperm of the man or of a male donor are mechanically introduced into the uterus of the woman at the time when conception is most likely to occur. When freshly donated sperm is used, pregnancies occur about 80 percent of the time. When the husband's sperm is used (where husband fertility is very low), pregnancy is successful in about 5 percent of the attempts.

Some physicians are now freezing sperm and storing it until needed. With frozen sperm, impregnation is successful in slightly over 50 percent of the cases. Repeated inseminations over several months are often necessary. Some men have requested prevasectomy storage of their sperm as insurance against unforeseen events. Although sperm stored for as long as 10 years has produced live births, frozen sperm loses much of its effectiveness if stored for more than 16 months. Frozen sperm has several advantages. Not only is sperm available at all times when tests show that ovulation is occurring, but parents can come back and request specimens from the same donor. There is also less chance of the donor meeting the recipient.

Donor artificial insemination may be looked upon as a type of semiadoption. There are often good reasons for requesting donor insemination over obtaining children through adoption. In the event the man is sterile, the child will at least be partially like one of the parents. It will, of course, inherit some of the characteristics of the woman. The woman knows this is her baby physically, psychologically, and legally. The man should look upon the child as his own child psychologically and legally.

The use of artificial insemination is slowly gaining acceptance. It requires a great deal of serious planning and discussion, between the prospective parents—to determine their emotional satisfaction with the process—and with the physician to determine the best method and to find an appropriate donor. Some couples have had more than one child by this technique.

Adoption Pregnancy for some couples wanting children is impossible or too dangerous for the mother. These couples may still have the pleasure of raising a family through adoption. Adoption has many advantages. It provides a good home for the child; it does not contribute to population increase; and it guarantees the parents a healthy child of the desired sex.

The availability of children for adoption varies from area to area and from year to year, but there are fewer available infants for adoption each year. This is caused by a variety of factors, including more effective use of birth control by unmarried persons, more readily available abortions, more unmarried women choosing to keep and raise their children, and more couples choosing to adopt a child rather than contribute to the population problem.

However, certain types of children are still readily available for adoption. These include children who are beyond infancy, children of certain ethnic minorities, and children with physical or mental disabilities. Many couples have found the adoption of such children to be a very rewarding experience.

About half of all adoptions involve the children of blood relatives (as in cases where both parents are lost through death or desertion). Adopting a child who is a blood relative is a rather simple matter and can usually be handled by a family attorney. Adopting an unrelated child is handled either through a licensed agency or privately through direct arrangements with the child's family. The great majority of children adopted by nonrelatives are the children born out of wedlock.

Determination of Eligibility The operations of adoption agencies are controlled by law; consequently, these agencies usually provide the best protection for the child, the natural parents, and the adoptive parents. The major element in this protection is the determination of eligibility. Though the standards do vary from agency to agency, certain points are commonly found.

Agencies attempt to place children in homes where the atmosphere, attitudes, financial circumstances, living conditions, and health of the family are conducive to a satisfactory adjustment of the child. The age of the prospective parents, their religious and racial background (though these factors are less important now than in previous years), their obvious attitudes towards the idea of adoption and the child in particular, and the stability of the marriage of the prospective parents are easily discernible and valuable indices.

Adoption Procedure Once the "match" between parents and child is made to the satisfaction of all parties concerned, the child enters the adoptive home, generally for a probationary period of one year. If the adoption proves suitable during this time, an adoptive decree will be issued for the child. A new birth certificate, giving it the family name of the new parents and their chosen first and middle names, will be drawn up. The original birth record is sealed by the court, never to be opened

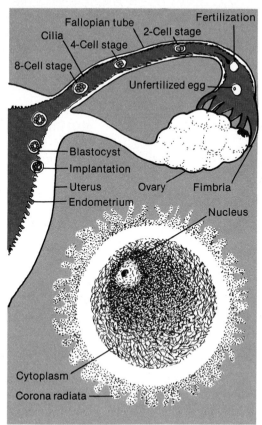

The human ovum (lower right) and its path during ovulation, fertilization, and finally implantation in the uterus.

again except on court order. From this moment, the adopted child is treated as a natural child of the couple. It is entitled to matters of inheritance as is a natural child and is so treated by the courts.

Pregnancy and Childbirth

Although many millions of sperm are deposited in the female genital tract, only one will penetrate the egg. This requires the efforts of many other sperm surrounding the egg, which give off an enzyme that detaches a covering over the egg, the corona radiata, allowing one sperm to enter.

As soon as the sperm has penetrated the egg, the membrane covering the egg thickens and prevents the entry of any other sperm. Following entry, the nucleus in the head of the sperm fuses with the nucleus in the egg, and fertilization has occurred. The united cell is now referred to as a *zygote*. The woman is now said to be pregnant.

Embryology (The Development of the Fertilized Cell) The zygote immediately begins to divide. From a 1-celled zygote, it divides to form 2 cells, 4 cells, 8 cells, and so on. It is now called an *embryo*. By the end of the first week it is a hollow ball of many cells. As cell division speeds up, one side of the ball of cells forms a depression or indentation. This is the first indication that specialized cells, tissues, and organs will be appearing. A fold develops called the *neural groove*, later to become the nervous system. The groove becomes a tube, and the head end of the tube enlarges to become a beginning brain. Blood vessels develop and spread out and by the twelfth day the primitive beginnings of the head, heart, and limbs are evident.

Implantation While this development is starting, the embryo is being carried down the fallopian tube towards the uterus. The embryo spends about three days within the fallopian tube. By the time it leaves the fallopian tube and enters the uterus, the mass of cells looks like a hollow ball, but is actually filled with fluid. Even though the cell mass consists of many cells by this time, the whole mass is no larger than the undivided zygote. (See figure on stages of development of zygote.)

For the next two or three days the cell mass, now called a *blastocyst,* floats around in the cavity of the uterus. Then, at a site chosen by chance, the mass attaches onto the endometrial lining of the uterus and begins to take root. The site of this attachment, or implantation, is usually some place in the upper half of the uterus.

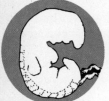 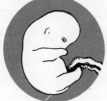 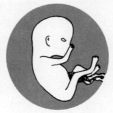 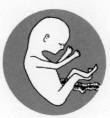 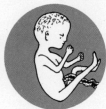

FIRST LUNAR MONTH	SECOND LUNAR MONTH	THIRD LUNAR MONTH	FOURTH LUNAR MONTH	FIFTH LUNAR MONTH
Embryo about ¼ in. long; mouth and jaws present; eyes, ears, and nose forming; arms and legs budding out; heart beating and pumping blood through simple vessels; head very large in proportion to body	Embryo about 1 in. long; face human; eyes, ears, nose visible; thin skin forming; hands and feet forming; fetus begins slight movements; external genitalia beginning to form	Fetus 3 in. long, weight 1 ounce; teeth forming under gums; fingers and toes well formed and bear nails; eyes covered by closed lids; kidneys working; fetus starts swallowing amniotic fluid; sex distinguishable; responds to stimuli; fetus moves easily—not felt by mother	Fetus 6¼ in. long, weight 4 oz; fine hair on body; fetal skeleton visible on x-ray; mother may feel fetal movements; wall of uterus begins stretching	Fetus 9½ in. long, weight 11 oz; buds for permanent teeth begin to form; hair on the head; fetal movements strong; heartbeat perceptible with stethoscope; breasts stop enlarging; uterus as high as navel

The blastocyst sinks in the endometrium, which closes over it. Here the embryo continues to increase in size, soon bulging into the cavity of the uterus, still completely surrounded with endometrial tissue, now called *decidua*.

Placenta Formation From the outer wall of the blastocyst, small fingerlike growths called *chorionic villi* now begin to project into the decidua. In the decidua between the blastocyst and the uterine wall, spaces filled with maternal blood are formed. This area of special tissue for the transfer of nutrients from the mother to the child and for the transfer of wastes from the child to the mother is called the *placenta*. Even though there is a very close relation between the villi of the embryo and the tissues of the mother in the placenta, there is never a direct connection between the two circulations. Blood does not cross directly from the mother to the embryo, and vice versa. The placenta actively transfers ma-

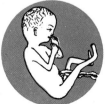
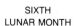
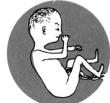
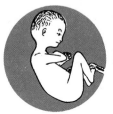
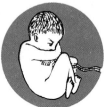
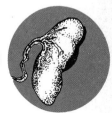

SIXTH LUNAR MONTH	SEVENTH LUNAR MONTH	EIGHTH LUNAR MONTH	NINTH LUNAR MONTH	PLACENTA
Fetus 12 in. long, weight 1½ lb; skin very wrinkled, fat forming underneath; growth now more rapid at head end; eyebrows and eyelashes forming; eyelids reopened; fetus sucks thumb, has hiccups, rolls freely in amniotic fluid	Fetus 14 in. long, weight 2½ lb; skin reddish; thin and scrawny; organs immature, but chance of survival if born	Fetus 16 in. long, weight 3½ lb; skin wrinkled; hair on head abundant; good chance of survival if born	Fetus 18 in. long, weight 6 lb or more; more fat beneath skin makes it plumper, less wrinkled; chances of survival excellent; tip of uterus near breastbone Term—fetus 20 in. long, weight 7¼ lb or more; skin smooth	Placenta—1 to 2 in. thick, 6 to 9 in. diameter at birth. Serves two purposes: (1) anchors fetus to the interior of the uterus through the gestation period; (2) includes a complex web of blood vessels through which nutrients pass from the mother to the developing fetus. Also called the *afterbirth*, and is expelled from the uterus as the final step of a normal birth.

terials from the end of the fourth week after fertilization.

Amniotic Fluid The embryo is attached to the placenta by the umbilical cord, and is surrounded by a double membrane that consists of the amnion and chorion. The space inside of these layers is often called the "bag of waters." The space is filled with amniotic fluid, which bathes the developing embryo. This fluid contains embryonic wastes that are exchanged with the mother's fluids. It also serves to give the embryo space in which to develop, protects it against injury, and keeps it at a constant temperature.

Lunar Months of Pregnancy During the first 8 weeks of pregnancy, the developing child is called the *embryo*. The rest of the time, it is known as the *fetus*.

A full-term human pregnancy usually lasts about 266 days from the time of conception, or about 280 days after the beginning of the last menstrual period (ovulation occurs about 14 days after the beginning of menstruation). The events of pregnancy are commonly subdivided into lunar months; 280 days represents 10 lunar months, each 28 days or 4 weeks in length (although the true lunar month is 29½ days long). Thus a full-term pregnancy would be expected to last about 40 weeks.

According to the calendar, pregnancy lasts a little over 9 months. These 9 calendar months are commonly divided into three parts of three months, each called *trimesters*. Each trimester is about 13 weeks. The chart on fetal development shows and describes the changes during each of the 10 lunar months of pregnancy.

Diagnosis of Pregnancy The determination of pregnancy can be based on symptoms a woman senses, signs the physician notes from physical examinations, and certain laboratory tests. The signs and symptoms of pregnancy are divided into three self-explanatory headings: presumptive, probable, and positive signs.

Presumptive Signs Presumptive signs are the least definite evidence of pregnancy. Each of these symptoms that the woman can detect may also result from causes other than pregnancy.

The first symptom noticed is a missed menstrual period. One missed period is questionable evidence, but two missed periods is strong indication. The breasts may increase in size and firmness and be more sensitive. The nipples may become larger and darker. Nausea and vomiting ("morning sickness") may be associated with early pregnancy. The need to urinate more frequently is common to both early and late pregnancy. Pregnant women tend to fatigue more easily.

Probable Signs The probable signs are discovered by a physician. Like presump-

tive signs, all of them may be simulated by nonpregnant conditions. Yet two or more probable signs occurring simultaneously provide strong evidence of pregnancy.

Near the end of the third lunar month, the uterus can be felt through the abdominal wall as an enlargement that gradually increases in size up to the end of pregnancy. Besides pregnancy, abdominal enlargement can also be caused by tumors, fluid, or rapid fat increase. Changes in the size, shape, and consistency of the uterus during the first three months of pregnancy are important indications of pregnancy, as is the ability to palpate the outline of the fetus. Sudden pressure against the fetus during the fourth and fifth months, causing it to rebound in a few seconds, is among the most certain of probable signs.

Positive hormonal tests for pregnancy are largely reliable. In the event of implantation, the chorion of the embryo gives off a hormone called *chorionic gonadotropin*. Carried by the bloodstream, some of it gets into the urine where tests may detect its presence about 10 to 14 days after the first missed menstruation or about the end of the first lunar month. There are several such tests for pregnancy.

1. *Immunoassay.* This procedure is based on an antigen-antibody response. The hormones present in the urine sample serve as the antigen and will react with the prepared antibody being used in the test. (Absence of agglutination is considered a positive test.) Results, which may be obtained in anywhere from a few minutes to two hours may be 99 percent accurate if the technician is well-trained.

2. *Bioassay.* Urine from a woman is injected under the skin of a female animal. In the event the woman is pregnant, her hormone-laden urine will cause follicular development and ovulation in the female animal, as indicated by the presence of the corpus

luteum. Various animals such as rats, frogs, rabbits, and mice may be used for such tests. The rat test is the most widely used, provides an answer in 16 to 24 hours, and is accurate 95 percent or more of the time.

3. *Hormone test.* In the event a woman has missed a menstruation, estrogen and progesterone hormones are given to her for two or three days. If she is not pregnant, a normal menstrual flow should occur within several days. In the nonpregnant woman, the hormones quickly build up the uterus lining; then with their discontinuance this lining is shed in bleeding. In the event she is pregnant, no unusual bleeding will occur.

Once more, none of these hormonal tests provides positive proof of pregnancy. Many obstetricians use them with reservations.

Positive Signs   There are three positive signs of pregnancy. All three arise from the fetus: fetal heartbeat, perception of active movements of the fetus, and ability to see the fetal skeleton by x-ray. Hearing and counting the fetal heartbeat is unmistakable evidence of pregnancy. The pulse rate will be about twice as fast as the mother's pulse. Fetal movements are commonly felt after the fifth month of pregnancy by placing the hand over the abdomen. The fetal skeletal outline will be visible sometime after the fourteenth week of pregnancy. X-rays are especially useful with obese women in order to distinguish between a tumor or a normal pregnancy.

Care of the Pregnant Mother   The care of the mother from conception to the beginning of childbirth is called *prenatal care.* This care is most important in order to ensure the good health of both the mother and the child. Unfortunately, many women are not able to obtain this

care. It has been estimated, for instance, that one-third to one-half of the women delivering children in major city public hospitals see a doctor for the first time when they are in labor.

Because of the demands a pregnancy places on the body of the mother, a disorder or disease that might normally have little effect on her can turn into a major complication. A condition affecting the mother can have a similar effect on the fetus. Careful medical supervision during this time can avert many damaging conditions.

When a woman suspects that she is pregnant, she should have a complete physical examination, including blood tests and pelvic examination. Follow-up examinations should be made every four weeks until the seventh calendar month of pregnancy; then every two weeks, or more frequently as indicated, until the final month; then once a week until labor begins.

Diet in Pregnancy   The diet of the pregnant woman will have lifelong implications for her baby. Proper nutrition is important in the development of the fetal brain, bones, teeth, and other tissues. The diet must contain increased amounts of proteins, vitamins, and minerals. While physicians usually prescribe special vitamin preparations during pregnancy, an adequate intake of proteins and minerals normally depends on the mother's diet.

In recent years, many physicians have relaxed their restrictions on how much weight the pregnant woman should be allowed to gain. There is evidence that the birth weight of an infant is strongly associated with and conditioned by the weight gain of the mother, and that restriction of diet during pregnancy may unfavorably affect the growth and development of the fetus. The higher the infant's birth weight, the better its growth and performance during the first year of life. The Committee on Maternal Nutrition of the National Research Council is now recommending an average weight gain of 24 pounds (or a range from 20 to 25 pounds). This is particularly important for the low-weight woman whose weight before pregnancy is under 120 pounds. Such women may need a physician's help to maintain sufficient weight gain during pregnancy. For other women, the objective in weight control during pregnancy would be to keep weight gain reasonably close to the 20- to 25-pound average.

Difficulties in Pregnancy Various conditions are the cause of complaint or concern during pregnancy. Some are typical or common, and are to be expected. Others, such as chronic or infectious diseases, are of particular concern both to the unborn child and mother and must be closely watched.

Nausea About 85 percent of all pregnant women experience a feeling of nausea or "morning sickness" during the first three months of pregnancy. Experienced on arising or at other times of the day, it may be accompanied by a distaste for food and vomiting. If the vomiting does not disappear during the day, it is known as *pernicious vomiting*. A physician can normally control this condition by the use of specific foods and drugs.

Diseases in Pregnancy Many diseases assume an increased importance in pregnancy. During the early months of pregnancy, when the fetus is most vulnerable, the woman should try to avoid exposure to contagious diseases of any kind. Virus infections are particularly damaging to the fetus. One of the most serious of these is rubella (German measles). German measles in the first six months of pregnancy may cause congenital disorders

such as cataracts, deafness, heart defects, or mental retardation. It is also thought to cause the death of the fetus in about one-fifth of cases where the mother contracts the disease early in pregnancy. Some states now require evidence of immunity to rubella (acquired through immunization or by having had the actual disease) before issuing a marriage license.

Among bacterial diseases, syphilis and gonorrhea may create serious conditions. The spirochetes of syphilis will be transmitted from the mother to the fetus during the last half of pregnancy unless an infected mother receives treatment. Untreated syphilis frequently causes fetal

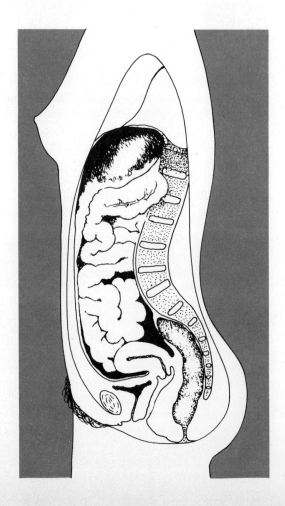

damage or death. Gonorrhea during pregnancy may lead to infection of the eyes of the infant during delivery. A germicide is dropped into a child's eyes immediately after childbirth to prevent this infection.

Toxemias   The term *toxemia*, as applied to certain conditions in pregnancy, is inaccurate, since no toxin, or poison, is found in the blood. The toxemias are characterized by hypertension (high blood pressure) and are sometimes associated with protein in the urine, swelling, convulsions, coma, or other signs, alone or in combinations. Acute hypertension may be called *preeclampsia*. Preeclampsia can be considered severe if symptoms include continued high blood pressure, protein in the urine (proteinuria), less than normal urine output (oliguria), cerebral or visual disturbances, blueness (cyanosis), or pulmonary edema (fluid in the lungs). Preeclampsia overwhelmingly occurs during a first pregnancy and then typically during the third trimester. In severe cases, the untreated patient may go into convulsions, or coma, and the baby may be stillborn. Treatment includes restriction in dietary

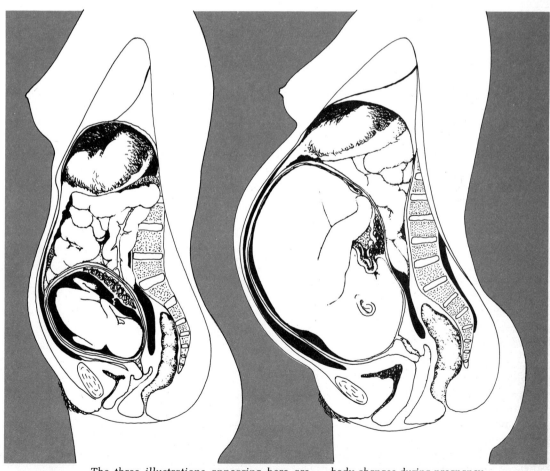

The three illustrations appearing here are cut-away views of the way in which a woman's body changes during pregnancy.

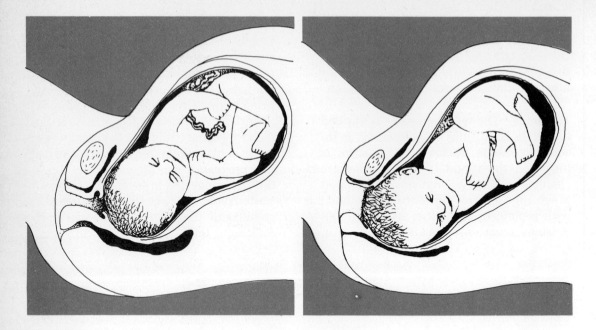

salt, complete bed rest, drugs to reduce swelling and quiet the mother, and prescribed amounts of water.

Drugs in Pregnancy Recent years have brought an increased awareness of the importance of minimizing drug intake during pregnancy. Many drugs have been shown to increase the incidence of congenital defects. In fact, many physicians discourage the use of any nonessential drugs.

In general, the greatest risk of damage occurs during the first three months of pregnancy. Unfortunately, during much of this time, a woman may not be certain that she is actully pregnant. Thus it is important to avoid drugs whenever pregnancy is suspected. This includes almost all drugs—street drugs, nonprescription drugstore remedies, and prescribed medications—unless the physician has specifically approved usage during pregnancy. It is important that any physician or dentist administering medications be told of the fact or possibility of pregnancy.

Although alcohol readily crosses the placenta, its use in moderation has not been shown to produce pathologic changes in the mother or fetus or to affect the course of pregnancy. Maternal chronic alcoholism, however, may lead to fetal underdevelopment. Moreover, growth retardation from such a cause is likely to persist after birth.

Smoking should also be avoided during pregnancy. The more a pregnant woman smokes, the less her baby will weigh at birth. As previously mentioned, the weight of a baby at birth is related to its chances of survival and helps determine how well it will thrive and develop during the first year of childhood.

Childbirth The events of childbirth are well-defined landmarks. An understanding of them not only will help the pregnant woman in closely following the counsel of her physician, but also is important in allaying her apprehensions.

Fetal Position As shown in the figures

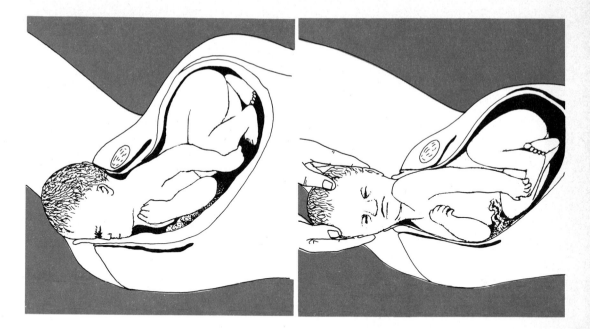

on the previous pages, by the end of pregnancy the upper point of the uterus has pushed up almost to the breastbone of the mother. As a rule, in the later months of pregnancy, the fetus forms a mass roughly similar to the shape of the uterine cavity, folded upon itself so that the chin is almost in contact with the chest, the thighs bent over its abdomen, the legs bent at the knees, and the arms either crossed over the chest or parallel to the sides.

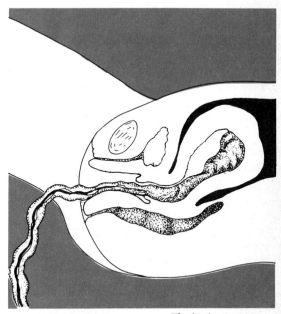

The lowest part of the fetal body or that part first seen in delivery is called the *presenting part*. The presentation is named according to the presenting part. When the head is lowermost it is a *cephalic presentation*. When the buttocks are lowermost it is a *breech presentation*. If the fetus is transverse, it may make a *shoulder presentation*. Almost all babies are born with the back of the head (the vertex) appearing first.

The birth of a baby.

Estimated Date of Delivery   A customary way of estimating the expected day of delivery is to count back three months from the first day of the last menstrual period and add seven days (Naegele's rule). For example, if a woman's last menstrual period began on June 10th, the expected day of delivery would be March 17th. Few mothers deliver on the expected day, but will commonly deviate only two weeks on either side.

False Labor False labor contractions may occur as early as three or four weeks before the termination of pregnancy. They are nothing more than an exaggeration of the irregular uterine contractions that occur through the entire period of pregnancy.

There are ways of distinguishing them from true labor. They occur chiefly in the groin rather than in the top region of the uterus. Their duration is short and they are rarely intensified by walking about (walking may even relieve them). They do not increase progressively in intensity, duration, and frequency. True labor contractions cause a dilation (expansion) of the cervix of the uterus within a few hours, whereas false labor does not.

Labor Labor is the process by which the products of conception are expelled by the mother (also commonly called *childbirth*, *travail*, or *parturition*). The word *delivery* refers to the actual birth of the baby. This is expected to occur at term, or the end of the fortieth week.

Labor is conveniently divided into three stages: the preparatory stage; the birth of the baby; and delivery of the afterbirth.

1. *Preparatory stage.* This period starts with the beginning of labor contractions and lasts until the cervix of the uterus is fully dilated and ready for the passage of the child. The initial contractions are short, mild, and separated by intervals of 10 to 20 minutes. The woman may walk around to remain comfortable between contractions. The

discomfort usually starts in the small of the back and then sweeps around to the front of the abdomen. As labor progresses the contractions become more frequent (every 3 to 5 minutes), become more intense, and last longer. The contractions preceding full dilation may be quite painful. The average duration of the first stage of labor is about 12 hours for the first child and about 7 hours for children born subsequently, although there is marked variation.

2. *Delivery of the child.* Delivery starts with the full opening of the cervix and ends with the completed birth of the child. Contractions are severe and may last 50 to 100 seconds, occurring at intervals of 2 or 3 minutes. The pressure of the contractions will usually cause the rupture of the amniotic sac during the early part of this stage (but also sometimes before or during the first stage). During the contractions the mother strains and bears down strongly.

When the cervix is open, the child begins to move down into the vagina. Each labor contraction moves the head down farther. With the cessation of each contraction, the head recedes somewhat. Just before the head emerges, it rotates to the side to pass the front part of the pelvic bone. With the next few contractions the neck and shoulders emerge. The body of the child is then quickly expelled. Immediately afterward the rest of the amniotic fluid gushes out. As soon as the child has emerged, the physician ties off the umbilical cord several inches from the navel. Immediately after birth he or she helps the child to begin breathing. The child usually begins breathing within one minute and follows this with a strong cry.

The average length of the second

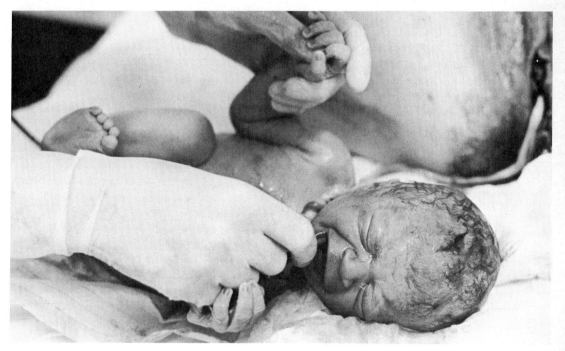

Photo by Suzanne Arms/Jeroboam.

stage is 50 minutes in the first delivery and 20 minutes in later ones.

3. *Delivery of the afterbirth.* Contractions stop for a few moments following passage of the child and then begin again at regular intervals until the placenta is separated and expelled. Placental separation lasts about 2 to 3 minutes. Its expulsion from the uterus will take 5 to 6 additional minutes.

Reducing the Pain of Delivery Pain is normally involved in the delivery of a child. The amount of this discomfort can be reduced by preparing the mother. This preparation should include an understanding of the physical and emotional aspects of delivery. Practicing controlled relaxation and breathing before delivery can reduce muscle spasms during labor. Such natural methods to reduce childbirth discomfort are referred to as *natural childbirth*. It entails education of the mother to eliminate fear, exercises to promote relaxation, muscle control and breathing, and careful management throughout labor by a physician or skilled nurse.

Drugs are commonly used if the pain becomes too severe. Some reduce the pain but allow the mother to remain conscious; others act only on specific parts of the body; some cause her to lose consciousness. Drugs may be injected into the spinal cord to deaden nerves coming from the uterus, but not affect her consciousness. The drugs used depend on the wishes of the mother and the choice of the physician.

With mothers who are receptive to it, hypnosis has been effective in allowing labor with little or no drugs. Although recognized by the American Medical Association, it has limited use. It requires time and patient response.

Handling the Newborn The completed delivery of the child is the official time of birth. As soon as the baby is delivered, it is grasped by the feet and held head down to drain fluids from the nose and mouth. The umbilical cord is clamped and cut (within a few days the cord drops off). The baby must now breathe almost immediately, in order to obtain its own oxygen. Some cry and take their first breath almost as soon as they are born; in most cases breathing starts within one minute. A strong cry indicates that the respiratory system is functioning well. In case of any breathing difficulty, resuscitation must be applied immediately to prevent asphyxiation (suffocation). Delay in breathing can cause damage to the brain cells or the death of the infant.

The child is quickly checked for normal heartbeat, regular breathing, good movement of arms and legs, nervous reflex, and healthy color. The infant's eyes are treated with a germicide to prevent possibility of gonorrheal infection, or ophthalmia neonatorum (this treatment is required by law in most states). The physician inspects the infant for any apparent abnormalities, such as birthmarks, clubfeet, or improperly formed body openings. He or she must also decide whether the infant needs incubator care or not.

To prevent confusing it with other babies in the nursery, the infant must be properly identified before it leaves the delivery room. Identification bands with numbers are commonly fastened to both the baby (wrist and/or ankle) and the mother. Some hospitals also take inked footprints. This can serve as positive identification.

Observation of the Mother The mother is now ready to be moved from the delivery room. She will need close observation for the next few hours to prevent any complications that may arise following delivery. She is exhausted and cold and will need to be kept warm. She should see her husband or a friend as soon as possible after leaving the delivery room. To insure rest and relaxation, she may need to be given a sedative.

Complications of Delivery Childbirth is not always a routine procedure. The following kinds of possible complications justify the services of a qualified physician.

Premature Birth Occasionally a pregnancy ends before the fetus is mature. Whether or not the fetus survives will depend on what point during the pregnancy the termination occurs, the causes, and the conditions of the termination.

By definition, a premature infant is one whose birth weight is less than 2,500 grams. Since no fetus weighing less than 400 gm has survived, and rarely so if less than 500 gm, a premature infant may be defined as one weighing between 500 gm and 2,500 gm (5½ pounds) at birth. Being born so early during the course of pregnancy that its organs have not reached full development, its chances of survival are poorer than that of a full-term infant.

The less an infant weights at birth, the less its chances of survival. The survival chance of a fetus at birth is often classified according to the following scale:

1. 499 gm (1 lb. 1 oz.) or less—no chance of survival (abortuses).
2. 500 gm (1 lb. 2 oz.) to 999 gm. (2 lb. 2 oz.)—poor chance of survival (immature infants).
3. 1,000 gm (2 lb. 3 oz.) to 2,499 gm. (5 lb. 8 oz.)—chances of survival range from poor to good according to weight (premature infants).
4. 2,500 gm (5 lb. 9 oz.) or more—optimal chances of survival (mature infants).

In terms of age of the fetus, the fetus may

weigh 500 gm (1 lb. 2 oz.) during the sixth lunar month (about 22 weeks), or 1,000 gm (2 lb. 3 oz.) at about the end of the 28th week. Generally the fetus becomes viable (will survive if born) at the beginning of the third trimester.

As many as half of all premature births are without explanation. However, suspected maternal causes include high blood pressure, placental problems, and untreated syphilis. Prematurity is the leading cause of infant mortality (death between the time of birth and the first year of age). The death of the infant may often be caused by respiratory difficulties or infections of various kinds.

Cesarean Section The delivery of the fetus through an incision in the wall of the abdomen and uterus is a cesarean section. About half of all cesarean sections are performed on women bearing their first child. The most frequent indication for cesarean section for a first delivery is a space limitation—too large child for the birth canal, a birth canal tumor, or pelvic contractions. Other reasons might be a breech presentation, maternal diabetes, placental or umbilical cord complications. It might also be done in an attempt to save the fetus in the event a mother late in pregnancy dies from other causes.

The other half of all cesarean sections are performed on women who have had cesarean sections before. In such cases the concern is over the rupture of the scar, especially during labor. Although women who have experienced a previous cesarean section may give birth to a fetus through natural labor, more commonly subsequent deliveries would also be by cesarean section. Accordingly, how often a mother could deliver in this manner would depend on the counsel of her physician. Most commonly a mother is counseled to limit her children to two or three, although some women have had more cesarean sections.

A physician will usually set a definite date for performing the operation if he can estimate the maturity of the fetus with confidence. Otherwise, he or she may wait until the patient goes into labor. In any event, the physician may not want to perform a section more than ten days before the calculated date of the delivery due to increased chances of undue prematurity.

Multiple Pregnancies A multiple pregnancy is one in which the uterus contains two or more embryos. Twins occur in about 1 out of every 86 pregnancies, and triplets in about 1 out of every 7,000 births. Twins occur more commonly among blacks than among whites.

Twins may result from the fertilization of either two separate eggs or a single egg. Twins developing from two separate eggs are called *fraternal twins*. Since they are from two separate eggs, fertilized by two separate sperms, they are the same as two different individuals born of the same parents, but at different times.

In about one out of every three cases of twins, one mature egg, fertilized by a single sperm, completely divides into two halves. Since both developing embryos are from the same egg and are fertilized by the same sperm, they are both alike genetically, or *identical*.

Triplets may arise from one, two, or three eggs. If from one egg, the egg has completely divided into three parts, in which case the triplets are identical. If from two eggs, one of the eggs has divided into two halves, two of the triplets are identical and one not. The same would hold true for quadruplets, quintuplets, or other kinds of multiple pregnancies. In one case, the Dionne quintuplets, it is believed that all five were from a single egg.

Sterility caused by lack of ovulation has

been treated with human gonadotropins and has not only successfully induced ovulation, but has also produced multiple eggs, often two or three. The common result has been multiple pregnancies. Efforts are being made to reduce this side effect from the use of these hormones.

Extrauterine Pregnancies Some pregnancies are located outside the uterus. Almost all of these occur in the fallopian tubes. This type of pregnancy is believed to be caused by slowed movement of the egg down the tube and by increased receptivity of the tube to the egg. Regardless of the place the egg lodges, the fetus usually aborts. The mother may feel severe abdominal pains and, if hemorrhaging occurs, may show vaginal bleeding. In any event, the affected tube must be removed. This does not preclude later pregnancies, since another fallopian tube is still available for egg transport.

Induction of Labor Where a pregnancy has developed medical complications, it may be necessary to terminate the pregnancy artificially in order to save the life of the fetus, the mother, or both. In a few cases a physician may decide to terminate the pregnancy for reasons of convenience—a mother who has had a history of rapid deliveries and who might not make it to the hospital in time or who lives a great distance from a hospital. The timing and techniques used to induce labor may present hazards to both the fetus and mother and must be decided on only by a qualified physician.

Changes in the Mother after Delivery
By the end of the first week after delivery, the tissues of the vagina and uterus have greatly contracted. Within six weeks, the uterus is virtually back to its prepregnancy condition. The abdominal wall ought to be back to original shape and firmness within 2 to 3 months.

Loss of Weight With delivery a weight loss of around 11 pounds occurs. Within the next several weeks the mother should lose an additional 4½ to 5½ pounds. Unless she has gained excessively during pregnancy, she should return to her nonpregnant weight within 6 to 8 weeks.

Menstruation Women who do not nurse their babies usually menstruate within 8 weeks after delivery. With those who do nurse them, menstruation is often delayed until the fifth or sixth month, although it may vary from 2 to 18 months. It may return before or after milk production by the breasts is ended. The first menstrual cycles may be irregular. Although ovulation is normally suspended while milk is produced, a nursing mother may become pregnant even though she has not yet menstruated since delivery.

Breasts Breasts begin enlarging early in pregnancy, during which time they may produce small amounts of colostrum, a yellowish fluid. On about the third day after delivery, the breasts become engorged with milk. At first they may feel uncomfortable, but within several days these feelings disappear as production becomes regulated. Frequent and complete emptying of the breasts stimulates production. If the baby cannot empty the breasts in the early days of nursing, it is sometimes necessary to empty the breasts artificially. The length of time a mother breast-feeds her child will vary. Discontinuing of nursing should be a gradual process allowing milk production to decrease.

A mother may choose not to nurse her baby. Milk production can be suppressed by stopping the production of milk-producing hormones. Failure to remove accumulated milk from the breasts will also inhibit further milk production. However, the breasts will become engorged with milk in the meantime and this may cause some discomfort for several days.

The Sex Education of Children

Sex education is often one of the most poorly handled duties of parenthood. The subject may be avoided entirely or handled on a "too little and too late" basis. Many children get most of their sex education from their friends, who are typically poor sources of information, since their own sex education has been just as poorly handled. Often many serious misconceptions are picked up from misinformed friends.

Even parents who have handled other phases of parenthood very well often fail in the area of sex education. The parents who have the most difficulty in sex education are those who, as a result of their own poor sex education, hold negative attitudes toward sex, feel uncomfortable about their own sexuality, or fear that the information will encourage further curiosity and experimentation. Out of embarrassment or a feeling that sex is "dirty," these parents delay giving factual information to their children. The questions of the child are either dodged with a hasty change of subject or else answered with outright lies or with a stern moralistic lecture ("Nice girls don't ask questions like that").

Successful sex education of children (whether by parents or by school teachers) requires that the instructor have correct factual knowledge about sex as well as positive, healthy attitudes toward sex. Sex education can be considered successful only if both correct facts and positive attitudes are learned by the child. Parents who feel uncomfortable about sex educa-

tion should start by examining their own knowledge and attitudes about sex.

A detailed explanation of sexual anatomy and physiology without reference to sexual attitudes and sexual behavior is not complete sex education. Nor is the negative approach—sitting a child down and telling it all the things the child must not do, accompanied by threats of retaliation if the child does. But all too often, sex education takes one of these forms.

How Much, How Soon? Parents (and even schools) are often in a quandary as to how much about sex should be taught to a child of a given age. Sex education should not be tied to any particular schedule because growth patterns vary from child to child and there can be several years difference in the emotional maturity of two children of the same age. But there are some guidelines to follow.

The first is to provide the child with honest answers for any questions asked at the time they are asked. The answers should not be postponed, for several reasons. The child is likely to detect a parent's feeling of embarrassment or uncertainty about sex if questions go repeatedly unanswered. An opportunity to reveal a positive attitude toward sex will be lost. Children should never be given a false answer. They will soon realize its dishonesty and turn to another source, such as their friends, for sexual information, which quite often will be wrong. Any reluctance of the parents to discuss sex honestly can only create doubts about sex in the mind of the child and will close the door to open and honest discussions of sexual problems in the coming adolescent years.

Another guideline is to be sure the child has necessary information before he or she will need it. For example, a girl should know the facts regarding menstruation and breast development in advance of the actual events so that she will not be frightened or embarrassed when they occur, which may be as early as age ten. A boy should similarly know about erection, seminal emission, masturbation, and ejaculation by age ten, to prevent his feeling frightened or guilty at the time they occur.

When discussing sex with children, it is best to concentrate on human sex, which is where their interest really lies, rather than dwelling on sex in various plants and animals ("the birds and bees") in which they are only moderately interested. Of course, animals can be drawn upon occasionally for purposes of illustration and comparison, such as in egg production and nursing. Similarly, when animals are observed mating, giving birth, or nursing their young, it is useful to tell the young child in frank and honest terms just what is happening, pointing out similarities to and differences from human reproduction, and honestly answering all questions raised by the child.

There are many intangibles in sex education. Attitude development, for example, is influenced every day as children detect their parents' attitudes toward sex, not just in "facts of life" talks. Even little things like the inflection given to certain words will betray the parents' true feelings. Children acquire concepts of masculinity and femininity largely through the daily observation of the roles taken by their parents.

Some Specific Considerations Certain aspects of creating a relaxed attitude in the home are perplexing to many parents. A solid background in sexual facts for the parents helps set the stage for a comfortable adjustment by the children.

Nudity in the Home Parents often wonder to what extent their child should see them or brothers or sisters in the nude. Certainly, an important part of the early sex education of any child is that realization that boys and men are different from girls and women and that this difference is perfectly natural.

Home nudity among young children and their parents can be quite harmless, and even useful, if neither the parent nor child is embarrassed by nudity and the nudity is in a normal context such as bathing or dressing. Parents should never flaunt their nudity before their children.

Older children and adolescents are likely to be self-conscious about their developing bodies and will probably wish privacy. Their wishes for privacy should be respected by their parents as well as their brothers and sisters.

Masturbation Another problem topic for many parents is masturbation. The parents may carry residual fears and guilt about masturbation as a result of the way their own parents cautioned or threatened them about masturbation. It is only in recent years that masturbation has been recognized as perfectly harmless and a normal part of both male and female sexuality. Parents should accept masturbation as a harmless way of relieving the powerful sexual tensions of adolescence. Threats should never be made nor fear or guilt created as a result of masturbation.

Terminology Many parents are reluctant to teach children words for sexual parts and functions that are proper in the sense that the children both understand their meaning and yet will not be condemned when they use them among their peers. A poor word selection may reflect the embarrassment of the parent or even doubt about what a preferable word would be. To a child the word may seem nonsensical or be almost impossible to pronounce correctly.

The best policy is to select a word on the

child's level of understanding that he can pronounce. The word should not be infantile, evasive, or inaccurate in the way the child perceives it. (The parents might try placing themselves in the child's situation and trying to imagine what the word might imply to the child.) The mother trying to toilet train her 2-year-old need not try to teach the child to say *urinate*, but when the child can pronounce the word, it should be taught and used.

Nonmarital Sex Parents should frankly and calmly discuss nonmarital sexual relationships with their early adolescents. Too often, the only real discussion comes after a 15-year-old daughter is already pregnant. Rather than centering around threats and accusations, the discussion of nonmarital sex should rationally discuss the issues mentioned at the beginning of this section.

Contraception An often neglected topic in sex education is fertility control. Some parents are actually afraid that a knowledge of contraception will encourage intercourse by their adolescents. But studies have shown that this is not the case. In fact, many adolescent sexual relationships include absolutely no precautions against pregnancy. Knowledge of contraception is seldom, if ever, the deciding influence in determining whether or not a teen-age couple engages in intercourse. But it is certainly desirable that those adolescents who do engage in intercourse make use of an effective contraceptive method.

Even more important than teaching the technique of contraception is teaching why nonmarital pregnancy may be undesirable, why pregnancy should be delayed in early marriage, why children should be spaced, and why the total number of children a couple produces should be limited.

Sexually Transmitted Diseases Adolescents should be given a thorough and factual knowledge of sexually transmitted diseases, not as a scare tactic to prevent nonmarital intercourse, but as a protection against several serious diseases that are now in an epidemic state among adolescents.

Syphilis and gonorrhea should be stressed—their early symptoms, and what to do in case these symptoms appear. The adolescent must feel free to seek treatment for the sexually transmitted diseases. Delayed treatment may result in permanent damage. Since symptoms appear late in many instances, teen-agers should be encouraged to visit clinics after intercourse in which infection may have occurred.

Homosexuality Parents should expect questions from their children regarding homosexuality and should be ready to give honest answers. Homosexuality is and will continue to be prominently featured in literature, theater, television, and popular music. Many adolescents pass through a stage where homosexual attractions are felt. This may cause mixed feelings that, when combined with lack of understanding from the parents, may lead to the irrational fear of homosexuality.

For Further Reading

Boston Women's Collective. *Our Bodies, Our Selves*. Boston: New England Free Press, 1972. A unique handbook on health for women.

Gillette, Paul. *The Pill and Other Birth Control Methods*. New York: Bantam, 1970. Explains the choices available to a woman who wants to control the number of children she would like to have.

Guttmacher, A.F., et al. *Complete Book of Birth Control*. New York: Ballantine Books, 1970. Written by one of America's foremost advocates of informed family planning; one of the best books on the subject.

Hamilton, Eleanor. *Sex Before Marriage*. New York: Bantam Books, 1970. Comments on the implications of sex before marriage; a good book for knowledgeable decision-making on an important personal topic.

Hettlinger, Richard F. *Human Sexuality: A Psychological Perspective*. Belmont, Calif.: Wadsworth, 1975. A contemporary look at psychological and social aspects of human sexuality.

Kinsey, Alfred C., et al. *Sexual Behavior in the Human Male*. Philadelphia: Saunders, 1948. Pioneering study of male sexuality.

_____. *Sexual Behavior in the Human Female*. Philadelphia: Saunders, 1953. Pioneering study of female sexuality.

Martin, Del, and Lyon, Phyllis. *Lesbian Woman*. New York: Bantam Books, 1972. An honest, open account of the difficulties encountered by a lesbian couple.

Masters, William H., and Johnson, Virginia E. *Human Sexual Response*. Boston: Little, Brown, 1966. A study of male and female physiological sexual response.

_____. *Human Sexual Inadequacy*. Descriptions of clinical procedures developed by the authors for the medical treatment of sexual inadequacy.

Rosenfeld, Jack. *Total Orgasm*. New York: Random House, 1973. A positive approach to helping people increase sexual enjoyment.

Weinberg, Martin, and Williams, Colin. *Male Homosexuals: Their Problems and Adaptations*. New York: Oxford University Press, 1974. Problems of male homosexuals in a heterosexual society.

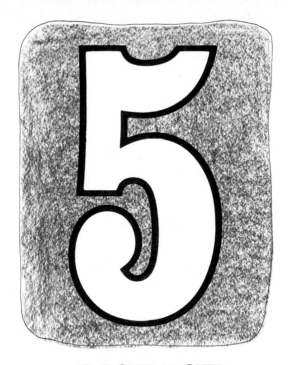

DISEASE

Chapter 18   Noncommunicable Diseases   405

Cancer
Other Major Noncommunicable Diseases
Heart and Circulatory Diseases

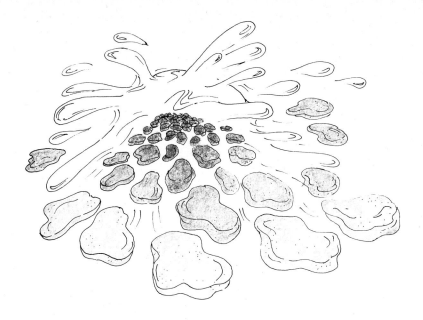

16

COMMUNICABLE DISEASES

The word *disease* has a very broad meaning, being properly applied to any process in which the physical or mental health is impaired. Within this framework would fall such diverse conditions as nutritional deficiencies, emotional problems, drug or alcohol dependence, allergies, noncommunicable degenerative conditions, and the communicable diseases. Throughout most of human history, the communicable diseases have been the principle limiting factor in life expectancy. Malaria, tuberculosis, pneumonia, smallpox, yellow fever, plague, cholera, and a host of other infectious conditions for centuries held the life expectancy to only 30 or 40 years.

In recent years, however, the communicable diseases have been largely controlled in many parts of the world, increasing life expectancies in those regions by 30 years or more. As a result, in the developed countries of the world, the noncommunicable degenerative diseases have emerged as the principle causes of death. Any further increase in life expectancy must now come from control of degenerative circulatory conditions, cancers, and other degenerative diseases.

Yet the communicable diseases still lurk in the background as potential killers of vast numbers of people. The germs that cause these diseases have not been eliminated from the face of the earth. They have only been controlled. Any of them could reemerge if sanitation, immunization, or other control measures were neglected. Also a constant threat is the development of a new disease or more resistant strain of an existing disease through mutation of its germ. Still another threat to our control of communicable diseases is the current explosive growth in world population, which is making adequate sanitation difficult or even impossible to maintain, allowing many of the formerly controlled diseases to reemerge.

Theories of Communicable Diseases

Communicable diseases are diseases that are caused by living organisms or their metabolic products. Other terms used to describe this class of diseases are *contagious* and *infectious*. Communicable diseases have a unique place in human history. They have been responsible for more suffering, death, and destruction than all the wars that have ever been fought. For many centuries, they were the primary natural population control device of several regions. And despite the great advances medicine has made against them during the past century, some diseases still have this dubious distinction in certain areas of the world.

The awesome power of diseases, such as the bubonic plague, cholera, and malaria, to debilitate their victims and seriously interrupt the normal functioning of entire nations kept understanding of the causes and control of these diseases inextricably tied up with myth and superstition. It appeared that only supernatural forces and demonic powers could cause such misery. The progress against these diseases made by European and American bacteriologists, chemists, and physicians during the eighteenth and nineteenth centuries seemed almost anticlimactic. It was based on the theory that minute, invisible life forms—pathogens—were responsible for these diseases. The obvious corollary of this theory is that the cure and treatment of such conditions as smallpox, tuberculosis, and yellow fever related directly to the control of these organisms.

Pathogens The first step in understanding communicable diseases is to gain some familiarity with pathogens and their role in the causation of these diseases. A disease is "caught" when a pathogen invades the body. The disease that follows is caused by some aspect of the parasitic life of the pathogen. (See table on the major pathogen groups.)

Pathogens cause disease in a variety of ways; identification of a particular organism as the causative agent of a disease does not necessarily explain which of these modes is involved. Many pathogenic bacteria, fungi, and protozoa release enzymes that destroy and digest the surrounding human tissues, making the products of their digestion available as food for the pathogens. Other pathogens, particularly bacteria, release powerful toxins (poisons), some of which destroy cells near the site of the infection and some of which are carried by the blood to work in other parts of the body, often on the nervous system, heart muscle, liver, or other or-

Illustrative Plate	Group and Size Scale	Description	Diseases Caused	Mode of Action
	Viruses (10 to 250 nanometers)	Minute, submicroscopic particles composed of nucleic acids and protein; intracellular parasites	Rabies, polio, yellow fever; colds, influenza	Disrupt protein synthesis of cells, sometimes kill cells
	Rickettsia (less than one micrometer)	Small bacteria always associated with insects and other arthropods	Typhus fever; Rocky Mountain spotted fever; Q-fever	Interfere with metabolism of host cells; all are intracellular parasites
	Bacteria (1 to 10 micrometers)	Single-celled, plantlike; abundant in the biosphere; secrete disease-causing toxins; are commonly found in rod, spiral or spherical shape	Tuberculosis, syphilis, pneumonia, scarlet fever, boils, meningitis	Produce toxins and enzymes that destroy cells or interfere with their function
	Fungi (A few micrometers to several inches)	Single-celled or multicelled plantlike organisms; consist of threadlike fibers and reproductive spores	Athlete's foot; most commonly diseases of the skin, hair and nails, and lungs	Release enzymes that digest cells
	Protozoa (A few to 250 micrometers)	Microscopic animals; each is single-celled	Malaria, amebic dysentery, and African sleeping sickness	Release enzymes and toxins that destroy cells or interfere with their functions
	Parasitic Worms (1/32 inch to 20 or 30 feet)	Multicellular animals; common types are round or flat	Pinworm, trichinosis, tapeworms	Release toxins; compete for foods; block digestive tract and blood and lymph vessels

A nanometer is one billionth of a meter; a micrometer is one millionth of a meter; a meter is 39.37 inches.

gans. Some of the bacterial toxins are among the most poisonous substances known to man.

Pathogenic viruses produce disease in an entirely different manner. When a virus enters a host cell, such as a human cell, the genetic material of the virus takes over the control of the host cell. The virus genes direct the protein-synthesizing mechanism of the cell to produce the protein needed for the reproduction of the virus, while neglecting to produce the proteins needed by the cell itself. This disruption of cell function leads to the symptoms of many virus diseases. After several hundred virus particles have been produced, they leave the host cell to infect other cells. Some viruses kill the host cell as they burst out, while other viruses leave the host cell capable of recovery.

Vectors The transmission of many diseases from an infected person or other reservoir of pathogens to a healthy person requires a *vector*. In its more general sense the word vector means a *carrier*. In reference to diseases it usually applies to an arthropod (insect, tick, mite, and so on) that carries the pathogen. The arthropod may or may not suffer from the disease it carries. In most cases it is the bite of the vector that transmits the pathogens, but some pathogens are transmitted through the feces of the vector or are carried on the feet or body of the vector.

Mosquitoes are among the most important vectors, transmitting malaria, yellow fever, encephalitis, filariasis, dengue fever, and other diseases. The piercing mouthparts of the female mosquito contain two ducts, one for sucking blood and one for injecting saliva. The saliva of a mosquito contains an anticoagulant to prevent clotting of blood and is always injected into the person or other animal being bitten before any blood is drawn out. This makes the mosquito an efficient vec-

tor of disease. (The male mosquito never bites, feeding instead on the nectar of plants.)

Other important vectors include ticks, mites, fleas, lice, flies, kissing bugs, and other arthropods. Each transmits specific diseases in specific ways. The pathogen-vector relationship is generally quite specific. For example, each of the diseases mentioned as being transmitted by mosquitoes is carried by only certain specific mosquitoes.

A worldwide conflict exists between public health workers, on the one hand, who seek to control vectors, especially mosquitoes, through the application of insecticides and elimination of breeding areas by draining swamps, and environmentalists, on the other hand, who feel that these measures are ecologically unwise. The outcome of this controversy may determine whether vast areas of the earth's surface are suitable for human habitation.

Stages of Communicable Diseases

Most communicable diseases progress through several definite stages. The identification of these stages in particular cases is of great importance for three major reasons: (1) some diseases involve stages during which no obvious symptoms are present, but the patient is still clinically in danger; (2) contagion control requires that those stages during which the disease can be transmitted be clearly identified; and (3) the possibilities of isolation and immunization frequently relate to the progress of the disease.

Transmission and Infection Transmission is the process whereby a disease is "caught." In this process the pathogen is carried in some way from its source and enters the body in an area where it can cause infection. Infection is the process establishing a pathogen as a parasite in the body. Transmission and infection require the following:

1. *Pathogen.* The pathogen, as discussed earlier, may be one of a number of viruses, rickettsia, bacteria, fungi, protozoa, or parasitic worms.
2. *Source.* The source, also called the *reservoir*, may be human or animal, soil, water, food, or an object that will allow the pathogen to survive.
3. *Method of transmission.* Pathogens are often passed from person to person or animal to person by direct or indirect contact. Transmission by direct contact can occur as a result of touching, kissing, or other close personal contacts. Indirect transmission takes place when pathogens are released during coughing, breathing, or talking. Transmission also can take place when contaminated food or water is taken into the body.
4. *Portal of entry.* The pathogen must get into the body. This occurs as the result of a vector bite, a wound, or entry through body openings such as the nose, mouth, eyes, genital openings, and skin and mucous membranes.
5. *Susceptible host.* A susceptible host is an individual who is unable to resist the pathogen and its effects.

Should all five links in the cycle be present, then infection will occur and the cycle may begin again. If any link in the cycle is broken, however, the disease will be prevented.

Incubation Period   Once a communicable disease has been caught, it progresses through an incubation period, the interval between the time of infection and the appearance of the first symptoms. During this time, the pathogen multiplies in numbers until it is abundant enough to overcome the body's defenses and produce its disease.

The incubation period may be as short as a few hours or as long as several months or years, depending on the disease. Most diseases have an incubation period of a few days to a few weeks. Generally, diseases are not contagious during the early part of the incubation period, but they do become highly contagious at the end of the period, just before the symptoms appear.

Prodromal Period   The prodromal period is the time during which vague, nonspecific symptoms of a disease appear. This period lasts from a few hours to several days and is characterized by fever, headache, and various aches and pains. Many diseases are highly contagious during this period.

Typical Illness Period   After the prodromal period a group of specific symptoms will appear. This is the typical illness period during which a recognizable disease is present. The term *syndrome* often is used to indicate a group of symptoms characteristic of a given disease. In this

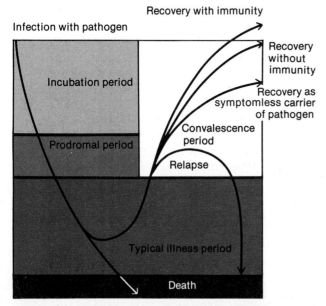

The stages of a communicable disease from infection to death or recovery.

period the person is usually ill enough to stay home, so many diseases are less contagious than during the late incubation and prodromal periods.

Recovery Stage The recovery stage begins when the body defenses start to overpower the pathogens and the symptoms disappear. It is important to remember that the pathogens are still present in the body during the recovery or convalescence stage. If a convalescent person resumes full activity too soon, the body defenses will be weakened, and there may be a relapse (return of the symptoms of the disease.) As is indicated in the figure showing the stages of communicable disease, there are degrees of recovery, each of which has long-range significance both to the future health of the patient and to contagion of the disease.

Protection Against Communicable Diseases

Not too many years ago, little could be done to control the spread and effects of communicable diseases. As we have seen, this was partly caused by the lack of knowledge about pathogens and how they cause disease. Another factor, however, was the need for collective (public) responsibility. Many protections against diseases are impossible or extremely difficult for the individual to carry out on his or her own. The responsibility for these protections, therefore, has been assumed by modern public health agencies.

The major emphasis in public health is on prevention. This is reflected in such functions as immunization, the inspection of such reservoirs of pathogens as food, water, and insect vector sources, and the discovery and isolation of carriers. Public health agencies have increasingly also served an educational function—

alerting the public to the symptoms of common and dangerous diseases, and encouraging anyone suspected of being ill to receive treatment. In many cases, public health agencies will provide treatment free of charge to those who cannot afford to pay.

Though it is becoming less common, public health agencies occasionally deal with the consequences of widespead epidemics. The "flu" epidemics of recent years have mobilized the facilities of health agencies across the country. The control of carriers of smallpox is a continuing function, the importance of which is dramatized by the constant possibility that a widespread epidemic of this disease could sweep the country within days of a break in this protection.

To a certain extent, the success or failure of public health facilities to control communicable disease hinges on the degree to which the individual's natural body defenses can be activated. The human body has a great ability to resist disease. We are constantly being exposed to germs. Most of the time we completely resist these germs, and no infection occurs. When infection does take place, recovery is often possible through the body's own unassisted defenses. Some of these natural defenses are:

Skin and Mucous Membranes The unbroken skin or mucous membrane keeps out most pathogens, even though a few can penetrate healthy skin.

Tears Tears, constantly flowing over the surface of the eyes, contain a substance (lysozyme) that inhibits bacteria. Without this substance, the eyes would have many more infections than they do.

Cilia The ducts of the respiratory system have an inner lining of cilia. These are millions of microscopic hairs that pick up

Typical Immunization Schedule

Age	Preparation
2 months	DPT (diphtheria, whooping cough, tetanus)
	Trivalent OPV (oral polio vaccine containing types I, II, and III)
3 months	DPT
4 months	DPT
	Trivalent OPV
12 months	Live measles vaccine[a]
12 months to puberty	German measles vaccine[a]
	Mumps vaccine[a]
15 months	DPT
	Trivalent OPV
Before school entrance	DPT
	Trivalent OPV
15 years	Td (adult type tetanus and diphtheria booster)
Over 15 years	Td boosters every 10 years for life

[a]Measles, German measles, and mumps vaccines may be combined into a single trivalent vaccine.

NOTE: This schedule is recommended as a flexible guide that may be modified within limits to meet the needs of the individual patient or physician.

Taken from *Public Health Service Advisory Commitee on Immunization Practices*, 1972 Recommendations, National Communicable Disease Center Morbidity and Mortality report, Vol. 21, No. 25, June 24, 1972.

inhaled bacteria, dust, and foreign matter on a thin layer of mucus. The cilia wave in such a manner that the foreign matter is carried up to the throat and swallowed. This action helps keep the lungs free of infection. In the heavy smoker these cilia are inactivated or completely disappear. The smoker then must cough frequently to clear foreign matter from the lungs. Years of coughing may contribute to emphysema, a serious condition in which the air sacs of the lungs break down.

Interferon Virus-infected cells release a chemical called *interferon*. Because this chemical protects other cells from invasion by viruses, it is thought to be important in our recovery from virus diseases.

White Blood Cells The white blood cells, or leucocytes, serve several important functions in defending the body against infections. Some of the white cells are able to surround bacteria and digest them, a process called *phagocytosis*. Other white blood cells play an important role in producing inflammation, which occurs when the concentration of white blood cells in an area increases. Still other white cells are important as the source of antibodies.

Antibodies The invasion of the body by pathogens or certain other foreign substances stimulates the production of antibodies. Antibodies are proteins that act against the foreign substances that stimulated their production, the *antigens*. Thus, antibodies are very specific in their action. Antibodies are the basis of immunity.

The antigen–antibody–immunity relationship is the basis of an artificial method of disease prevention, immunization. Through immunization, a person can develop immunity to a disease without having to suffer from the disease first. There are two basic methods of immunization. Active immunity is obtained by injecting or otherwise exposing a person to an antigen, which causes the person to produce antibodies. The resulting immunity is usually long lasting. That is, it is effective for several years or even for a lifetime. Passive immunity is obtained by injecting a person with antibodies extracted from the blood of an animal or from another person. Passive immunity is instant immunity, but it has a short duration. The injected antibodies break down in a few weeks without stimulating the person to produce antibodies. Only exposure to antigens can give long-term protection.

Some Major Communicable Diseases

Name of Disease	Caused By	Usual Age Infected	Mode of Transmission	Incubation Period	Early Signs	Length of Disease
Common Cold	Over 50 types of viruses	Any age	Direct or indirect contact with nose or throat discharges (cough or sneeze) of infected person	12 to 72 hours, usually 24 hours	Sore throat, running nose, chills, aches, classical prodromal period	2 to 7 days
Influenza or "flu"	Many strains of viruses that fall into three types, A, B, and C. New strains always developing	Any age	Direct or indirect contact with nose or throat discharges (cough or sneeze) of infected person	Quite short, usually 24 to 72 hours	Very rapid onset of fever, chills, headache, muscular aches, and severe coughing	1 to 3 days
Chickenpox	*Varicella virus.* Same virus causes herpes zoster (shingles) in adults	Childhood disease, 2 to 8 years	Direct or indirect contact with discharges from skin or nose or throat lesions of infected persons. Virus may also be airborne	10 to 21 days, usually 14 to 16 days	Slight fever, skin eruptions (lesions)	9 to 14 days
Poliomyelitis or "polio"	Three types of polio viruses	Any age, most common among children (called *childhood disease*)	Direct contact or close association with infected person. Indirectly by fecal contamination or nose or throat discharge of an infected person	3 to 28 days, usually 7 to 12 days	Fever, headache, sore throat, nausea, muscle pain, and general weakness	Highly variable—up to several months
Smallpox	*Variola* or Smallpox *virus*	Any age	Direct or indirect contact with throat or skin discharges of lesions of infected persons; airborne transmission of virus over a short distance	7 to 16 days	High fever, headache, prostration, skin eruption	1 to 7 weeks

Contagious Period	Permanent Aftereffects	Immunity	Prevention	Additional Information
From 24 hours before onset of symptoms until 3 to 5 days after	None	Little or none	Avoid infected persons	Very serious side effects may result from the improper care of colds. When a high fever accompanies cold symptoms, a secondary infection may be present and a physician should be consulted
One day before onset until 4 days after	Rare, but predisposes elderly or weakened persons to pneumonia. The general death rate goes up during flu epidemics	Infection produces immunity of unknown duration to the type of virus infecting you; but not necessarily to other influenza viruses	Annual immunization with vaccine based upon prevailing strains of virus	True influenza is an infection of the respiratory tract. Many other types of viral, or even bacterial, infections are commonly, though incorrectly, called "flu"
From 1 day before eruption of lesions until 6 days afterward	Very rare; deaths from encephalitis or pneumonia do occur	One attack confers long immunity	No effective prevention has yet been developed	The same virus, when contracted by adults who have not had chickenpox, sometimes causes an infection of the nervous system called *shingles*—a painful inflammation of the skin is produced
Maximum period from 1 week before symptoms to 3 months after onset of symptoms; usually from 3 days before to 10 days after onset	Two to 10% fatality rate in paralytic cases; or paralysis may be permanent	Most cases are nonparalytic and result in immunity to the specific type of virus responsible, but not to the other two types	Oral polio vaccine (OPV) currently given in a mixed form containing all three types of weakened polio viruses; called *trivalent OPV;* should be taken 4 times during childhood for lifetime immunity	Polio is completely preventable by proper immunization. However, cases continue to occur in the United States among people who have had only partial immunization or whose parents were not interested enough in their welfare to even have them immunized
From 4 to 5 days before rash appears until rash disappears	From 1 to 40% of cases die; blindness, brain damage, scars	Second attacks are very rare	Vaccination when traveling outside the U.S.	A campaign for the worldwide eradication of smallpox has confined this disease to isolated areas of India and Bangladesh. Routine immunization has been discontinued in the United States except for certain foreign travel

Some Major Communicable Diseases (Cont.)

Name of Disease	Caused By	Usual Age Infected	Mode of Transmission	Incubation Period	Early Signs	Length of Disease
Measles "red measles" (Rubeola)	*Rubeola virus*	Childhood disease, 2 to 8 years	Direct or indirect contact with nose or throat discharge of infected person; also airborne	7 to 14 days, usually 10 to 12 days	Gradually increasing fever, cold symptoms, severe cough, conjunctivitis, running nose; rash appears on third or fourth day	6 to 12 days
German Measles "three-day measles" (Rubella)	*Rubella virus*	Childhood disease, 2 to 15 years	Direct or indirect contact with nose or throat discharge of infected person; also airborne	10 to 28 days, usually 14 to 21 days	Slight fever, swelling of lymph glands, rash	1 to 4 days
Diphtheria	*Corynebacterium diphtheriae,* the diphtheria bacillus	Childhood disease, under 15 years of age	Contact with nose or throat discharges of a patient or carrier	1 to 6 days	Sore throat, mild fever, running nose	Highly variable; possibly several weeks
Whooping Cough (Pertussis)	*Bordetella (Hemophilus) pertussis,* the pertussis bacillus	Childhood disease, birth to 10 years	Direct or indirect contact with nose or throat discharges of infected person	5 to 16 days, usually 7 to 10 days	Gradually increasing *dry* cough	2 to 10 weeks, usually 4 to 6 weeks
Tetanus "Lock jaw"	*Clostridium tetani,* the tetanus bacillus	Any age	Tetanus spores in dust or dirt infect the body through an open wound or cut	Commonly 4 days to 3 weeks	Painful contractions of the body's muscles	Variable; several weeks
Mumps	Mumps virus	Childhood disease, 2 to 14 years	Direct or indirect contact with nose or throat discharge of infected person	12 to 28 days, usually 16 to 20 days	Fever, swelling of salivary gland	4 to 10 days
Tuberculosis	*Mycobacterium tuberculosis,* the tubercle bacillus	Any age	Contact with patients, indirect contact through contaminated articles, unpasteurized milk; bacillus may be airborne	4 to 6 weeks	None (may go undetected for long periods of time)	Indefinite

Contagious Period	Permanent Aftereffects	Immunity	Prevention	Additional Information
From 4 days before until 5 days after rash appears	Occasional death or brain damage due to encephalitis	Congenital immunity lasts a few months. The disease usually confers permanent immunity	Immunization with live measles vaccine	A single injection gives an active immunity against measles for life. Some states require immunization before registering for school. This disease can cause death and disability. All children should be immunized
From 1 week before until end of rash	Rare, except to fetus of an infected expectant mother	One attack usually confers permanent immunity	Immunization with German measles vaccine	There is a high chance of permanent damage to the fetus of a woman who is in the first six months of pregnancy when contracting German measles. This vaccine should not be given to a pregnant woman or one who may become pregnant within two months after the shot. All girls should be immunized before their first menstrual flow
Variable; usually from 3 days before until 10 days after onset of symptoms	Five to 10% of cases die; toxin may permanently damage heart or nervous system	Congenital immunity lasts for several months. The actual disease usually confers a lasting immunity	Immunization with DPT shots	Diphtheria bacteria release a toxin that, when carried by the blood, has serious destructive effects on many parts of the body
Variable; usually first two weeks	In infants, death or brain damage	No congenital immunity; second attacks rarely occur	Immunization with DPT shots	In the United States today, whooping cough occurs mainly among young children from low-income families where proper immunization practices are not always followed. It is very dangerous to young children, especially those under six months of age
Not contagious from human to human	Fatality rate about 50% of cases; usually no permanent damage to someone who recovers	Second attacks are known to occur.	Immunization with DPT shots	When tetanus infection occurs, the toxin released by the bacteria is picked up by the blood and acts upon the central nervous system. The muscles contract fully, become rigid, and convulsions occur. Death is usually because of failure of the muscles needed for breathing
Seven days before swelling until end of swelling	Very rare; brain damage, atrophy of one testis in some adult males or ovarian involvement in some females	The disease usually confers lifelong immunity	Immunization with live mumps virus vaccine	An effective vaccine is available and should be given to all children over one year of age and to any adult who has never had mumps. After puberty there is a chance (25%) that one testis of an infected male may degenerate. In mature females ovarian degeneration may occur
As long as disease is active	Death; destruction of lungs, bones, kidneys and skin	Immunity conferred by healed infection is very limited	Avoidance of crowding, proper nutrition, chest X ray, skin test, BCG vaccine for high-risk individuals	Tuberculosis is a disease of poor health conditions, poverty, and crowding. Adequate health conditions can overcome it

Name of Disease	Caused By	Usual Age Infected	Mode of Transmission	Incubation Period	Early Signs	Length of Disease
Infectious Hepatitis	A virus infection of the liver	Any age	Contact with feces, urine, blood, and probably nose and throat discharges of infected persons	2 to 7 weeks, commonly 3 to 4 weeks	Fever, mild headache, chills, fatigue and jaundice	Variable, often 2 to 4 weeks
Infectious Mononucleosis	A virus infection centered in the lymph nodes	Can be a childhood disease, 2 to 20 years of age	Unknown—believed to be direct contact with nose or throat discharges of infected persons; some implication of cats as a reservoir	2 to 6 weeks	Fever, sore throat, fatigue, enlarged lymph nodes	Variable; 1 week to several months

A special type of passive immunity is congenital immunity. During pregnancy, antibodies pass across the placenta from the body of the mother into the blood of the child. These antibodies give the newborn child an immunity to many common diseases. But since this is passive immunity, it lasts only for several months. The proper protection of an infant requires a series of injections given at regular intervals during the first few years of life. It is the responsibility of parents to see that their child receives these immunizations. The first injections are usually given when the infant is about two months old. Every child born in the United States should be immunized against seven diseases: diphtheria, tetanus, whooping cough, polio, measles, German measles, and mumps. (See table on typical immunization schedule.) It should be remembered that continued protection against diphtheria and tetanus requires booster immunizations every ten years throughout adult life.

Immunizations against several other common diseases are still being developed, and may eventually become part of the standard immunization series. In addition, immunizations against many other diseases are already available for use in special cases, such as before travel into foreign countries.

Treating Communicable Diseases

The use of drugs to treat diseases is called *chemotherapy*. In general, the drugs developed so far have had the greatest success against bacterial diseases, moderate success against protozoan, fungal, and parasitic worm diseases, and little or no effect on the viral diseases. A few antiviral drugs have been developed, however, and there is good probability that others will follow.

The discovery of sulfa drugs (sulfonamides) in 1935 was the first major step

Contagious Period	Permanent Aftereffects	Immunity	Prevention	Additional Information
Unknown; believed to be from 1 week before onset until 1 week after	Rarely death or permanent liver damage	Second attacks are rare	None	This disease is more severe in adults than in children. It is often transmitted through traces of blood remaining in or on an injection needle, through blood transfusions, or by shared needles when abusing drugs.
Probably from several days before symptoms until end of sore throat	None	Infection with or without symptoms is believed to confer lasting immunity.	None	This disease is most severe among young adults. It is rarely fatal but a period of general weakness may last for several months

NOTE: For a more complete listing of the communicable diseases see: Kenneth L. Jones, Louis W. Shainberg, and Curtis O. Byer, *Health Science* (New York: Harper and Row, 1974).

toward the control of bacterial infection. Sulfa drugs prevent the multiplication of bacteria by interfering with the bacterial metabolism. People taking sulfa drugs must drink plenty of fluids. Otherwise, the drugs may crystallize in the kidneys and cause damage.

Antibiotics, such as penicillin, are substances that are produced by soil-inhabiting microorganisms in order to inhibit the growth of competing soil organisms. Antibiotics are made for drug use by growing the organisms that produce them in large vats. The liquid growth of these organisms is released from the vats. From this liquid, antibiotics are extracted and then purified. Most antibiotics are given by injection, but some are effective if taken by mouth.

Antibiotics are generally effective only against bacteria. They have no effect on viruses. Antibiotics cannot cure a cold, influenza, measles, mumps, or other common viral diseases.

When people are taking drugs, they should follow these precautions:

1. Follow instructions exactly.
2. Use a drug only for the illness for which it was prescribed. Do not keep leftover drugs for future use. Many drugs break down in storage and may become worthless or even harmful.
3. Avoid borrowing or lending prescriptions. Entirely different diseases may have very similar symptoms, and a borrowed prescription may be very dangerous. (It is also illegal to possess a prescription drug without having a prescription.)
4. Keep all drugs out of the reach of children.
5. Avoid unnecessary use of antibiotics. The indiscriminate use of antibiotics has two undesirable effects. First, it can cause the development of allergic reactions to the antibiotic, which can later be serious or even fatal. Second, it speeds the development of drug-

resistant strains of bacteria. Such bacteria have already become a critical problem in public dealth, since by definition they are not susceptible to our major weapon against disease.

Some Major Communicable Diseases

The major communicable diseases include several diseases commonly called *childhood diseases* because the greatest number of cases are in the age group of 1 to 15 years. Since these diseases usually confer lifelong immunity, repeated infection is not common. It is not unusual, however, for a person to escape infection during childhood and then catch one of these diseases as an adult. Frequently, the consequences of an adult case of a "childhood" disease can be more serious than that occurring in earlier years.

In addition, the common diseases include the common cold and influenza, neither of which confer any long-term immunity. Thus, they can be contracted many times. (See table of major communicable diseases.)

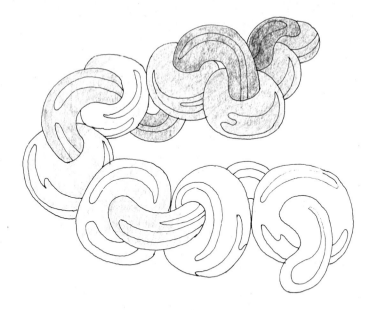

17

THE SEXUALLY TRANSMITTED DISEASES

The sexually transmitted diseases are a paradoxical medical problem. They are basically easy to detect and diagnose, and the drug industry offers a wide and effective range of treatments. Yet, these serious, painful, and often devastating diseases are now occurring in epidemic proportions. Why?

The problem is not really a medical one. Rather, social and cultural factors conspire to prevent detection and treatment. The major reason, of course, is the association of these diseases with human sexuality. It is understandable that guilt and uncertainty interfere with our acceptance of these diseases as the treatable, communicable diseases that they actually are.

A New Name for an Old Problem

The traditional designation *venereal diseases* has been in use for over 300 years. Yet, it has recently come in for criticism as an inadequate and troublesome label. The World Health Organization began in the spring of 1975 to introduce the term *sexually transmitted diseases* (STDs) in the hope of changing the popular attitudes that have long hampered control of these diseases.

Changing the name does not, of course, alter the problem in any way, but hopefully it will help lead to more open and realistic attitudes about these diseases. Such attitudes could contribute greatly to their control.

Why STD?

Except for having similar methods of transmission, the various sexually transmitted diseases are all different. What they do have in common is an affinity for the mucous membranes, such as those lining the reproductive organs, as well as relatively weak resistance to adverse environmental conditions such as dryness and cold. Transmission of the STDs generally requires the direct contact of warm, moist body surfaces. Sexual contact is ideal for this purpose.

No animals besides humans are commonly known to carry any of the sexually transmitted diseases; the pathogens apparently evolved from harmless inhabitants of the human body or perhaps even of soil or water. Nor is it logical to view STD as punishment for "sin." Too many innocent people, such as newborn babies and spouses of unfaithful mates, are infected to make this idea plausible. It is best to think of these diseases as potentially dangerous infections that happen to be commonly transmitted through sexual contact and that should receive prompt treatment before others are infected or permanent damage results.

History of STD

The early history of the sexually transmitted diseases is obscured by the confusion and lack of knowledge that surrounded diseases in general until fairly recently. However, diseases fitting the descriptions of STD can be traced back as many as 3,000 years. Hippocrates wrote of gonorrhea in 460 B.C., and several chapters of the Bible describe diseases that accurately correspond to the various stages of syphilis. The first recorded epidemic of syphilis swept through Europe late in the fifteenth century, possibly having been brought back from the New World by Columbus' crews. There was widespread death and disfigurement throughout much of Europe.

At one time gonorrhea and syphilis were thought to be the same disease. This erroneous idea was corrected in 1879 by the German bacteriologist Neisser, who identified the bacterium causing gonorrhea.

Both gonorrhea and syphilis have had a variety of names. Gonorrhea has been called "clap," "dose," "strain," and "G.C." Syphilis has been called "scab," "pox," "French pox," "Gallic disease," "Spanish sickness," "German pox," "Persian fire," "lues," and "syph." Syphilis received its present name in 1530 in a poem by a physician named Fracastoro about an afflicted Greek shepherd boy named Syphilus, who had offended the sun god.

Today's Incidence of STD

The number of cases of gonorrhea and syphilis exceeds the number of cases each year of strep throat, scarlet fever, mumps, measles, hepatitis, and tuberculosis *combined*. There are now well over 900,000 new cases of gonorrhea officially reported each year, but it is estimated that only one case out of every four actual infections is reported. For this reason, the actual incidence is probably more than 3 million per year. An estimated one-half million people in the United States suffer from untreated syphilis, and it is estimated that over 90,000 new cases are added each year. The cases of genital herpes infection probably number in the millions.

Other studies indicate that even these estimates may be too conservative. For example, during the 12-month period ending June 30, 1973, gonorrhea screening programs cultured specimens from almost 5,000,000 women in the United States, of which 4.9 percent were positive for gonorrhea. The *Weekly Morbidity and Mortality Report* of the U.S. Center for Disease Control noted, on October 10, 1973, that although the highest gonorrhea rates (18.9 percent) were found predictably in visitors to STD clinics, only 12 percent of the tests were performed in such clinics. The remaining 88 percent were in other settings.

Who Gets STD?

STD is in no sense a class phenomenon, that is, restricted to any one level in society. It has permeated all social levels; infections cross all lines of age, income, and ethnic group.

Most gonorrhea infections occur in the young, between the ages of 15 and 24. According to Dr. Walter Smartt, former chief of the Los Angeles County Venereal Disease Control Division, "the probability that a person will acquire VD by the time he's 25 is about 50 percent." Victims are, understandably, fairly equally divided between male and female. Yet, most *patients* are male because men more often show symptoms that lead to seeking of medical treatment. For every two women who are treated for gonorrhea, there are seven men treated. The difference is accounted for by the large number of undiagnosed women whose disease does not produce apparent symptoms (*asymptomatic*). Tests for gonorrhea conducted on female patients seeking treatment for purposes of birth control at public and private clinics indi-

cate that about one in ten women between the ages of 15 and 25 has gonorrhea and does not know it.

According to the World Health Organization, certain groups are particularly susceptible to these diseases. For example, military personnel, highly mobile businesspeople and vacationers, sexually active young people, homosexually oriented people, and members of "free living" communities are more likely, statistically, to encounter this epidemic health problem.

Why the Increase in STD?

Throughout most of history, no specific cure for the sexually transmitted diseases was available. The introduction of sulfa drugs in the 1930s and penicillin in the 1940s promised a cure for both gonorrhea and syphilis with no more than a single office visit. Thus treatment moved from chronic care institutions into the private physician's office. Following the introduction of antibiotics, physicians began to rely solely on such treatment to eradicate STD. Treatment is vital because it may cure the infected individual. But it does not lead to the eradication of the disease from the population. (In the words of Dr. Smartt, "Treatment alone cannot, will not, and has never *eliminated* a communicable disease.")

After 1947, STD dropped steadily for a decade through the use of penicillin and other antibiotics. Then a blanket of complacency settled down over government agencies, the medical profession, and the public. Funds for STD control diminished, and STD began its spectacular resurgence. Late in the 1940s, patients were not even being interviewed for information on sexual contacts from or to whom the infection may have passed. Medical schools underemphasized its importance, and the general public became largely apathetic. Research on STD halted, there were few attempts to produce appropriate vaccines or to develop a better method of diagnosing gonorrhea. Physicians were content to "spot-treat" isolated cases showing up in their offices. This neglect, particularly by the medical profession in developing better control procedures, is essentially the cause for the current gonorrhea epidemic (see graph on incidence of STD).

According to some authorities, an important factor in the current STD epidemic is the birth control pill. The pill has largely eliminated fear of pregnancy, thus encouraging greater freedom in sexual activity. Further, it has reduced the use of condoms, the only birth control method of value in preventing the transmission of STD. More than this, the pill increases the alkalinity and moisture of the female genital tract, thus encouraging the rapid growth of gonorrhea organisms. Other contraceptive aids for females, such as vaginal jelly and foam, are acidic and thus provide an environment antagonistic to the growth of infectious organisms. The estimated risk of contracting gonorrhea for a woman engaging in a single act of unprotected intercourse with an infected partner is 40 percent. For a woman taking the pill, it is almost 100 percent.

The life-styles of young people have incorporated greater freedom of sex and greater personal mobility, both of which are favorable to the spread of infections. There are three other important changes in sexual behavior that may bear on the increase of incidence. They include (1) sexual relationships beginning at earlier ages; (2) greater variety in sexual partners; and (3) possibly less concern over the welfare of sexual partners.

Eradication of gonorrhea does not seem likely for some time because of several factors:

1. The so-called sexual revolution has had a profound influence and shows no signs of abating.

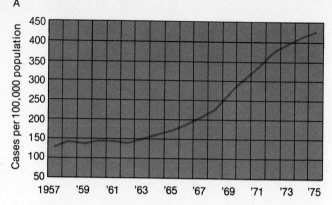

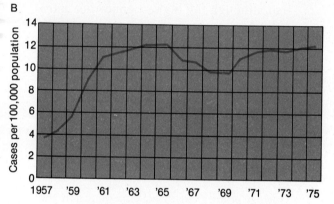

Reported incidence of STD in United States, 1957–1974: (A) gonorrhea, (B) primary and secondary syphilis.

Taken from U.S. Center for Disease Control, Morbidity and Mortality Report, 1973 Annual Supplement (July, 1974) and Weekly Morbidity and Mortality Reports for 1974 and 1975. Figures for 1974 and 1975 are preliminary estimates.

2. There are apparent weaknesses in the medical lines of defense. Some physicians still think either that STD, in the presence of penicillin, is no more significant than the common cold, or that STD patients are second-rate patients, and as such do not merit proper treatment. Many physicians are simply not aware of the possibilities in STD and

the various forms it takes and do not *expect* their patients to get it.

3. The gonorrhea germ is constantly growing more resistant to penicillin. Treatment requires periodic increases in amount and use of different kinds of drugs for complete effectiveness.

4. The public attitude has not been conducive to control. It is extremely difficult to alter public attitudes, since there is a persistent association of STD and sex with "sin." Wittingly or unknowingly, there is constant reinforcement of the idea that STD is evidence of sexual transgression. Some people look upon the infected person as an undesirable member of society who is getting what he or she deserves.

5. There is no vaccine yet available for any sexually transmitted disease. The ideal preventive measure for STD would be a vaccine administered early in life.

Gonorrhea   Gonorrhea is the *most common sexually transmitted disease* in the United States today. It is the second most common communicable disease in the United States, surpassed only by the common cold. Although less lethal than syphilis, gonorrhea is far more widespread and harder to control.

Gonorrhea is caused by a diplococcus (see illustration) called *Neisseria gonorrhoeae*, also called the *gonococcus*. *Neisseria gonorrhoeae* is extremely selective about where it grows, requiring just the right temperature, humidity, and nutrients. It dies or is inactive when exposed to cold or dryness. For this reason, the transmission of gonorrhea requires contact between warm, moist body surfaces. Inanimate objects such as toilet seats hardly ever help transmit gonorrhea.

Source and Transmission   Humans are the only natural reservoir of gonorrhea. The organism occurs in the moist substances from mucous membranes of infected persons. The gonococcus may be transmitted through various kinds of sexual contact—heterosexual or homosexual—including genital, oral-genital, and anal-genital.

Nature of the Disease   The gonococcus has an affinity for membranes. It most commonly infects the mucous membranes of the genitals, throat, anus, or the eye. If this organism enters the blood, it may infect the membranes lining the heart or the joints.

Gonorrhea in the Male   In most males, symptoms appear in two days to a week after exposure. Many, however, remain free of obvious symptoms. The disease begins with a painful inflammation of the urethral canal in the center of the penis. This causes a scalding pain during urination. The inflammation begins at the tip of the penis and works up the urethra. The result is a "drip" of pus from the penis. In

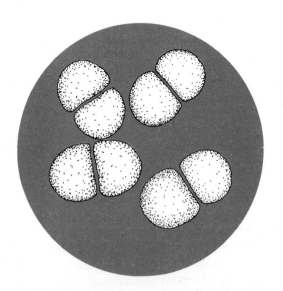

Neisseria gonorrhoeae, the cause of gonorrhea.

early acute infection, the discharge tends to be watery or milky. Later it becomes thick greenish-yellow, often tinged with blood.

The burning sensation upon urination may subside after two or three weeks. By this time the infection may have reached the prostate gland and testicles, as well as the bladder and kidneys. Permanent damage can include urinary obstruction, *chordee* (downward, painful curvature of the penis on erection), inflammation and abscesses of the prostate, or sterility caused by blockage of the vas deferens and epididymis. Infection of the throat occasionally occurs following oral-genital contact. Rectal gonorrhea may follow anal-genital intercourse.

Gonorrhea in the Female Gonorrhea may produce no painful symptoms in women. In fact, about 80 percent of women infected do not realize they have the disease until their male partners discover their own infections. Infected women are therefore more likely to transmit the disease. The prevalence of asymptomatic carriers is an important part of the history of the gonorrhea epidemic. Public Health Service studies show that up to 5 percent of all women in the United States may be asymptomatic carriers of the gonococcus. Investigators are now reporting frequent discovery of gonococci in the urethras of males who reveal no symptoms.

The symptoms of gonorrhea in the female (when they exist) are different from those in the male. The usual symptom of a woman is irritation or "smarting" of the vagina accompanied by discharge. Unfortunately, such discharge is an unreliable sign in the female, since she may ordinarily experience vaginal discharges unrelated to gonorrhea. In the female the gonococcus prefers the cervix and fallopian tubes. In about 10 percent of cases the infection is found wholly in the rectum.

A gonorrhea infection generally moves methodically up the genital tract. In the vagina its effects are usually asymptomatic, or at least unclear. As it reaches the upper tract—the uterus, fallopian tubes, and ovaries—a pus discharge occurs and complications begin to set in, usually not until after at least one menstrual cycle. However, if the woman is on the pill, complications may show up as quickly as 3 to 5 days after exposure.

Gonorrhea in Newborn Children Untreated gonorrhea in pregnant women may be responsible for *conjunctivitis* (an inflammation of the conjuctiva of the eye) in newborn children, acquired at the time of delivery. This condition, which can lead to blindness, is prevented by drops of either penicillin or silver nitrate, required by law to be placed in the eyes of every newborn infant. Infection of the infant's external genitalia may also result, especially in breech deliveries. In addition to the child, physicians have become infected when gonococcal-contaminated amniotic fluid has splashed into their eyes during a delivery.

Complications Gonorrheal complications may include gonococcal arthritis characterized by pain, heat, swelling, and redness; abscesses in the fallopian tubes and ovaries; and a spreading of infection out of the fallopian tubes into the abdomen, giving rise to a massive abdominopelvic infection called *pelvic inflammatory disease* (PID). Symptoms of PID include extreme pain (often mistaken for appendicitis), fever, and abdominal swelling.

One study has shown that at least 12 percent of all females with gonorrhea suffer from some degree of invasion of the fallopian tubes. This can result in sterility or ectopic pregnancy (a fertilized egg implanting itself in the fallopian tube rather than in the uterine wall) because of scar tissue that may block the free passage of the egg. Pus material may also collect into an abscess, which may rupture painfully. Gonorrhea-produced sterility is increasing and is presently the leading cause of sterility in the female.

Gonorrhea occasionally progresses into a serious, even fatal, systemic (blood-borne) infection. Systemic gonorrhea may attack the joints (causing arthritis), heart lining (causing endocarditis), heart muscle, brain, membranes covering the brain (causing meningitis), lungs, kidneys, veins, and skin. A common group of symptoms of systemic gonorrhea includes fever, arthritis, and sores on the skin. Even though the gonococcus is fragile outside the human body, its potential for tissue destruction and widespread complications within humans is great.

Diagnosis of Gonorrhea A blood test has recently become available for the detection of gonorrhea. At the time of this writing its distribution is still limited and its effectiveness still being established. Other diagnostic methods involve demonstrating the presence of *Neisseria gonorrhoeae* organisms in stained microscope slides and in cultures on special growth media. For either slides or cultures, the sources of bacteria include swabs from the urethra of the male, cervix of the female, the anus, and the throat. Since females usually notice no symptoms of gonorrhea, periodic laboratory tests for gonorrhea are advisable even in the absence of symptoms if there is any chance of exposure to the disease.

Very often a patient may be infected with both syphilis and gonorrhea at the same time. While examining for gonorrhea, a physician should also be alert for symptoms of syphilis.

Treatment of Gonorrhea The gonococcus has a long history of developing resistance to everything that has been used for its treatment. Some of the drugs that have gradually lost their effectiveness are potassium salts, silver compounds, sulfa drugs, and most recently, penicillin. Penicillin is still the drug most commonly used against gonorrhea, although much larger doses are now required than when the drug was first available. A typical dosage is now 4.8 million units of penicillin compared with 1.5 million units in the early 1960s. Even at this high level, penicillin often fails to cure gonorrhea completely. Fortunately, other drugs may be used when penicillin fails or the patient is hypersensitive (allergic) to penicillin.

It must be emphasized that *there is no effective home remedy for gonorrhea*. Nothing can be mixed up or bought from a drug store or by mail that will cure this or any other sexually transmitted disease. The infected person must see a private physician or his or her local public health department for effective treatment. It is most important that gonorrhea be treated promptly before any permanent damage, such as sterility, can occur.

There is no vaccine that will prevent gonorrhea. Similarly, no immunity results from a case of gonorrhea. After a penicillin treatment wears off in a few days, reinfection can occur.

Syphilis Syphilis is the most serious sexually transmitted disease. While gonorrhea is usually confined to the urogenital system in men and to the reproductive organs in women, syphilis spreads to the blood stream and is thus a systemic infection. The main similarity between these two diseases is that both are transmitted primarily by sexual contact.

The organism that causes syphilis is the spirochete (spiral bacterium) *Treponema pallidum* (see drawing). This germ is very frail and cannot survive drying or chilling. It is killed within a few seconds after its

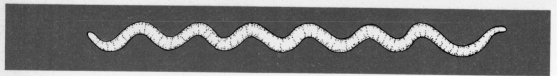

Treponema pallidum, the cause of syphilis.

exposure to air. Since the germ is so easily killed by air, it is easy to see why syphilis must be transmitted by sexual intercourse, kissing, or other intimate body contacts. The germ requires warm, moist skin or mucous membrane surfaces for its penetration into the body. After the spirochetes burrow through the skin or mucous membrane and enter the blood, they are carried throughout the body. Because its symptoms are so varied that they can resemble any one of many other diseases, syphilis has been called the "great imitator." It progresses through definite stages, which are explained in the following sections.

Primary Syphilis After infection with syphilis, there may be a symptomless incubation period of 10 to 90 days, although the usual period is 3 to 4 weeks. During this time the spirochetes multiply in the body.

The first symptom that appears is the *primary lesion* or *chancre* (pronounced "shanker"). This is a sore that appears at the exact spot where infection took place. The typical chancre (see illustration) is pink to red in color, raised, firm, and painless. It is usually the size of a dime, but it may be so small that it resembles a pimple. The chancre is *swarming with spirochetes.* Any contact with it is likely to result in a syphilitic infection.

The usual location of the chancre is on or near the sex organs, but it can be on the lip, finger, or any part of the body. In females, the chancre is often within the vagina and,

since it is painless, it goes unnoticed.

Even if primary syphilis is not treated (which it definitely should be), the chancre will disappear spontaneously in 3 to 6 weeks. But this disappearance of the chancre does not mean that the disease is cured. It is just progressing to the next stage. At about the time the chancre disappears, blood tests for syphilis become positive.

Secondary Syphilis In *secondary syphilis*, the true systemic nature of syphilis becomes obvious. Symptoms may appear throughout the body, starting 1 to 6 months after the appearance of the chancre, though in many cases this stage is skipped over. The most common symptom of secondary syphilis is a rash that does not itch. This rash is variable in appearance and may cover the entire body or any part of it. Common sites of this rash are on the palms of the hands or the soles of the feet. Large, moist sores may develop on or around the sex organs or in the mouth. These moist sores are loaded with syphilitic germs. Contact with them, through sexual intercourse or even kissing, may cause syphilitic infection. Secondary syphilis is, therefore, extremely contagious.

Other symptoms that may occur in secondary syphilis include sore throat, headache, slight fever, red eyes, pain in the joints, and patches of hair falling out. When a person has these symptoms and thinks he or she may have been exposed to syphilis he or she should explain this fact to a physician. Because syphilis can easily be mistaken for one of many other diseases, it is difficult to diagnose. Without an accurate diagnosis, it may not be properly treated. Syphilis at this secondary stage is best diagnosed by means of specific blood tests for the disease.

The symptoms of secondary syphilis last from several days to several months. Then, like the chancre of primary syphilis, they disappear even without treatment. Syphilis has then entered the latent stage.

Latent Syphilis Latency begins with the disappearance of untreated secondary symptoms; it may extend from a few months to a lifetime. Latency may be divided into two stages—a potentially infectious stage, *early latent syphilis*, and a noninfectious later stage, *late latent syphilis*.

Early Latent Syphilis If the disease remains untreated, there may be a series of recurring infectious lesions of the skin or mucous membranes for the first 2 to 4 years. Because of these new lesions the disease is considered communicable throughout its early latency. During the long latent period the disease loses some of its infectiousness; after the first 2 years, a person can rarely transmit syphilis through sexual intercourse, although a syphilitic pregnant woman can still transmit it to her unborn child (*congenital syphilis*) for an additional 2 years.

Late Latent Syphilis When the individual has lost all ability to infect, the disease has entered the period of late latent syphilis, lasting anywhere from several months to a lifetime. During this period there are no discernible signs of illness. If routinely examined, the individual *will* show a positive blood test but will have no further signs. In this latent stage, progressive degeneration of the brain, spinal cord, hearing, sight, or bones may be occurring

unnoticed. If and when the symptoms of this degeneration appear, the individual then slips into the last and most destructive stage.

Late Syphilis Many people, having contracted syphilis and having allowed it, through neglect or ignorance, to progress untreated, may develop a late stage that will incapacitate or kill them. Although almost any part of the body may be affected, only the most common manifestations will be discussed below.

Cardiovascular Syphilis The damage in most cases of cardiovascular syphilis is located in the thoracic aorta. The elastic tissue is destroyed and the aorta stretches, producing an aneurysm (saclike bulge). The infection may also involve the aortic valve, causing an insufficient flow of blood. The symptoms of cardiovascular syphilis do not differ from other heart and vascular disorders.

Neurosyphilis The symptoms of neurosyphilis arise from widespread destruction of the tissues of the brain and spinal cord by large numbers of *Treponema pallidum*. The brain damage of late syphilis is called *paresis* or *dementia paralytica*. The mental changes vary but most commonly become manifest in gradual changes of personality, decreased ability to work, and impairment of concentration and judgment. These changes produce abnormal behavior, including delusions, loss of memory, lack of insight, apathy or violent rages, convulsions, and disorientation. Neurosyphilis is responsible for many deaths, as well as for many of the chronic invalids seen in mental institutions.

The most common outcome of the progressive destruction of the spinal cord by large numbers of spirochetes is impaired muscle control. Occasionally all reflexes may be lost, including the ability to vary pupil size (affecting vision), general sense of balance, and various elements of muscular coordination. Considerable paralysis may eventually result from untreated syphilis.

In treated cases life can be prolonged, but permanent care may be necessary because of extreme degeneration that may have taken place prior to treatment.

Loss of Vision Syphilis can cause degeneration of the optic nerve, usually first noticed as a loss of peripheral vision. Central vision may be lost in advanced cases, leaving the individual completely blind.

Syphilis in Pregnancy If a woman is infected with syphilis at the time of conception or shortly thereafter, the primary chancre appearing on her may be very mild or completely suppressed. Secondary symptoms in her skin are likely to be absent, and *if she has not had blood tests during her pregnancy* she may have no indication that she has syphilis until the birth of her child. Infection of a fetus takes place when the spirochetes of syphilis cross the placental membranes within the womb. Such infection of the fetus apparently does not occur before the fifth month of fetal life. Consequently, adequate treatment of a previously syphilitic pregnant woman *before the fifth fetal month* should insure the child's safety. Treatment given the mother after the fifth month may also cure the syphilitic fetus. Because of the conditions just discussed and because syphilis can also be acquired during pregnancy, blood tests during the first half of pregnancy and during the seventh month are considered adequate for detecting this disease.

In a majority of instances, infection of the fetus takes place quite late in pregnancy. The more recent the mother's syphilitic infection, the greater probability that the child will be born with syphilis. A severe infection is very likely to lead to death of the fetus before birth, and syphilis is a common cause of stillbirth. Among the infants born alive to untreated syphilitic mothers, approximately 50 percent have syphilis at birth (congenital syphilis).

Congenital Syphilis A syphilitic infant may show secondary lesions at birth, may appear normal at birth and develop lesions within a few months or may remain without symptoms until adolescence, when the symptoms of late syphilis may appear. As a rule, the earlier the symptoms appear, the more severe the infection. Syphilis is capable of producing many different types of lesions, but never do all of them occur in one infant.

Of the various secondary symptoms appearing at birth, *snuffles*, an inflammation of the nose with a discharge of *Treponema pallidum* spirochetes—is most frequent. This discharge may interfere with breathing, is extremely infectious, and accounts for many infections of individuals who handle such children. During fetal development the growth of the nasal bones may be disturbed, resulting in the deformity known as "saddle nose." Skin lesions at birth are frequent and are often similar to the rash seen in secondary stages of sexually transmitted syphilis. In a high proportion of children, the palms of hands, soles of feet, or skin about the mouth may be reddened, inflamed, and thickened at birth or shortly after birth. When this occurs around the mouth, fissures may radiate in all directions. After healing, these lesions leave radiating scars about the mouth known as *rhagades*.

Following the secondary lesions, the course of untreated congenital syphilis is similar to that of sexually transmitted syphilis. These late symptoms may appear in a few months, at 6 or 7 years of age, or in the late teens. Some of the more common are "Hutchinson's teeth" which are "notched" or screwdriverlike permanent central incisors; *keratitis,* a condition of the eyes uncommon in young children but very common in older children and capable of causing permanent blindness; and injury to bones and body joints.

Diagnosis of Syphilis Early diagnosis followed by prompt and adequate treatment can completely cure syphilis.

Microscopic Examination The lesions of early syphilis are rich in *Treponema pallidum.* This fact provides the best means for conclusive diagnosis of the disease. *Treponema pallidum* taken from such a chancre of primary syphilis or from skin lesions of secondary syphilis can readily be seen under a microscope by what is termed darkfield illumination.

Blood Tests for Syphilis Blood tests become positive only after a general invasion of the body by the spirochetes. The underlying principle of a blood test is appearance in the blood after syphilis infection (and occasionally following some other conditions) of an antibodylike substance called *reagin.* All of the blood tests for syphilis based on reagin in the blood are modifications of the original Wassermann test, an older test for determining blood reagin that was much less sensitive than present tests.

Besides the reagin tests, there are others for *Treponema pallidum* spirochetes and specific antibodies produced by the body in response to syphilis infection. They are positive for syphilis only, are quite expensive, and involve complicated procedures that cannot be used as easily as the reagin tests for screening large numbers of individuals.

Syphilis Therapy The purposes of treatment are to destroy all spirochetes, to initiate the healing of existing lesions, and to prevent further damage to the body. Treatment of syphilis also serves to prevent the spread of the disease to others. The earlier this treatment is begun, the more effective it is in accomplishing these purposes. Once the organisms are present in the cerebrospinal fluid (as determined by a spinal tap), there is a good chance that neurological impairment will follow.

In the mid-1940s penicillin began to replace the lengthy, expensive, and difficult treatment of syphilis with arsenic products and bismuth preparations. Since that time the use of penicillin alone in the treatment of syphilis has become a worldwide standard.

The primary consideration in treatment is maintenance of a high penicillin level in the blood and tissues for a period of time sufficient to destroy all spirochetes present in the body. Consequently, treatment varies with progressive stages of the disease. Unfortunately, the widespread use of penicillin for treatment of a variety of other disorders has frequently added some difficulties to the diagnosis of syphilis. Syphilitic infection may be masked completely or its course altered by smaller doses of penicillin than are necessary to eliminate all the spirochetes. Larger doses of penicillin are needed to treat syphilis than for most other diseases. When a patient's allergy to penicillin precludes the use of this preferred drug, *erythromycin* and *tetracycline* are good alternatives. No matter what drug is used, inadequate therapy may lead to a relapse. There is no home remedy, mail-order cure, or nonprescription drugstore product that will cure syphilis. It must have professional treatment by a physician.

Genital Herpes Virus Infections

Some of the most common, troublesome, and persistent genital infections are caused by viruses from the *herpes simplex* group. Herpes simplex viruses are apparently carried by most people at all times, though usually in a state of latency (dormancy). Some 70 to 90 percent of adults carry antibodies against herpes simplex, but these antibodies do not prevent occasional activiation of the virus. In addition to genital sores, herpes viruses are associated with cold sores, fever blisters, eczema, corneal infection, meningitis, encephalitis, and possibly uterine and other cancers. Two types of herpes viruses, type 1 and type 2, have been identified to date. Type 1 more typically attacks the upper parts of the body while Type 2 more typically attacks below the waist, but there are many exceptions to these generalizations.

Most people receive their initial infection with herpes virus during childhood. The antibodies carried by most adults are transferred across the placenta to the fetus during pregnancy so most infants are protected from infection during the first few months after their birth. If the mother acquires her first infection during pregnancy, however, and the child is born before sufficient maternal antibodies can be transferred across the placenta, severe infection of the newborn may occur, often with fatal consequences. The virus may be widely distributed in infant tissues, producing severe lesions in skin, mucous membranes, liver, and brain.

Much more typically, infection occurs during childhood and without serious complications. Children are usually infected through contact with the virus in the saliva of other children or adults or through contact with the eczema or other lesions in infected persons. About 90 per-cent of initial childhood infections are symptomless. About 10 percent of children suffer a mild illness of fever and general discomfort (malaise) lasting only a few days. Following initial infection, herpes virus usually is carried in the body cells in a latent state, being periodically reactivated by various stimuli such as fever, mechanical irritation, and certain foods.

Genital herpes simplex sores in adults may result from either the reactivation of latent herpes infections or from newly acquired virus transmitted through genital or orogenital sexual contact. These sores may occur on the labia or within the vagina in females or on the penis or within the urethra in males.

In someone not already carrying the virus, the symptoms of genital herpes usually appear about 6 days after sexual contact with an infected person. Subsequent attacks are caused by reactivation of the virus, which apparently stays in the nerve endings between attacks. The average person may have four or five recurrences in the first year and two or three in subsequent years. The infection is contagious whenever there is a recurrence of lesions.

Genital herpes usually starts with some minor itching or a slight rash. Then a cluster of small blisters forms. This then breaks open to form one or more red, eroded lesions that are extremely painful, especially during sexual intercourse. In a few cases, the pain may radiate into the legs, and there may be severe swelling, which may make urination difficult. In a first attack, the sores usually disappear in 2 to 4 weeks, while subsequent attacks usually clear up in 1 or 2 weeks.

Unlike gonorrhea and syphilis, there is no specific treatment for herpes simplex viruses. Viruses in general are not susceptible to control by antibiotics or other drugs. Various treatments have been tried, but none is universally effective or accepted as safe by all physicians. The fact that genital herpes lesions clear up with the passage of time even if untreated tends to make any form of treatment appear to work at least part of the time. One of the more common treatments has been to paint the lesions with a red dye and then expose the area to light, which appears to shorten the duration of the outbreak. This treatment, however, in experiments with animals, has appeared to increase the cancer-causing tendencies of the herpes viruses. Many authorities thus discourage its use. Some doctors feel they are able to prevent recurrent genital herpes attacks with repeated smallpox or tuberculosis vaccinations, but other doctors doubt the effectiveness of this approach. What is really needed is a specific herpes vaccine. Several laboratories are working on such a vaccine, but its successful development appears to be several years in the future.

Uterine Cancer—A Sexually Transmitted Disease?

A possible although still unproven association has been suggested between a herpes simplex virus (type 2) and cancer of the cervix or the uterus. The virus is often found within cancerous cells, but no cause-and-effect relationship has been established. Preliminary studies do indicate that women who suffer herpes type 2 infections are eight times more likely to develop cervical cancer than those who are free of the disease.

A possible correlative statistical association has been proposed by some cancer researchers (and disputed by others) in which the incidence of cervical cancer may be statistically related to a patient's sexual history. According to those who accept this association, the incidence of cervical cancer is higher among women who begin sexual intercourse at younger ages and among those with a history of many sexual partners. Conversely, the incidence of uterine cancer has been reported to be low among virgins, women experiencing intercourse at a later date, and women with a history of few sexual partners.

Assuming the statistical relationship between early coitus and uterine cancer is valid, such a relationship would be compatible with the role of a sexually transmitted herpes simplex virus as a causal agent for such cancer, since the herpes viruses are noted for their ability to lie dormant for many years. The incidence of uterine cancer increases with age, although it is possible that the cells of some particular younger woman might be more susceptible to infection by a virus.

Other factors might also account for an association between early intercourse or multiple sexual partners and cervical cancer, again assuming that such an association exists. Genetic mutation of the cervical cells is one such possibility. The cause of such mutation might be repeated mechanical trauma during coitus or perhaps some carcinogenic (cancer-causing) chemical in semen, although the latter seems extremely unlikely. Still another possibility is that the stimulus for cancer production might be irritation and weakening of the cervical tissues by chronic infection with one or more of the many sexually transmitted pathogens.

Three Uncommon Sexually Transmitted Diseases

The following three diseases occur throughout the world, but are uncommon in most parts of the United States. Each is almost totally preventable by merely washing with soap and water immediately following exposure. Together, they amount to about 1,600 reported cases per year in the United States, mainly in the southern states.

Chancroid Chancroid, also known as "soft chancre" or "soft sore," is a localized infection usually acquired by sexual contact and caused by a bacillus called *Haemophilus ducreyi*. About 3 to 5 days after exposure to the bacillus, a small red area appears at the site of infection. This enlarges into a pimplelike growth that soon breaks down, forming an ulcer (open sore) with ragged edges and exuding pus. If a cut or abrasion of the skin exists at the time of exposure, the lesion may appear within 24 hours. The ulcers bleed easily and are soft and very painful.

In roughly half of all cases, the disease is self-limiting and heals by itself. In the other half, in about a week the lymph glands near the ulcer may swell, accumulate large amounts of pus, and rupture spontaneously. Also, if a lesion is located in a body area that is hard to keep clean, is hidden, or does not receive prompt treatment, rapidly destructive ulcerations can destroy much of the local tissue. The bacillus can be spread to surrounding areas of the body, causing multiple lesions to develop. Systemic reactions are rare, pain is the most frequent complaint, and extreme tissue destruction is the most severe complication.

Chancroid has been confused with the chancre stage of syphilis. Chancroid can be readily distinguished because its lesions are usually multiple and tender (instead of firm or hard) with a slightly grayish base.

Various antibiotics are used to treat chancroid. Chancroid is mainly a disease of people who do not use soap and water frequently enough to keep the genital areas clean. The key to prevention of chancroid is cleanliness. The use of soap and water immediately after sexual exposure is a reliable preventive measure. As with many other STDs, symptomless carriers, particularly females, are an important source of infection.

Granuloma Inguinale Granuloma inguinale causes small, rounded, fleshy masses of pus-filled ulcerations that occur on the skin covering the external genitals and groin (inguinal) region of the body. It occasionally spreads to the lymph nodes in the area. It is a chronic and progressive disease, caused by a bacillus called *Calymmatobacterium granulomatis*.

This disease is not necessarily transmitted by sexual contact only. It may be spread by contaminated objects as well. It is a disease of those who do not, or cannot, maintain standards of cleanliness.

The incubation period of granuloma inguinale is apparently quite variable, ranging from 8 to over 100 days. If untreated, the infection spreads peripherally and may involve a large area of skin and mucous membrane of the genital region. It may be successfully treated with antibiotics.

Lymphogranuloma Venereum Lymphogranuloma venereum is a sexually acquired infection of the lymph channels and lymph glands near the genital organs. It is caused by a very small bacterium of the *Chlamydia* group.

The disease starts as a small, painless, primary lesion (sore) at the site of entry of the bacteria, usually on the genitals. This lesion appears about 7 to 12 days after infection has taken place and disappears soon thereafter. It is often of such short duration that it escapes notice. About 10 to 30 days after exposure the lymph nodes in the groin region enlarge, fill with pus, and may rupture and drain continuously. Fever, chills, headache, and joint pains may be present. Chronic infection of the pelvic lymphatic ducts may block drainage of fluid from this region, causing swelling of genital tissues. Lymphogranuloma venereum may be successfully treated with sulfa drugs or antibiotics.

Other Infections of the Reproductive and Urinary Organs

In addition to the true STDs, the reproductive organs are susceptible to several other kinds of infections. These infections are not usually classified as STDs because they are very commonly transmitted through nonsexual means, although each of these infections may also be contracted through sexual contact.

In recent years there has been a great increase in these infections. This may be related to an increase in casual sexual contacts and definitely is related to modern birth control methods. As previously mentioned, birth control pills change the vaginal environment, creating a more moist, alkaline condition, favoring infection by *Candida*, *Trichomonas*, and herpes viruses, as well as gonorrhea. At the same time, pills and IUDs have somewhat replaced birth control methods such as condoms and vaginal foams that actively help prevent the transmission of infections.

Candida One of the more troublesome infections of the sexual organs, and especially the vagina, is caused by a yeastlike organism called *Candida albicans*. This organism is a normal inhabitant of the mouth, digestive tract, and vagina, but it is usually held in check by the other organisms present and by the body's natural defenses.

Various factors can act to reduce normal defenses against *Candida* (also called a "yeast" infection), allowing it to erupt into a serious infection. One of these factors is intensive antibiotic therapy for some other infection. During such therapy the normal bacterial "flora" of the intestine and vagina may be reduced in numbers, allowing *Candida* to flourish instead. Poor nutrition may also lead to *Candida* eruption, as may any general weakening of one's health.

Diabetes, which impairs the body defenses against most kinds of infections, is frequently associated with severe *Candida* infections. Hormone therapy, including use of birth control pills, as well as pregnancy may alter the vaginal environment to favor growth of *Candida*. A moist environment also encourages the organism. Spending many hours in a wet swim suit or in clothing that does not "breathe" freely, such as nylon underwear or pantyhose, sometimes leads to severe *Candida* infections, especially of the vagina and labia.

Vaginal candidiasis (the medical name for *Candida* infection) is most troublesome of the *Candida* infections. The characteristic symptoms of vaginal candidiasis include burning and itching and a whitish discharge, which can be quite abundant. There may be patches of white *pseudomembrane* (false membrane) on the vaginal lining. In treating vaginal candidiasis, there are several considerations. First is keeping the vaginal area dry and correcting any contributing conditions such as poor nutrition. A variety of effective oral and vaginal medications are available by prescription. It is important that male sex partners use condoms during the period of infection to avoid "ping-pong" infections in which the male is infected and later reinfects the female.

Other sites of *Candida* infection include the penis, vulva, and mouth cavity. Infection of the mouth cavity is called "thrush" and occurs most commonly among infants, elderly persons, or patients on intensive antibiotic therapy over long periods of time. *Candida* rarely enters the blood, but once within blood plasma it may cause serious or even fatal kidney or heart damage if not treated.

Trichomonas Another common cause of vaginitis is infection by the protozoan (or one-cell animal) *Trichomonas vaginalis*. *Trichomonas* lives in the vaginas of many women without producing noticeable symptoms. Symptomless infections of the male prostate gland, urethra, and seminal vesicles are also common. Under certain conditions, however, *Trichomonas* can multiply enormously in either the male or female reproductive organs. Symptoms in the female can include intense itching and burning of the vagina, small rashlike spots on its lining, and a profuse discharge of a thin, foamy, yellowish discharge that may have a foul odor. Symptoms in the male, though they rarely occur, include urethritis or, even more rarely, inflammation of the prostate or seminal vesicles.

Trichomonas is a common infection among adult females throughout the world. The organism is transmitted from person to person by contact with vaginal and urethral discharges of infected persons during sexual contact, during birth, and possibly by contact with infected articles. Symptomless vaginal infections are often converted into troublesome vaginitis through modification of the vaginal environment produced by the hormonal changes associated with birth control pills or pregnancy.

Trichomoniasis can be successfully treated by medically prescribed oral or vaginal medications. Simultaneous treatment of sexual partners is important in preventing reinfection. Even though a partner may be symptomless, he or she may well carry the organism.

Cystitis Cystitis is inflammation of the urinary bladder. Any of a variety of bacteria and other organisms may cause this problem. The symptoms include frequent, burning, or painful urination, chills, fever, fatigue, and, infrequently, blood in the urine. Bladder infections occur more often

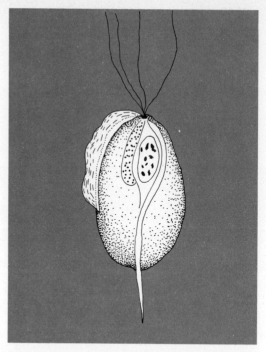

Trichomonas vaginalis *of humans.*

in females than in males, because the shorter urethra of the female makes it easier for bacteria to reach the bladder.

Cystitis should be treated promptly with medically prescribed drugs. Untreated it may become a chronic problem or spread to the kidneys. Cleanliness, frequent urination, and drinking adequate water helps prevent this infection. Vigorous sexual activity tends to force bacteria up through the urethra to the bladder, especially in women. Urinating immediately following intercourse helps to prevent cystitis from this cause.

Nonspecific Urethritis *Nonspecific urethritis* (NSU), also called *nongonorrheal urethritis* (NGU), is a term often applied to any inflammation of the urethra other than by gonorrhea. Numerous pathogens have been associated with urethral infections. In many specific cases, the infecting agent is never definitely identified.

NSU is often transmitted through sexual contact and is more common among people having a variety of sexual partners. Most cases can be cleared up with the combination of prescribed medication, avoidance of alcohol and caffeine, and moderation in sexual activity until the infection is healed.

Pubic Lice Pubic lice, commonly called "crab lice" or "crabs" because of their crablike appearance, are small, gray insects (1/16 inch long) that live as external parasites on the body. They live in body hair, holding onto the shaft of the hair with their crablike pincers. They prefer pubic hair but will also live in the hair under arms and in eyebrows and beards, but never scalp hair (which is too fine in texture). Crab lice do not really pinch with their claws, but they do feed on human blood, causing an intense itching and discoloration of the skin. They often remain attached for days, with their sucking mouthparts inserted into the skin of an unfortunate host. Female lice attach eggs, called *nits*, to the body hair. These eggs hatch in 6 to 8 days. Since sexual maturity is reached in only 14 to 21 days and each female lays up to 50 eggs, a crab louse infection can grow to alarming proportions in just a short time. Heavy infestations may result in fever and other disorders caused by toxins injected by the feeding lice.

Pubic lice may be transmitted through sexual intercourse, but they can also be spread through less intimate physical contact with infested people or by use of contaminated clothing, toilet seats, bedding, or other materials.

Crabs can usually be killed by washing the affected body parts with a special shampoo, such as Kwell, available by pre-scription. Several applications are required. Contrary to popular belief, infested hair need *not* be shaved, and exposed clothing need not be thrown away. However, it should not be worn until it is cleaned or thoroughly washed in hot water.

Preventing the Sexually Transmitted Diseases So far, our discussion of STDs has centered upon recognition of their symptoms and the importance of obtaining prompt treatment if infection occurs. But from both personal and public health standpoints, it is much more desirable to prevent any disease than to treat it. The prevention of these diseases requires action by both the individual and public health personnel.

Personal Prevention As with most other diseases, the ultimate responsibility for the prevention of the sexually transmitted diseases lies with the individual. The most important personal preventative measure is the avoidance of sexual contact

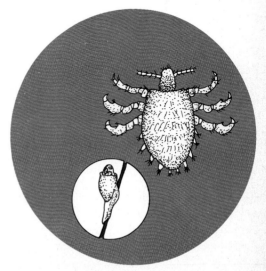

The pubic louse, Phthirus pubis. Egg attached to hair, lower left.

with anyone who is likely to be infected. Considering today's high incidence of sexually transmitted diseases, that would include anyone who has sexual contact with a variety of partners or who has sexual contact with another sexual partner who, in turn, has a variety of sexual partners. Remember that these diseases can be transmitted through either heterosexual or homosexual contact and through either genital-genital, oral-genital, or anal-genital sex, and even through certain "petting" practices.

The prime mechanism for prevention of the sexually transmitted diseases, then, is selective sexual behavior. Unfortunately, for the public as a whole, this mechanism has failed because it has never been widely practiced. The current STD epidemic is glaring evidence of this failure. Thus, for the person who chooses to be somewhat less discriminate in the choice of sexual partners, it becomes important to make maximum use of other personal preventive (prophylactic) methods to reduce the chances of infection. Note that we use the word *reduce* rather than *eliminate*, since even the best of the currently available prophylactic methods are far from totally effective.

The single most important personal preventive method is probably the liberal use of soap and water immediately after sexual contact. The pathogens of the diseases that enter the body through the skin can often be killed or removed in this manner. The three less common diseases, chancroid, lymphogranuloma venereum, and granuloma inguinale, can be almost entirely eliminated by this simple technique.

Urination by a male immediately after sexual contact and prompt douching by a female may help reduce the chance of infection with gonorrhea. (It should be pointed out that douching is not effective as a birth control measure and that fre-

quent douching often results in vaginal irritations and infections. Thus, douching should be reserved for disease prevention or for special situations upon the recommendation of a physician.)

The use of a condom (rubber) over the penis of the male will help prevent the transmission of STD, especially gonorrhea, in either direction—from male to female or from female to male. To be effective, the rubber must be applied onto the erect penis at the very start of any sexual activity, before any sexual contact is made. Even when a condom is used, it is still important to wash with soap and water immediately after contact because the condom covers only the penis, and several of the diseases, especially syphilis, can enter the body through the skin at any point whatsoever. The condom thus affords limited protection against syphilis. In its favor, however, it should be noted that the condom is the only commonly used device that is effective both as a prophylactic against gonorrhea and as a contraceptive. Carefully and consistently used, it can be reasonably effective for both purposes. Although it has traditionally been a male responsibility to make sure of its availability for coitus, a woman might want to keep a supply of condoms available to protect herself against STD and, if she is not otherwise protected, against pregnancy as well.

Antibiotics have been used on a prophylactic basis, administered either before or after possible exposure to STD, but this practice cannot be recommended for routine use because it tends to breed antibiotic-resistant strains of pathogens, including but not limited to those that cause the sexually transmitted diseases, and because it tends to build allergies to the antibiotics in those who receive them.

The ideal personal preventive would, of course, be a vaccine for each disease. Few communicable diseases have ever really been controlled until effective vaccines have been developed against them.

Public Health Measures Many methods are used by public health agencies in their fight against the sexually transmitted diseases. And while STD is still rampant, it seems certain that the incidence would be even greater than it is without the efforts of dedicated public health workers.

Most public health departments carry out programs of education concerned with prevention and symptoms of sexually transmitted diseases and the importance of prompt treatment. The media used often include newspapers, billboards, radio, TV, and posters in public places. Some public health departments assist local schools in their STD education programs, providing classroom materials and teacher training for effective STD instruction.

Clinics for the diagnosis and treatment of STD are also common functions of public health departments. The services of clinics are usually offered at little or no cost to the individual. Laws in most states have been revised to allow the treatment of minors, often as young as 12 years of age, without obtaining permission from their parents or otherwise notifying them. It has been found that when parental permission must be obtained prior to treatment, many young people will avoid treatment out of fear of reprisal from parents, thus tragically risking permanent damage from infection.

Another important public health function in STD control is case finding. In many localities, each patient treated for a sexually transmitted disease, especially for syphilis, is interviewed to determine from whom the disease might have been caught and to whom it may have been transmitted. These people can then be con-

tacted, notified that they may be infected, and asked to visit the public health department or their private physician for STD testing. Since so many cases of STD are symptomless, this is the only way in which many infected people can learn of their disease before serious damage is done.

One of the real barriers to effective case finding is that while by law every case of STD a physician treats must be reported to the local health department, in reality the majority of cases are not reported. The reporting rate for privately treated gonorrhea is especially low, even though gonorrhea reports are essentially for statistical purposes rather than for case finding. Many public health departments lack adequate funds for thorough case finding even for deadly syphilis.

While it may seem obvious, the STD patient should be warned to refrain from sexual contact with previous partners until they have been tested and, if necessary, treated. It is common (and frustrating) in STD clinics to find that a newly cured patient has gone back to the same partner and becomes reinfected again and again.

A technique that has revealed thousands of cases of syphilis is compulsory blood testing for certain people, such as applicants for marriage licenses, pregnant women, military personnel, hospital patients, and new employees of many corporations. Most of the cases so detected are in the symptomless latent period and, without detection and treatment, many would progress into late syphilis, with its irreversible damage to vital organs and even death.

It is an excellent idea for anyone who has a variety of sexual partners to obtain *an annual blood test for syphilis*. Many cases progress directly into the latent and eventually the late stages without ever exhibiting any noticeable symptoms. Yearly blood tests can reliably detect such cases, and the cost of such tests is minimal or even free if they are obtained through public health departments or free clinics.

In summary, while public health departments are making great efforts to control STD, syphilis, gonorrhea, and genital herpes remain as epidemic diseases. It is imperative for the individual to take reasonable precautions against infection, to know the symptoms of these diseases, and to seek prompt treatment if these symptoms develop.

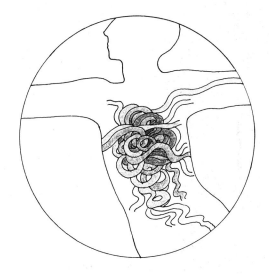

NONCOMMUNICABLE DISEASES

During the first half of the twentieth century, advances in preventive medicine vastly altered the pattern of disease in the United States and many other countries. The table of the leading causes of death in the United States shows the shift in importance from communicable to noncommunicable diseases.

Improvements in diagnosis, treatment, sanitation, nutrition, housing, and working conditions, as well as more specific preventive measures, such as immunizations, have played important roles in the conquest of the communicable diseases. Drugs, such as antibiotics and sulfas, have greatly reduced premature deaths from communicable diseases.

The increase in noncommunicable diseases has been due in large part to the

Leading Causes of Death in the United States—1900 and 1975

| 1900 (Life Expectancy 46.3 Years For Males, 48.3 Years for Females) | | 1975 Estimate (Life Expectancy 67.6 Years for Males, 75.3 Years for Females) | | |
Rank	Cause	Rank	Cause	Percent Of All Deaths
1	Tuberculosis	1	Heart and circulatory disorders	51%
2	Pneumonia	2	Cancer	18%
3	Intestinal infections	3	Accidents	6%
4	Heart diseases	4	Pneumonia and influenza	3%
5	Diseases of infancy	5	Diabetes	2%

increased life expectancy. Many of these diseases are cumulative and degenerative in nature. They require relatively long periods of time to develop and some of them are apparently related to the general aging processes. In just one hundred years—from 1870 to 1970—the proportion of persons in the United States over 45 years of age climbed from 13 percent to over 30 percent of the population and this percentage continues to increase. This increase in older-age groups is currently changing the whole field of preventive medicine. Whereas previous efforts were directed largely toward the control of communicable diseases of early life, efforts are now being directed increasingly toward the noncommunicable diseases—those common in middle and later life.

Cancer

Throughout a person's life the cells in many parts of his or her body are constantly dividing to provide replacements for worn-out or damaged cells. In cancer the normal, orderly division and growth of the cells is replaced by rapid, uncontrolled division and growth. In most cases cancer seems to start when a single cell goes "wild."

The general term *cancer* includes a group of related diseases that are characterized by the abnormal growth and spread of body cells. Considered as a group, the various types of cancer are the *number two* cause of death in the United States today. Approximately one in every four Americans will develop cancer sometime during his or her life. Currently, approximately 18 percent of all deaths in this country are attributed to some form of cancer.

Generally, a cancer cell can be distinguished from a normal cell principally by its nucleus. The nucleus of a cancer cell is usually larger than that of a normal cell, and differs in the number and appearance of its chromosomes, and in the number of nucleoli present (see figure of a cancer cell and a normal cell). The earliest detectable sign of cancer is an increase in the number of chromosomes in a cell. Not only are these numbers odd and irregular, but also the chromosomes may be abnormally shaped.

An outstanding characteristic of cancer cells is their invasive ability. Normal cells are slowed in dividing by close contact with surrounding cells. But cancer cells do not show such a response. They continue to divide and push into and invade the surrounding normal tissue.

Another important characteristic of cancer is metastasis, the transfer of disease from one organ to another. Cancerous growths tend to shed living cancer cells.

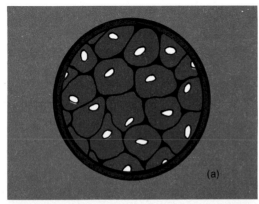

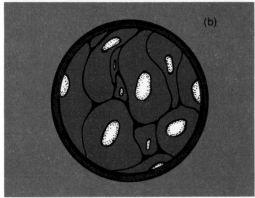

Cancer cells and normal cells as they might appear under the microscope. Cancer cells have large irregular nuclei, and the cells often take strange shapes: (a) microscopic view of Pap smear to detect cervical cancer, showing normal cells; (b) microscopic view of Pap smear to detect cervical cancer, showing cancer cells.

These cells can be picked up by the blood or lymph and be carried to remote parts of the body. Wherever these cells happen to lodge, they begin to grow, divide, and invade. Thus, through the process of metastasis, the body of the cancer victim may become riddled with dozens of growths at many locations.

Any mass of new tissue that persists and grows without serving any useful purpose is called a *tumor* or *neoplasm* ("new tissue"). The growth of tumors is characteristic of many, but not all, kinds of cancer. Tumors are divided into two classes—benign (non-cancerous) and malignant (cancerous).

Benign tumors tend to grow more slowly than malignant tumors and are usually surrounded by a fibrous membrane that prevents them from invading surrounding tissues. They may, however, reach such an enormous size that they exert dangerous pressure on the surrounding organs. Benign tumors commonly occur on the skin as warts or birthmarks, inside the body as fibrous tumors or cysts, or on the skeleton as growths of bone tissue. Some benign tumors, if exposed to certain harmful irritations, may become malignant.

Malignant tumors are cancerous growths. Kinds of cancers may be recognized by their names, which often end in the suffix -oma. Some examples: Carcinomas are malignancies of epithelial tissues; melanomas, of pigment cells; lymphomas, of lymph tissues; sarcomas, of connective tissues, and so forth.

Although cancer can kill in many ways, three conditions most often lead to the death of the cancer victim—anemia, infections, and debility.

Anemia is the inability of the blood to carry sufficient oxygen in the body. In some types of anemia there is an insufficient production of red blood cells, or red blood cells are produced but do not survive long enough. In other cancers there is internal bleeding that results in a dangerous loss of red blood cells.

Infection often results from the inability of the white blood cells to destroy infection germs. In some types of cancer few white blood cells are produced. In other cancers, such as leukemia, vast numbers of white cells are produced, but they are malformed and unable to fight germs.

Debility, the lack or loss of strength, is common in almost all forms of cancer. It may result from simple undernutrition, such as might occur when there has been damage to some part of the digestive system. Debility may also be a side effect of treatments such as surgery, drugs, or radiation.

Symptoms of Cancer The degree of success in treating cancer depends largely on how early the disease is detected and treatment is begun. (See table on some major cancer sites.) It is extremely important for everyone to recognize the early symptoms of cancer. They are:

1. Any sore that does not heal, regardless of its appearance or location.
2. Any lump or thickening anywhere on or in the body.
3. Any unusual bleeding or discharge from any body opening.
4. Any change in a wart, mole, or birthmark, such as a change in its color or size.
5. Persistent indigestion or difficulty in swallowing.
6. Persistent hoarseness or cough.
7. Any change in bowel or urination habits.
8. Any unusual pain—seldom a symptom of early cancer, but not to be ignored.

If any of these symptoms appear, either singly or in combination, a physician should be seen as soon as possible. Any of these symptoms can be produced by many conditions other than cancer, but prompt treatment of cancer is so essential that it is foolish to take a "wait and see" attitude. If cancer is found, it can be promptly treated. If cancer is ruled out as a cause of the symptom, needless worry can be avoided.

Diagnosis of Cancer A physician can definitely confirm the presence of cancer in several ways. Some of these methods are applied when a patient notices one of the early symptoms of cancer. Others are used on a routine, periodic basis to detect generally symptomless forms of the disease.

X Rays Certain cancers, such as lung cancer, may be detected through X rays. It is important that smokers have chest X rays frequently. Some authorities recommend chest X rays every six months for smokers.

Smear Tests Since many kinds of malignant tumors shed cancer cells from their surface, it is often possible to detect cancer through a microscopic examination of certain body fluids. This is accomplished by smearing the fluid onto a glass microscopic slide, staining it, and examining the slide under the microscope.

The most commonly used smear test is the Papanicolaou ("Pap") smear test for cancer of the uterus. In this simple procedure, a microscope slide is prepared from the secretions of the upper vagina. Since most uterine cancer begins on the cervix, which extends into the vagina, cancerous cells may be present in the vagina while the uterine cancer is still in its early development.

Uterine cancer usually remains on the cervix for one to two years before it begins its devastating spread through the entire uterus and the surrounding organs. If the cancer is detected through a Pap smear during this early period, the chances of a successful cure are excellent. It is strongly recommended that every woman have a Pap test every year, without fail, starting in her late teens. After age 45 the test should be made every six months.

Blood Tests   Leukemia and other cancers of the blood-forming organs are normally diagnosed through a count of the blood cells on a stained microscope slide. Some progress has been made toward the development of blood tests for other forms of cancer, but it must be emphasized that there is currently no way of detecting many forms of cancer through blood tests.

Rectal Examinations   The lower portion of the large intestine is a common place for cancer to develop. Cancers in this area are usually symptomless in their early stages. But a physician often can detect rectal cancers through a visual inspection of the inner walls of the lower large intestine.

Biopsy   A biopsy is the microscopic examination of cells removed from a living organ for the purpose of diagnosis. This procedure is normally applied when an organ or tumor is suspected of being cancerous. A small slice of the suspected tissue is removed and examined, often while the patient waits in the operating room. If the tumor is cancerous, extra care is taken to ensure the complete removal of all accessible cancerous tissue.

Theories of Causation

Several important factors distinguish research into the causes of cancer from analogous research on other diseases. First, dominating much of this research is the basic premise that underlying the answer to the riddle of cancer causation is the understanding of the functioning of the normal cell. By studying the chemistry and physiology of normal tissues, scientists hope eventually to learn by comparison between normal growth patterns and abnormal, cancerous ones.

Second, there is the as yet poorly understood relationship between causes and "triggers" of cancer. Certain external stimuli are apparently related to the development of the disease, but more basic "causes" also appear to be involved.

And third, further complicating all this is the fact that there are indications that some animal cancers are caused by viruses. As yet, no human cancers have been definitely connected with a specific pathogen, though some suspicious associations do exist.

The Basic Causes

The focus of much cancer research has been at the cellular level. The following basic causes of cancer are associated with defective or diseased cellular function.

Heredity   Only a few uncommon forms of cancer are definitely hereditary. One type of cancer of the eye follows a predictable hereditary pattern. Several other forms of cancer, while not yet proven to be hereditary, do seem common in certain family lines, suggesting that the tendency toward these cancers may be inherited. Examples of these cancers include colon cancer, thyroid cancer and breast cancer.

Mutations   In addition to the possibility that some cancers are hereditary in nature, scientists are looking at another aspect of the genetic causation of the disease. When a cell becomes cancerous, definite changes occur in the chromosomes. It is possible the effect of certain chemicals is to alter the hereditary material and "dictate" a new, cancerous growth pattern.

Viruses   In recent years, considerable evidence has accumulated associating at least some forms of human cancer with viruses. While a definite cause-and-effect relationship is yet to be proved, the presumptive evidence is strong enough to warrant an intensive research effort to determine the role, if any, that viruses play in causing cancers.

Site	No. of New Cases Per Year By Site And Sex		No. of Cancer Deaths By Site And Sex		Warning Signal—When Lasting Longer Than Two Weeks—See Your Doctor
	Male	Female	Male	Female	
Lung	72,000	19,000	63,500	17,600	Persistent cough or lingering respiratory ailment
Breast	700	88,000	300	32,600	Lump or thickening in the breast
Colon and Rectum	48,000	51,000	23,800	25,400	Change in bowel habits; bleeding from the rectum; blood in the stools
Prostate	56,000		18,700		Difficulty in urinating
Uterus (Cervical)		46,000		11,100	Unusual bleeding or discharge from vagina
Pancreas	12,000	9,500	10,900	8,600	Nausea, feeling of fullness, abdominal discomfort
Lymphomas (cancers of lymph tissues)	15,700	13,100	10,000	8,600	Painless enlargement of lymph nodes; pain in abdomen and back; persistent sore throat; trouble in swallowing
Ovary		17,000		10,800	Abdominal discomfort and pain; pressure, constipation, swelling of abdomen
Stomach	14,000	8,900	8,500	5,900	Persistent chronic indigestion; aversion to rich food and meat; decreasing appetite; dark, tarry stools
Leukemia (cancer of the blood-forming tissues)	12,000	9,200	8,500	6,700	Weakness; loss of weight; fatigue; bleeding from mucous membranes; enlarged liver and spleen
Bladder and Urethra	30,000	13,200	11,000	5,500	Blood in urine; frequent painful urination
Oral (including pharynx and larynx)	16,600	6,700	5,900	2,300	Sore that does not heal; difficulty in swallowing; hoarseness
Skin	4,300	4,700	2,900	2,100	Sore that does not heal, or change in wart or mole

Safeguards	Additional Information
Best safeguard is prevention by not smoking; annual physical checkup and chest x-ray series for smokers	The leading cause of deaths among males and is increasing in females as more females smoke. Is preventable by not smoking. Commonly metastasizes to the brain, bones or liver.
Annual checkup; monthly self-examination	Uncommon in males. Develops most frequently in females who have not lactated. This is the leading cause of cancer death in women.
Annual checkup, including protoscopy	Considered a highly curable disease when annual physical check-ups include proctoscopic examination for early detection.
Annual checkup including palpation of prostate gland and urinalysis	One of the most common types of cancer in males. Usually develops in males past age 60.
Annual checkup including pelvic examination and Papanicolaou (Pap) smear; avoid casual sexual contacts (?)	Uterine cancer deaths have declined 50 percent during the last 25 years, with wider application of the Pap smear; many thousands more lives could be saved. This cancer is increasingly being linked to a virus causation that may be spread to the female by the male. Most often develops in women who have had children.
Annual checkup including urinalysis	Only detected by physical checkup. Is usually fatal when it develops.
None known	These diseases arise in the lymph system and affected individuals often lead normal lives for years. *Lymphosarcoma* is frequently found in children. These diseases are found throughout the body in the lymph system including lymph nodes.
Annual checkup and notification of a physician when swelling in abdominal area is noticed	The growth may become quite large before producing any pain or discomfort. Woman often feels a necessity to urinate when there is no need.
Often is thought to be a peptic ulcer at first. Any persistent chronic indigestion should be brought to attention of a physician	Most wait too long for treatment; has been decreasing in last few years but is still a major cause of death in the United States.
	Acute leukemia mainly strikes children and is treated by drugs which have extended life from a few months to apparent cures. *Chronic leukemia* strikes usually after age 25 and progresses slowly. Cancer experts believe that if drugs or vaccines are found which can cure or prevent cancers they will be successful first for leukemia and lymphomas.
Annual checkup with urinalysis; do not smoke tobacco	There is some linkage with cigarette smoking. Consequently, not too common in females except in smoking females. One urination may be bloody while the next is entirely clear, or the bloody urine may slowly change to a normal color over a period of days; blood may not reappear for several months—any blood in the urine (except during menstrual flow in females) should be brought to the attention of a physician.
Annual checkup, including mirror laryngoscopy; do not smoke tobacco	Many more lives should be saved because the mouth is easily accessible to visual examination by physicians and dentists.
Annual checkup, avoidance of overexposure to the sun	Skin cancer is readily detected by observation, and diagnosed by simple biopsy; there are few deaths considering the large number of cases each year. These figures represent invasive cases only. Superficial cases amount to another 300,000 to 600,000 per year.

Adapted from *1975 Cancer Facts and Figures*, American Cancer Society, Inc., 1975.

It seems likely that cancer-causing viruses (if they exist) have long periods of latency during which they are present in the human body cells in an inactive state. Perhaps certain irritants, such as chemicals or radiation, act to "trigger" cancer by activating these viruses.

If cancer-producing viruses can be isolated and cultured (grown in tissue culture) this might open the door to the production of anticancer vaccines, which would seem to be the ideal solution to the cancer problem.

It is logical to wonder whether cancers are contagious, if viruses do cause cancer. The only current evidence of communicability is in the case of cervical cancer, which is rather strongly associated with the presence of a form of herpes simplex (type II), presumed to be transmitted through sexual intercourse (see discussion in chapter 17). While males rarely suffer cancer of the penis, they apparently do carry the herpes simplex type II virus.

There is no definite evidence that any other form of human cancer is ever "caught" from another person.

Deficiency in Immune Mechanism Many authorities now feel that isolated cancer cells appear from time to time in most or even all persons. Normally, these cancerous cells are quickly destroyed by specialized white blood cells that constantly patrol the body. According to this theory, at least certain types of cancer would only be able to develop beyond a few isolated cells when the "immune surveillance" mechanism was deficient. Supporting this theory is the established fact that the incidence of certain types of cancers increases dramatically in persons whose immune mechanism has been intentionally suppressed to prevent rejection of organ transplants.

None of these theories on the cause of cancer is mutually exclusive. It seems likely that each may apply to certain types of cancer or to certain individuals and that, in fact, a particular case of cancer might result from a combination of two or more of these factors. The combination of hereditary predisposition, virus infection, and immune deficiency, for example, could all contribute to the development of a case of cancer.

Cancer Triggers Several factors are known to produce cancer with prolonged exposure to human tissues. These forces are often referred to as *causes* of cancer ("Does smoking cause cancer?"), but the term *triggers* better relates these factors to the influences mentioned above.

Chemical Carcinogens Hundreds of chemicals have been definitely proved to be carcinogenic (cancer-triggering), either to man or to experimental animals. Some of these carcinogens are contained in tobacco smoke and the smoke from other burning vegetation. Others are carried by various petroleum derivatives such as tars, asphalts, and oil; coal derivatives; and soot.

Sunlight The factor in sunlight that causes skin cancer is its ultraviolet radiation. Since ultraviolet has little penetrating power, it is not associated with cancers of the deeper tissues.

External Irritation Some cases of cancer seem to be the result of a prolonged irritation such as the constant rubbing of a tight belt or brassiere strap over a wart, mole, or birthmark or the rubbing of loose dentures and bridges against the jaw.

Extreme Heat Prolonged exposure to very hot objects seems to be an occasional cause of cancer. The high temperature of a pipe stem may be a factor contributing to lip cancer that often develops in pipe smokers.

Radiation It has been well established that exposure to excessive X rays and other forms of radiation increases the chances of cancer. It has been found that either a single exposure to a high level of radiation or the repeated exposure to more moderate levels increases the risk of leukemia. It must be stressed that medical and dental X rays present very little risk. The risk involved in these X rays (which may be used to detect tuberculosis, fractured bones, dangerously infected teeth, and so on) is far less than the risk in not taking them.

Treatment of Cancer Many people have the mistaken idea that a cancer diagnosis is the same as a death sentence. In fact, this notion keeps many people away from doctors altogether when they fear they have cancer. Actually, with prompt medical treatment the chances of survival are good with many types of cancer. Even when the disease cannot be completely cured, proper treatment often can extend a patient's life.

We have already discussed the relationship between pathogens and the treatment and cure of communicable diseases. Until the pioneering work of Robert Koch and Louis Pasteur in the nineteenth century, doctors treating a communicable-disease patient could only try to make the patient comfortable, for the ability to cure depended on understanding of the cause.

Thus, in comparison with the history of the treatment of communicable disease, we have the paradoxically fortunate situation of cancer cures and treatment despite our lack of knowledge of the disease's cause. The methods of treatment of cancer deal not with eliminating the (unknown) causative agent, but rather with eliminating the cancerous cells and/or interrupting their growth pattern. There is no absolute standard for evaluating the success of a cancer cure. A cancer patient is generally considered "cured" only after he or she has shown no sign of the disease for at least five years after treatment.

In a sense, a doctor treating a cancer patient works "backwards." He or she studies the location, pattern, size, effects and symptoms of the cancerous growth and plans treatment accordingly. He or she might use a single method of treatment, or might combine a few different methods to effect a cure. The three basic methods of cancer treatment in use today are surgery, radiation, and chemotherapy.

Surgery The key to successful treatment of cancer is to diagnose it at a stage when the cancer can be removed entirely from the body. The major use of surgery in the treatment of cancer is to attempt to remove completely all of the cancerous tissue in the involved area. Because of the spreading nature of cancer, varying amounts of normal tissue are often removed along with the malignant growth. Surgery may be used to remove certain endocrine glands (ovaries, pituitary, or adrenal glands) in an effort to check the spread of cancer in organs that depend on the hormones produced by these glands for growth. It is also used to relieve pain in cases of incurable cancer by severing nerves serving the area of pain.

Surgery, radiation, and chemotherapy are being combined in an effort to find the most effective cancer cures possible. Chemicals are now being fed directly into surgical wounds to prevent the spread of any remaining cancer cells into the blood or lymph. Preoperative radiation to prevent implantation and growth of tumors in tissue surrounding the surgical area is also being used.

Radiation Radiation has been used as a cancer treatment for about fifty years. Amounts of radiation that seem to have no effect on normal cells cause considerable damage to cancerous cells, and sometimes even destroy the cancer completely. Some types of cancer, however, are not affected by doses of radiation that are safe for normal tissue. Three sources of radiation are used in cancer treatment—high-voltage x-ray machines, radioisotopes (elements such as cobalt that release energy and nuclear particles as they change to other elements at a predictable rate), and laser radiation.

X Rays X rays are controlled beams of electrons at variable high-energy levels. X rays of extremely high-energy levels readily penetrate tissues and can be used to arrest the growth of or kill cancerous cells in deep internal organs. Low-energy X rays are used for superficial cancers such as skin growths.

Radioactive Cobalt Radioactive cobalt releases a much more penetrating beam than does X ray. Used in a procedure similar to that used with X rays, cobalt therapy involves a placement of the patient in such a position that either the patient or the cobalt can be rotated during exposure to the radiation beam so that the tumor is at the center of rotation. This placement and rotation permit maximum amount of radiation without unnecessary damage to nearby healthy tissue.

Radioisotopes The advantage of radioisotopes is that they are picked up by the body through the digestive system, like many other chemicals. Physicians may select the appropriate radioactive isotope on the basis of the area or organ they wish to reach. Certain glands and organs tend to collect specific chemicals. As small, harmless doses of a radioisotope are introduced into the body, they accumulate at the area of the tumor. The thyroid gland, for instance, tends to collect and accumulate iodine. Consequently, in the treatment of

cancer of the thyroid, a radioisotope of iodine (I^{131}) is introduced into the body and accumulated by the thyroid gland. Its destructive energy is thus concentrated in a strategic spot to attack the tumor.

Laser Radiation Laser radiation is a relatively new type of light energy that was first made available for biomedical research in the late 1950s and early 1960s. In cancer therapy, beams of laser light are focused on a tumor. (They may be focused internally through special glass rods). This radiation has produced death in certain types of cancerous cells. After laser radiation the cells have also shown chromosomal changes. This indicates that the cellular changes induced by lasers may be more than just heat reactions.

Chemical compounds are now being used in conjunction with radiation. These drugs markedly increase the radiosensitivity of cancer cells. Under some conditions, doses of radiation in combination with drugs are much smaller than those required when radiation is used alone.

Chemotherapy Although surgery or radiation can often remove or arrest localized cancers, rarely can they cure cancers that have spread beyond their point of origin. Surgery cannot be used to cure cancers of the blood or blood-forming tissues that are widespread from the beginning. For many years scientists felt that the only way to treat such cancers would be with drugs or chemicals that would destroy cancer cells and yet not harm normal tissues. Prior to the 1940s, however, there was no evidence that such drugs could be produced. Today, however, many drugs are being used in the treatment of cancer, and in the past few years progress has been made in the chemotherapy of certain types of cancer, such as leukemia.

Much progress has been made in treating leukemia. New drugs and combinations of drugs are constantly being tested. Some drug combinations have prolonged the life of leukemia patients for more than ten years. In some medical centers, remissions are being achieved in up to 90 percent of childhood leukemia cases. In 1960, only a few patients could be expected to live for five years following the onset of leukemia. Today, about 25 percent of treated patients live that long, and new drugs are constantly extending the life expectancy of leukemia patients.

These effective drugs, as used by research medical centers and practicing physicians, should not be confused with the unproven cancer remedies that have been marketed for many years. Having failed to gain Food and Drug Administration approval for sale of these remedies in the United States, their promoters have established clinics in Canada, Mexico, and other countries. Many cancer patients travel to these countries to obtain unproven remedies such as Krebiozen and Laetrile. Too often, the time spent trying worthless cancer treatments delays effective treatment until a cure is impossible.

Depending on the type of cancer and its extent, drugs may be used alone or in combination with surgery or radiation. Some drugs attack cancerous cells directly, hormones are important in slowing the growth of certain cancers, and pain relievers are often necessary in advanced cases.

Immunotherapy One of the newer and more promising approaches to treating cancers is through stimulating the patient's immune mechanism to attack the cancerous cells. This approach is consistent with the theory that at least some cases of cancer are the result of deficient immunity.

Several means of stimulating immunity are being tested. None of these is yet considered to be a proven treatment for cancer. One treatment that has shown some promise for certain cancers is the injection of BCG vaccine (for Bacillus Calmette-Guerin, named after the Frenchmen who developed it). BCG is a weakened (attenuated) strain of living tuberculosis bacteria that is routinely used to immunize against tuberculosis in some European countries. It is seldom used in the United States. BCG is not an anticancer drug as such, but it does appear to stimulate the immune system. When injected directly into cancer lesions, it can cause the immune system to send white blood cells to the scene to fight the invaders. In some patients, these cells apparently attack the cancers as well.

Other experiments have involved vaccines made from tumors similar to those of the patient, injecting the substance into cancer victims in the hope of triggering an immune reaction that is specifically directed against the cancer. Still another immunologic approach has been the transplant of lymphatic (antibody-producing) tissue from healthy persons to cancer patients.

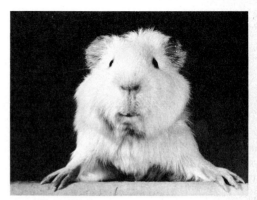

The unsung hero of cancer research—the guinea pig.

Photo by Ewing Galloway.

As more and more evidence accumulates linking viruses to at least some forms of cancer, the chance of producing effective specific vaccines against those cancers increases. If specific cancer-causing viruses are isolated, it will probably be only a matter of time until vaccines against them can be produced.

Survival Prospects for Cancer Patients

The survival of cancer patients depends on many factors. One of the most important is the location of the tumor. Other factors include the degree to which the tumor had spread when treatment was begun, the age and general health of the patient, and the method of treatment. (See figures on cancer survival rates and types of cancer by age groups.) Because of the larger number of men who have lung cancer, the survival of males in general is somewhat below the survival rate of females.

Chances for survival are also closely related to the size of the tumor and how

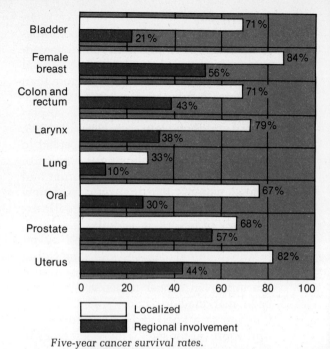

Five-year cancer survival rates.

Adapted from 1975 Cancer Facts and Figures, American Cancer Society (New York, 1975), p. 6.

Most Frequent Types of Cancer by Age Groups

Age	Most Frequent Types of Cancer
0–15	Leukemia, cancer of brain, lymphosarcomas, cancer of bone, kidney
15–34	
male	Leukemia, Hodgkin's disese, cancer of brain, testis, lymphosarcomas
female	Cancer of breast, leukemia, uterus, Hodgkin's disease, cancer of brain
35–54	
male	Cancer of lung, colon and rectum, pancreas, brain, stomach
female	Cancer of breast, uterus, lung, colon and rectum, ovary
55–74	
male	Cancer of lung, colon and rectum, prostate, pancreas, stomach
female	Cancer of breast, colon and rectum, uterus, lung, ovary
75 and over	
male	Cancer of prostate gland, lung, colon and rectum, stomach, pancreas
female	Cancer of colon and rectum, breast, stomach, uterus, pancreas

NOTE: Cancer of the skin is omitted from this table since there is seldom adequate reason for failure to diagnose it correctly and early.

Adapted from 1975 Cancer Facts and Figures, American Cancer Society, Inc., 1975.

much tissue is involved. Patients with strictly localized tumors generally have the best survival rates. The rates usually decrease in direct relation to the advancing tumor stage. Some people, however, with extremely small and localized cancers, die quickly despite apparently adequate treatment while a very few people with widespread metastasis live for many years with no treatment at all. This phenomenon, like many in cancer research, is unexplainable as yet.

Other Major Noncommunicable Diseases

In addition to cancer, there are many other noncommunicable diseases to which humans are subject. Included in the following discussions are some of the most prevalent of such diseases. Although these diseases bear little resemblence to each other, all are debilitating to a greater or lesser extent, and some are even life threatening.

Arthritis *Arthritis* is a general term for any inflammation of the joints. Its symptoms commonly include stiffness in the joints and mild to extreme pain, especially when affected joints are moved. In some types of arthritis, the joints become twisted and deformed.

About 100 types of arthritis are known today. Among the more important forms are *osteoarthritis* (degeneration of the joint) and *rheumatoid arthritis* (inflammation and swelling of the joint). A less common form, *gout*, is the painful deposit of urate crystals in and around the joints.

Arthritis is the number one crippler in the United States today. Over 17 million people suffer from some form of arthritis. For more than 3 million of these people, the symptoms are severe enough to limit their activity. Arthritis becomes more common and more severe as people grow older. Over 80 percent of people over age 65 are affected by some degree of arthritis. Rheumatoid arthritis is also fairly common among younger people. The measurable cost of arthritis in this country, including treatment and loss of earning power, is over $4 billion a year.

Considerable progress has been made in the treatment of arthritis. While there is still no permanent cure for most forms of arthritis, many victims who five years ago would have been immobilized or restricted drastically in their activity can now enjoy a normal life. Treatment involves drugs, directed at both the basic cause of the problem and the relief from pain; total joint replacement with joints of plastic and metal; and a variety of less drastic surgical methods. Bed rest, special exercises, and possibly acupuncture, all under medical supervision, may help in mild forms of arthritis. Early detection and treatment of arthritis is important in the prevention of its progression into a crippling form.

It is important to consult with a reputable physician for the treatment of arthritis. One of the most prevalent forms of quackery today is the dispensing of fraudulent or unproven treatments for arthritis. This field is lucrative to quacks because of the great numbers of people affected and the fact that no complete cure yet exists for many types of arthritis. Arthritic persons should be cautioned to avoid unproven treatments, whether sold by mail order, in stores, or administered by unethical practitioners.

Diabetes *Diabetes mellitus* is a disturbance of the metabolism (body chemistry), resulting from a deficiency of the hormone *insulin*. Insulin is produced in the pancreas by special clusters of cells called the *islets of Langerhans*. Insulin has the important function of increasing the rate of movement of glucose (blood sugar) through the membranes of most of the cells of the body. In diabetes, the blood sugar is unable to enter the cells in adequate amounts.

Diabetes is a rapidly increasing health problem. In the 25 years between 1950 and 1975, the number of diabetics in the United States increased more than 300 percent while the population increased only about 50 percent. The reasons for this increase are unknown. The number of diabetics in the United States is now estimated as between 5 and 8 million. Many people, perhaps half of all diabetics, have this dangerous disease without even knowing it. In spite of treatment with insulin, strict diets, and oral antidiabetic drugs, diabetes is still a major cause of death in the United States and the second leading cause of blindness. Periodic testing for diabetes is important for everyone, especially for relatives of known diabetics.

The tendency toward diabetes may be inherited. Not everyone who inherits the genetic tendency actually develops the disease, however. Diabetes is most common among older people, especially those who are overweight. Less commonly, it is a problem during youth. There are two forms of diabetes mellitus, apparently caused by different genetic factors. *Juvenile-onset* diabetes, developing during childhood, is usually much more severe than the *maturity-onset* form developing during adulthood. Many adults who carry the hereditary tendency for the maturity-onset form can avoid the disease entirely by merely controlling their food consumption.

Recently, viruses have been implicated as possible factors in the development of juvenile-onset diabetes. Mumps virus, along with a host of other common viruses, has been associated with the onset of diabetes, but a cause-and-effect relationship has not yet been proved. It is clear, though, that a genetic predisposition plays a major role in juvenile-onset diabetes and is the predominant factor in the maturity-onset form.

There may or may not be noticeable symptoms of diabetes. The most common symptoms that do appear include frequent urination, excessive thirst, craving for sweets and starches, and weakness. The most common medical test for diabetes is analysis of the urine for the presence of sugar. If sugar is present, a test is made for the level of sugar in the blood. The blood-sugar level is abnormally high in diabetics, a condition called *hyperglycemia*.

Some cases of adult-onset diabetes can be controlled with modification of the diet or increased exercise. The diet should be lower than average in carbohydrates (sugars and starches). Exercise increases the movement of blood sugar into muscle cells, thus helping to control the disease.

Many cases of diabetes, particularly those of juvenile-onset, require treatment with insulin or other drugs. For many years insulin was the only effective drug for the treatment of this disease. If the dosage of insulin is properly balanced with the intake of carbohydrates, most of the consequences of diabetes can be prevented. This is not a cure for the disease, merely a control. The drug must be taken indefinitely.

One disadvantage of insulin is that it must be taken by injection since, being a protein, it is digested if taken by mouth. Several other drugs are available which can be taken by mouth. These drugs stimulate the cells of the pancreas to produce insulin. Such drugs are effective only in adult-onset diabetics whose cells have retained some ability to produce insulin. If this ability has been totally lost, as in many severe juvenile-onset cases, insulin by injection is still the only effective treatment.

If diabetes is not adequately controlled, severe dehydration and acidity of the body fluids may occur. The result may be *diabetic coma* (unconsciousness), which is almost always fatal unless the patient receives immediate medical treatment. The breath smells of acetone (like most nail polish remover) and breathing is rapid. Another situation that requires immediate medical treatment is *insulin shock,* the result of an overdose of insulin. In insulin shock, the blood-sugar level is too low (*hypoglycemia*) for proper functioning of the central nervous system. As the blood-sugar level drops progressively lower, the person first trembles and seems nervous, then goes into convulsions, and finally drops into a state of coma. This coma can be distinguished from the diabetic coma by the absence of acetone breath and rapid breathing.

If an overdose of insulin has been administered to a diabetic and the person is still conscious, sugar or some product containing sugar, such as candy or orange juice, should be given. If he or she is already unconscious, the diabetic should receive immediate medical attention.

In addition to diabetic coma, untreated diabetes may lead to early death from heart disease or infection, or to blindness, kidney disease, or stillbirth or infant death of babies born to diabetic women.

The key steps in preventing such damaging results of diabetes are, in summary:

1. *Avoid becoming overweight.* This alone will prevent many potential cases of diabetes from ever developing.
2. *Have periodic medical examinations* that include blood or urine tests for diabetes.
3. *Seek medically supervised treatment* of a diagnosed case, including proper diet, exercise, and drugs.

A much less common condition, *diabetes insipidus,* results from improper functioning of the posterior lobe of the pituitary gland. Damage to the posterior pituitary is usually the result of an injury or a disease, such as syphilis. The anti-diuretic hormone (ADH) released by this gland is suppressed, causing excessive production of urine (polyuria). Unless water is continually replaced, dehydration develops rapidly, leading to acidosis, unconsciousness, and death.

Noncommunicable Respiratory Disorders

Severe respiratory disorders are among the most disabling of human diseases since they interfere with the oxygen supply that is so vital to all living tissues. The noncommunicable respiratory disorders, such as asthma, chronic bronchitis, and emphysema, therefore rank high as causes of human discomfort, disability, and death.

Asthma *Asthma* is a disease in which there are periodic attacks of difficulty in breathing. During an attack, wheezing and shortness of breath may be mild or so severe as to require medical treatment in order to prevent death.

The choked breathing that accompanies an asthma attack is caused by a narrowing

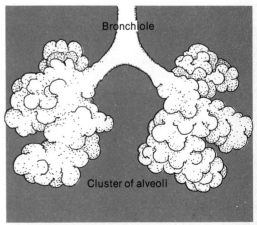

Microscopic structure of the lungs. Each lung consists of millions of microscopic air sacs (alveoli) supplies with air by small ducts (bronchioles).

of the *bronchioles*, small tubes inside the lungs (see drawing). This narrowing can be the result of a swelling of the membrane that lines the bronchioles, a spasm (constriction) of the tubes, or mucus blockage of the tubes.

There are many causes of asthma, among which allergic reactions are prominent. Asthma related to allergy is called *extrinsic asthma*. About 75 percent of the people who have asthma are allergic to one or more substances. Many cases of asthma are associated with bacterial infections of the sinuses, throat, and nose (*intrinsic asthma*). Most of these cases improve if the infection clears up. In some asthmatic patients, attacks are brought on or made worse by emotional stress that may lead to constriction of the bronchioles.

It is important that asthma sufferers receive the best available medical treatment, since prolonged or repeated attacks can cause permanent damage to the lungs and heart. Forced breathing can stretch the lung tissue, leading to the very serious condition known as *emphysema*, to be discussed below.

The treatment of asthma must be under the supervision of a physician. No one should try self-diagnosis or self-treatment. The exact cause of the attacks must be determined in order to decide the proper type of treatment. If an allergy is involved, the substance causing the allergy can sometimes be avoided, or, in some cases, the patient can be desensitized by a series of injections. If an infection is involved, it should be promptly treated. Ways may have to be found to reduce emotional stress, if this is the cause of the attacks. A change of climate may or may not be useful. The decision to move to another area should be made only after consultation with a physician. Various drugs are prescribed to provide relief from asthma attacks.

Chronic Bronchitis The inside of the bronchiole is lined with a highly specialized membrane. This membane secretes a layer of mucus to trap the foreign matter that enters the lungs. Millions of hairlike cilia constantly sweep the layer of mucus with its trapped foreign particles upward to the throat where it is swallowed.

Repeated irritation of this ciliated mucous membrane can paralyze the action of the cilia, eventually destroy them, and stimulate excessive production of mucus. This is the condition known as *chronic bronchitis*. Since the cilia can no longer clear the lungs of mucus, it accumulates until the flow of air through the bronchioles is obstructed. This obstruction then triggers a spell of coughing that helps clear the lungs. Frequent coughing is the most prominent symptom of chronic bronchitis. Other symptoms may include shortness of breath and wheezing. Chronic bronchitis often leads to emphysema and other forms of lung damage.

The main treatment of chronic bronchitis consists of eliminating the irritation that causes it. The source of irritation is often a chronic infection or smoking tobacco. The so-called smoker's cough is in reality a symptom of chronic bronchitis. The first step in treating any lung disorder is to *stop smoking*. If the source of irritation is an infection, this should receive prompt treatment. Coughing itself can contribute to the irritation of the bronchioles, thus creating a self-perpetuating condition. Coughing should be avoided unless absolutely necessary, and then it should be as gentle as possible. Above all, chronic bronchitis should receive the treatment of a physician.

Emphysema *Emphysema* is a deterioration of the lungs that develops gradually over a period of years. It is therefore more common among older persons, although it may begin to develop during youth. In emphysema, the thin walls of the tiny air sacs lose their elasticity and tear. This reduces the ability of the lungs to exhale.

The lungs swell up permanently, creating a "barrel chest" appearance in the victim of emphysema. Exhaling becomes extremely slow and difficult. The blood circulates with difficulty through the damaged lung tissue, creating a great burden on the heart, which must pump all the blood through the lungs before it can circulate to the body. Emphysema is an extremely disabling disease and often leads to fatal heart failure.

The development of emphysema often can be traced to prolonged asthma or chronic bronchitis. The most common link between emphysema victims is a history of heavy smoking. The disease is far more common among smokers than among nonsmokers. Air pollution and metabolic disorders are also believed to be associated with emphysema.

There is no real cure for emphysema. A physician may prescribe certain measures, such as mild exercise, drugs and special breathing techniques, but these mainly help the patient to live with the condition; they do not cure it.

Immune Disorders Many people suffer from disorders of the immune mechanism. We will briefly consider three important forms of these disorders.

Allergy An allergy (hypersensitivity) results when an immune response is stimulated by some substance in the diet or environment. The allergic symptoms are a "side effect" of the immune reaction. Once the exact substance (the allergen) causing the reaction is discovered, perhaps through skin tests, a person can sometimes be desensitized (have the immune re-

sponse deactivated) through a series of injections of minute amounts of the allergen. The symptoms in some allergies are produced by histamine, a body chemical released during certain immune reactions. Thus antihistamine drugs sometimes give symptomatic relief in such allergies.

A massive, life-threatening allergic reaction, called *anaphylaxis*, may occur in response to insect stings or allergy to penicillin or other drugs. Blood vessels dilate and the permeability of their walls increases; fluid leaks out of the blood vessels; little or no blood returns to the heart; blood pressure drops to nearly zero; breathing and pulse become rapid, but very weak. Death results from both circulatory and respiratory failure. Anaphylaxis may lead to rapid death if the victim is left without immediate medical attention. Some people who are known to have strong insect-venom allergy carry epinephrin (adrenalin) with them at all times to inject as an antidote for this reaction. Since people with marked allergy to insect stings may not have the time and/or ability to inject themselves with adrenalin there is a simple "Epe-inhaler," which is easier to use and just as effective.

Autoimmune Disorders Several degenerative conditions are known or believed to be caused by the failure of the immune system to recognize one of the body tissues as "self." In effect, a person is attacked by his or her own immune system. Some examples of such conditions include rheumatoid arthritis, in which the membranes lining the joints are attacked; rheumatic fever, in which the membranes of the joints, heart, and kidneys are damaged; multiple sclerosis, in which the central nervous system is attacked; myasthenia gravis, which is not well understood, but which impairs nervous stimulation of the muscles; lupus erythematosus, in which antibodies attack the kidney, spleen, and skin; and damage to the kidneys, liver, or thyroid gland. There are many more examples.

One way to treat an autoimmune problem is to suppress the immune system. Unfortunately, this cannot be done in a selective manner. The general suppression of immunity leaves the person without protection from germs of all kinds and fatal infections are a frequent result.

Immune Deficiency Some people suffer from an inadequate immune response. As a result, they have many serious infections. In its most complete form, immune deficiency is fatal unless the problem is predicted in an infant and the infant is kept in a sterile environment from birth. To date, no really successful treatment has been developed for such total immune deficiency. Immune deficiency may be a hereditary problem or it may result from exposure to radiation or certain drugs.

Epilepsy The name *epilepsy* is applied to a group of related disorders in brain function in which there are recurring sudden attacks of violent muscle contraction, loss of consciousness, or both. Between ½ and 1 percent of the population suffers from some form of epilepsy.

Despite the fact that many epileptics can now completely control their seizures with drugs, there is still much misunderstanding about epilepsy. Employers may still be reluctant to hire anyone with a history of epilepsy. Some states refuse to issue a driver's license to epileptics, even though they may not have suffered a seizure for years.

There are many different types of epilepsy, but most of these can be included in the following categories.

Grand Mal Epilepsy This is the most violent type of epilepsy. A typical grand mal seizure begins with an involuntary crying out as air is forced from the lungs. The victim loses consciousness, falls to the ground, and has repeated contractions of all the body's voluntary muscles. The attack typically lasts from 2 to 5 minutes and may be followed by deep sleep or confusion. Assistance given during grand mal attacks should be limited to preventing the victims from injuring themselves. Guidelines to follow would include:

1. Keep calm. There is nothing you can do to stop a seizure.
2. Do not try to restrain the patient.
3. Clear the area around the patient to avoid injury.
4. Try not to interfere with the victim's movements in any way.
5. Do not force anything between the teeth. If the mouth is already open, you might place a soft object between the side teeth.
6. Generally it is not necessary to call a physician unless the attack is followed almost immediately by another major seizure or the seizure lasts more than 10 minutes.
7. Treat the incident in a calm, matter-of-fact manner. After the seizure is over, let the patient rest.

Petit Mal Epilepsy This is a mild form of epilepsy in which the attacks consist of brief lapses in consciousness. Victims suddenly stop any activity in which they are engaged and then resume it when the attack is over. The attack lasts for only 1 to 30 seconds. There is usually no change in the state of the muscle tone, so victims usually do not fall down. During the attack they are not aware of their surroundings, and after the attack they often do not even realize that it has occurred. For example, victims may suffer attacks while talking to someone. They may pause for a few seconds while the attack is in progress, then continue logically from where they stopped, totally unaware of the seizure.

Psychomotor Epilepsy Psychomotor epilepsy can be classified between the petit mal and the grand mal forms of epilepsy in the severity of its attacks. In an attack of psychomotor epilepsy, there are physical and mental disturbances. These attacks last about 1 to 2 minutes. During this time, victims are conscious but are out of touch with the environment. They may suffer from hallucinations, anxiety, fear, or rage. They speak incoherently or make meaningless sounds. They do not understand what is said to them. Usually they do not fall down, but stagger around, performing automatic, useless movements, and often lose bladder control.

Our understanding of the causes of epilepsy is still somewhat limited. It is believed that epilepsy can be caused by any of several types of brain damage, particularly physical injury, as well as by hereditary factors or tumors. Most commonly, seizures begin in childhood or adolescence. There seems to be no relationship between the incidence of epilepsy and the intelligence, sex, or socioeconomic level of the victim.

Epilepsy usually is treated through medication with one or more of a variety of drugs in use. Once the proper dosage of the most effective drug or combination of drugs is established, often through a process of trial-and-error, seizures can be completely controlled in over half of all cases. About another 30 percent of all cases gains partial control and experiences seizures only infrequently. A few persons are helped through surgery, though this method is used only when every other alternative has already been tried.

Epilepsy patients whose condition is adequately controlled so that seizures seldom or never occur should be able to live an active, normal life. Most can work, participate in sports, go to school, drive a car (if they have complete seizure control), marry, and have children. For many, the only obstacle is lingering public fear and misunderstanding of the true nature of epilepsy.

Anemias Although the word *anemia* literally means "lack of blood," it is actually used to describe any condition in which the oxygen-carrying capacity of the blood is reduced. Anemia can result from a variety of conditions, including loss of blood (hemorrhage), deficient red cell production, excessive red cell destruction, nutritional inadequacies, or genetic disorders.

Nutritional Anemias The most common anemia, *deficiency anemia,* is the result of an iron-deficient diet and is most frequently seen in females. This type of anemia can be corrected with proper diet planning or with the use of iron supplements in pill or liquid form. Occasionally iron injections are given when the deficiency is severe.

Another important nutritional anemia, *pernicious anemia,* is associated with a lack of vitamin B^{12} (cobalamine). Cobalamine functions as a coenzyme in the formation of red blood cells. B^{12} is usually present in the diet, but the intestines of some people lack a substance necessary for its absorption into the blood. The tendency toward this problem is hereditary. In pernicious anemia the red cells are characteristically larger and have less pigment (hemoglobin) than normal red cells. Their oxygen-carrying capacity is severely decreased. Without injections of B^{12}, death is the eventual outcome.

Aplastic Anemia *Aplastic anemia* is associated with impairment of the blood-forming functions of the bone marrow. It is most common in adolescents and young adults. While aplastic anemia is sometimes a result of chromosomal defects, it is usually the result of ingesting a toxic

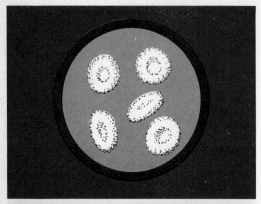

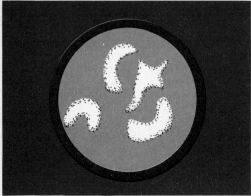

Sickle-cell anemia. Top, normal red blood cells; bottom, sickled cells.

sickle-shaped, instead of the normal round shape (see drawings of normal and sickled cells). Since sickled cells tend to flow through the smaller blood vessels with more friction, they bunch up in some of the tiny capillaries so that blood clots form. Typically, symptoms begin to appear between the ages of 2 and 4 years, including weakness, poor appetite, frequent illnesses and infections, pain in the joints and elsewhere, sores on the ankles, and anemia. The most characteristic symptom of the disease is the "sickle-cell crisis," during which there is high fever, excruciating pain, and the possibility of death from blood clots forming in the lungs, kidneys, or brain.

A child may inherit the recessive gene for sickle-cell anemia from one or both parents. The difference between a single dose and a double dose of sickle-cell anemia usually means the difference between health and disease. Someone who has inherited the trait from only one parent is called a "carrier." Such carriers seldom have sickle-cell anemia, but will carry a gene for the disease and may pass it on to their children. A few sickle-cell crises have been reported among carriers.

About 1 in 10 black Americans is a carrier of sickle-cell disease. About 1 in 100 black couples are *both* carriers, and they risk a 1 in 4 chance of having a child with sickle-cell anemia each time a pregnancy occurs. Thus, about 1 in 400 black babies born in this country has sickle-cell anemia. Currently, about half of these people die before age 20, though improved treatment methods are extending the lives of sickle-cell anemia victims.

Sickle-cell disease also occurs among black peoples of Africa, the Caribbean, Latin America, and southern India, and it occurs occasionally among whites of Mediterranean origin. The sickle-cell trait evolved in a malaria-ridden area of the

chemical agent. The bone marrow produces a deficient number of red cells, and these cells exhibit atypical structural formations. The general symptoms are severe, including waxy pallor of the skin and multiple internal hemorrhages throughout the body. Administration of whole blood transfusions is the main therapy and may prolong life, but the condition is usually fatal.

Sickle-Cell Anemia   A hereditary type of anemia of special importance to black people is *sickle-cell anemia*. In this disorder, a minor chemical abnormality in the hemoglobin of the red blood cells causes them to appear elongated and sometimes world. In that setting, it is actually a valuable characteristic, since it provides resistance to malaria.

Considerable research is taking place on treatments for sickle-cell anemia. The incidence and severity of the crises can now be reduced through medication. Also, several simple and inexpensive tests are available for detecting individuals who are carriers of the gene. They can then be counseled on the advisability of selecting mates who are not also carriers of the gene or the risk of sickle-cell anemia among any

children they might produce. Extreme care must be exercised that a diagnosis of sickle-cell anemia is not used as a basis for discrimination such as restricted job opportunities.

Heart and Circulatory Diseases

Diseases of the heart and blood vessels (cardiovascular diseases) are the number one health problem in the United States and account for more deaths than all other causes of death combined. At any given time, almost 25 percent of the adult population of this country has definite or suspected cardiovascular disease. Cardiovascular ailments are by far the chief causes of illness, disability, and death among both middle-aged and elderly people in this country. Among these, coronary heart disease, illness of the blood vessels supplying the heart, is responsible for the greatest number of deaths (over 50 percent of all cardiovascular deaths). Other cardiovascular problems causing numerous deaths are strokes and hypertension (high blood pressure). These three conditions are responsible for more than 80 percent of all cardiovascular deaths.

Like cancers and emphysema, heart diseases appear to be related to the extension of the average life expectancy, which permits degenerative diseases the decades they may require to develop. However, certain other factors are definitely involved in the high incidence of heart disease—the stresses of personal accomplishment, diets high in saturated fats, the tendency toward obesity with age, lack of sufficient physical exercise, and the use of tobacco. These factors appear to relate to a higher incidence of heart disease in this country than in societies lacking these characteristics.

The severity and danger of heart and artery diseases cannot be minimized. A disease in an arm or leg may cripple a

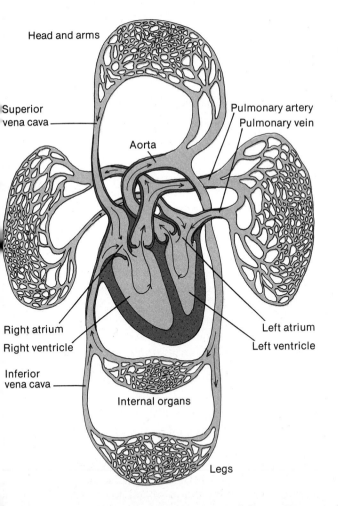

Head and arms

Superior
vena cava

Aorta

Pulmonary artery
Pulmonary vein

Right atrium
Right ventricle

Inferior
vena cava

Left atrium
Left ventricle

Internal organs

Legs

Adult circulation.

person, but a disease of the heart may lead to death.

Congenital Defects

Abnormalities in the development of the heart often occur during the first three months of fetal life. Although the specific causes of many congenital malformations of the heart are unknown, some of the causes are known to include certain maternal illnesses or bodily upsets or drugs taken during the first three months of pregnancy.

Among the more common types of congenital defects are valve defects, which may allow a reverse flow of blood, heard through the stethoscope as a "murmur"; holes in the internal walls (septa) of the heart, allowing leakage between chambers; and inadequate flow of blood to the lungs. Any of these problems may result in inadequate oxygenation of the blood and a "blue" baby (named after the bluish color of underoxygenated blood). Effects of congenital disorders may range in degree from insignificant to fatal. Many severe congenital heart ailments may be successfully corrected surgically, often within hours of birth. The activity of many people has unnecessarily been restricted by parents, teachers, or others who have heard that a child has a heart murmur. Many murmurs are unimportant in terms of heart function and require no restriction of activity.

Degenerative Disorders

Although the heart is very resistant to many disorders, certain conditions can seriously reduce its efficiency. The total effects are cumulative, becoming more and more serious as they go without correction or treatment. Heart disease may be the result of infections, toxins (poisons), injuries, poor nutrition, inactivity, emotional problems, use of tobacco, or other disturbances that weaken the heart.

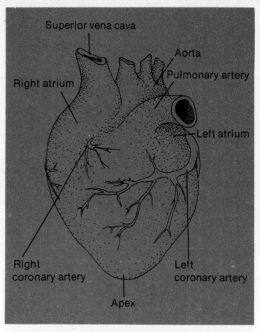

The heart, showing the coronary arteries.

Rheumatic Heart Disease

Much heart disease in childhood is the result of rheumatic fever, which usually first attacks the individual between the ages of 5 and 15.

A small percentage of persons suffering from certain streptococcal infections develop the symptoms of rheumatic fever (a swelling and pain in the joints, accompanied by fever). The original infection may be in any part of the body, but it is usually strep throat, scarlet fever, or middle-ear infection. Rheumatic fever is actually an allergic autoimmune response to a streptococcal infection. In about 60 percent of the cases the heart is inflamed, and in about 25 percent of the cases it may be permanently damaged.

Although other layers of the heart may be infected, the most common damage is done to the endocardium (the inner lining of the heart). Inflammation of this lining causes the heart valves to become scarred.

Blood deposits on such scarred valves. They thicken and either lose their flexibility or stick together.

Open-heart surgery has been increasingly effective in relieving such damage. Antibiotics have lowered the death rate. As a preventive measure, all streptococcal infections should be promptly brought to the attention of a physician. Anyone with a history of rheumatic fever must be particularly prompt in seeking treatment for infections, as one attack leaves a person highly susceptible to repeated attacks.

Heart Murmurs   Heart murmurs are abnormal sounds produced by vibrations that result from improperly working heart valves. They may be due to the endocarditis of rheumatic fever or other causes. The "murmur" sound heard through a physician's stethoscope results from an incompletely closing valve. Blood flows back across a valve into a heart chamber as it relaxes, producing the characteristic sound.

Murmurs are occasionally heard in hearts that are actually normal. A young person may engage in such strenuous exercise that the flow of blood through the valves creates a temporary turbulence, or murmur.

Atherosclerosis   Atherosclerosis is an artery disease. The walls of the arteries become thickened and hardened. A mixture of cholesterol and other fatlike materials is deposited in the arterial walls. This deposit is called *plaque*. The arteries gradually become hardened with deposits of calcium and other minerals. The end result of atherosclerosis is that the inside diameter of the artery is reduced and the inner lining of the artery is rough and irregular.

One of the major dangers of atherosclerosis is that of blood clotting. The damage to the inner surface of the artery may cause a clot (thrombus) to develop. Such a thrombus may cause the partial or complete obstruction (occlusion) of the blood vessel at this particular spot and shut off the blood flow. On occasion such blood clots may break loose in the bloodstream, and be carried to another point in the circulatory system.

Although such damage may occur in any blood vessel, it is more serious in certain places than in others. If it blocks an artery in the heart, the individual will have a heart attack; if it is in the brain, a stroke; if in the foot, gangrene; if in the kidney, high blood pressure; if in the eye, blindness.

The consequences of hardening of the arteries usually appear during old age, but there is growing evidence of it in young adults. The full-blown disease in older people is probably the result of a lifetime of fat deposition within the arteries.

Cholesterol, a major component of animal fats, appears to be one factor causing this condition. A certain amount of cholesterol is necessary for certain body functions, but an excess may be deposited in the walls of arteries, resulting in a hardened condition.

Some authorities now suspect that large quantities of table sugar (sucrose) in the diet may be a factor in the development of atherosclerosis, perhaps even more important than animal-fat intake. Other factors that may be involved include emotional stress, lack of exercise, diabetes, and perhaps most important of all, heredity. The tendency to atherosclerosis often follows family lines.

Hypertension   Hypertension simply means high blood pressure. As a normal heart pumps blood through the body, a certain degree of pressure is exerted against the blood vessels. With each beat of the left ventricle, a wave of pressure starts at the heart and travels along the arteries. This wave is called the *pulse*. The pulse can be felt on any arteries that are close to the surface of the body, such as on the wrist, the sides of the throat and the temple. The pulse results from peaks in the blood pressure. The blood pressure at the moment of contraction is the systolic pressure; it should normally be sufficient to displace about 120 mm of mercury in a glass tube. The blood pressure at the moment of relaxation of the heart is the diastolic pressure. It normally displaces about 80 mm of mercury. Blood pressure readings are presented as the systolic pressure over the diastolic pressure—for example, 120/80. Systolic pressures of 110 to 140 and diastolic pressures of 70 to 90 are usually considered within a normal range.

Hypertension is very common. It is believed to affect about one out of every five Americans at some time and is one of the nation's leading causes of death. It is a major contributor to heart disease, strokes, and kidney disease. Someone with untreated hypertension is four times as likely to have a heart attack as someone with normal blood pressure and twice as likely to develop kidney disease. It is the leading cause of strokes.

Anyone may suffer from high blood pressure. Males and females are about equally susceptible. While the incidence increases with age, a surprising number of cases exist among young people. For some reason, blacks are affected about twice as often as whites.

Modern medicine can now control virtually every case of hypertension, usually through one or more of a variety of drugs and reduced salt intake. Yet hundreds of thousands of people are still dying each year as a direct result of hypertension. Less than half of all people with hypertension are even aware of their condition. Of those who are aware, only about half are under treatment and many of those are in-adequately or improperly treated. It is among the most neglected of all health problems.

Hypertension is damaging in several ways. It forces the heart to work harder, pumping against increased resistance. The overworked heart may enlarge, requiring more oxygen than the coronary arteries can provide, and permanent damage to the heart muscle may occur. The prolonged excess pressure within the arteries gradually weakens their walls. An artery may rupture or, due to the damage to the arterial wall, a clot may form. Ruptures and clots in the vessels of the brain and kidneys are particularly destructive.

Several factors have been implicated as causes of hypertension. Kidney disease, while sometimes the result of high blood pressure, is also a cause of the condition. Kidney function depends upon an adequate blood pressure and the kidneys release a blood-pressure-raising hormone called renin to help provide this pressure. Diseased kidneys may release excessive renin. Obesity is another important cause. More fat means more blood vessels, which means more blood pressure to supply the additional volume of blood. Heredity plays a role. Those whose parents are hypertensive are far more likely to have the problem than those whose parents have normal blood pressure. Excess salt in the diet is a common causative factor. Most doctors agree that Americans eat far too much salt. Salt holds water in the body, causing swelling, a high fluid volume, and hypertension. Emotional stress is another well-established cause of hypertension, probably as a result of constriction (narrowing) of small arteries. The reasons for the high rate of hypertension among black people are still being determined. Some possibilities include a high salt diet, emotional pressures of being black in America, and hereditary predisposition.

WAYS IN WHICH STROKES OCCUR

HEMORRHAGE (Bleeding)

The wall of an artery of the brain may break, permitting blood to escape and thus damage surrounding brain tissue. Such escape reduces the flow of blood to other brain parts

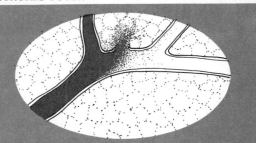

THROMBOSIS (Clot formation)

A clot of blood may form in an artery of the brain and may stop the flow of blood to the part of the brain supplied by the clot-plugged artery

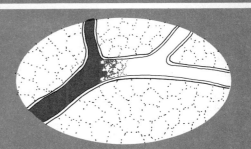

floating in the blood-

y be pumped to the ries

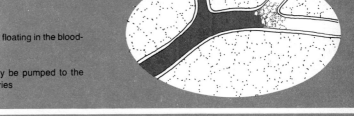

sure)

clot from another ves- d stop its flow of blood

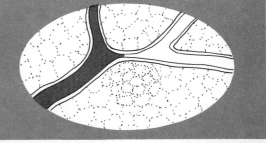

he walls of an artery)

hus reduce the flow of m is of short duration

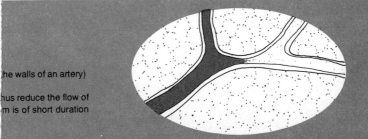

Many people have dangerously high blood pressure without experiencing any symptoms whatsoever. Crippling or fatal consequences can occur without any prior warning. Thus it is important to have one's blood pressure checked periodically, a quick, simple, and totally painless procedure. If high blood pressure is found, it should be regarded as a serious condition, despite any lack of symptoms, and should receive prompt treatment by a physician.

Cerebrovascular Accidents (Strokes)

The brain receives over one-fifth of all the blood pumped by the heart. As with the heart, any interruption in the normal flow of blood to the brain can have serious consequences. Such interruptions, commonly called *strokes*, may come about in several ways (see figure for ways strokes occur). Three-fourths of these accidents result from arterial hemorrhage and one-fourth from clots forming in the cerebral arteries. Depending on which part of the brain is destroyed, either of these kinds of accidents may cause speech impediments, loss of memory or mental confusion, some degree of paralysis, blindness, or even death.

Considerable progress has been made both in the treatment and rehabilitation of stroke patients. While some individuals lead a restricted life because of the permanent loss of some essential brain function, others recover quickly, depending on the site and extent of the brain damage.

Varicose Veins In the previous discussion of veins, it was mentioned that some of the veins of the body, such as those in the limbs, are provided with valves to prevent the backflow of blood as it is raised to the heart. These valves may be destroyed when veins are overstretched by an excess amount of blood for a prolonged period of time. This sometimes occurs in pregnancy or when a person stands much of the time.

Stretched veins become larger in diameter, but the valves do not stretch accordingly. Such valves fail to prevent the backflow of blood. The result is increased blood pressure in these veins. Circulation in surrounding muscles is inadequate, and nutrients fail to diffuse into such tissues properly. Muscles often become painful and weak, and the skin may become ulcerated.

Therapy for varicose veins includes elevating the legs to heart level, or binding them tightly. The legs may also be injected with certain agents that harden and plug the most protruding veins. The weakened sections of veins may be removed surgically. The blood then will be carried by other veins.

Coronary Heart Disease The coronary blood vessels surrounding the heart derive their name from the fact that they encircle the heart like a crown, or corona (see figure showing coronary vessels). These vessels transport almost a half pint of blood every minute over the surface of the heart. Any sudden blockage of one of the coronary arteries deprives that section of the heart of its blood supply. Cardiac cells die, heart contractions may cease, and circulation may come to a standstill. If a coronary artery is completely plugged, the condition is called a *coronary occlusion* or *heart attack*. If the obstruction is only partial or is in one of the smaller coronary tributaries, prompt treatment often leads to the individual's recovery. An occlusion in a main coronary artery is very serious and may cause sudden death. Other causes of the coronary diseases include inadequate exercise, aging, dietetic habits, obesity, smoking, or hypertension. Heavy physical exercise may serve as the precipitating factor for a heart attack for someone who is out of condition or who has coronary disease.

Pain from the heart may be due to a

blood-flow deficiency in the coronary vessels. This is referred to (actually, felt in) the left arm and shoulder. Such pain from the heart is called *angina pectoris*. Angina pectoris may not actually be noticed until the work load is too great in relation to the blood flow in the coronary vessels. People who experience it repeatedly often do not feel pain unless they exercise or experience strong emotion. Others experience it much of the time.

Fortunately, the great majority of coronary disease patients recover and are able to lead active, useful lives, providing they receive proper treatment under good medical supervision. Approximately one-fourth of all deaths in the United States, however, still result from coronary artery diseases. Also, it is estimated that more than one out of every ten Americans suffers some degree of insufficiency of blood supply to the heart.

Factors Relating to Heart Disease Increased understanding of American life-styles and their influence on heart disease has contributed to some reduction in the death rate from these illnesses. (See table on factors relating to heart disease.)

Symptoms of Heart Disease Symptoms vary according to the exact illness. Even though they may be absent, heart disease itself can be present. When symptoms are present, they can sometimes be mistaken for those of other body dis-

Factors Relating to Heart Disease

Factor	Explanation	Risk Involved
Serum cholesterol	Refers to cholesterol carried in liquid portion of blood. The amount of cholesterol in the blood is believed to relate to diet and heredity	A person with serum cholesterol over 240 mg. % has more than three times the risk of a person with less than 200 mg. %
Age		A person in the 50s has four times the risk of of attack as a person in the 30s
Blood pressure	Refers to elevated levels of blood pressure, or hypertension	A person with systolic blood pressure greater than 160 has four times the risk of an individual with SBP of less than 120
Cigarette smoking	Although referring to any cigarette smoker, the greater the amount and the longer the smoking history the greater the risk. Pipe and cigar smoking do not appear related	A cigarette smoker has nearly twice the risk of the nonsmoker
Vital capacity	Refers to amount of air a person can forcefully inhale and exhale	An individual with low vital capacity has about twice the risk of an individual with high vital capacity
ECG abnormalities	Refers to recording of electrical activity related to the contraction of cardiac muscle	An individual with an ECG abnormality has two and a half times the risk of an individual with normal ECG

NOTE: Miscellaneous suspected factors include gross obesity, insufficient physical activity, and inheritance.

Possible Symptoms of Heart Disease

Symptom	Explanation
Breathlessness	Unusual shortness of breath associated with moderate exertion might be an early symptom of a weakened heart muscle. It signals a marked oxygen shortage somewhere in the body. If, for instance, people are out of breath after climbing one flight of stairs, they should see their physician
Chest pains	Pain or a tight feeling in the chest during or after exertion or excitement may be due to oxygen deficiency. Cardiac pain is often in the center of the chest, very pressing, and may move to the shoulders and arms. Chest pains may also result from other causes, but it is best to be safe and consult a physician when such pains occur
Swelling of feet and ankles	If the heart fails to pump with usual vigor, the blood flow slows down and fluid may gather in the tissues (*edema*). This may be noticed first in the feet and ankles. It also may occur from other causes
Persistent fatigue	Frequent tiredness without apparent reason may be a sign of heart difficulty or hypertension. Other possible symptoms of heart disease may include a heavy feeling in the limbs, a weakness, and a lack of vigor during or following exertion
Miscellaneous symptoms	Other symptoms that may occur in some cardiac patients include *cyanosis* (blueness of skin due to insufficient oxygen in blood), loss of consciousness (fainting), recurrent bronchitis, and heart palpitations

orders. For example, dizziness and chest pains are common to many conditions. Legitimate symptoms of coronary heart disease are often overlooked. Breathlessness, for example, may be mistakenly attributed to bronchitis, or coughing to smoking. Generally, however, there are certain important symptoms that should be looked for and referred to a physician. (See table on symptoms of heart disease.)

Treatment of Heart Disease The treatment selected for a heart patient will depend on the nature of the disease and how critical the case is. A chronic illness (one slowly affecting the individual) usually permits time for a more deliberate diagnosis and treatment. Surgery for the repair of congenital conditions, for exam-

ple, may be planned some time in advance. In a critical, sudden heart attack case, however, prompt diagnosis and treatment are needed.

Emergency Care The person who has just had a heart attack is in need of immediate emergency care and should be taken to a hospital at once. The first medical treatment is usually to provide the oxygen that the weakened heart is unable to supply. This may involve the use of oxygen, drugs (such as nitroglycerin) to dilate the obstructed blood vessels, or electric or drug stimulators to revive the faltering heart. Next, measurements are needed for pulse and blood pressure, electrocardiograms to record the electric impulses of the heart, or x-ray and fluoroscopic examinations to measure the size and outline of the heart. All efforts must be made as soon as possible to reduce the blood-pumping load placed on the heart by reducing the patient's physical exertion and emotional excitement.

The first week (and especially the first 48 hours) after a heart attack is the most critical period. The largest number of deaths from heart attacks occur during this time. The danger of death is reduced as time goes on. With coronary patients, new blood vessels gradually form around the obstructed vessels, setting up new circulation, and an adequate oxygen-food supply is slowly restored to the deprived cells. Scar tissue forms over the affected area, and slowly, as the heart returns to normal, the patient can resume many normal activities.

Long-term Care   The cardinal rule of all treatment for heart patients is to prevent chest pains. Absence of such pain is a good indication that the heart muscle is receiving adequate circulation. To help circulation, drugs are often used: digitalis for a fuller heartbeat; drugs such as nitroglycerin to dilate coronary blood vessels and reduce pressure; antiocoagulants to reduce the possiblity of clotting; sedative drugs to quiet the body; and other drugs to cause certain actions to take place in the kidneys to help relieve pressure on the heart. A diet is planned that includes all essential foods in adequate amounts. The person must learn to rest and limit activity, if necessary. Schedules of moderate exercises must be established. Physicians usually insist that their patients lose any excess weight and stop smoking.

Through careful treatment by their physicians, many patients are able to resume much or all of their previous routine and may expect to live a nearly normal life. Longevity will depend, however, on properly understanding one's condition, faithfully using all medicines prescribed, and preventing situations that might cause another attack.

Prevention of Cardiovascular Diseases   Whether or not cardiovascular disorders are preventable largely depends on their causes. Diseases due to infection or malnutrition are often preventable. Heart damage caused by rheumatic fever can be prevented by reducing the incidence and severity of rheumatic fever with proper and prompt use of antibiotics in treating streptococcal infections. On the other hand, we are unable to predict or prevent many of the congenital malformations of the heart and blood vessels.

Circulatory problems can be greatly reduced by a reduction in cigarette smoking. The prevention of atherosclerosis appears to depend upon a reduction of cholesterol in the blood. Excessive blood pressure, underlying many cardiovascular problems, can often be reduced by regular physical exercise.

Smoking and Cardiovascular Diseases   It has been suggested for years that smoking has adverse effects on the cardiovascular system. Studies of large groups of people reinforce this suggestion by showing that cigarette smokers, in particular, are prone to die earlier (in middle age rather than old age) of certain cardiovascular disorders than are nonsmokers. Chief among these disorders is coronary artery disease.

The cardiovascular effects of smoking are caused by nicotine and carbon monoxide. Low concentrations of nicotine, as obtained from the smoking of one or two cigarettes, cause in most persons an increase in the resting heart rate of 15 to 25 beats per minute (30,000 extra beats per day), a rise in blood pressure, and an increase in the heart output. As the number of cigarettes smoked increases, there is also a dangerous decrease in blood flow to both the coronary arteries and the arteries of the rest of the body. Such a decrease is easily noted in the fingers after smoking (temperature drops because of a lack of blood). Such decreased blood flow accounts for the association of cigarette smoking and the increased incidence of coronary disease.

If as few as eight cigarettes are smoked within a period of one day, the carbon monoxide inhaled may cause an impairment of the oxygen-carrying mechanism of the blood. Such oxygen reduction in the body reduces the body's ability to produce adequate energy. This affects the total performance of the individual and is particularly damaging to the heart muscle.

Physical Exercise The heart of a person who gets regular, adequate physical exercise usually beats more slowly than the heart of someone who gets little exercise, as each heartbeat moves a greater volume of blood. Also, the blood pressure of the regular exerciser is usually lower. Exercise increases the blood-carrying capacity of the blood vessels, allowing more efficient circulation of the blood to take place at a lower pressure. The combination of reduced heart rate and lowered blood pressure, along with improved condition of the blood vessels, helps considerably in reducing the incidence of circulatory disorders of many kinds.

The National Heart Institute and the American Heart Association agree that one of the major causes of atherosclerosis, a major cardiovascular disease, is lack of exercise. Many studies indicate that the chemical cholesterol is greatly responsible for atherosclerosis. Exercise helps the body to maintain normal levels of cholesterol despite relatively high intakes of fat.

Vigorous physical activity 3 days per week for 5 weeks produces significant decreases in plasma cholesterol. Such decreases are linked to the reduced blood pressure attained through exercise. High blood pressure stimulates the production of cholesterol in the liver. This, in turn, increases cholesterol levels in the blood that accelerate the formation of cholesterol plaques and lead to atherosclerosis.

There are many factors (diet, heredity, smoking, obesity, lack of physical activity) linked to the enormously widespread incidence of degenerative cardiovascular conditions. It is difficult to single out any one factor and say that it is the major cause of such conditions. However, the individual who seems to have a good chance of suffering a heart attack is one who is male, eats too much, smokes too much, worries too much, and gets insufficient exercise. Such a person, especially if he comes from a family with a history of heart conditions, is "a heart attack waiting for a place to happen."

Ways of Preventing Cardiovascular Illnesses The incidence of cardiovascular disease could be substantially reduced if more people followed these simple guidelines:
1. Eat the proper foods in reasonable amounts. Reduce intake of animal fats.
2. Avoid infections or secure adequate treatment of infections.
3. Avoid excessive emotional stress and upsets.
4. Get adequate and regular rest.
5. Exercise regularly and in keeping with your general level of fitness.
6. Have regular physical examinations.
7. Do not smoke, or at least cut down your daily use of tobacco.

For Further Reading

Benenson, Abram S., ed. *Control of Communicable Diseases in Man* (12th ed.). New York: The American Public Health Association, 1975. Comprehensive reference on infectious diseases in compact paperback form.

"Conquering the Quiet Killer," *Time* (January 13, 1975), pp. 60–64. Good review of current information on hypertension.

Jones, Kenneth; Shainberg, Louis W.; and Byer, Curtis O. *Disease.* San Francisco: Canfield Press, 1975. Information on both communicable and noncommunicable diseases.

_____. *Total Fitness.* San Francisco: Canfield Press, 1972. Thorough background on fitness and specific activity programs.

_____. *VD.* New York: Harper and Row, Publishers, 1973. Includes information on common genital infections as well as the sexually transmitted diseases.

World Health (published by the World Health Organization), May, 1975. Special issue devoted entirely to sexually transmitted diseases.

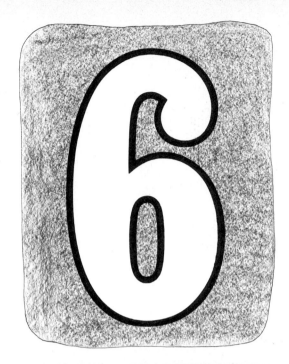

ENVIRONMENTAL HEALTH

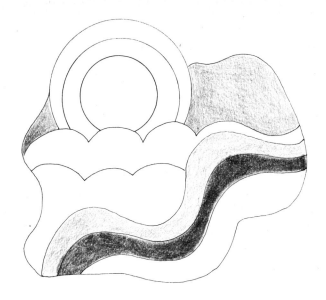

ENVIRONMENTAL QUALITY

A critical issue facing us in our struggle for a long, healthful, and fulfilling life is the quality of our environment. In many areas, serious environmental problems already exist. In many other places, they are rapidly developing. Several major world trends are contributing to environmental deterioration. Some of these trends include the rapid growth of world population, the acceleration of world industrialization, and the increasing world per capita consumption of resources—all resulting in increased pollution and other environmental deterioration.

Unfortunately, popular interest in environmental quality "peaked" several years ago, then declined somewhat as pressing world political and economic realities assumed a high priority. Yet since all of us continue to be dependent on the environment for survival, environmental quality is everyone's concern and an examination of the interactions between environmental quality and human health remains an important part of contemporary health science.

Politics and Environment

In the late 1960s and early 1970s, environmental quality was a hot political issue. Large numbers of people were gaining new environmental awareness and were demanding and getting environmental legislation. For officeholders, it was politically advantageous to be known as an environmentalist. But the mood of the public rapidly changed when two related problems hit the country: a shortage of expensive energy and rising unemployment. Suddenly, strip-mining for coal, shale-oil mining, and offshore drilling found renewed favor. As a political issue, protecting the environment became secondary to getting the economy moving again and gaining independence from foreign energy sources. Tightening of air pollution standards was delayed or abandoned and other environmental quality standards were compromised for the expediency of economic and political concerns. Thus, in many respects the environmental movement has suffered serious setbacks in recent years. Yet, in the long run, environmental problems still need to be solved if the quality of life is to be maintained.

The Quality of Life   An essential step in our study of ecological relationships is to consider the general nature of our surroundings. The concept of environment includes much more than just the physical side—land, air, water, and so forth. It encompasses every living and nonliving thing that in any way influences the form, quality, or length of our lives. Thus, even social and cultural conditions are included in the concept of environment.

Thinking first about the physical aspects of our environment, the idea we hope to convey is the very finite or limited nature of the land, air, and water. While the continents once seemed vast and the air and water unlimited, we are increasingly aware of the really restricted nature of these resources. Most of the earth's surface that is really suitable for living or raising food is already being put to one of those uses. The remaining unexploited landmasses are mostly too hot, cold, wet, dry or otherwise unsuitable for use without tremendous expenditures of already scarce resources and further disruption of the world's physical balance. The atmosphere is actually made up of a very thin layer of gases, which cannot always tolerate the quantities of pollutants that are dumped into it. The oceans are important living systems in which small amounts of various pollutants can upset vital life cycles. The entire environment is not just a passive sink that can tolerate everything poured into it. It is a dynamic system, reacting to every abuse heaped upon it.

We must think of the healthful environment not only as one that is devoid of harmful substances, but as one that includes a wide variety of favorable factors as well. We must not be content with an environment that merely makes life possible, but must concentrate on maintaining or developing an environment that makes life worth living. A healthful environment allows the individual to achieve full physical, emotional, and social potential. It contributes to emotional well-being through beautiful scenery, clean and orderly communities, and quiet surroundings for the enjoyment of leisure time. It provides for the needs of families and individuals, including adequate housing and educational and economic opportunities. It offers a variety of life-styles and the opportunity to choose among them. It provides a social and technological environment within human adaptive capacity.

Thus, the concept of a healthful environment involves much more than the mere absence of pollutants. It raises basic questions about the design and size of metropolitan areas and about the effectiveness of social, economic, and political systems.

Pollution   Foremost among the environmental health hazards today is pollution, the introduction into the environment of substances and forms of energy that unfavorably alter our environment. They are the by-products of human activities—the residues of things we make, use, and throw away. They include the excretory wastes from humans and domestic animals, industrial sewage and gases, pesticides, automobile exhausts, empty cans and bottles, radiation, and even heat and noise.

Since most of these wastes have been with us for many years, one might wonder why pollution has only recently emerged as a major problem. One important reason is the recent increase in human population. An environment that could easily assimilate the wastes and by-products from a smaller population can be completely befouled by the proportionately increased pollutants from a larger population. In addition, new pollutants are constantly being introduced into our environment as a result of continuing technical advance. An estimated 400 to 500 new chemical substances are being created for our use each year. The long-term effects of these new chemicals on our environment and us are virtually unknown.

It must be remembered that many pollutants are the unavoidable consequences of our human nature as biological organisms and as creative, social beings. These are the wastes from our metabolic processes and from our efforts to feed, house, clothe, and transport ourselves. Some pollutants will always be with us. They will increase in abundance as our population increases and as the world standard of living (hopefully) rises. They will become more concentrated as urbanization continues and more people live in less space.

It is obvious, then, that we cannot eliminate all pollutants. Therefore, our goal must be to minimize the production of pollutants, particularly those with serious environmental consequences, and to manage the disposal of pollutants so that they can be effectively assimilated into the environment.

Air Pollution   We can live without food for weeks and without water for days, but we can live without air for only a few minutes. Accordingly, air is the most immediately vital resource.

For many years people have been treating the atmosphere as if it were a sewer, exhausting different kinds of waste products into it—gases, dusts, fumes, vapors, and smoke. Since the amount of contamination until recent years was small in relation to the vastness of the atmosphere, little trouble resulted. In the last few decades, however, continuing contamination is producing concentrations that are harmful to people, animals, and plants.

Air pollution is produced by different air contaminants in different areas. By general definition, air pollution is the introduction of hazardous material into the atmosphere as the result of human activities. This definition would exclude air contaminants produced by such natural phenomena as volcanoes, hot springs, and dust storms. Some pollutants, such as smoke from forest fires, may stem from either natural or human causes. Pollution, as discussed here, will imply the possibility of control.

In order to understand the problem of air pollution more fully, let us briefly examine the nature and size of our atmosphere. "Pure" air is, of course, a mixture of many kinds of gases, including about 78 percent nitrogen, 21 percent oxygen, less than 1 percent argon, 0.03 percent carbon dioxide, traces of several other gases, and varying amounts of water vapor. So far, contrary to popular belief, the percentage of oxygen in the air has not been reduced significantly with the advent of air pollution. However, human activities are reducing the world supply of green plants (our only sources of oxygen) at an alarming rate. An acre of food-crop plants produces far less oxygen than the acre of forest it may have replaced. An acre of pavement produces no oxygen at all. Thus, some authorities feel we may eventually run into oxygen depletion problems with the elimination of green plants, though other air problems are more pressing at this time.

About 95 percent of the earth's air mass is concentrated in a layer about 12 miles thick around the earth's crust. This represents an area no deeper, proportionately, than the skin of an apple to the apple itself. Thus, it is indeed necessary to regard the earth's air supply as limited.

The problem of air pollution is further complicated by the existence of inversion layers over many of the world's major cities. An inversion layer is a layer of warmer air over a cooler surface layer of air, and results from an area's topographical character and proximity to water. This inversion layer acts as an air trap, preventing air pollutants from mixing with upper layers of air. Thus, instead of pollutants being diluted through 12 miles of atmosphere, they may be held within several

hundred feet of the ground. In some western cities, such as Los Angeles, inversion layers may be present on as many as 340 days of the year.

Sources of Air Pollutants   The majority of the thousands of human air-contaminating activities can be grouped into three general categories: attrition, vaporization, and combustion.

Attrition means the wearing or grinding down by friction. Have you ever wondered what becomes of the tread rubber from the millions of tires that are worn out each year? And the asbestos from millions of brake shoes? Much of this worn-off material drifts into the air as microscopic dustlike particles. Additional sources of particulate pollutants include sanding, sand blasting, drilling, grinding, and a multitude of other industrial processes.

Vaporization is the change of a substance from the liquid to the gaseous state. Vaporization is a major source of air pollution. Such materials as gasoline and many industrial solvents vaporize freely at normal air temperatures and are troublesome air polluters. Other materials will vaporize only under the less common conditions of increased heat and pressure. Some of the most noxious pollutants result from vaporization of industrial chemicals.

Combustion is the process of burning. Combustion is never complete or perfect, regardless of where it takes place. The fuel may not be a pure hydrocarbon; there may be too much or too little air; or the temperature may be too low or too high. The by-products of combustion may include unburned bits of carbon, carbon monoxide gas, and products from impurities in the fuel. When sulfur is present, it is converted into sulfur dioxide and sulfur trioxide. In addition to being undesirable by themselves, these gases can combine with water vapor to form sulfuric acid.

Another pollutant results from what

might be considered perfect combustion conditions—very high temperatures and an air supply beyond that needed for complete combustion. Under such conditions, the high temperature causes the nitrogen and oxygen of the air to combine into nitric oxide, which further oxidizes to form nitrogen dioxide, one of the most troublesome components of air pollution. Nitrogen dioxide irritates the eyes and mucous membranes, damages vegetation, and contributes to *photochemical smog*.

Photochemical Smog   *Smog* is a coined word, combining "smoke" and "fog." It is a phenomenon common to many metropolitan areas, particularly those along sea coasts. Photochemical smog results when air pollutants trapped beneath an inversion layer are changed to more noxious chemicals by the action of sunlight.

The basic ingredients of photochemical smog include nitrogen dioxide and incompletely burned hydrocarbons from auto exhausts. Carbon monoxide is not involved. When nitrogen dioxide (NO_2) absorbs energy from sunlight, it separates into nitric oxide (NO) and atomic oxygen (O). The normal atmospheric oxygen is in the form of molecular oxygen (O_2). The atomic oxygen unites with the molecular oxygen to form ozone (O_3). Ozone induces much eye irritation and is also thought to cause lung damage (pulmonary fibrosis) after long exposure. Ozone also reacts with other air pollutants (especially hydrocarbons) to form literally hundreds of undesirable compounds. Among the worst offenders of photochemical smog are PAN (peroxyacetylnitrate) and various aldehydes. Both PAN and the aldehydes are highly irritating to the eyes and respiratory tract and are harmful to vegetation as well. In the mountain ranges of Southern California, thousands of acres of prime forest are currently being killed by photochemical smog.

The Fluorocarbon Controversy   In 1974, controversy erupted when a scientific journal carried a report that the chlorofluoromethanes, also known as fluorocarbons and sold under the DuPont trademark, Freon, were suspected of damaging the layer of ozone (O_3) that lies in the stratosphere, many miles above the surface of the earth. Fluorocarbons are the principal gases used in refrigeration and air conditioning units and are used as a propellent in some spray cans. The importance of the ozone layer is that it screens most of the ultraviolet radiation from sunlight. Without this layer, life as we know it on earth would be impossible. The present concern is that even a slight reduction in the amount of ozone would result in many additional cases of human skin cancer each year and might have still-unknown effects on other plants and animals such as an increase in mutations.

On a world basis, over 800,000 *tons* of fluorocarbons are manufactured and used each year. Most of this amount eventually finds its way into the atmosphere. In the United States, about half the fluorocarbon production goes into spray cans; about 35 percent is used in refrigeration; and about 15 percent is used in production of foam for cushions and insulation, in fire extinguishers, and as cleaning solvents. Hair spray and deodorant cans often contain fluorocarbons while most shaving cream, paint, and insecticide spray cans do not. The labels usually do not indicate what propellent is used.

Many scientists favor a halt in fluorocarbon production, at least until more information is available on the extent (if any) of damage to the ozone layer. To be effective, such a ban would have to include all uses of fluorocarbons and would have to be worldwide in its scope. United States manufacturers account for only about half of the world's production and international cooperation on this matter would seem difficult or impossible to attain. The biggest problem would be in replacing fluorocarbons for refrigeration; no adequate substitute is available. Other propellents are available for spray cans and, of course, many products commonly sold in spray cans can be packaged in other types of containers.

The Effects of Air Pollution   Some of the effects of air pollution are immediately obvious to even the most casual observer. Our eyes sting, our throats burn, the view is spoiled, we may suffer from a vague state of emotional depression. But the more serious effects of air pollution are insidious. Occurring over a period of years, they often go unnoticed until permanent damage has been done. In the following paragraphs we will survey some of these more serious effects of air pollution.

Smog damage to vegetation is creating an alarming situation. At a time when the world food supply is growing ever more scarce, many important food plants are showing increasing damage—and subsequent reduction in yield—due to air pollution. In addition, the world's only oxygen supply—photosynthesis in green plants—is being impaired by air pollution. However, though it may not be much comfort, most authorities say that even if air pollution goes uncontrolled, we will starve to death before we run out of oxygen.

The effect of air pollution on animals is of double concern. In addition to the illness and death of the animals themselves, there is the ominous portent that the same fate lies ahead for us. Among the many alarming examples of the effects of air pollution on animals are cases where arsenic from smelting operations has settled on vegetation and poisoned grazing animals; where fluorides from aluminum fertilizer plants have so crippled grazing animals

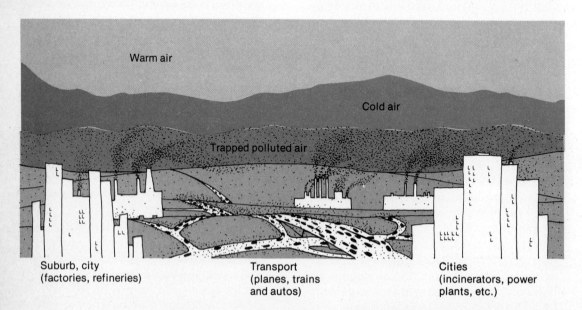

Warm air

Cold air

Trapped polluted air

Suburb, city
(factories, refineries)

Transport
(planes, trains
and autos)

Cities
(incinerators, power
plants, etc.)

The activities of modern urban and suburban communities include many practices that produce air pollution. When natural phenomena, such as temperature inversions, are added, a situation like that shown above can result. This is particularly dangerous for living things because the pollutants emitted into the lower atmosphere will stay close to their sources until the temperature pattern is altered by weather changes.

that they had to be killed; and where cattle grazing several miles from lead and zinc foundries have been poisoned.

The economic loss from damage to various materials is almost incalculable. Few, if any, materials are totally impervious to air pollution. Materials that commonly show smog damage are such metals as steel, iron, zinc, brass, copper, nickel, lead, tin; and such building materials as marble, slate, mortar and paint. Particularly susceptible to damage are such organic materials as rubber, leather, paper, and both natural and synthetic fibers.

When we live day in and day out in a pall of air pollution, it is only the rare clear day that reminds us what we are missing. In addition to the obvious problems of reduced visibility for driving or flying, there are the subtle psychological results of foul air. Every mountain view blocked by air pollution, every flower soiled by smog, and every expanse of blue sky turned gray destroys a portion of our identity with nature and leaves the quality of life diminished by the loss.

The most disastrous result of air pollution is its effect on human health. In addition to the more obvious effects, such as eye and throat irritation, air pollution is believed to cause more serious harm to the respiratory system and heart. Air pollution levels have been correlated to chronic bronchitis, asthma, emphysema, lung cancer, and, through impaired lung function, to heart disease. Initially there is an acute inflammation of the lungs, with fluid partially filling the tiny air sacs, or alveoli, of the lungs. The normal breathing reflex is affected. Breathing becomes shallow, and the usual rate of oxygen consumption is decreased. Over the long term, an irreversible disease known as *emphysema* may result. Asthma or heavy cigarette smoking can cause emphysema. Toxic air pollutants, sulfur dioxide, and ozone are other known causes. The walls between the al-

veoli break down. The walls of the respiratory tubes become fibrous and constricted, and breathing becomes harder and harder. Other long-term or chronic effects are suspected but as yet have not been conclusively identified. Air pollution is particularly harmful to infants, the elderly, and those suffering from chronic respiratory disorders. Some scientists warn that residue from the internal combustion engine results in high levels of lead capable of affecting human behavior.

Because so much definite evidence of the harmful effects of air pollution has been compiled, many public health authorities now recommend curtailing vigorous outdoor activities during intense smog attacks. In Los Angeles County, ozone levels are monitored daily as indicators of photochemical smog levels, and schools are advised to keep pupils indoors during recess and lunch periods when ozone levels exceed 0.35 part per million—a condition occurring several times each year in parts of the county.

Many people hold exaggerated ideas about the ability of humans to "adjust" to a poisoned environment, feeling that so long as pollution levels increase gradually, we will be able to accommodate to almost any level of pollution. During the 1971 "mercury scare," a representative of the fishing industry was quoted as stating that the American public might have developed such a level of tolerance to mercury-contaminated fish that it might be dangerous to discontinue eating such fish, perhaps resulting in some kind of "withdrawal" symptoms. Needless to say, his fears were unfounded and just might have been influenced by his concern for the "health" of the fishing industry.

Obviously, the human species must have some ability to adapt to adverse environmental conditions or we would not have survived this long. But our ability to tolerate any particular poison is definitely limited and regardless of how gradually its level in the environment increases, a point would be reached at which continued human life would be impossible. Unfortunately, it seems that for certain poisons in certain areas this level is approached from time to time, or even exceeded.

Suppose that in your city the level of some air pollutant reached the point where medical authorities agreed that it had become hazardous to engage in any outdoor activities whatsoever! This hypothetical situation is probably already an unrecognized reality in many cities today. Imagine what life would be like if all outdoor activities were forbidden. Children would rush from sealed, air-filtered homes to sealed, air-filtered schools, perhaps wearing gas masks while in transit. Adults similarly would live in fear of the unfiltered air. This joyless situation could become a reality if air pollution is not effectively controlled.

Control of Air Pollution The control or prevention of air contamination is a complex, and often expensive, problem. Some authorities believe it is now possible to eliminate such pollution almost entirely, but each locality must decide how clean its air should be and how much it is willing to pay for smog control. At the present time, toleration levels can be determined for only a few contaminants. Ideally, pollution should be eliminated at the source.

In some places the answer is to reduce the source of pollution by using cleaner-burning home-heating fuels, such as switching from coal to oil, or better, to natural gas or electricity. In other cases—for example, motor vehicles—the problem requires reduction of private auto use by developing better rapid transit systems and by stricter control of auto emissions. The reduction of car size and horsepower also contributes to cleaner air, as will the development of new types of engines.

Also involved are the legal and regulatory aspects of pollution control. We must be free to use our property, yet at the same time we must be prevented from doing harm to others. The atmosphere must be kept clean enough for humans to breathe safely and to insure the growth of food crops. Conflicts of interest must be overcome. The "right" to dischard waste products into the atmosphere must be made subordinate to the "right" to breathe safe air. Such priorities must be established and they will require the modification of certain practices by both corporations and individuals. Does anyone really have the "right" to pollute the air that others must breathe in order to live?

Government Controls Traditionally, the regulation of pollution has been left to state and local governments. But it has become increasingly clear that such regulation is not always adequate. State and local agencies hesitate to enact or enforce regulations that would restrict the activities of corporations that contribute significantly to the employment tax rolls within their jurisdiction. These same corporations may make sizeable contributions for the election of "reliable" candidates. The citizens within an area are reluctant to push for pollution control when it might affect their "bread and butter."

Pollution obviously does not confine itself to the political jurisdiction in which it originates. Polluted air drifts freely from county to county. Polluted rivers may flow through many states. Untreated refuse dumped into the ocean by one city may easily wash up on the beaches of another. Thus, the control of pollution rightfully becomes an interstate problem, subject to federal control.

Federal control of pollution has evolved slowly, over a span of several decades. Until recently, federal efforts were often ineffective, as responsibilities were fragmented among many different agencies and departments of the government. There have been instances where the policies of two federal agencies were directly contradictory—one agency actively polluting the environment with the same pollutant another agency has sought to control.

In a move to coordinate and strengthen the environmental control activities of the federal government, President Nixon in 1970 authorized the formation of the Environmental Protection Agency (EPA). This agency consists of units transferred from other federal agencies, including the departments of the Interior, Agriculture, Health, Education, and Welfare, and the Atomic Energy Commission. Thus, the federal agencies dealing with air and water pollution, the regulation of pesticides, atomic radiation, and solid waste control were brought under one roof. The EPA operates with a budget in excess of $2 billion per year. Among the specific activities and powers of the EPA are the setting of air-quality standards for all sources of air pollutants, with authority to assess penalties up to $25,000 per day for first violations, and up to $50,000 per day and up to 2 years in prison for second offenses.

Other EPA activities include control over all industrial waste discharges into bodies of water, though the elimination of such discharges will be a gradual process. Local government agencies are being given financial and technical aid in the construction of sewage treatment facilities. Another goal is the closing down of 5,000 open dumps scattered across the country.

Water Pollution Water, in its natural state, is never 100 percent pure. As soon as it condenses as rain, water begins gathering impurities that it carries until purified or until it evaporates. Much of this impurity is not sufficient to spoil the usefulness of water. Some materials and substances, however, do limit its usefulness.

By definition, *water pollution* means the presence in water of any substance that interferes with any of its legitimate uses—for public water supplies, recreation, agriculture, industry, the preservation of fish and wildlife, and esthetic purposes.

The principal forms of water pollution are domestic, industrial, and agricultural wastes, and silt. Domestic wastes include sewage, detergents, and everything else going down the drains of a city into its sewer system—used water from toilets, bathtubs, sinks, and washings from restaurants, laundries, hospitals, hotels, and other businesses. Industrial wastes are the acids, oils, greases, other chemicals and animal and vegetable matter discharged by factories. These wastes are discharged either through some sewer system or through separate outlets directly into waterways. Agricultural wastes include pesticides (insecticides, fungicides, and herbicides), fertilizers (mainly nitrates and phosphates), and animal wastes. Silt includes the soil that is washed into streams that muddies waters and fills up reservoirs and waterways. In addition to these principal forms, other pollutants, such as heat and radioactive substances, can contribute to water pollution.

Pollution in a body of water can be measured several ways. Most common pollutants are organic. Bacteria break them down into simpler compounds, and in doing so, need oxygen. With more organic material, the bacteria population increases, and a greater demand is placed on oxygen in the water. The demand for oxygen by bacteria is called *biological oxygen demand* (BOD). BOD is an indicator of organic pollution. It also determines which forms of life can best survive in the stream. Large water animals need more oxygen and therefore have a higher BOD than invertebrate animals and bacteria, which have a

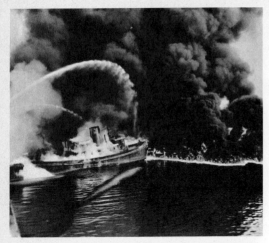

As a result of years of use as a dumping ground for the major industries of Cleveland, Ohio, the once-beautiful Cuyahoga River is now designated a fire hazard. A single match can set off the type of blaze shown here.

Photo by The Cleveland Plain Dealer.

much lower BOD. In fact, certain invertebrate animals living in bottom mud of freshwater streams occur in inverse proportion to the oxygen content of the water. One, a small worm, *Tubifex*, has an occurrence as high as 20,000 individuals per square foot in badly polluted water, but may be absent altogether in clean water. Not all water pollutants are broken down by bacteria. Radioactive substances, silt, pesticides, detergents, and certain oil products are more difficult to clean up.

Wide-Range Effects of Polluted Water
Not only is clean water needed for domestic uses, but water is also the most extensively used of all raw materials in industry. Since the availability of good-quality water determines the location of many industries, having good water becomes an economic asset for most communities. Correspondingly, lack of good water may turn into an economic liability.

There are other economic considerations. Crops irrigated with polluted water

may transmit disease. Certain forms of industrial pollution in irrigation waters may damage crops. Heavy metals such as mercury and arsenic and certain hydrocarbons such as DDT are particularly difficult to keep out of water resources. As natural sediments flow into a body of water, nitrate and phosphate concentrations begin to build up. Algae and other plants flourish. While algae is an oxygen-producer during daylight hours, it is an oxygen-consumer during the nighttime. With great "blooms" of algae, the oxygen level of the water may fall below the level required for respiration of higher forms of animal life. As increased bacterial action depletes the supply of dissolved oxygen, the water no longer supports animals requiring high levels of dissolved oxygen. Trout and salmon disappear, and are replaced by carp. Eventually these coarser fish disappear and are replaced by worms or other animals requiring low levels of oxygen. Decay progresses. Hydrogen sulfide and other odorous gases are produced. The water tastes bad, and is unfit for swimming. "Polluted Water" and "Beach Closed" signs appear. Boating becomes undesirable, and outdoor water recreation limited. As lakeside businesses are affected, the economy of polluted localities is depressed.

Future demands on our country's water may well outstrip the supply. Many experts believe that only through increased reuse of water will future needs be supplied. Reuse cannot occur, however, if the water has been irreversibly damaged. Thus, it is of the utmost importance that we find answers to deal with the present pollution problems.

Purification Processes There are two primary methods of purifying water—either by natural processes or by specific treatment of domestic and industrial sewage.

Natural Processes   Water can purify itself by natural means up to specific points of capacity. The time required for self-purification will depend on the degree of pollution and the character of the water.

Since the infiltration of sunlight is minimized in polluted water, few water plants will grow in it; thus the oxygen supply is reduced. This reduction leads to fewer bacteria that can break down organic wastes, which increases the pollution problem. The result is foul-smelling, unattractive water that cannot support fish or other aquatic life. The solution to such instances is to reduce incoming wastes sufficiently so that the stream can handle them through self-purification. The amount of reduction necessary differs from stream to stream, depending on its specific characteristics.

Sewage Treatment   Sewage treatment is designed to reduce the polluting effect of wastes before they are discharged into public waterways. Such treatment may be carried out by industries or by municipalities. Industrial treatment may be an in-plant process where the water is treated for reuse.

In municipal sewage treatment, the process may involve either a primary treatment or a primary-secondary treatment. In the primary process, about 35 percent of the pollution is removed. The organic material is first settled out. The water is then chlorinated to kill bacteria and discharged into a stream. The settled sludge is removed or dried, made harmless by heating, and then used for fertilizer, soil conditioners, or land fill.

Further purification is necessary when the water is to be reused by humans. In such instances, a further settling-filtering process is involved. The amount of pollution reduction required determines the intensity of this secondary treatment. However, even secondary treatment fails to remove dissolved minerals, such as nitrates and phosphates, which cause excessive growth of algae in lakes and other bodies of water.

In addition to their stimulation of the growth of algae, nitrates can be detrimental to human beings. Damage results when nitrates, themselves relatively nontoxic, are converted to the more toxic compounds (nitrites). These nitrites combine with the blood's oxygen carrier, hemoglobin, in the red blood cells to form methemoglobin, a compound incapable of carrying oxygen. Thus the oxygen-carrying ability of the blood is reduced. This condition is especially dangerous to infants, elderly people, and those with heart or respiratory disorders.

Phosphate levels are the determining factor in the growth of algae in most bodies of fresh water. (Nitrate levels are the critical factor in marine environments.) In recent years, we have seen a great increase in the phosphate levels of most American surface waters. The principal sources of these phosphates are agricultural runoff, domestic wastes, and industrial wastes. The major source of phosphates in domestic wastes comes from household detergents, which have contributed hundreds of millions of pounds per year. Fortunately, beginning in 1970, consumers became increasingly aware of the significance of phosphates in detergents and many began selecting products on the basis of phosphate levels. In response, the detergent manufacturers were forced to alter the composition of many cleaning products. Some localities even passed ordinances banning the sale of high phosphate detergents, because to remove them from the sewage would require entirely new treatment processes.

Oil Spills   Oil spills are, in the public mind, a particularly alarming form of water pollution. They are highly visible, and they foul beaches for recreational use. Thus, even people of limited environmental awareness become disturbed when oil coats their favorite beach. There are many sources of oil spills. They may be accidents, as in collisions of oil tankers, or incidents involving offshore drilling rigs. As the size of oil tankers has increased, so has the threat of massive spills from their collision or breakup. Even more distressing are intentional discharges of oil when oil tankers dump a mixture of ballast water and residual oil from their tanks before reloading.

All oils contain some volatile substances that evaporate readily. As much as 25 percent of the volume of spilled oil evaporates during the first several days. Bacteria work to decompose the remaining mass. After three months on the surface of the sea, only about 15 percent of the original volume of spilled oil remains. This is a thick, asphaltlike lump of tar that often washes up on beaches. If the spill is close to shore, there is no time for this breakdown process to occur, and a thick layer of oil is deposited onto any object coming into contact with it.

Oil covers swimming and diving birds. Their buoyancy is reduced and they cannot fly. The feathers no longer insulate and the birds die of exposure. Some people believe, aside from damage to seabirds, that oil spills are more of an aesthetic pollutant than a biological one.

In any case, oil spills are undesirable and every effort must be made to reduce their frequency. Due to its visibility, oil was one of the first pollutants to receive governmental attention. The Oil Pollution Control Act of 1924 was designed to regulate the discharge of oil from ships in coastal waters. Since then, progressively more stringent laws have been passed. In 1970 a law was passed that imposes absolute financial responsibility on those guilty of causing oil spills in United States waters. The law also provides for fines that could run into millions of dollars for the polluters, and for prison sentences for officers of violating corporations. With today's increased awareness of pollution problems, we can expect to see even more effective antipollution legislation passed.

The Subtle Pollutants—Radiation and Toxic Chemicals If anything positive can be said for the problems of air and water pollution, it is that they are, at least in most cases, obvious. Their impact on our senses of sight, smell, and taste tells us that something is drastically wrong. In contrast, radiation and toxic chemicals may be entirely unnoticeable to the unequipped observer, even at extremely dangerous levels. They are detectable and measurable only with sophisticated instruments.

In addition, the effects of radiation and toxic chemicals may take years, or even generations, to become noticeable. While large doses of either will result in rapid death, the dosages more commonly encountered in the environment produce subtle damage, such as mutations, which may not become apparent for several generations, or cancers, which appear after many years.

Not only may the effects of radiation and toxic chemicals be remote in time, but in distance as well. Either of these factors may be carried thousands of miles from their source by air or water currents.

Radiation in the Environment Since the beginning of the "atomic age" over 30 years ago, there has been considerable concern about the effects of excessive radiation in our environment. Actually, there has always been some radiation present, referred to as *natural background radiation*. All forms of life have been subjected to low levels of radiation from natural sources throughout their evolution. In fact, such natural radiation is believed to be important in producing the mutations on which evolution is based. Natural background radiation comes from radioactive substances in the ground, air, and water, as well as from space in the form of cosmic radiation.

In recent decades, however, people have also been subjected to radiation of their own making. The intensity of such radiation ranges from high doses, such as result from a nuclear weapon, reactor accident, or from radiotherapy, down to low doses comparable to natural background radiation. Some of the major sources of human-created radiation are outlined below.

1. *Radiotherapy.* This is the use of radiation (usually x-ray and gamma radiation) as a means of diagnosis and treatment in medicine and dentistry. This is the major source of human-made radiation in the world today, and its value, in each case, should be weighed against its potential hazards.

2. *Radioactive isotopes.* These are atoms of radioactive elements used in research, in medical diagnosis and treatment, and in industry.

3. *Industrial X rays.* These are X rays used in industry for radiography of welds, castings, and products where flaws could impair the usefulness of the product.

4. *Radioactive fallout.* This is the result of the explosion of nuclear devices, as in the testing or use of nuclear weapons.

5. *Radioactive wastes.* These are produced from the use and processing of radioactive materials, fission products, and the possible accidental release of radioactive substances. Some of these affect only individuals who are subjected to radiation because of their occupation. But there are also radioactive wastes that constitute a hazard to the whole population through pollution of the environment.

Effects of Radiation on the Body Tissues
Large doses of all types of radiation will kill cells. With smaller doses of radiation, recovery is possible, and cells can continue to function. However, recovery may not be complete, causing malignant changes later. In general, certain cells are more readily affected by radiation than are others. Tissues that are actively regenerating with constant cell division and multiplication—such as embryonic tissue, intestinal mucosa, blood-forming tissue, gonadal germ cells, and skin—are more vulnerable. These various types of tissue damage may be simplified into two main classes: somatic tissue effects and genetic effects.

1. *Somatic tissue effects.* Somatic cells compose all body tissue, except for the eggs in the ovaries and the sperm in the testes. Large doses of radiation destroy somatic tissue, leading to the death of the individual. Lesser doses of radiation may show no immediate effect, but they will accumulate until cell function may be altered, possibly producing leukemia or another form of cancer.

2. *Genetic effects.* Genetic effects are the changes produced in the germ or reproductive cells. No damage will appear in the individual exposed to the radiation, but the effects will show up in descendents as abnormalities of form and function. Such genetic effects may be caused by small doses of radiation. Therefore, all radiation must be considered deleterious to one degree or another.

Radioactive Fallout Fallout is the return to earth of radioactive material that has been carried up into the atmosphere by the detonation of a nuclear device or as a result of a nuclear accident. The term also refers to any resulting contamination of food, drink, soil, air, or building materials caused by such fallout. Environmental contamination produced by the worldwide dispersion of radioactivity from nuclear weapon tests has been a source of both internal and external radiation.

Distribution of a fallout pattern is determined by yield, height, and location of the detonation, and by meteorological conditions. The dose rate (the amount of radiation absorbed by an individual) and the accumulated dose from fallout depend not only on the amount of radioactive fallout but also on the ionization effects of the radiation products.

For every megaton of fission involved in the detonation of a nuclear device, yield will be about 100 pounds of intensely radioactive substances. Fortunately, many of the substances formed have extremely short half-lives (period of time during which one-half of a substance's radioactivity decays) and thus have little significance other than in terms of local fallout. The isotopes remaining 1 hour after detonation decay approximately by a factor of 10 for every sevenfold increase in time

after detonation time plus 1 hour. Thus, as is shown in the table on fading radiation hazard, 7 hours after a nuclear explosion, the radioactivity has decreased to one-tenth of what it was at 1 hour. In 49 hours, the radioactivity is only one one-hundredth of what it was at 1 hour, and so on.

It has been shown that the total dose to bone marrow from artificial sources of radiation in technically advanced countries is approximately equal to the typical natural background dose. In children under 5, fallout probably accounts for some 5 to 10 percent of the artificial dose to bone marrow. With the advent of a test ban treaty, the dosage will decrease in younger children. Fallout during atmospheric testing periods has been responsible for about one-fifth of the total artificial dose.

Disposal of Radioactive Waste Radioactive wastes from industry vary so much that there is no single preferred method of management and disposal. The solution depends on such factors as the specific nature (radioactive half-life or type of radiation), concentration (quantity of radioactive material involved), and the environment in which disposal is being considered. The problem of disposal of radioactive wastes stems from the fact that there is

Fading Radiation Hazard

Contamination In Curies of Radio-Active Material	Time After Formation of Fission Products	Radiation Intensity From Fission Products (Roentgens Per Hour)
1,000	1 hour	10,000
100	7 hours	1,000
10	49 hours (2 days)	100
1	14 days (2 weeks)	10
0.1	14 weeks (3 months)	1

Adapted from C. W. Shilling. *Atomic Energy Encyclopedia* (Philadelphia: W. B. Saunders, 1964).

no way to destroy the radioactivity immediately. Time alone renders the waste stable and harmless or at least reduces the level of radioactivity to the point that it is nontoxic.

The magnitude of the waste disposal problem far outweighs the problem of fallout or the operation of a reactor. Waste disposal is potentially the greatest hazard to public safety. And the time for concern is now! Many reactors are not currently in use, or are being run at reduced capacity, because of the many tons of high-level radioactive waste already stored. Yet no satisfactory method for disposal has been developed. As the nuclear power program builds up, the disposal of fission products in a manner that will not be injurious to health must have particular attention.

Spent fuel elements are now removed from reactors and shipped to one of the major United States Atomic Energy Commission processing sites. Here they are "cooled" for 90 days to allow decay of radioactive isotopes with short half-lives. They are classified as having high, medium, or low energy levels and are disposed of accordingly.

High-energy radioactive wastes must be handled by containment in tank storage to allow time for radioactive decay. Suggestions for final disposal of high-level wastes include conversion of liquid wastes to solids and permanent storage in geological strata, with salt beds serving as major sites. Or, liquids could be put directly into geological strata, either in deep wells or salt beds. Or, both solids and liquids could be disposed of in the sea.

Medium-energy radioactive wastes are usually held in trenches, in artificial ponds, or in tanks to allow radioactive wastes to decay to a level where they may be discharged into the environment. Some wastes with radioisotopes of reasonably short half-lives (weeks to months) are discharged directly into the ground. Some

medium-energy wastes have been incorporated into concrete, poured into steel drums, and buried in trenches or dumped at sea.

Low-energy radioactive wastes are defined as having a radioactivity concentration in the range of one-millionth of a curie (a unit of measure of radioactive decay) per gallon. They are disposed of by dilution with water and released directly into the environment—into air, land, or sea. These wastes include the reactor-cooling water used in nuclear-powered ships and submarines.

Various other forms of waste processing, including chemical treatments, are being used or experimented with in an attempt to find a more economical and satisfactory method of waste disposal.

Pesticides in the Environment The era of the synthetic organic pesticides dawned in May, 1943, with the opening of the first commercial plant for the production of DDT. Production was soon measured in millions of pounds per year. For centuries before this, pesticides had been in use, but they were of entirely different types. Earlier pesticides consisted mainly of inorganic compounds, such as arsenicals, fluorides, and compounds of copper, sulfur, and mercury; or botanically derived, natural organic compounds, such as nicotine, pyrethrum, and rotenone.

The synthetic organic pesticides met with a tremendous reception. They offered a toxicity to insects far surpassing that of the older chemicals, and they were available in unlimited quantities at relatively low costs. They arrived on the scene at a time when rising populations demanded every possible means of increased food production. For several years it seemed that our insect control problems had been solved.

Then some unsettling problems began to arise. Many insect species began showing

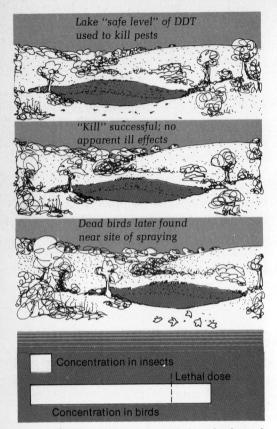

Lake "safe level" of DDT used to kill pests

"Kill" successful; no apparent ill effects

Dead birds later found near site of spraying

Concentration in insects

Lethal dose

Concentration in birds

One of the "hidden" dangers of poorly planned pesticide use. The natural food web, connecting insects with the birds that feed on them, multiplies the amount of DDT in the birds' diet, and can have the lethal effect shown here. The birds are killed by a concentration of the pesticide far greater than that which was first used to clear the lake of insects.

resistance to the effects of the new insecticides, stubbornly refusing to die. This situation was met by the development of more powerful poisons. Then traces of pesticides were found to remain in food products after harvest. Of course, this was not really a new problem. It was known that arsenic, for example, also had this unfortunate tendency. The pesticide residue problem resulted in a proliferation of government regulations limiting the quantity of a given pesticide in a given food product. Of course, it was not known for certain what the long-range effects of these "legal" residues would be, but at least no one was going to be poisoned outright.

Another unnerving problem was that a crop often showed evidence, exceeding the legal quantity, of some chemical with which that crop had never been treated. Perhaps the only previous use of that chemical had been miles away. It became apparent that pesticides were drifting rather freely through the environment. Not too long after that, traces of pesticides were detected on islands thousands of miles from the nearest site of pesticide application.

One of the original major selling points of certain pesticides was their persistence—or resistance to being broken down. They could control insects months or even years after their application. Less apparent was the fact that these persistent pesticides were gradually building up throughout the environment to levels where not only insects were killed but where many other kinds of organisms were being affected as well.

Widespread public attention was first drawn to this problem in 1962 with the publication of the now-classic *Silent Spring* by the late Rachel Carson. Even though Carson was initially laughed off by agricultural and agrichemical interests as a "crank" or "sensationalist," her observations on the effects of pesticides on birds, fishes, and other wildlife have been largely substantiated.

Among the proven ill-effects of various pesticides are:

1. *Destruction of natural enemies (parasites and predators) of insects, leading to massive "rebound" pest populations.* Most agricultural pests are held to generally low population levels by their natural enemies,

though there might be occasional de-structive outbreaks of pests. This is part of the dynamic "balance of na-ture," but this problem is aggravated by the practice of monoculture—the cultivation of large blocks of a single species of crop plant. There is fre-quently a "lag" period during which pest populations increase explosively before predator or parasite popula-tions catch up. Further complicating the situation is the fact that many pest species have been accidentally im-ported from other parts of the world, while their enemies have been left be-hind. Thus, a reasonable position on the use of pesticides is that some use of pesticides is probably unavoidable if current and future world populations are to be fed. Yet the first application of pesticide to a particular crop should be avoided unless there is a clear and present threat of destruction of a major portion of the crop. Then the pesticide to be applied should be chosen on the basis of a minimum of destruction of beneficial insects and other environ-mental damage. It should be borne in mind that the decision to make the first application of pesticide to a crop will usually commit the grower to further applications during the sea-son.

2. *Outright killing of birds, fishes, and other wild animals.* Sometimes the cause and effect relationship here is quite obvious, as when pesticide con-tamination of a river results in mil-lions of dead fish washing ashore. In other cases, the cause of death may be obscured. For example, the pesticide may be concentrated through the food chain, so that the bird or other animal killed may be quite remote from the point of application of the pesticide, either in distance or in time.

3. *Interference with the reproductive processes of birds, fishes, and other wildlife.* It has been clearly estab-lished that certain pesticides interfere with shell formation in bird eggs or with the sex hormones of both birds and mammals. Such reproductive in-terference by persistent pesticides in the environment has apparently al-ready doomed several species of birds to near extinction. Even if all use of such pesticides stopped immediately, it is likely that they would persist in the environment longer than some of the threatened bird species could sur-vive.

4. *Inhibition of photosynthesis in plants.* The exact mechanism of this inhibi-tion is not known.

5. *Concentration of pesticides in fishes to unsafe levels for human consump-tion.* This occurs through the many steps of the food chain, with about a tenfold concentration with each step. We may eventually have to curtail consumption of the larger fish species, turning instead to the smaller species, which, being the product of a shorter

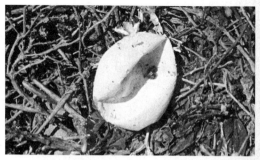

Another side effect of pesticide use is the threat to the natural life processes of some species. Along the West Coast of the United States, the number of brown pelicans is rapidly declining because of DDT-induced weakening of the shells of newly hatched eggs.

Photo by Joseph Jehl, Jr.

food chain, should have lower pesticide levels. A parallel situation resulted in the high levels of mercury in swordfish, which led, in 1971, to the virtual elimination of this fish as a part of the American diet.

6. *Presence in cow's milk of levels beyond legal tolerance for human consumption.* Production of pesticide-free milk requires pesticide-free hay and other feeds, the procurement of which has become extremely difficult. Large areas of many states are now unsuitable for the growth of hay for milk cows because of the high levels of pesticide used in those areas—the drift of pesticides onto hay crops being inevitable.

7. *Birth defects in animals (and humans?) attributed to commonly used herbicides (weed killers).* The herbicide, 2,4,5–T has enjoyed widespread use as a brush killer. Typical applications have included clearing of brush from rangeland and defoliation in jungle warfare. While this herbicide was, for years, considered safe, birth defects similar to thalidomide damage were noticed in animals in areas treated with 2,4,5–T. These results were confirmed in laboratory studies with mice and other animals. Whether such defects are also caused in humans is not known, but the possibility has led to the curtailment of use of 2,4,5–T.

8. *Acute and chronic impairment of the health of workers who apply and otherwise handle pesticides.* Each pesticide presents its own particular set of hazards to its handlers, ranging from the risk of swift death if only a few drops are spilled on the skin to such obscure possible hazards as genetic mutations that may affect future generations.

9. *Illness and death of farmworkers laboring in treated crop areas.* Following the application of any pesticide, there is a period of time during which workers should stay out of the treated area. This period varies greatly, depending on the chemical used and such environmental conditions as temperature, wind, and rainfall. Too often, growers have sent crews into recently treated fields for thinning, weeding, and similar operations, resulting in illness and occasionally death for the workers.

10. *Development of pesticide resistance in over 200 species of insects.* Continuing to show the great adaptability that has enabled them to survive for millions of years, most pest species have developed resistance to any pesticide to which they have been exposed over a period of several years. For example, the common housefly, once easily controlled with DDT, can now withstand a dose over 1,000 times as great as that which once proved fatal in every case.

Inevitably there are other serious problems yet undiscovered and unforeseen that will arise from the use of pesticides.

Alternate Methods of Pest Control It is obvious that continued haphazard and reckless use of pesticides will result in worldwide environmental destruction and the extinction of countless species of organisms, perhaps even human beings. Yet, the abrupt abandonment of all pesticides would result in widespread starvation and insect-borne disease. The answer to pest control must lie somewhere between these two extremes.

An imperative first step is to shift immediately from the persistent chlorinated-hydrocarbon pesticides to the more rapidly decomposing organic phosphates and carbamates. Even the less persistent pesticides should be used with caution, however, since their generally higher acute toxicity may result in immediate ecological changes caused by massive wildlife death. In addition, the effects of long-term human exposure to these chemicals are not really known. The table on common pesticides gives the acute toxicity level and other information on various pesticides.

Chemical pest control should be integrated into the many other effective methods of control and used only as a "last resort" when all other methods fail. Some of the alternatives to chemical control include relying on predators and parasites, insect-disease-producing organisms (bacteria, fungi, and viruses that cause insect diseases only); releasing sterilized insects (especially effective in species that mate only once); developing pest-resistant crop varieties; and using cultural control practices, such as rotating crops and timing plantings and harvests to escape insect attacks.

Consumers and government agencies have contributed to the pesticide problem by demanding that insect damage to fruits and vegetables be kept to unreasonably low levels. Some relaxation of the standards for insect damage or contamination could allow a great reduction in pesticide usage.

Pollutants in Food   One of the favorite topics among people concerned with maintaining overall health standards is the matter of substances added to food. On one side are people who claim that all types of dangerous chemicals are being added to food without due regard to the consequences. On the other side, food-industry spokesmen are quick to point out that purposely added substances are used with justification and safety. These chemicals re-

tard spoilage, enhance flavor, improve color, improve consistency, retard drying, or help to retain crispness. Some are added as nutritional supplements, such as thiamine to bread, iodine to salt, fluoride to water, and vitamins A and D to milk.

Some substances, including insecticides, hormones, antibiotics, and disinfectants, enter food accidentally and unintentionally. Some of these enter from the wrappers or containers that touch the food.

Certain federal agencies are going to great lengths to protect the consumer against injurious substances. Before we point out these areas of concern, however, we should define several terms. A *food additive* is a substance, other than a basic foodstuff, which is intentionally present in food as a result of any aspect of production, processing, storage, or packaging. This definition does not include chance contaminants. *Toxicity* is the capacity of a substance to produce injury. *Safety* is the practical certainty that injury will not result from use of a substance in a proposed quantity and manner. *Hazard* is the probability that injury will result from use of a substance in a proposed quantity and manner. An *adulterant* is a foreign or inferior substance added to a food product in place of a more valuable substance. The adulterant might be actually harmful when consumed, or merely deceptive, such as the inclusion of horsemeat or cereal in hamburger. A *residue* is a quantity of a pesticide or other contaminant remaining unintentionally on a food product as a result of treatments made during its growing or processing. A *tolerance* is a quantity of residue, presumed to be safe for consumption, legally permitted to be present in food.

Pesticide Residues in Foods   Modern food-production practices include the use of hundreds of pesticide chemicals—

Some Common Pesticides

Pesticide (Other Names)	Relative Acute Toxicity[a]	Comments
Chlorinated Hydrocarbon Group (*Characterized, in general, by long-term persistence in the environment.*)		
DDT	Toxic[b] $LD_{50} = 250$ mg/kg	Has been world's most used insecticide
DDD (TDE, Rhothane®)	Slightly toxic $LD_{50} = 3400$ mg/kg	A breakdown product of DDT
Dicofol (Kelthane®)	Moderately toxic $LD_{50} = 575$ mg/kg	Used to kill mites
Methoxychlor	Essentially nontoxic $LD_{50} = 6000$ mg/kg	
Benzene Hexachloride (BHC, Lindane)	Toxic $LD_{50} = 125$ mg/kg	Very stable
Chlordane	Toxic $LD_{50} = 225$ mg/kg	Very stable Absorbed through skin
Heptachlor	Toxic $LD_{50} = 90$ mg/kg	
Aldrin	Toxic $LD_{50} = 55$ mg/kg	
Dieldrin	Toxic $LD_{50} = 60$ mg/kg	Absorbed through skin Has been very damaging to wildlife
Endrin	Highly toxic $LD_{50} = 5\text{-}45$ mg/kg	Absorbed through skin Very poisonous to birds Very stable
Endosulfan (Thiodan®)	Toxic $LD_{50} = 110$ mg/kg	Absorbed through skin
Toxaphene	Toxic $LD_{50} = 69$ mg/kg	Less persistent than others in group
Organic Phosphate Group (*Generally less persistent than chlorinated hydrocarbons, but often of greater acute toxicity. Same mode of action as nerve gases of warfare.*)		
Azodrin®	Toxic $LD_{50} = 21$ mg/kg	Reportedly very harmful to beneficial insects
Bidrin®	Toxic $LD_{50} = 22$ mg/kg	
Ciodrin®	Toxic $LD_{50} = 125$ mg/kg	Rapid decomposition in environment
Diazinon (Spectracide®)	Toxic $LD_{50} = 150$ mg/kg	Widely promoted for home use
Dichlorovos (DDVP, Vapona®)	Toxic $LD_{50} = 56\text{-}80$ mg/kg	Widely promoted for home use
Malathion	Moderately toxic $LD_{50} = 900\text{-}5800$ mg/kg	Relatively safe for home use
Parathion	Extremely toxic $LD_{50} = 3\text{-}15$ mg/kg	Readily absorbed through skin. Too toxic for home use. Cause of many deaths
Phorate (Thimet®)	Extremely toxic $LD_{50} = 2\text{-}4$ mg/kg	A systemic insecticide, translocated through vascular system of plant. Not for home use
Mevinphos (Phosdrin®)	Extremely toxic $LD_{50} = 6\text{-}7$ mg/kg	Readily absorbed through skin. Many professional applicators refuse to work with this chemical

Pesticide (Other Names	Relative Acute Toxicity[a]	Comments
Carbamate Group (*Not persistent in the environment*)		
Baygon®	Toxic LD_{50} = 95 mg/kg	Has been widely used by exterminators
Sevin® (carbaryl)	Moderately toxic LD_{50} = 500 mg/kg	Relatively safe for home use. Extremely toxic to honeybees and beneficial to wild bees
Bux®	Toxic LD_{50} = 170 mg/kg	
Botanical Group (*Extracted from plants*)		
Nicotine (Black Leaf 40®)	Highly toxic LD_{50} = 10 mg/kg	Absorbed through skin Long a standard for home garden use
Pyrethrum	Slightly toxic LD_{50} = 2000 mg/kg	Among least toxic to man Safely used around foods and as "fog" for quick kill without residue
Rotenone	Toxic LD_{50} = 300 mg/kg	Extremely toxic to fish

[a] *Acute toxicity* refers to the amount required to cause immediate death, but does not take into account any possible long-term effects such as accumulation in tissues of body, carcinogenesis (cancer production), mutagenesis (stimulus of mutations), or any other long-term effect.

[b] LD_{50} is the *median lethal dose,* the amount required to kill 50 percent of the test animals. Figures given are for oral doses for rats. Human toxicity is generally comparable.
Adapted from Sun, Yun-Pei, *Pesticide Reference Standards,* Bulletin of the Entomological Society of America 14 (September 1968): 238–248.

insecticides, miticides, herbicides, nematocides, fungicides, and so on. There is now mounting concern about the possible immediate and long-term adverse effects of the consumption of food containing residual traces of various pesticides.

All pesticides must be registered with the EPA before application to crops is allowed. Such registration is granted only after extensive safety testing, which includes feeding the pesticide in measured quantities to test animals over long periods of time, as well as analyzing treated crops for the amount of pesticide residue. Registrations are quite specific in the quantity of pesticide that may be applied and in the conditions of the application, such as the interval between application and harvest. Pesticide registrations have been granted on the basis of a "zero tolerance" (no trace of residue permitted) or on the basis of a specific tolerance (generally a few parts per million permitted). In the case of specific tolerance the government insists on a residue safety margin of a hundredfold. In other words, only one one-hundredth of the presumed safety level of residue is allowed in consumer foods.

Fearing the possibility of yet unknown effects of long-term consumption of even small amounts of pesticides, some authorities now question the wisdom of allowing any tolerance. They often cite possible genetic damage, cancer, and metabolic disorders as effects that might show up after many years of exposure.

A more immediate danger lies in the occasional cases of improper use of pesticides. Excessively heavy or frequent application, improper formulation, or application too close to harvest times are examples of practices that may result in residues above the legal tolerance. Although many such cases are detected by EPA inspectors—with the subsequent destruction of the contaminated foods—it must be assumed that much food carrying illegal residues is reaching the consumer.

Some, though not all, pesticide residues can be removed from foods in the home by thorough washing, peeling, removing outer leaves, and similar processes. Foods showing visible residues or having unusual smells should not be purchased.

Intentional Food Additives Shifting our attention now to chemicals purposely added to foods, we find that some of the prepared "convenience" food products contain up to a dozen or more chemical additives. As with pesticides, new food additives must undergo intensive testing before their use is approved. Food additives are approved by the Food and Drug Administration (FDA) of the Department of Health, Education and Welfare. However, many additives that were introduced prior to 1958 did not receive the safety testing now required, yet they have been permitted to remain in use. The withdrawal of cyclamates from general use in 1969 illustrates that some of the older additives may not be as safe as had been presumed.

Increasing numbers of authorities are questioning the wisdom of our consumption of substantial quantities of food additives. While it is unlikely that the amount contained in one food product presents any great threat to health, the individual or family relying on convenience foods could potentially consume quantities and combinations of additives that might disturb the metabolism or result in genetic damage, cancer, or other serious disorders. It seems only sensible to minimize the intake of additives by selecting simple, basic food ingredients rather than premixed, additive-laden prepared foods.

The Urban Environment

The United States is an urban nation. When the first national census was taken, in 1790, only 5 percent of the people lived in cities of over 2,500 people, whereas 95 percent lived in the country or in very small villages. By 1970, the last year for which figures are available, 73.5 percent of the people lived in urban areas and the trend toward urbanization continued strongly. Thus, both numerically and by percentage, more and more Americans are living in cities. (See the table on urban and rural populations.)

Surprisingly, the western states are the most urbanized, with 82.9 percent of their population concentrated into the cities. California is the nation's most urbanized state, with 90.9 percent of its population living in urban areas.

While there is no clear-cut line between urban and suburban areas, the suburbs are, in general, the ring of younger and smaller cities surrounding the older central city areas. Census figures show that in recent years the greatest population growth has been in such suburban areas. For example, between 1960 and 1970, the entire United States population grew by 11 percent. However, this growth was concentrated in the suburbs, where population grew by about 25 percent. During this same period, the central cities grew by only 1 percent.

Another problem in population distribution is that the coasts seem to have a magnetic attraction for people. For many years the nation has experienced a migration of population out of the central states and into the coastal areas. By 1970, 53 percent of all Americans were living in counties lying at least partly within 50 miles of a seacoast. This trend continues today

Urban and Rural Populations, United States, 1790-1970

	1790	1910	1920	1930	1940	1950	1960	1970
By Millions of People								
Urban	0.2	42	54	69	74	96	125	149
Rural	3.8	50	52	54	57	54	54	56
Total	4.0	92	106	123	131	150	179	205
By Percentage of Total								
Urban	5	45.7	51.2	56.2	56.5	64.0	69.9	73.5
Rural	95	54.3	48.8	43.8	43.5	36.0	30.1	26.5

NOTE: *Urban population* is defined as those persons residing in cities of over 2500 persons.

Taken from U.S. Bureau of the Census. *Statistical Abstracts of the United States: 1970* (91st ed.) (Washington, D.C: U.S. Government Printing Office, 1970).

with no end in sight. We are becoming a nation of people jammed into strip cities extending the length of each coast, with relatively few people living in the vast spaces between.

Without adequate planning, certain problems can develop in this intense urbanization. Environmental quality problems can become overwhelming, including air pollution, sewage disposal, acquisition of safe water, noise abatement, space for outdoor recreation, substandard housing, and a host of other problems. For some city dwellers, especially those at lower income levels, emotional stress can be great. Yet the social, cultural, and economic advantages of city life continue to hold a powerful attraction for the majority of Americans today. Cities can and must be designed to avoid most or all of these problems.

Noise Pollution One of the more recently "discovered" pollutants in the modern environment is noise. For many people, noise may be the most significant environmental pollutant. They are constantly buffeted by the noise of aircraft, trains, motorcycles, buses, sirens, and machinery at home and at work. (See table on the intensity of some common sounds.)

Intensity of Some Common Sounds

Sound	Intensity in Decibels
Human whisper	30
Normal conversation	60
City traffic	80
Garbage disposal unit	80
Vacuum cleaner	85
Garbage truck	85
Food blender	93
Subway train	95
Jackhammer	95
Power lawnmower	96
Printing press	97
Farm tractor	98
Punch press	105
Boiler shop	105
Textile looms	106
Motorcycle	110
Riveting gun	110
Rock band (amplified)	114
Drop hammer	130
Jet airplane	135 to 150

NOTE: A *decibel* is the smallest difference in intensity of sound that the human ear can detect. The scale is logarithmic; a difference of ten decibels represents a tenfold increase in energy.
Adapted from *Medical World News* 10 (June 13, 1969), pp. 42–47, and other sources.

One study showed that the average noise level in residential areas rose as much as 9 decibels between 1954 and 1967. (The decibel scale is logarithmic—an increase of 10 decibels indicates a tenfold increase in energy.)

Some of the effects of noise have been known or suspected for years. Fatigue, emotional stress, and permanent loss of hearing acuity are well-documented effects of excessive noise. Noise, either prolonged or sudden, produces involuntary responses by the circulatory, digestive, and nervous systems. Noise can cause adrenalin to be shot into the blood, as during stress and anxiety periods. It can cause the heart to beat rapidly, the blood vessels to constrict, the pupils to dilate, and the stomach, esophagus, and intestines to be seized by spasms. A three-year study of university students showed that noise of only 70 decibels consistently caused constriction of the coronary arteries supplying oxygen to the heart muscle. Permanent hearing loss occurs with prolonged exposure to sounds over 90 decibels. High-decibel sounds destroy the hair cells of the inner ear.

Probably the most damaging effect of noise on the quality of human life is its disruption of our psychic balance. Loud, harsh, or persistent noise robs us of our peace of mind, puts our nerves "on edge" so that our personal relationships are strained and often explosive, interferes with our concentration, and impairs the efficient functioning of our minds. Noise must be regarded as far more than just an annoyance. It is a serious threat to the quality of our lives.

In our concern with other forms of environmental decay, we have largely overlooked the importance of noise control, and noise levels continue to creep upward. Like any other form of pollution control, noise control will require legislated limits on noise levels, strict enforcement of those limits, and a personal concern for the rights of others to live in a decent environment.

Substandard Housing About 34 million Americans are now living in some 11 million dwelling units that are either grossly overcrowded or have serious structural or plumbing deficiencies. Such dwellings occur most often in large cities or rural areas, less commonly in suburban areas.

The infant mortality (death in first year of life) in such housing is from three to five times the national average. Accidental injuries, burns, and poisonings occur five to eight times more frequently than the national average. In addition, more than 14,000 rat bites are officially recorded each year in such surroundings—certainly a much larger number is never reported.

Lead poisoning of children is a particular problem in families forced to live in substandard housing. In older, uncared-for homes, woodwork, walls, and furniture are often covered with multiple coats of old lead-based paint. Babies and young children often chew on furniture and woodwork, ingesting large amounts of lead. In addition, old paint may flake off walls and ceilings, falling into food and entering the body in the form of dustlike particles.

Lead poisoning can cause serious brain damage, mental retardation, and even death. Even in mild cases, a child's learning ability may be impaired.

Lead poisoning usually does not result in dramatic, sudden changes in a child's health. Instead, the child gradually becomes lethargic, loses appetite, and is less attentive to the environment. Later, the child may vomit, complain of vague stomach or arm or leg pains, and become irritable. Eventually, symptoms of brain damage, such as convulsions, appear. By then, the brain has suffered permanent damage.

If a specific check is not made for lead poisoning in the early stages, the symptoms are so vague that they will likely be overlooked. If the poisoning is detected in its early stages, however, the child can often be treated successfully. Of course, lead poisoning will recur unless the home environment is changed to remove this hazard.

Of the 12,000 to 16,000 cases reported every year in the United States, about 200 children die of lead poisoning. Thousands more are left with mental retardation and other impairments. The loss to the individual and to society from impaired learning ability due to lead poisoning is really incalculable.

Other results of substandard housing are more difficult to translate into figures. The psychological and sociological implications of poor housing are overwhelming. For example, privacy may be nonexistent. Quiet reflection, important to emotional stability, or successful schoolwork may be impossible in crowded living conditions. Marital relationships, sexual and otherwise, may be severely strained by lack of privacy, contributing to the decay of the family unit. Insufficient sanitary facilities (as results when several families are sharing one bathroom) make personal cleanliness and grooming difficult or impossible, putting residents of substandard housing at a social and health disadvantage.

To date, efforts toward upgrading housing on a national basis have had only limited success. In many cases, substandard housing has been removed in urban renewal projects, only to be replaced with units beyond the financial means of those who previously lived there. In addition, we are now facing the paradoxical situation of renewal projects postponed because sufficient housing on a temporary basis for the displaced residents is not even available.

While there are no simple answers to the national housing crisis, an immense need does exist for upgraded housing units. It seems likely that this need will have to be met through the combined efforts of government and private enterprise. Obviously, the basic problem is poverty; any long-term gains in housing quality must be the result of improved family economic units.

Stress As was discussed in the section on emotional problems, prolonged stress can have severe damaging effects on both the physical and emotional health of a person. Just a few among the many urban stressors are the problems of high-density housing, with its attendant noise, lack of privacy, and lack of play areas; substandard housing, with its rats and inadequate sanitation; deficient and crowded urban transportation; strikes, blackouts, and other service problems; ethnic tensions; and the ever-present fear of crime.

Many of the physical effects of stress can be objectively measured, such as increases in pulse rate and blood pressure, dilation of the pupils of the eyes, sweating, respiratory rate, and so forth. Studies have shown that the typical commuter, driving home at peak rush hours, experiences more of the deleterious effects of stress than have some of the astronauts during reentry into the earth's atmosphere.

Urban Planning The growth pattern of many cities has, in general, been haphazard, with little or no master planning. The almost formless lateral spread of many cities has been determined largely by the predominant form of transportation—the automobile. Development has simply spread along the paths of major traffic arteries. Sociological and ecological factors have been largely ignored.

Almost all population growth in metropolitan areas has been concentrated at their suburban edges. Suburbs of metropolitan areas now often meet back-to-back. We are currently witnessing the development of several "strip cities," one extending from San Francisco to San Diego, one from Chicago to Pittsburgh, and one from Boston to Washington, D.C.

The concept of the "planned city" is gaining popularity. Considerable evidence suggests that there is a maximum desirable size for any type of system, above which efficiency is decreased. This principle seems to apply to living organisms, machines, factories, schools, and to cities. Rather than encouraging further expansion of existing cities, communities might be planned in terms of maximum population, educational and public service facilities, businesses, wide-open areas, and quality housing.

City life offers many social, educational, and cultural advantages. From the stimulating intellectual climate of the city have come many of the world's cultural and scientific advances. With adequate planning, cities can provide a life-style combining all of these advantages with an environment that is favorable to optimum physical and emotional health.

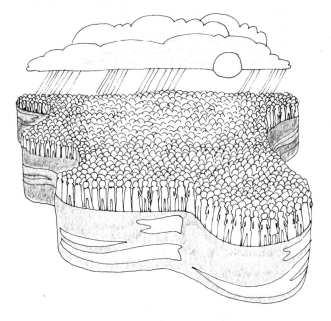

POPULATION DYNAMICS

Throughout human history, the increase in the number of human beings has been governed by three regulators—disease, war, and famine. As a result, each major upward step in population followed some major discovery or development that acted to control one of these regulators—the advent of agriculture, the initiation of urban life and trade, the harnessing of nonhuman power, or the progress of modern medicine. In addition, the human race, unlike animals, which breed until limited by one of the three regulators, has the unique ability to limit both its death rate and its birth rate. Thus as a more sophisticated and economically responsible group of societies developed, the ability to maintain a higher population level became a reality.

The Mechanism of Population Control   There has been little correlation between population growth and the ability of a region to support that growth. This imbalance has dictated widely varying standards of living for human beings. However, consistent patterns of population dynamics do appear, patterns which are of concern to us because they might indicate what the future holds in store.

The Past   Only fragmentary data are available to indicate the past growth rate of the population of the world. A regular census of population was not conducted before 1800, although registers were maintained for small groups prior to that time. Therefore, the commonly accepted population figures of the world before 1800 are only informed guesses. Nevertheless, it is possible to piece together a consistent series of estimates for the past two centuries. This information, supplemented by rough guesses of the number of persons alive at selected earlier periods, provides

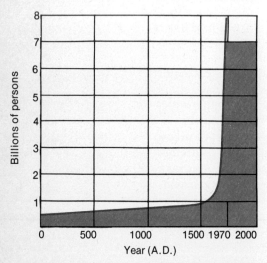

Estimated world population, 0 to 2000 A.D.

Based on estimates of the Population Reference Bureau and other sources.

the background for a graphic estimate of the world population from 1 to 2000 A.D. This graph reveals a spectacular spurt during recent decades (see graph on estimated world population).

World population is estimated to have reached its first billion mark sometime between 1810 and 1850 A.D. The second billion mark was reached in 1925, the third in 1960, and the fourth in 1975. It took most of man's history to reach one billion, about 100 years to reach two billion, 35 years to reach three billion, and an estimated 15 years to reach four billion.

According to two early reports on world demography (Carr–Saunders and Willcox), the population of Europe increased more than fourfold between 1650 and 1900, whereas the population of Asia increased only about two and one-half times. Moreover, the population in the area of European settlement, including Europe and the Americas, increased about five times. As a result of these different rates of growth in Asia and Europe, the proportion of the world's population living in Asia declined from around 60 percent in 1650 to about 53 percent in 1900. But since 1900, the proportion of the world's population living in Asia has been increasing and, according to the Population Reference Bureau figures, by 1975 it climbed to over 57 percent (*1975 World Population Data Sheet*, Population Reference Bureau, Inc., Washington, D.C.). The proportion living in Europe and North America has been declining and by 1975 it constituted only about 18 percent of the world's total.

The discoveries of sulfa drugs, antibiotics, insecticides, and other means of combating disease-carrying organisms radically altered the situation of population dynamics. It became possible to lower mortality rates irrespective of economic development. This was our first major vic-

Life Expectancy at Birth

Years	Life Expectancy at Birth In Years
1840	41.0
1900	50.5
1930	61.7
1940	64.6
1955 to 1975	73.0+

NOTE: The average of six European countries and one state in the United States. The countries are Denmark, England and Wales, France, the Netherlands, Norway and Sweden; the state in the United States is Massachusetts.
Taken from *1975 World Population Data Sheet*, The Population Reference Bureau, Inc. (Washington, D.C.: 1975).

tory over death. Within a few years, this victory was to be responsible for the rapid population explosion that now jeopardizes the economic growth of all developing nations.

In the developed countries of the West, the reduction in the death rate came slowly. Its effect on population growth was influenced by factors that reduced the birth rate, namely, a rising standard of living and industrialization. This meant that children were no longer an economic asset because many menial tasks were assumed by machines. The death rates per year in many advanced countries have been reduced from the traditional 35 to 40 per thousand to less than 10 per thousand. The average life span (life expectancy at birth) has almost doubled in the West since the mid-nineteenth century. It now stands at over 70 years in Europe and North America. This part of the world had time to adjust to lowered death rates while also accepting factors that lowered birth rates as well. In contrast, lowered death rates in developing countries occurred so fast that they have not had time to undergo a simultaneous rise in living standard and industrialization. Thus their populations have

mushroomed. The table shows how longer life spans have evolved in many regions of the world.

During the early years of the United States, the high rate of population growth was a source of great pride. With seemingly limitless resources and room for westward expansion, the fertility rate reached levels seldom exceeded anywhere on earth. During the colonial period the average family included about eight children. Even with the high death rate, the population more than doubled every generation. At that time, a large family was considered a definite asset. The more children a family produced, the more help it had to clear and cultivate land.

In addition to this high fertility rate, the United States for many years practiced an open-door policy of immigration. Prior to the 1921 Immigration Act, about 35 million immigrants entered the country, accounting for about one-third of the population growth up to that time. Since 1921, immigration has accounted for less than 10 percent of the population growth.

But long before 1921, the women of the United States slowly began to limit the size of their families. Actually, neither the government nor the women had yet become concerned about the threat of overpopulation. The government restricted immigration because of the diminishing need for unskilled labor. The women restricted their family size because their interests were beginning to extend beyond the farm, kitchen, and nursery toward the city, school, and labor force. By the middle 1920s the average family size had dropped to 2.5 children.

During the 1930s, the birth rate dropped still further to a low of just over two children per family. Although the low birth rate characterized those years, the trend toward it actually had started in about 1880. Actually, then (as now) poor economic conditions were only a slight deterrent to large family size. Traditionally, the poorest families have the most children. At what point the birth rate might have leveled off without the Depression is purely a matter of speculation. But even with this low birth rate the population of the country continued to grow, because of a diminishing death rate.

After World War II, a temporary surge in the birth rate was expected in order to make up for births "postponed" during the war years. But the birth rate, rather than rising and returning to "normal," continued to rise year after year until, in 1957, it reached a peak that resulted in an average family size of almost 3.8 children. Station wagons and four-bedroom houses suddenly became very popular. After 1957, the birth rate started dropping, at first slowly, then sharply during the 1960s. Possible future trends will be discussed later in this chapter. During the 1950s and 1960s the death rate has stayed virtually constant.

The Present The world population continues to grow at an accelerating rate. According to the Population Reference Bureau, the world population in 1975 was increasing by over 1.44 million per week. By 1975 the world population had surpassed 4.0 billion, fully five years ahead of the 1965 predictions. Current growth rates, if continued, will result in a world population of 6.5 billion by the year 2000, now less than 25 years away.

In general, the fastest growing countries are those with the lowest standard of living, the "have-not" nations—variously called the emerging or developing nations. The growth rate of many of these countries averages 2.5 percent per year, in contrast with an average of under 1 percent in the wealthier countries such as Europe and North America. Of the babies born each

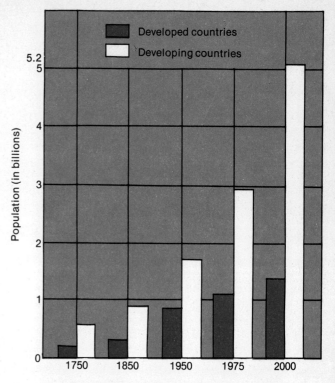

World population increase in developed and developing countries, 1750–2000.

Courtesy of the Population Reference Bureau, Inc., Washington, D.C.

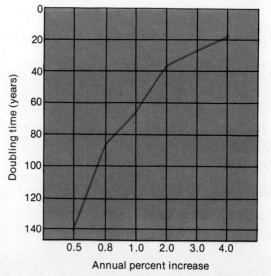

Time needed for a population to double.

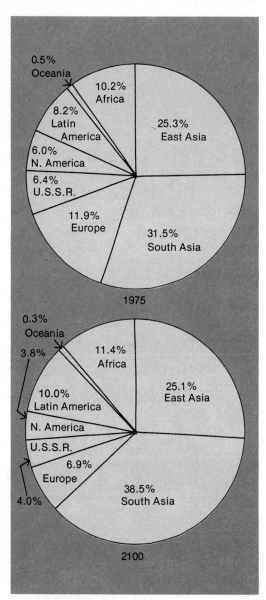

0.5%
Oceania

10.2%
Africa

8.2%
Latin
America

6.0%
N. America

6.4%
U.S.S.R.

11.9%
Europe

25.3%
East Asia

31.5%
South Asia

1975

0.3%
Oceania

3.8%

11.4%
Africa

10.0%
Latin America

N. America

U.S.S.R.

6.9%
Europe

4.0%

25.1%
East Asia

38.5%
South Asia

2100

Percentage distribution of world population, 1975 and 2100.

Courtesy of the Population Reference Bureau, Inc., Washington, D.C.

day now, over 83 percent are in Asia, Africa, and South America, as shown by the chart. If a 2.5 percent annual population growth rate does not sound very high, let us point out that such a rate doubles a population in just 28 years.

During the past decade, six out of every ten persons added to the world's population were born in Asia; another two out of ten were born in Latin America and Africa. According to the chart, by the year 2100 North America, the U.S.S.R., and Europe are expected to account for only 14.7 percent of the world's population (as compared to 24.3 percent in 1975). Undoubtedly, this increase will change the world's balance of power, and influence world affairs in coming years.

Equally important is the population growth potential of a country. This is reflected in the percentage of a population now under 15 years of age. In Africa, Asia, and Latin America, almost 40 percent of the population is under 15 years of age. This compares with 27 percent for the United States, the U.S.S.R., and Europe. The greater proportion of people in their pre-reproductive years in the developing nations represents an explosive growth potential. As these young people grow up and move into their reproductive years, the size of the childbearing fraction of the population will increase automatically. Even though significant progress is made immediately in reducing the number of births per female in these countries, it will be at least 30 years before such birth control could significantly slow population growth due to the large number of females of childbearing age.

The reduction of the death rate in the developing countries of the world was introduced with startling speed. Ancient diseases were brought under control or totally abolished in the space of a few decades, or even a few years. But the initiation of effective birth control measures on a national basis generally lags by many years (about a generation) after the accomplishment of "death control." In the interim, the birth rate remains very high because the majority of the children being born are, for the first time in the history of the nation, maturing and having children of their own. Consequently, the developing countries are now in a stage of explosive population growth. There are many factors contributing to the birth control lag. One belief held by many developing countries is that their emergence as world powers depends on producing and maintaining very large populations. In addition, there are powerful religious sanctions against birth control in many countries, and there is the lingering belief that many children must be born to insure the survival of a few to maturity. There are strong social or cultural influences favoring large families. There are still countries in which the status of women is so low as to preclude their having any authority over the number of children they produce. There are people so poor that the cost of many birth control methods seems prohibitive. There are countries whose availability of health services is so sparse that many women lack access to effective birth control methods. There are countries where the education level is so low that the majority of the people are either unaware of the need for birth control, unaware of the availability of effective methods, or lack the knowledge or motivation to use them effectively.

According to the Population Reference Bureau, the interests of a country's population are enhanced through slower growth. There is less difficulty in maintaining a viable ecological balance. It makes a modern society more manageable. Problems of nutrition, housing, education, health, sanitation, transportation, recreation, and so on, are easier to tackle. The providing of well-baby, prenatal, and pediatric clinics *is* important. Higher levels of maternal and infant mortality *do* deserve attention. Sufficient quality education to enable young people to realize vocational liberation from the patterns of the past *is* worthy of the expenditure of resources. Each of the above aspirations is more easily addressed by a society that grows more slowly.

The rate of human reproduction in any part of the globe directly affects the health and welfare of the rest of the human race. The birth rates in Africa, Asia, and Latin America are presently around 40 births per thousand population, whereas their death rates are about 10 to 20 per thousand. (See table on world birth and death rates.) The most rapid increase of population in the world today is in Kuwait, where a birth rate of 47.1 per thousand and a death rate of 5.3 per thousand is causing an increase of almost 7.1 percent per year, which means that the population of Kuwait will double in 10 years. Similar rapid increases are taking place in Latin America, where the population is expected to double within the next 26 years if the present rate of increase continues.

Such population increases intensify the existing imbalance between the distribution of the world's population and the distribution of wealth, resources, and the use of nonhuman energy. Probably for the first time in human history, there is universal aspiration for rapid improvement in the standard of living and a growing impatience with conditions that appear to stand in the way of its attainment. Millions of persons in Asia, Africa, and Latin America now are aware of the standard of living enjoyed by Europeans and North Americans. They are demanding the opportunity to attain the same standard and resisting the idea that they must be permanently content with less. But continuation of the present high rate of human multiplication in these areas will act as a brake on the already painfully slow improvement in the level of living. Just to maintain their current standard of living, let alone improve it, Latin America with a doubling time of 26 years will need to double *all* services (schools, roads, offices, hospitals, stores) within this time. This is patently impossible. This factor will increase political unrest and possibly bring about changes in governments.

The development, both population and economic, in the countries of Israel and Japan during the past 25 years needs a word of explanation. The development of Israel was accomplished only by the infusion of gigantic amounts of outside capital—as gifts, not loans—and by a massive wave of immigration of well-trained individuals. The development in Japan was accomplished through the United States, which rebuilt and updated Japan's entire industrial base after World War II. Without such outside help, although these countries were already very literate, such a development over so short a period of time would have been impossible.

The capital and technological skills that Africa, Asia, and Latin America require in order to produce enough food and to raise per capita income simultaneously exceed their existing national resources and abilities. A short-term supply of the necessary capital may be available, but only from wealthier nations. These nations, at the same time, may decide to protect their own domestic and world interests, or not be able to support the economic development of less advanced nations on the level they desire. It is not as clear how long the wealthier nations would be able to support the uncontrolled propagation of the populations receiving assistance. General application of such a foreign-aid program will postpone for only a few decades the inevitable reckoning with the results of unregulated human multiplication.

The complexities of the United States growth rate are worth our attention here. The birth rate in the more affluent countries reflects the influences of social and economic differentiation not found in the forces in the developing nations. In those countries, the population is generally skewed either toward the very high or the very low borders of the economic scale. In the more affluent nations, the existence of

World Birth and Death Rates, 1973

	Birth Rate[a]	Death Rate[b]	Current Annual Growth Rate[c]	Doubling Time	Population Under 15 Years
World	31.5	12.8	1.9%	36	36%
United States	16.2	9.4	0.9	77	25
Europe	16.1	10.4	0.6	116	24
USSR	17.8	7.9	1.0	69	36
Asia	34.9	13.6	2.1	33	38
Africa	46.3	19.8	2.6	27	44
Latin America	36.9	9.2	2.7	26	42

[a]Births per thousand population.
[b]Deaths per thousand population.
[c]Net rate, including immigration and emigration.

Taken from *1975 World Population Data Sheet.* Population Reference Bureau, Washington, D.C., 1975.

Birth Rates in the United States By Race

Race	1950	1955	1960	1965	1970	1972 (preliminary)
Nonwhite	33.3	34.7	32.1	27.6	25.1	21.8
White	23.0	23.8	22.7	18.3	17.4	14.8
Total	24.1	25.0	23.7	19.4	18.4	15.6

NOTE: Number given is the number of children born per 1000 population.

Taken from U.S. Bureau of the Census, *Statistical Abstracts of the United States, 1974*, 95th ed. (Washington, D.C.: U.S. Government Printing Office, 1974).

Family Size and Income

Family Income	Age 25–34		Age 35–44	
	White	Nonwhite	White	Nonwhite
Under $3000	2.74	3.69	3.23	4.57
$3,000 to $4,999	2.66	3.19	3.89	4.47
$5,000 to $7,499	2.38	2.98	3.50	4.10
$7,500 to $9,999	2.20	2.77	3.30	3.60
$10,000 to $14,999	2.15	2.41	3.06	3.45
$15,000 to $25,000	1.78	1.92	2.97	2.92

NOTE: Numbers given are for the average number of children ever born per woman of two age groups, by family income and race. As of June 1972.

Taken from U.S. Bureau of the Census, *Current Population Reports: Population Characteristics*, Report P–20 (248), Table 20 (Washington, D.C.: U.S. Government Printing Office, 1973).

Family Size and Education

Women's Educational Level	White	Nonwhite	All Races
Not high school graduate	2.65	3.53	2.76
High school graduate	1.99	2.29	2.01
College, one year or more	1.52	1.67	1.53

NOTE: Numbers given are for the average number of children ever born per woman, 14–39 years of age. As of June 1972.

Taken from U.S. Bureau of the Census, *Current Population Reports: Population Characteristics*. Report P–20 (248). Table 9 (Washington, D.C.: U.S. Government Printing Office, 1973).

a large middle class introduces other factors. The middle class consumes more of the world's resources. Its members buy more, travel more, dispose of more materials than lower classes. Increased use of these limited resources offsets the "safe" lower birth rate of middle-class families.

In addition to the total rate of population growth, it is significant to compare the relative birth rates of various segments of the population. Some of the groups we should examine for possible differences are those of differing racial composition, financial level, and educational background.

Birth Rate and Race   Let us first consider birth rate in relation to color, ignoring possibles differences in education or income between the groups. According to figures published in 1974 by the U.S. Census Bureau, 87.7 percent of the population in the United States is white, about 11.1 percent is black, and 1.2 percent is composed of other nonwhites, including primarily North American Indians and Asians.

In the table comparing the birth rates (number of births per one thousand population) of white and nonwhite women in different years, it can be seen that in the last two decades, nonwhite women had more children than white women. These figures, of course, do not indicate whether the greater rate is due to greater inherent fertility, desire for a larger family, or less effective use of contraceptive measures.

Some members of the black community express fears that advocacy of fertility limitation among blacks may be aimed at limiting their numbers and strength, and even possibly at total extermination or genocide. While the nation, in addressing itself to future population levels, must find solutions to unemployment, poor housing, poor health services, and poor education, it is still possible that fertility reduction necessary for attaining and maintaining zero population growth may not come

about on a totally voluntary basis. Yet available data indicates that as minority groups participate more fully in the total society, their fertility rates begin to decline drastically.

Birth Rate and Income   In the United States, low income is often accompanied by large family size ("the rich get richer and the poor get children"). This is shown in the table on family size and income. In 1969, the last year for which such figures are available, those families with the lowest income had the most children. As incomes increased, family size decreased until an income of over $15,000 was reached. At this level there was an upturn in family size. The apparent significance of these figures is that the middle-income groups desired smaller families and made more effective use of contraceptive measures than did the lower income groups. Possible reasons may include greater motivation to control family size; better education, enabling more efficient use of contraceptives; household conditions more favorable to contraceptive use; and income sufficient to engage medical assistance in the selection and prescription of contraceptives. Another possible reason is the high infant-mortality rate of the poor (three to five times the national average). The resulting feeling of uncertainty whether each child will survive may act to motivate a higher birth rate. Until living conditions are improved, the poor will probably continue to conceive more children.

Birth Rate and Education   Another table relates the number of children born to the educational level of the woman. The relationship here is similar to that between income and number of children. The higher the level of education, the fewer children produced. Unlike the income comparison, no upturn in number of offspring exists at the upper end of the scale. The racial breakdown is also similar to that found in the income comparison. The poorly educated nonwhite woman has more children that the similarly educated white woman. Among women who finish high school, the number of children produced by the two racial groups is about equal.

These sets of data have been the subject of serious analysis by political scientists, sociologists, demographers, and historians. Information of this type can be used to produce an organized view of American society and its priorities.

In the writings of Rufus E.Miles, Jr. ("Whose Baby is the Population Explosion?" Population Bulletin 16 [February 1970]), we find good examples. He is Chairman of the Board of the Population Reference Bureau and has specified seven major influences that promote large families in the United States. He calls these the "pronatalist" influences:

1. Large numbers of adult Americans, both male and female, feel that procreation is the best way for them to find self-fulfillment.

2. For many parents—primarily mother—large families are a psychological defense against lack of interesting employment, lack of a sense of belonging to a satisfying social group, or lack of other forms of self-realization.

3. Smaller numbers of people—mainly those in or near poverty areas—lack the knowledge or medical services available to higher-income people that would facilitate the control of their family size.

4. Large numbers of parents desire a child of a particular sex and will keep trying until they produce such a child, regardless of how many children they have in the process.

5. Many people are influenced by the "growthmania" of the American way of life. They believe that any system that is growing is healthy and good, while any that is not growing is stagnant and bad.

6. Government policies have reinforced the pronatalist influences of society and have partially offset the economic disadvantages of children through such provisions as high taxes on single people, tax deductions for children, provision of public housing and public assistance only for families with children, and other measures that provide similar encouragement to childbearing.

7. Too little educational information has come from leadership sources or from the mass media to counteract the effects of the six pronatalist influences listed above. Most of the information presented always seems to imply that population problems are in "other" countries, or that the problem is most serious among the poor.

The rate of population growth for the United States declined during the 1960s. As the table on population growth shows, in 1960 the population increased only by 1.8 percent. By 1975 the annual rate of increase has dropped to less than 1 percent. In spite of the trend in declining birth rates, the total U.S. population will probably continue to increase for some years due to the large number of women just now reaching reproductive age. If the downward trend continues, however, there appears to be a good chance of eventually achieving population stability in this country.

The Future Is the present spurt of worldwide population growth a temporary phenomenon, or will it continue until the former biological regulators—war, disease, and famine—once again take control?

Future populations of individual nations, of regions, or of the entire world cannot be predicted with any degree of

Recent Population Growth in the United States

Year	Fertility Rate[a]	Birth Rate[b]	Death Rate[c]	Total U.S. Population On July 1 (Millions)	Percent Annual Population Growth[d]
1960	119.1	23.8	9.5	179.3	1.7
1961	118.4	23.5	9.3	183.1	1.7
1962	113.2	22.6	9.4	185.9	1.5
1963	109.4	21.9	9.6	188.7	1.4
1964	105.8	21.2	9.4	191.4	1.4
1965	97.3	19.6	9.4	193.6	1.3
1966	91.8	18.5	9.5	195.7	1.1
1967	88.1	17.9	9.4	198.8	1.1
1968	86.1	17.6	9.7	201.2	1.0
1969	86.2	17.8	9.5	203.1	1.0
1970	88.0	18.3	9.4	205.2	1.0
1971	82.6	18.2	9.3	207.1	1.1
1972	77.2	15.6	9.4	208.2	0.8
1973[e]	69.3	15.6	9.4	210.3	0.8
1974[e]	68.8	16.2	9.4	211.9	0.9

[a]Fertility rate is the number of births per 1000 women ages 15 through 44
[b]Birth rate is the number of births per 1000 total population
[c]Death rate is the number of deaths per 1000 total population
[d]Includes immigration and emigration

[e]Figures for 1973 and 1974 are estimates
Adapted from U.S. Department of Health, Education and Welfare, *Monthly Vital Statistics Report, Provisional Statistics* (April 1975) and *1975 World Data Sheet*, Population Reference Bureau, Inc. (Washington, D.C.: 1975).

accuracy for more than a few decades at a time. Just as Thomas Malthus could not foresee the tremendous changes that have taken place in Europe since the eighteenth century, we really cannot foresee the future extent and consequences of population growth.* There are too many unpredictable influences on population. In addition, it is usually difficult to predict what

*Robert Thomas Malthus (1766–1834), an English economist and theologian, was among the first to foresee overpopulation as a major world problem. His basic thesis, very unpopular at the time, was that human population increases by a geometric progression (2, 4, 8, 16, 32, 64, 128, and so on) while food supplies can increase only by an arithmetic progression (1, 2, 3, 4, 5, 6, and so on). Malthus was, surprisingly, an outspoken foe of contraceptive techniques, urging, rather, late marriage and "moral restraint" as a means of controlling population. It should be remembered, however, that in the eighteenth and early nineteenth centuries there were few other reliable methods of controlling the birth rate.

the exact effect of a particular event or condition will be. Starvation, political turmoil, natural disasters, industrialization and agricultural improvement have caused both higher *and* lower population growth rates at different times.

The basic tendency in population prediction unfortunately has been to steadily underestimate future population levels. It is difficult to choose those specific factors that can reliably be extrapolated into the future. For example, the average annual rate of population growth in the United States from 1790 to 1964 (174 years) was 2.2 percent. Simply projecting this rate for another 174 years (until the year 2138) would have given this country a population of 8.8 billion, better than twice the current population of the entire world.

Since the annual rate of growth in this country is now below one percent, it's obvious this level will not be achieved. Actually, the level at which the population of the United States will stabilize might be as low as 300 to 400 million people. Yet this too is far larger than our present population.

Our most immediate concern is with the "boom babies" born between 1950 and 1960. In 1960 there were 11 million women in the 20 to 30 year age group.. In 1980 there will be 20 million women in this prime reproduction group. This statistic is not just a guess or a rough speculation—these females have already been born and are now growing up. The only question remaining is the rate at which they will reproduce. Will the current trend toward smaller families continue, or will a larger family again become "fashionable"? If the latter takes place, the baby boom of the 1950s will compare to the boom of the 1980s like a cap gun compares to a cannon.

The future may witness a dramatic increase in our ability to control our environment. We have been able to modify or control many natural phenomena, but we have not yet discovered how to evade the consequences of biological laws. No species has ever been able to multiply without limit. Fundamentally, there are only two methods of population control—high mortality or low fertility. We can choose which of these checks will be applied—but one of them *must* be. Whether or not we use scientific knowledge to guide the future of man on this planet, some control will be instituted—possibly only by the blind forces of nature.

The Boundaries of Population Growth

Unfortunately, discussion of the population problem often centers on two issues—space and food—as though finding enough standing room and enough food per person to allow survival would resolve the problem. Such oversimplification misses the vastness of the problem for many reasons:

1. Most of the world's people are already living under such poor conditions that it is not sufficient for food production merely to keep pace with population growth. A great increase in food production would be necessary just to feed the *current* population properly.

2. Many of the methods that have been proposed to increase food production (such as insecticides, fertilizers, and land reclamation) are, even at their current level of application, proving harmful to the total environment.

3. World production of many commodities (not only food) must be increased sharply to meet the reasonable needs and demands of people seeking an adequate existence.

4. The production of waste products (pollutants) increases with the population. The ability of the environment to "absorb" pollutants is limited. Even the disposal of human wastes becomes a serious problem at high population densities.

5. Frustration of the growing desires among all people for decent living conditions, education, and economic opportunity is creating tremendous political and social tensions throughout the world.

6. The world is not one big, unified reservoir of space, skills, resources, knowledge, and capital from which nations can procure their respective needs for unlimited time.

7. There is a wide gap between what is technologically or theoretically possible and what can be applied with safety and at reasonable cost.

The population problem is based on the procurement and distribution of resources. The alarming differentials in consumption of resources between different nations and regions of the world cause additional problems. Furthermore, a society devoted to supporting maximum numbers of people at a bare subsistence level is incompatible with any humane standards of civilization. To what extent are we willing to sacrifice quality of life in order to attain quantity of life? And if the quality of life is sacrificed, how long will we be able to maintain the quantity? Our environment could be so severely damaged in the process that it might eventually be able to support only a small number of people at a very low level of existence.

Some people argue that we really do not have to worry about population control—that "nature" will take care of the problem. Unfortunately, however, nature's population control methods are often inimical to the quality of life. Those who would rely on starvation, drought, natural disasters, suicide, and the other serious consequences of population excess show a callous disregard for humanitarian values. The question of quality must be a major concern in our approach to world population problems.

In the following pages, we are going to consider the various factors that are either potential or actual brakes on population growth. It is time to take a careful look at these factors and determine which can be useful or detrimental to the quality of human life.

The Fixed Factors Some of the factors that control population growth have already been established for us. Regardless of our needs or efforts, the amounts and availability of these materials cannot be increased.

Space In relating space needs to population, it is essential that our thinking go beyond the question of how many people could survive on the land surface of the earth. Most people are concerned about the quality of life, rather than the attainment of a minimal level of survival.

Space is needed for decent living conditions, without the constant sight and sound of neighbors. Space is needed for recreation and for the opportunity to enjoy solitude from the ever-present crowds. Space is needed for food production. Natural watershed area is essential for replenishment of water supplies. Undeveloped wilderness area is required for the maintenance of such natural cycles as the oxygen cycle and for the total ecological balance of the earth.

With regard to space for living or agriculture, some experts point to the deserts of the world as room for expansion. But most people do not want to live in a hot, dry desert climate. If people really wanted to live on the deserts, these areas would have been settled some time ago.

The use of the deserts for agricultural purposes on any large scale is still only a theoretical possibility. The cost, both in terms of dollars for irrigation and transport and in terms of environmental damage from widespread irrigation, is staggering. For the deserts are not vacuums in the ecological system of this planet. They are an important element in the earth's natural balance, and cannot be tampered with.

Resources We are living in a world where a rapidly increasing number of people must share a fixed, or in some cases decreasing, supply of natural resources. The world population problem is the total of all the population problems of the major countries of the world. Through modern transportation and communication, the world has become so "small" that a population problem in any one country may have serious effects in other countries.

The earth's capacity to provide raw materials is limited. Many minerals and most of the presently used energy sources are nonrenewable. In some places the scarcity of forests limits the use of wood and wood products. More and more cities are finding it necessary to curtail their water service or to make use of new, and more remote, sources of fresh water.

If the entire world were to develop industrially on a level comparable to that of the United States and Europe, our known reserves of coal, petroleum, and natural gas would not be sufficient for the proportionately increased energy requirements. It has been forecast that the high point in petroleum production will be reached in the relatively near future—sometime before the year 2000. The pressure to produce petroleum in increasing amounts is pushing the oil companies toward more and more ambitious and possibly ecologically catastrophic systems, such as the Alaska pipeline and the huge oil tankers now being built. The fossil fuels (natural gas, petroleum, and coal) are expected to provide the world's energy needs for no more than several hundred years.

Our traditional sources of energy are water (which provides about 4 percent of our electrical power), coal, gas, and oil. In fulfilling an ever-increasing demand for power by burning the fossil fuels, we are depleting stores that cannot be replaced. These are nonrenewable natural resources, and in time (an alarmingly short time if the demand keeps growing as it has in the past quarter of a century) these fuels will be gone. However, there are two energy sources that may be substitutes for fossil fuels. One is radiation from the sun (solar energy) and the other is nuclear energy— that derived from the fission (splitting) of heavy atoms and the fusion (union) of light atoms.

Considering the inherent dangers of atomic energy, it would seem that capturing solar energy directly is preferable to utilizing nuclear energy. An increasing number of companies are coming out with workable units for individual homes, although still on a small scale.

The adoption of fission power will be slow and its rate of development will depend ultimately on the exhaustion of fossil fuel reserves. Fusion power, while potentially having many advantages over fission power, including an inexhaustible fuel supply of negligible cost, has not yet been established as feasible and its costs cannot be readily assessed.

The two major problems with the adoption of atomic power as a major energy source are the problems of waste heat disposal and the possibility of nuclear accident. While great precautions are taken, there is always the danger of improper engineering or workmanship in the design and/or construction of a reactor. While not unsafe, present-day reactors can be made far safer, starting with greater care in site selection. One reactor was nearly constructed on top of the San Andreas Fault in northern California. Because of the possibility of a "leak" and the resulting public pressure against the building of nuclear power stations near populated areas there is continuing resistance to the adoption of this method of power production.

The waste disposal problem is probably more significant. The water circulating through the nuclear power plant picks up the excess heat given off by the operating nuclear reactor. Unless cooling bins are installed, the heated water then flows directly into a living community of fish, birds, and aquatic plant life. The effects of continual "washing" by heated water have not been competely evaluated, but most ecologists predict that the effects can be serious indeed.

It might seem strange that heat is considered a pollutant. After all, heat is a form of energy and a potentially useful one. A recent study of Oak Ridge National Laboratory in Tennessee has presented encouraging evidence that this same "thermal pollution" can be cycled directly in the heating system of a city the size of Philadelphia and thus reduce the possibility of ecological damage. The most important point, however, is that careful study is required before nuclear power plants can be safely incorporated into the environment.

Since the most easily obtained minerals and sources of energy have already been used, the continuing mining of less accessible deposits will cost this country considerably in the future. Yet, even this low-yield extraction has its limits. Each of the acts just mentioned represents an unnecessary borrowing on the future, or solving the problems of today while creating potential problems for our grandchildren.

Borrowing on the future is taking place with the resources of the United States, as well as those elsewhere in the world. Although North Americans compose only about 6 percent of the world's population, they consume half of the world's production of major minerals. They consume twice as much commercial energy per person as the British and four times as much as the people of India. It is estimated that each year the average American utilizes an amount of natural resources equal to that used by 25 to 30 Indians.

The average American needs twenty times the energy available to an Asian to support himself or herself in the style to which we have grown accustomed. And our energy appetite is increasing by 10 percent per year. Aside from solar energy, it takes 35 percent of the world's available energy, mostly from fossil fuels, to supply America's energy needs.

Conservation of Energy With a stable or decreasing supply of some conventional fuels, and with a rising demand for energy, Americans must now consider stopping the excessive energy waste that has characterized our culture. There has been adjustment to the reduced supply and/or increased cost of gasoline in spite of cries that it could not be done. Total gasoline consumption has, as a result, declined at least temporarily. It should also be possible to reduce the demand for other forms of energy.

All of us can participate. Recycling can be increased, reducing both solid waste and the use of natural resources. More efficient trains, barges, and mass transportation can replace less efficient trucks, cars, and planes. Buildings can be constructed to conserve energy, both in design and in materials used. Synthetics, plastics, and aluminum require far more energy to produce than steel and wood. Doubling the insulation may as much as halve the energy requirements of heating and cooling. Elimination of frost-free refrigerators, pilot lights on appliances, and incandescent lamps, the closing of unused fireplace flues, and the lowering of thermostats would conserve enormous amounts of energy. The voluntary changing of life-styles may be adequate to meet the shortage, but if unduly postponed, obligatory changes in our way of life will undoubtedly become necessary.

In relation to these facts, the increase of this country's population appears frightening. In light of the aspirations of many parts of the world for better living standards, it is questionable whether 6 percent of the population is justified in continuing this extraordinary level of consumption.

The Absorption of Pollution As previously discussed, the environment has a limited ability to absorb and assimilate pollutants. But the quantities of many population-related pollutants *now* being dumped into the environment exceed this ability. Disposal of one of the most directly population-related pollutants, human sewage, has become a particularly critical problem. Even after treatment, sewage still contains large quantities of inorganic nitrates and phosphates that overstimulate the growth of algae, leading to "dead" rivers and lakes, such as Lake Erie. But much sewage in the United States, and most sewage on a world basis, does not receive any treatment. It is dumped into the most convenient lake, river, or ocean as raw sewage—teeming with living disease organisms and laden with nitrates and phosphates. Consequently, since 1960 there has been a great world increase in the incidence of sewage-borne diseases, particularly cholera and other dysenteric (diarrheal) diseases.

The gap between sewage production and sewage treatment is growing, not closing, as world populations increase. It is easy to offer the solution of increased sewage treatment facilities, but the reality of the situation is that such facilities are economically impossible for much of the world at this time. How can the developing countries hope for adequate sewage treatment when this goal cannot be attained by even the wealthy United States?

In addition, the quantity of almost every other pollutant also relates to population levels. The more people, the more need for transportation, food, power, housing, and so forth, all of which contribute to environmental decline. Thus, it is obvious that population control is the first requirement for the maintenance of a livable environment on this planet.

The Flexible Factors

Other factors affecting population growth are subject to expansion to some degree. If there is any prospect of bringing order to the quandary of population growth, the greatest hope lies with these factors whose potential we can influence and increase.

Food Production

Most people do not have enough food to eat. As the table on food consumption shows, more than half of the people in the world today live on 2,100 calories per person per day, although the Food and Agricultural Organization (FAO) of the United Nations recommends a daily minimum of 3,200 calories per man, and 2,300 calories per woman. By 2000 the average daily intake is estimated to be 1,340; 1,350 per day is starvation level. The amount of calories in food is only one consideration. Equally important is how well the diet is balanced with various kinds of foods. The low-calorie diets of the world consist primarily of plant foods and cannot be considered balanced. Though the majority of Americans enjoy adequate diets, millions of people in this country suffer from diets deficient in quantity, quality, or both.

Most of the world's population increase is occurring in poorly developed areas that are already short of food—Asia, Africa, and Latin America. The basis for most food production is land. But an increasing population itself requires even more land

Levels of Daily Per Capita Consumption of Food by Regions and Groups of Countries

Regions	Calories	Total Protein (Grams)	Animal Protein (Grams)
Far East	1910	54	6
Near East	2190	70	14
Africa	2100	61	15
Latin America	2380	67	29
Europe	2870	91	31
Northern America	3120	90	60
World	2260	66	18

NOTE: The postwar levels of consumption were used.
Taken from Stuart Mudd, ed. *The Population Crisis and the Use of World Resources* (Bloomington, Inc.: Indiana University Press, 1964)

for housing, industries, businesses, roads, schools, and all the other services necessary for a satisfactory standard of living. In too many places, the choicest agricultural land is being taken out of production to provide for increasing populations. As a result, farming operations must move onto less suitable land where the production of adequate crops requires greatly increased expenditures for land leveling, irrigation, and fertilization. Although this adjustment can usually be made in the United States with relative ease, the more limited economies of most of the world's countries cannot bear an increased cost for food.

The most important techniques for increased food production have included extensive use of insecticides and mineral fertilizers. Only through their use is the world being fed as well as it is, though that is not really very well. But insecticides cannot be used in limitless amounts without inflicting severe damage on our environment and perhaps on ourselves, as well. Evidence now indicates that excessive nitrates from fertilizer applications are present in food and water supplies at levels that may be harmful to humans, especially infants, and are contributing to the pollution of rivers and lakes.

Thus, it seems that the cost of greatly increased food production will be much higher than predicted and that this cost will be measured not only in economic terms but also in damage to the environment. Optimistic viewpoints should be further dampened by the fact that during the last 60 years, food production has actually increased much more slowly than has the population.

How much food could be produced throughout the world? Only about 40 percent of the earth's total land area is capable of productive use of cropland, grazing, or timber production. The other 60 percent is unavailable as ice and snow, mountains, and desert. Of the potentially cultivable land, only 25 percent could reasonably be brought under cultivation, and only one third of this land is in Asia, where six out of every ten humans live. The table shows the production of organic matter per year by the vegetation of the earth. Thus it indicates the earth's potential food-producing

Annual Production of Organic Matter

Type of Vegetation	Area In Millions of Square Kilometers	Net Production Per Year	
		Grams Of Carbon Per Square Meter	Millions of Tons of Carbon
Cultivated	13.31	204	2,728
Forest	44.41	874	48,100
Grassland	36.90	103	3,286
Other (desert, swamp, and so on)	53.90	178	2,706
Total			
Land	148.5	373 (mean)	56,820
Sea	371.0	90 (mean)	33,400

Adapted from data in "The Human Population" by Edward S. Deevey, Jr., *Scientific American* 203 (September 1960), p. 203.

capacity based on current standards of cultivation.

Cultivated vegetation is shown to be less efficient than forests in producing organic matter, yielding a smaller overall output. Yet despite its impracticality, this type of vegetation will replace all others for the production of food. Also, total land vegetation leads sea vegetation in efficiency and in net tonnage. This comparison implies that reaching into the sea is not the ultimate answer to food production problems.

Since the most easily cultivated land—both in terms of cost and energy—is already in use, higher yields, as well as conservation of existing lands, offer the best means of increasing food production. However, efforts made to feed the present hungry people of the world will mean little if the world's population continues to grow unabated. The best hope combines increased food production and a reduction of birth and death rates to replacement levels.

Population and Health Public health agencies have been highly successful in their battle against long-established infectious diseases. Through measures such as antimalarial programs, it has been possible (in Sri Lanka, formerly Ceylon, for example) to open huge areas for habitation and cultivation that were formerly uninhabitable. Public concern over health problems has resulted in improved sanitation, purer and more adequate water supplies, and prevention and control of communicable diseases through immunization, insecticides, antibiotics, and increased attention to nutritional disorders. These improvements have contributed toward a lowered death rate and an increased life expectancy.

It is mistakenly assumed by some that the present world population problem is due solely to the great efficiency of health programs. It is true that as countries develop economically, better living conditions and improved nutrition usually result. These in turn lead to a drop in death rates. After a lag of several generations, however, the birth rate also tends to decline. In the past, owing to infant mortality, parents conceived more children than they expected to raise to maturity. For example, parents may have conceived six children in order to raise three to maturity. As medical services improve and as they are made available to larger numbers of people, infant mortality drops. But it takes time for parents to realize that they can be assured of the survival of most of their children. If this lag could be reduced from several generation to a single generation, the total population growth in economically developing countries could decrease.

Health programs, therefore, may prove to be one of the best prospects for solving the population problem, especially if a corresponding emphasis on family planning is also provided. Ideally, parents would feel secure enough about the health of their children to decide upon, and practice, birth control measures. As a result of the logical relationship that can and does exist between health programs and population control, national family planning programs are commonly assigned to health services. These have pioneered in Japan, India, Korea, Taiwan, Pakistan, Egypt, Turkey, Czechoslovakia, and Poland.

As we have implied, the success of family-control programs lies in sufficiently motivating the entire population. Historically, when food or living conditions became too bad, people voluntarily controlled population through methods they would normally consider objectionable or immoral. During the potato famines in Ireland a century ago, the excessive population was decreased by late marriages, emigration, and inheritance legislation favoring eldest sons in addition to the natural forces of infectious disease, malnutrition, and starvation. Japan currently legalizes abortion as a principal method of population control—with the number of abortions exceeding the number of live births. In mainland China they provide free contraception, sterilization, and abortion. Family planning services are taken out to the homes of the people. These examples of population controls lead some authorities to doubt that the "standing room only" prophecies will ever become a reality. In preference to such practices as infanticide, people must be motivated to accept the use of contraceptives in family planning.

The Underlying Problems Many people look to science for the answer to world population problems, believing that when the "ideal" means of fertility control is developed, population control will automatically follow. Unfortunately, there is very little evidence to support this belief. The methods of fertility control now available (sterilization, contraception, and abortion) are more than adequate for the purpose of stabilizing world population. The problem is that even with ready access to family-planning methods, many couples will plan to have three, four, or even more children. Thus, controlling population is primarily an economic, cultural, and political problem, not a scientific one.

The United Nations Declaration of Population states, "The opportunity to decide the number and spacing of children is a basic human right." The intent of the statement was to encourage the availability of birth control information and facilities, but it can be, and has been, interpreted as an approval of large families and high birth rates.

In the past, the official policy of the United States government has been limited to family planning assistance for those who would like to restrict family size. It was not until 1971, when the Commission on Population and the American Future issued its interim report, that the need for an "explicit U.S. population policy" was indicated. The report brought home the question of excessive population growth, and how it contrasts with the long-range goal of achieving a good standard of living for all Americans.

To date, most birth control programs have been oriented toward low-income families. But studies show that poor families account for less than one-third of all births in the United States. Although "unwanted" births pose a major problem in all income groups, the real problem, in relation to population control, is not the unwanted but the *wanted* child. There is a definite distinction between "family planning" and "population planning." Family planning by millions of couples may have no effect at all in terms of world wide population control.

Personal Responsibilities Any hope for controlling the population explosion must lie in motivating individual couples to limit their families to two children (actually, an average of 2.1 children would achieve stability, since some persons never marry or else die in childhood).

Millions of couples today who could afford (financially and emotionally) more children are voluntarily limiting their family size out of concern for the population crisis. Many couples who want to raise more than two children are adopting additional children.

Couples who are not motivated by a concern for world population can perhaps be reached through an appeal to their more selfish interests. For example, the cost of raising a child to the age of eighteen should be widely publicized. It now costs the family of average income over $30,000 to raise each child through high school graduation, not to mention the cost of college. In making the decision whether to have another child, it is very difficult for a couple to foresee the cost of food, clothing, shoes, medical and dental care, school expenses, and so forth, that would be required to raise that child. For the great majority of couples, the choice is simply between raising a small family in relative comfort or a larger family in relative hardship, with the children "doing without" such advantages as vacation trips, orthodontia, and adequate medical care.

Social and Governmental Factors The status of women in society is, according to Rufus E. Miles, Jr., Chairman of the Board of Population Reference Bureau, one of the key determinants of the birth rate. He feels that the more satisfying the employment opportunites for women, the less likely it is that they will want large families. Women who lack the satisfactions that come from decent employment—a sense of belonging to a group, a sense of self-esteem from being able to express a talent or make a contribution to society and be paid fairly for it—must find self-fulfillment in some other way. If, in addition to lacking satisfactory employment, women lack membership in any social group with which they have rapport, they are strongly motivated to create a social group of their own by producing babies.

If Miles' assumption is true, and there is considerable proof that it is, then greatly enlarged employment opportunities for women may be one of the most important factors in reducing average family size. There is much evidence that many if not most women of childbearing age prefer employment at decent jobs to being fulltime homemakers. If our society genuinely desires to lower its birth rate, it must find more numerous, more satisfying, and better-paying opportunities for women, particularly those of childbearing

age. An important step in freeing women for meaningful employment is the creation, either by government or by private enterprise, of expanded neighborhood child-care centers. In many areas, such centers are either nonexistent, prohibitively expensive, or of such poor quality that concerned mothers are reluctant to leave their children there.

As previously mentioned, the real problem in relation to population control is not the unwanted child, but the wanted one. Yet unwanted children do add significantly to the birth rate, as well as to a multitude of social and psychological problems. According to several surveys, it's believed that at least one American child in five is unwanted. Certainly, most out-of-wedlock babies (about 1 out of 12 births in the United States) can be considered unwanted, as can the majority of infants born to mothers under 17 years old. Preventing the birth of unwanted children would reduce the birth rate to below 2.1—the level of zero population growth.

The obvious solution is to make contraceptives and abortion cheaper and easily available. It is imperative that every woman have access to family planning assistance, regardless of her age, marital status, or financial condition. It has been estimated that there are about 5 million women in the United States who need publicly supported family planning services.

Although current forms of fertility control could decrease population growth if properly utilized, new methods are also needed. None of the currently available methods is entirely satisfactory, either in relation to its safety, effectiveness, or ease of use. Fertility-control research must be given high priority in the allotment of federal funds.

Finally, there must be a reversal of the numerous social and government pressures and incentives favoring marriage and childbearing. Unmarried women have been made to feel that they are social failures, when in reality a person of either sex can live a personally satisfying, socially useful life without marriage. Tax laws have generally penalized single people, while heavily favoring those with large families. Welfare programs, public housing projects, and many other government policies clearly display a bias in favor of the social norm, which holds that everybody should marry and have children. Not only are such policies damaging from the population standpoint, they are sociologically and psychologically destructive as well.

It is our emphatic belief that humans, as intelligent beings, can and must maintain their population at such a level that every individual is able to achieve full biological potential for a long and worthwhile life. It is obvious that if our population continues to increase at its present rate, each individual's "slice of the pie" of life is going to get smaller and smaller until life becomes a burden to be borne rather than a joy to live.

For Further Reading

Anderson, Walt, ed. *Politics and Environment*. Pacific Palisades, Calif.: Goodyear, 1970. A collection of some of the most important papers on the ecological crisis.

Chamberlain, Neil W. *Beyond Malthus*. New York: Basic Books, 1970. The business and economic views of world population growth and its impact on economics and trade.

Dasmann, Raymond. *The U.S. Environment: A Time to Decide*. Washington, D.C.: Population Reference Bureau, 1968. A factual basis for action to improve the environment.

Ehrlich, Paul R., and Ehrlich, Anne H. *Population-Resources-Environment*. 2nd ed. San Francisco: W. H. Freeman, 1972. A probing examination of our environmental crisis together with suggested political and personal solutions.

Fraser, Dean. *The People Problem: What You Should Know About Growing Population and Vanishing Resources*. Bloomington, Ind.: Indiana University Press, 1971. Explains the biological and mathematical laws regulating population growth and what can be done.

Odum, Eugene P. *Fundamentals of Ecology*. 3rd rev. ed. Philadelphia: Saunders, 1972. A thorough, updated treatment of basic ecological concepts.

Paddock, William, and Paddock, Paul. *Famine Nineteen Seventy-Five: America's Decision, Who Will Survive*. Boston: Little, Brown, 1968. An excellent book tracing the projected effects of unchecked population growth in the United States.

Sears, Paul B. *This is Our World.* Norman, Okla.: University of Oklahoma Press, 1971. First published in 1937, now a classic exploring how society's values and standards will determine what is done concerning the environmental problems of today.

Wagner, Richard H. *Environment and Man.* 2nd ed. New York: W. W. Norton, 1974. A systematic review of today's environmental problems with suggestions on what we can do to survive.

Waldbott, George L. *Health Effects of Environmental Pollutants.* St. Louis: Mosby, 1973. The nature and sources of pollutants and their actions on human systems.

Wilson, Richard, and Jones, William J. *Energy, Ecology, and the Environment.* New York: Academic Press, 1974. A concise examination of the conflicting interests of people in their use of energy and their preservation of natural resources.

GLOSSARY INDEX